Nutrigenomics and Nutrigenetics in Functional Foods and Personalized Nutrition

Nutrigenomics and Nutrigenetics in Functional Foods and Personalized Nutrition

Lynnette R. Ferguson

CRC Press
Taylor & Francis Group
Boca Raton London New York

CRC Press is an imprint of the
Taylor & Francis Group, an **informa** business

CRC Press
Taylor & Francis Group
6000 Broken Sound Parkway NW, Suite 300
Boca Raton, FL 33487-2742

Printed on acid-free paper
Version Date: 20130507

International Standard Book Number-13: 978-1-4398-7680-0 (Hardback)

Library of Congress Cataloging-in-Publication Data

Nutrigenomics and nutrigenetics in functional foods and personalized nutrition / editor, Lynnette R. Ferguson.
p. ; cm.
Includes bibliographical references and index.
ISBN 978-1-4398-7680-0 (alk. paper)
I. Ferguson, Lynnette R.
[DNLM: 1. Nutrigenomics--methods. 2. Diet Therapy--methods. 3. Individualized Medicine--methods. 4. Nutritional Physiological Phenomena--genetics. 5. Nutritional Requirements--genetics. QU 145]

RM217
615.8'54--dc23 2013007249

Visit the Taylor & Francis Web site at
http://www.taylorandfrancis.com

and the CRC Press Web site at
http://www.crcpress.com

Contents

SECTION IV Bringing Nutrigenomics to Industry, Health Professionals, and the Public

Preface

A balanced diet, with a good range of foods to cover the population nutrient requirements and thereby optimize metabolism, is generally considered to equate to good population health. By these means, the risk of disease and its progress may be effectively reduced. Food should not only be nutritious but also enable satiation without excess energy and weight accumulation that is now so prevalent, especially in Western societies. But a food that is tasty, attractive, and beneficial to one individual may not be so for another. There are clear examples of some people who appear to thrive on a particular diet and lifestyle, while others may be disadvantaged. Nutrigenetics, that is, the way in which genotype determines nutrient requirement, may explain some of these individual differences.

If a food company wishes to bring a new food onto the market, or a new dietary regime is being developed, there are increasing pressures to prove human efficacy. This is increasingly an area where the aligned discipline of nutrigenomics (sometimes called foodomics if it is primarily food orientated) comes into its own. Omics technologies can be used as endpoints of cell culture, animal model, or human studies. They enable relatively accurate and cost-effective studies, which do not require a starting hypothesis, and can be done with small study numbers in a relatively short time. While not yet directly acceptable for human-orientated European Food Safety Authority health claims, they can point efficiently to the way forward. That is, they can suggest, but cannot definitively prove, an appropriate biomarker for a larger and more rigorous clinical trial.

While functional foods have become a reasonably well-established concept, especially in countries such as Japan, personalized nutrition is still being treated with skepticism by certain populations and population groups. The recognition that some people would have different nutrient requirements, and/or perceive different foods in different ways, raises several concerns, some real and some not so real. This is a logical follow-on from the recognition that nutrients will be absorbed, utilized in biochemical reactions, metabolized, and excreted to varying extents among different individuals.

This book addresses nutrigenetics and nutrigenomics from a range of perspectives, ranging from purely scientific to ethical, consumer-driven, and public health aspects. It contains up-to-date information in a number of areas that are becoming essential for those trained in nutrition, including both nutritionists and dieticians, as well as other health professionals, including pharmacists and clinicians. It will also provide useful background information for those in the food business and food regulators.

Section I covers some of the best characterized examples of key gene–diet interactions. While referencing nutrigenomics, nutrigenetics is especially important in this section. An overview example of several key genetic variants that influence dietary response and how this might impact the teaching of the dietary pyramid is covered in Chapter 1. Chapters 2 and 3 focus on some transporter mutations that are particularly likely to influence micronutrient requirements, and some apolipoprotein gene variants that affect the amount and nature of fat that is desirable. Chapter 4 takes an interesting example to show how nutrigenomic tools, this time being applied to studies of a novel fat, can reveal a novel mechanism of action thereby leading to intellectual property that can benefit the food industry.

Several examples of the way in which studies on nutrigenetics and nutrigenomics can help modulate disease risk are described in Section II. Four important chronic diseases are singled out here—cardiovascular disease, obesity, diabetes, and inflammatory bowel disease (IBD)—initially as good examples, where relevant gene variants can respond to very specific nutritional interventions. The latter example is also a very good one in which another environmentally responsive factor—the microbiome—also interacts in a number of gene–diet interactions. Indeed, this is increasingly recognized as a major factor in several key diseases. That is, nutrients influence the expression of bacterial genes, which then in turn affect human gene expression. Chapter 9 also focuses on IBD, this time showing how transcriptome profiling studies can significantly augment an understanding as to how nutrients affect the expression of genes of particular importance for IBD susceptibility.

Chapter 9, arguably, could have been included in Section III, which focuses on technologies. Transcriptomics is an increasingly valuable tool, whose cost has decreased and efficiency increased over the past 10 years. An example of its application to a human dietary intervention study is provided in Chapter 13. One of the increasing challenges in nutrigenomics research is the size and complexity of the datasets generated. Data mining and network analysis are of increasing importance to this field. Other technologies of importance are metabolomics, epigenetics, and genotyping.

Section IV of the book considers some of the benefits—and challenges—of taking nutrigenetics and nutrigenomics beyond being largely science-led endeavors. They are now moving out of the laboratory and into the food industry, as well as out to health professionals and the public. The dangers of going directly to industry and the importance of industry–academia partnerships are emphasized as necessary, but nevertheless, something of a challenge.

As described in Chapter 16, commercialization of these fields is increasingly occurring with a range of different models prevailing. In terms of nutrigenetics, many of the initial ventures that used direct-to-consumer testing have floundered. While some had genuine bases, others were little more than costly excuses for price premiums on micronutrient supplements or functional foods. Those companies that continue to flourish are those that include a health professional, such as a dietician or physician (Chapter 18). There is an increasing number of demonstrable benefits—both to individual health and company finances—of such ventures.

Chapters 19 through 21 consider the implications of these new fields to the public and to the individual. The original title for Chapter 19 was "Is Contemporary Society Ready for Nutrigenomics?" This reflects the degree of skepticism being shown by individuals as to whether or not they want to understand their genotype or effects of their favorite foods on the expression of those genes. Chapters 20 and 21 consider these questions more generally, in the context of public health.

I hope you enjoy reading this book and that it gives you the same amount of pleasure it gave me in receiving chapters from many of the key players in these developing, and extremely important, fields.

Editor

Lynnette R. Ferguson, DPhil, DSc, QSO, FNZIFST earned her DPhil from Oxford University, working on the subjects of DNA damage, DNA repair, and mutagenesis in yeast. After her return to New Zealand, she began working as part of the Auckland Cancer Society Research Centre, using mutagenicity testing as a predictor of carcinogenesis, with particular focus on the New Zealand situation. In 2000, she took on a 50% role as head of a new discipline of nutrition at the University of Auckland. In more recent years, Dr. Ferguson has considered the interplay between genes and diet in the development of chronic disease, with particular focus on inflammatory bowel disease, a cancer-prone condition, and also in prostate cancer. As program leader for the multidisciplinary, multiorganization Nutrigenomics New Zealand, she is working with a range of others to bring nutrigenomics tools and potential to the New Zealand science scene.

Dr. Ferguson has supervised more than 30 students to the successful completion of a BTech, MSc, or PhD. Her laboratory regularly supervises two to three summer students each year. She is the author or coauthor of more than 300 peer-reviewed publications as chapters in books or articles in international journals. She serves as one of the managing editors for *Mutation Research: Fundamental and Molecular Mechanisms of Mutation*, as well as on the editorial boards of several other major journals.

Contributors

Maria Agelli
Department of Health and human Services
National Institutes of Health
National Cancer Institute
Bethesda, Maryland

Matthew P.G. Barnett
Food & Bio-Based Products Group
AgResearch Limited
The Liggins Institute
The University of Auckland
Grafton, Auckland, New Zealand

Shalome A. Bassett
Grasslands Research Centre
AgResearch Limited
Palmerston North, New Zealand

Emma N. Bermingham
Food & Bio-Based Products Group
AgResearch Limited
Palmerston North, New Zealand

David Castle
ESRC Innogen Centre
University of Edinburgh
Edinburgh, UK

Javier Delgado-Lista
Lipids and Atherosclerosis Unit
Reina Sofia University Hospital
University of Cordoba
Cordoba, Spain

Colleen Fogarty Draper
Nestlé Institute of Health Sciences SACampus EPFL
Quartier de l'innovation, bâtiment G
Lausanne, Switzerland

Peter Eck
Human Nutritional Science
University of Manitoba
Winnipeg, Manitoba, Canada

Stephanie Ellett
Faculty of Medical and Health Sciences
The University of Auckland
Auckland, New Zealand

Isobel R. Ferguson
Faculty of Medical and Health Sciences
The University of Auckland
Auckland, New Zealand

Lynnette R. Ferguson
Department of Nutrition
Faculty of Medical and Health Sciences
The University of Auckland
Grafton, Auckland, New Zealand

Antonio Garcia-Rios
Lipids and Atherosclerosis Unit
Reina Sofia University Hospital
University of Cordoba
Cordoba, Spain

Peter J. Gillies
New Jersey Institute for Food, Nutrition, and Health
Rutgers, The State University of New Jersey
New Brunswick, New Jersey

Dug Yeo Han
Faculty of Medical and Health Sciences
The University of Auckland
Auckland, New Zealand

Daniel Hurley
Department of Molecular Medicine and Pathology
Faculty of Medical and Health Sciences
University of Auckland
Auckland, New Zealand

Jim Kaput
Nestlé Institute of Health Sciences
Lausanne, Switzerland

Nishi Karunasinghe
Faculty of Medical and Health Sciences
The University of Auckland
Auckland, New Zealand

Joerg Kistler
Institute for Innovation in Biotechnology
The University of Auckland
Auckland, New Zealand

Bianca Knoch
Illawarra Health and Medical Research Institute
University of Woollongong
New South Wales, Australia

Michiel Korthals
CSG—Centre for Society and the Life Sciences
Radboud University Nijmegen
Nijmegen, the Netherlands

and

Chair Group Applied Philosophy
Wageningen University
Wageningen, the Netherlands

Wen J. Lam
Faculty of Medical and Health Sciences
The University of Auckland
Auckland, New Zealand

Hui-Ming Lin
Garvan Institute of Medical Research
Sydney, New South Wales, Australia

Jose Lopez-Miranda
Medicine, Lipid and Atherosclerosis Unit
Department of Medicine
Reina Sofia University Hospital
University of Cordoba
Cordoba, Spain

Elizabeth H. Marchlewicz
Department of Environmental Health Sciences
University of Michigan School of Public Health
Ann Arbor, Michigan

Gareth Marlow
Faculty of Medical and Health Sciences
The University of Auckland
Auckland, New Zealand

Warren C. McNabb
AgResearch Limited
Grasslands Research Centre
Palmerston North, New Zealand

John A. Milner
Beltsville Human Nutrition Research Center
United States Department of Agriculture
Agricultural Research Service
Beltsville, Maryland

Angharad R. Morgan
Faculty of Medical and Health Sciences
The University of Auckland
Auckland, New Zealand

Gilbert S. Omenn
School of Public Health
University of Michigan Center for Computational Medicine and Bioinformatics
Ann Arbor, Michigan

Virginia Parslow
Department of Nutrition
Faculty of Medical and Health Sciences
The University of Auckland
Auckland, New Zealand

Bart Penders
Department of Health, Ethics & Society (HES), School of Primary Care and Public Health (CAPHRI)
Maastricht University
Maastricht, the Netherlands

and

CSG—Centre for Society and the Life Sciences
Radboud University Nijmegen
Nijmegen, the Netherlands

Francisco Pérez-Jimenez
Lipid and Atherosclerosis Unit
Department of Medicine
Reina Sofia University Hospital
University of Cordoba
Cordoba, Spain

Pablo Perez-Martinez
Lipid and Atherosclerosis Unit
Reina Sofia University Hospital
University of Cordoba
Cordoba, Spain

Jason S. Peters
AgResearch Limited
Grasslands Research Centre
Palmerston North, New Zealand

Karen E. Peterson
Environmental Health Sciences
University of Michigan School of Public Health
Ann Arbor, Michigan

Catherine Phillips
HRB Centre for Diet and Health Research
Department of Epidemiology and Public Health
University College Cork, Ireland

Helen M. Roche
UCD Conway Institute
University College Dublin
Dublin, Ireland

Daryl Rowan
Plant & Food Research Ltd
Palmerston North, New Zealand

Nicole C. Roy
AgResearch Limited
Grasslands Research Centre
Palmerston North, New Zealand

Anna E. Russ
Food & Bio-Based Products Group
AgResearch Limited
Grasslands Research Centre
Palmerston North, New Zealand

Ralf C. Schlothauer
Comvita New Zealand Limited
Tauranga, New Zealand

Artemis P. Simopoulos
Center for Genetics
Nutrition and Health
Washington DC

John P. Vanden Heuvel
Department of Molecular Toxicology
Pennsylvania State University
University Park, Pennsylvania

Vijayalakshmi Varma
Division of Systems Biology
National Center for Toxicological Research
U.S. Food and Drug Administration
Jefferson, Arkansas

Wayne Young
Food & Bio-Based Products
Food Nutrition & Health
AgResearch Limited
Grasslands Research Centre
Palmerston North, New Zealand

Shuotun Zhu
Faculty of Medical and Health Sciences
The University of Auckland
Grafton, Auckland, New Zealand

Section I

Examples of Some Key Gene–Diet Interactions

1 Nutrigenetics and Nutrigenomics

Importance for Functional Foods and Personalized Nutrition

Lynnette R. Ferguson

CONTENTS

INTRODUCTION

Classic research on nutrition considered the effects of macronutrients (lipids, proteins, carbohydrates), or micronutrients (vitamins, minerals), defining physiological requirements for these, and determining the implications of either a deficiency or excess. The primary objective of these studies was to prevent signs of either nutrient deficiencies or of dietary excess. However, it is now apparent that nutrient intakes at levels that prevent classic symptoms of nutrient deficiency may still be inadequate for long-term health and wellness. As new methods for judging these optimal levels are developed, the recommended daily amounts (RDAs) of many nutrients are changing, and are likely to continue to do so [1]. Most studies on nutrient requirements are limited by studying effects of nutrients one at a time. Nutrient–nutrient interactions and effects of the food matrix are also critical. Furthermore, much of the research to date has implied that all people have the same dietary requirements. It is increasingly clear that not all individuals will benefit from an identical dietary regime, that is, they have a different nutritional phenotype. Although this may be partly a result of early dietary exposures and enzyme induction, as for example, with lactase deficiency [2], or other factors such as stress or concomitant disease, it may also relate to individual genetic variations.

"Nutrigenetics" describes how human genetic variation results in distinct nutritional requirements. Interindividual differences in genetics, resulting in different effects of nutrients on metabolism, were recognized early in nutrition research. A classic example of this may be folate metabolism, whereby a common single nucleotide polymorphism (SNP) exists for the gene that encodes the enzyme, methylenetetrahydrofolate reductase (MTHFR). Around 10% of the human population is homozygous for this SNP. Such individuals require higher than average amounts of dietary folic acid to minimize blood levels of homocysteine [3]. Other examples are given in Chapters 3 and 6 through 8. Although some key genetic variants are likely to be amenable to personal genotyping, practically, many will not. Even if they are, nutritional remedies may not also be immediately obvious. The general principle in setting RDAs has been to ensure that these have a sufficient margin of error to cover population variability.

For nutrients such as folate, there are probably wide gaps between the minimum level required and an excessive dose, so that the approach described earlier is appropriate. But there are several nutrients that have a relatively narrow window of efficacy, below or above which is deleterious to human health. Selenium (Se) provides such an example [1,4]. This micronutrient is important for DNA repair and enabling the cell to cope with oxidative stress. However, there is a relatively narrow window where it is effective, and too much is as damaging as too little. Furthermore, this window changes according to variants in a number of genes. How to combine information on the various affected genes may be beyond the current scope of knowledge in nutrigenetics.

Although the term "nutrigenomics" describes how diet modulates the expression of genes, it is often conceived as the application of high-throughput genomic tools in nutrition research. When such high-throughput screening is applied to nutrition research, it enables the study as to how nutrients affect the expression of the thousands of genes comprising the human genome. This field is increasingly being acknowledged as essential for understanding the role of diet in maintenance of homeostasis (wellness), prevention of risk of chronic disease, or slowing of disease progression. Its considerable potential for the future of food may currently be underrated.

HUMAN GENETIC VARIATION

No two humans are genetically identical. Even monozygotic twins, developed from a single zygote, have occasional genetic and epigenetic differences occurring during development. SNPs are a common source of genetic variation among people (Table 1.1).

TABLE 1.1
Some Useful Terms in Describing Human Variation

Allele: a particular configuration of a locus with a particular DNA sequence (can be many alleles for a particular locus, depending on its size)
Genotype: measured DNA sequence at a locus
Haplotype: a set of SNPs on a single chromosome of a chromosome pair that are statistically associated
Locus: an arbitrary region of the genome that can have mutations/polymorphisms
Mutations: differences in DNA sequence in an individual that are rare and may be unique to the individual (or their family line)
Polymorphisms: differences in DNA sequence that are found in many individuals, at a specified frequency (usually 1% or greater of a population)
Single nucleotide polymorphisms (SNPs): DNA sequence variations occurring when a single nucleotide, that is, adenine (A), thymine (T), cytosine (C), or guanine (G), differs between individuals or paired chromosomes in an individual. An SNP is defined as occurring at least in 1% of the population. There are several types of SNPs:

- Synonymous SNP: one in which both forms lead to the same polypeptide sequence (sometimes called a silent mutation)
- Nonsynonymous SNP: one that leads to a different polypeptide sequence (may either be missense or nonsense)
- Missense change: results in a different amino acid
- Nonsense change: results in a premature stop codon

SNPs occur once in every 300 nucleotides on average, making approximately 10 million SNPs in the human genome. Commonly, these variations are found in the DNA between genes. When SNPs occur within a gene, or in the gene's regulatory region, they may affect the gene's function. Most SNPs have no direct effect on health or development, but somewhere between 3% and 5% are functional, influencing phenotypic differences between humans [5]. Knowledge of SNPs may help predict an individual's response to certain diets or drugs, susceptibility to environmental toxins, and risk of developing particular diseases. Genome-wide association studies are becoming increasingly important in identifying SNPs associated with susceptibility to complex chronic diseases, such as cancer or cardiovascular disease (CVD).

Recent evidence suggests that non-SNP variation accounts for even more human genetic variation than SNPs. This variation includes copy number variation (CNV), and results from deletions, inversions, insertions, and duplications [6]. It has been estimated that approximately 0.4% of the genomes of unrelated people differ with respect to copy number. Including this figure, human-to-human genetic variation is estimated to be at least 0.5%, implying 99.5% similarity. CNV may be inherited or may arise during development. A variable number tandem repeat is a chromosomal location where a short nucleotide sequence is repeated in a tandem manner. Tandem repeats are found on many different chromosomes and often show variations in length, even between closely related individuals.

Epigenetics is another major source of genetic variation (Chapter 12). This is the study of heritable changes in gene expression or cellular phenotype caused by mechanisms other than changes in the underlying DNA sequence. Examples of such changes are DNA methylation and histone modification [7]. It is also becoming increasingly important to recognize the interplay between human and microbial genes (Chapter 5). Microorganism genomics is redefining our previous understandings of microbial food safety and the role of microbes in human health [8].

DESIRABLE HUMAN DIET

Most people, in most countries, will turn to their health department–approved dietary pyramid for healthy eating advice. In 2001, the epidemiologist, Walter Willett, debunked the U.S. Department of Agriculture (USDA) food guide pyramid, which serves as a model of desirable eating behavior for many Western countries. "At best, the USDA Pyramid offers wishy-washy, scientifically unfounded advice on an absolutely vital topic—what to eat. At worst, the misinformation contributes to overweight, poor health and unnecessary early deaths. In either case, it stands as a missed opportunity to improve the health of millions of people." With the help of his Harvard coworkers, he developed his own Healthy Eating Pyramid (Figure 1.1). The main recommendations of this are as follows [9,10].

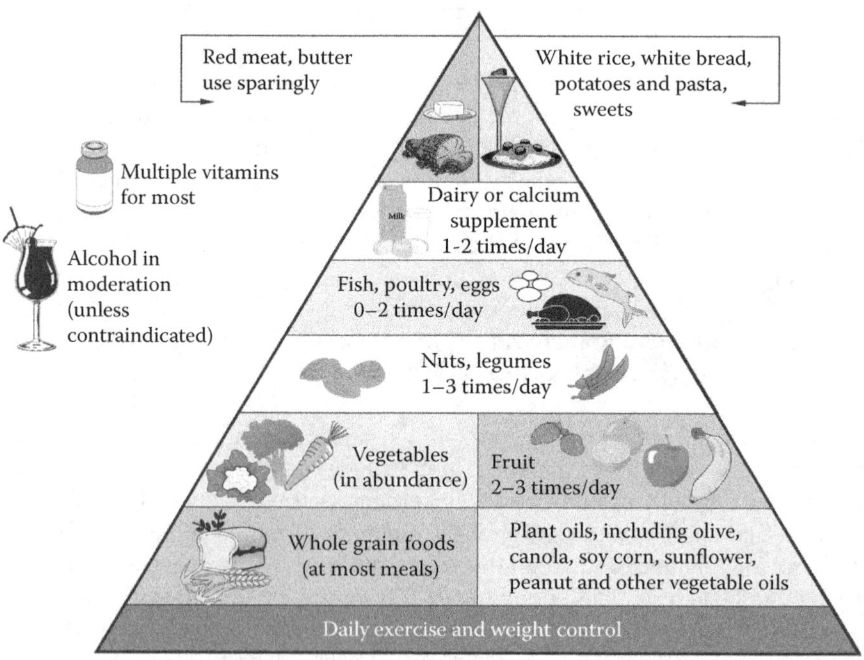

FIGURE 1.1 Healthy eating pyramid. (From Willett, W.C. et al., *Eat, Drink and Be Healthy: The Harvard Medical School Guide to Healthy Eating*, 299, Simon & Schuster Source, New York, 2001.)

At the base of the Healthy Eating Pyramid is regular exercise and weight control. In practice, this will usually involve conscious caloric restriction. Restriction of fats is commonly recommended as a means of caloric reduction. While recognizing their high energy density, Willett also points to the importance of certain types of fat in the diet. That is, he claims that, providing total energy balance is attained, nonhydrogenated plant oils are desirable in the diet, and indeed come low in his pyramid. He acknowledges some confusion about the benefits of carbohydrates and concludes that instead of recommending complex carbohydrates, the pyramid should reinforce the choice of minimally refined whole grains (WGs) in preference to refined starches and simple sugars. Vegetables and fruits should be consumed in abundance, with green leafy and orange vegetables being consumed daily. Red meat should be consumed rarely, with nuts, legumes, fish, and poultry being consumed in moderation as alternative protein sources. Dairy products may be optional and calcium (Ca) may be conveniently supplied as a supplement. Salt intake should be low, while regular intake of a multivitamin tablet and moderate alcohol consumption may be desirable.

Although several versions of this pyramid are now available, a generally agreed version appears in Figure 1.1.

EVIDENCE FOR A DESIRABLE HUMAN DIET

A major advantage of the Healthy Eating Pyramid is its strong evidence base, which is continually being reevaluated. The basis of the Healthy Eating Pyramid is mostly epidemiological and clinical studies, in particular, access to data from several large prospective cohort studies, such as the Nurse's Health study in the United States or the European Prospective Investigation into Cancer and Nutrition (EPIC) study across Europe [11]. Although the sheer size of these studies helps in statistical power, they suffer from well-recognized problems of imprecision of dietary recall. In addition, people tend to eat in patterns, so establishing the importance of a single food or nutrient becomes difficult.

The most compelling evidence that a certain level of a certain food or supplement benefits health comes from a controlled clinical trial that feeds large numbers of people, in two comparable groups, either the nutrient in question or a placebo, over enough time for disease to develop. However, the perils of such an approach have been brought into focus by large studies such as the SELECT (the Selenium and Vitamin E Cancer Prevention Trial) [12].

Animal and epidemiological studies had suggested that Se and vitamin E (alone or in combination) might reduce the risk of developing prostate cancer (PC). The randomized, placebo-controlled SELECT trial studied 35,533 men from 427 participating sites in the United States, Canada, and Puerto Rico, randomly assigned to four groups (Se, vitamin E, Se + vitamin E, and placebo) in a double-blind manner, between August 22, 2001 and June 24, 2004. However, an initial analysis of data at 5 years showed that, instead of the predicted and desired trends, there was a small increase in the number of PC cases in men taking only vitamin E and the number of cases of diabetes in men taking only Se [12]. After an average of 7 years (5.5 years on supplements and 1.5 off supplements), there were 17% more cases of PC in men taking only vitamin E than in men taking only placebos.

Surrogate biomarker endpoints to such trials provide a compromise that enables a smaller number of subjects to be used, over a shorter time. The important point is that if the dietary item being tested has an opposite effect to that desired, it is still possible to stop taking it in time to reverse the trend. For example, many recommendations on diet typically recommend that total fat intake should be 30% of energy, or less, to decrease CVD and cancer. Many studies on which these recommendations are based have assumed that total serum cholesterol levels predict CVD risk, thus serum cholesterol functioned as a surrogate biomarker. For example, much data were summarized in the early 1980s [13], suggesting that compared to carbohydrates, saturated fat increases and polyunsaturated fat decreases serum cholesterol, while monounsaturated fat has no effect. However, differentiating high-density from low-density lipoprotein enables more precise predictions of risk, pulling out more accurate and predictive descriptions of dietary desirability [9]. Biomarkers continue to be developed, providing increasingly more accurate dietary feedback. Nutrigenomics is one approach to biomarkers that may further refine current information.

DESIRABLE HUMAN DIET AND HUMAN GENETIC VARIATION

One disadvantage of the Healthy Eating Pyramid is that it still assumes a "one size fits all" approach to nutrition. Genetic polymorphisms will affect the relative importance of the various nutrient classes, at the level of an individual. Thus, going through the key points identified in the Healthy Eating Pyramid:

- Regular exercise and weight control: The effects of exercise and attempts at portion control will be affected by several genes that have been associated with obesity. For example, carrying certain variants in the *FTO* gene affects dietary selection and the amount of food needed for satiety, especially in children [14]. This may in part be overcome by substantial increases in physical activity levels [15]. The influence of the selection and total intake of fats in the diet will also interact with these polymorphisms. Red meat and dairy products make those individuals carrying an *FTO* variant even more likely to have a high body mass index [16].
- Rational selection of lipid source: In terms of risk of chronic disease, it is the nature of the lipids and their concentration in plasma that is likely to be more important than their overall intake in determining the risk of chronic disease. Variants in a number of genes, such as *PPARa*, *PPARg*, or others identified in Chapters 3, 6, and 7, will substantially modify the nature of the lipid being transported through the body [17].
- Rational selection of carbohydrate source: Varma et al. [18] used a data mining approach to suggest a significant role of various genes in carbohydrate metabolic pathways in the risk of obesity and, to a lesser extent, T2DM. This suggests that the implications of high-carbohydrate diets will vary among the population. The efficacy of high WG consumption in protecting against T2DM has been shown to interact with variants in the transcription factor 7-like 2 (*TCF7L2*) gene [19].

- Abundant fruits and vegetables, with daily consumption of green leafy and orange vegetables: Many green leafy vegetables are in the family Cruciferae. As well as containing a range of recognized nutrients, these vegetables have other phytochemicals, such as glucosinolates, with recognized roles in prevention of chronic diseases, especially cancer. The enzyme coded by the glutathione S-transferase mu 1 (*GSTM1*) gene functions in the detoxification of electrophilic compounds, and a high intake of glucosinolates is associated with upregulation of this gene. However, this function will not occur in individuals carrying a *GSTM1* null variant [20]. The particular value of orange vegetables is that the color indicates significant levels of the micronutrient, beta-carotene. Again, the efficacy of this nutrient will be determined by circulating levels of carotenoids in the plasma, and these levels depend not only on total intake, but also on the presence or absence of a common SNP in the beta-carotene 15,15′-monooxygenase 1 gene [21].
- Occasional or no red meat and dairy product consumption: Both red meat and dairy products are major dietary sources of saturated fatty acids, which are considered as one of the most undesirable types of fat in the human diet. Phillips et al. [22] concluded that dietary saturated fat and gender predict the development of metabolic syndrome when certain genetic variants in the *TCF7L2* gene are taken into account. The other concern relating to high red meat consumption is in relation to a possible iron overload. This would be a particular problem for individuals carrying variants in the hemochromatosis (*HFE*) gene, who are prone to iron overload, liver cirrhosis, and cardiomyopathy.
- Nuts, legumes, fish, and poultry as preferred protein sources: A particular justification for using these as protein sources, as opposed to red meat and dairy products, is that they have a more desirable lipid profile. The interactions of these lipid sources with common genetic variants in a number of genes are detailed elsewhere (Chapters 2, 3, 6, and 7). The interactions between dietary fish oil intakes and common variants in a number of genes are also reviewed in relation to the response of biomarkers of CVD risk [23].
- Ca supplied as a supplement: A variant in the Ca-sensing receptor A986S is associated with higher serum Ca and higher urinary Ca excretion [24]. In addition, Ca supplements have been associated with an increased risk of CVD [25].
- Salt intake should be low: Although there is general agreement on this principle as a preventive measure against CVD risk, there is considerable variability among the population in terms of salt sensitivity, partly through polymorphisms in genes related to the renin–angiotensin–aldosterone system [26].
- Regular intake of a multivitamin tablet: Simple single gene–single nutrient examples, such as that given previously for MTHFR/folate, are probably rare. Even for that example, knowing that an individual is homozygous for a functional SNP in the *MTHFR* gene will indicate a dietary requirement for

higher than average levels of folate, but not the exact amount. Other genes and dietary factors impact on this pathway (Figure 1.2).

- There is good evidence linking key genes with multiple effects on micronutrient and lipid handling in the body. Genetic variations in the genes involved in folate metabolism have multiple effects. Micronutrient and macronutrient interactions are also important. SNPs in MTHFR increase the risk of chronic diseases such as cancer and CVD through more than one mechanism, and respond to nutrients other than folate, albeit indirectly. The micronutrient genomics project provides a range of examples [27].
- Minerals: Although vitamins often have a relatively wide range of tolerances, a number of minerals are also considered to be essential micronutrients because of their role as cofactors for key enzymes. Typically, these have a somewhat narrow dose range of efficacy, as compared with toxicity. Examples include Ca, for which high-dose supplementation has been associated with increased risk of CVD [25], Se, and zinc (Zn). For each of these examples, SNPs in key genes may significantly affect the appropriate dose range for efficacy, and the desirability of supplementation may be disputed. Se provides a well-characterized example. Glutathione peroxidase (GPx) is the general name of an enzyme family whose main biological role is to protect the organism from oxidative damage through peroxidase activity. Their biochemical functions are to reduce lipid hydroperoxides to their corresponding alcohol and free hydrogen peroxide to water. Since the human GPxs are Se-containing, their function and activity depend significantly on the body Se level. SNPs in the genes for GPx can modify GPx4, GPx1, and GPx3 protein expression or activity, in response to Se supplementation. Thus, depending on the particular variants carried by an individual, as well

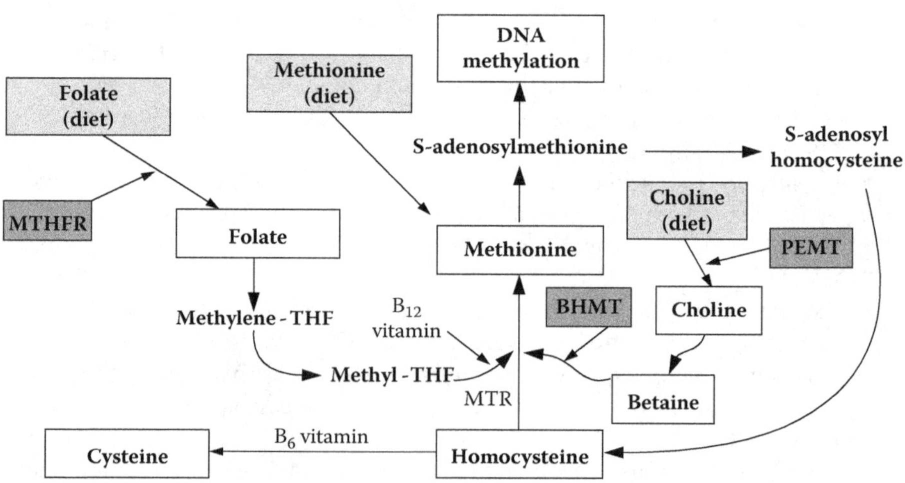

FIGURE 1.2 Examples of genes and gene products, and their effects on dietary items, in the pathway leading to accumulation or removal of homocysteine and DNA methylation. *Note*: PEMT: phosphatidylethanolamine N-methyltransferase; BHMT: betaine–homocysteine S-methyltransferase; MTR: 5-methyltetrahydrofolate-homocysteine methyltransferase.

as the starting plasma Se level, Se supplementation may be beneficial, have no effect, or be detrimental [4,28]. Similar examples can be found for Zn.
- Alcohol consumption may be desirable in moderation: Certain groups may find even low levels of alcohol to be undesirable, and alcohol may exacerbate the effects of other known genetic variants. For example, a high alcohol intake may increase still further the need for extra folate in those carrying variants of the *MTHFR* gene [29].

A more striking example, relevant to functional foods, is where knowledge of SNPs in a gene has been used to tailor remedial dietary preparations to specific groups. Kornman and coworkers [30,31] stratified subjects by genotype before a nutritional intervention. Their proof-of-concept trial considered the effects of a specifically formulated botanical mixture on inflammation in individuals stratified according to genetic variations that predispose to overexpression of interleukin-1β (IL-1β) and early CVD. They selected healthy adults with elevated C-reactive protein (CRP), a biomarker of inflammation, and genotyped them for variations in the *IL-1* gene that have previously been found to have a higher risk of heart disease. These subjects were then randomized to the candidate botanical formulation that included rose hips, a blueberry and blackberry mixture, and a grapevine extract, or placebo. The participants supplemented their normal diet with this mixture for 12 weeks, then provided samples for the study of *IL-1β* gene expression in stimulated peripheral blood mononuclear cells. The botanical mixture significantly reduced expression of this gene, and the effect was greater in higher risk than lower risk subjects. There was, however, no significant change in serum CRP levels. This study was important, not only in showing the effects of stratifying subjects for such trials, but also in justifying nutrigenetic and nutrigenomic approaches to study endpoints.

The gut microbiota also adds another dimension to individual dietary requirements. For example, the desirable human levels of vitamin H (biotin) are contentious. The U.S. dietary guidelines claim that biotin deficiency is rare because, in general, intestinal bacteria produce biotin in excess of the body's daily requirements [32]. For that reason, they do not prescribe an RDA of biotin. This conclusion neglects, however, the variations in microflora known to occur between healthy individuals and those with certain diseases, such as inflammatory bowel diseases [33], or between population groups with different dietary practices. It also neglects the impact of infections and use of antibiotics. Thus, biotin deficiency may be a significant problem in certain population groups.

NUTRIGENOMICS TOOLKIT

Although genomics has successfully identified associations between genetic variants and the risk of specific diseases, the biological mechanisms by which gene variations interact with one another and with the environment, including diet, to influence disease development and severity, are often not fully understood. It is important to realize that there are possibly thousands of genetic polymorphisms that may result in minor deviations in nutritional biochemistry, where only marginal or additive effects would result from these deviations. The tools to study the physiological impact were not available until now and are only now becoming available enabling the development of nutrigenomics. Such tools include those that measure the transcriptome—DNA microarrays, exon arrays, and tiling arrays. Methods to measure the proteome are less developed. These include methods based on gel electrophoresis, chromatography, and mass spectrometry (MS). Finally, the tools that measure the metabolome include methods based on nuclear magnetic resonance (NMR) spectroscopy and MS, often in combination with gas chromatography (GC) and liquid chromatography (LC).

Transcriptomics

As an example, the demonstration of functional effects due to variations in the concentrations of micronutrients in our diet is difficult, unless they are at such low levels as to lead to a risk of deficiency disease. It is even more complicated to estimate optimal levels of bioactive food components. The transcriptome, that is, the total set of RNA transcripts in a given organism, may be helpful. Transcriptomics measures the expression level of RNAs in a given cell population, providing information on relative amounts of RNA. Increasingly sophisticated methods to estimate gene expression, including whole-genome transcriptome analysis, are highly suitable to obtain unbiased information on potentially affected biological processes, at a whole-genome level. Transcriptome analysis is playing an increasingly important role in benefit–risk assessments, helping to identify functional effects and appropriate levels of micronutrients and bioactive food components.

Proteomics

Unfortunately, RNA levels are not directly proportional to the expression level of the proteins. In addition, transcripts may be translated into more than one protein. Proteomics reveals more details of molecular processing, and thereby potentially leads to a more comprehensive molecular understanding of the health benefits of micronutrients and bioactive food components. Identification and quantification of bioactive proteins and peptides, using proteomic technologies, can more precisely address questions of nutritional bioefficacy. However, a given cell type may produce different proteins at different times, and under different conditions. Also, any protein can undergo a wide range of posttranslational modifications. Thus, although genomics, transcriptomics, and proteomics may suggest a potential phenotypic response to a given dietary intervention, they cannot definitively predict this.

Metabolomics

Metabolomics (or metabonomics) may provide an answer to the problem. The metabolome consists of all the low-molecular-weight molecules or metabolites in a cell, tissue, or organism, thereby providing a functional readout of cellular biochemistry. Thousands of metabolites can now be measured quantitatively from relatively small amounts of biological material. Global metabolite profiling (untargeted metabolomics) enables new discoveries linking cellular pathways to biological mechanism in ways not previously suspected. In contrast, targeted metabolomics is defined by the identification and quantification of sets of structurally characterized and biochemically annotated metabolites, utilizing current knowledge of most biochemical pathways. Most enzymatic reactions and their end products are relatively well characterized, allowing early signs of disease processes to be identified, and targeted remedies, including tailored diets, to be developed. Targeted metabolomics generally provides quantitative information on the molar concentrations of metabolites in a pathway. Thus, deviations from normal are relatively easy to interpret, whether the study considers healthy versus diseased or treated versus untreated. Such methodology is well suited for high-throughput and routine applications. It has at least three important applications:

- Stratifying population groups (phenotyping): Metabolomics technologies are often appropriate to distinguish those individuals most likely to respond positively to a dietary intervention from those who will not.
- Biomarkers of disease risk: Many diseases, including cancer and inflammatory bowel diseases, have distinctive metabolomic signatures that increase as the disease progresses. In this case, metabolomics can provide a biomarker to consider whether a given dietary intervention can enable a reversal of the progression to advanced disease, or at least a slowing of the disease process.
- Validating dietary intake: It has been repeatedly found that many human subjects show a selective memory for dietary intake. There is no perfect method of dietary assessment in human populations. Metabolomics technologies, using sensitive measurements, such as GC–MS, LC–MS, capillary electrophoresis, or NMR, may help to characterize markers of nutrient exposure or detect relatively subtle shifts in dietary patterns.

The large multidimensional datasets that result from such studies must be processed and analyzed to render the data meaningful. Thus, bioinformatics tools are essential for the efficient processing of huge datasets, the characterization of the detected signals, and to align multiple datasets and their features.

Next-generation sequencing technologies are cost-effective ways of producing millions of short DNA or RNA sequence reads in a high-throughput manner. Their applications include whole-genome sequencing and resequencing, SNP and structural variation discovery, noncoding RNA profiling, and protein–nucleic acid interaction assays. Case studies in structural, functional, and comparative genomics, including metagenomics and epigenomics, provide a comprehensive picture of genomic structures and functions. They are highly appropriate for solving complex biological problems in diet and nutrition.

NUTRIGENOMICS AND THE MAINTENANCE OF HOMEOSTASIS

Nutrients are detected by cellular signaling molecules and may be seen as signals that tell a specific cell in the body how to react to a specific dietary factor. By this means, the cell obtains information about its environment, which is the diet. The sensory system that interprets information from nutrients about the dietary environment includes transcription factors together with many additional proteins. Once the nutrient interacts with such a sensory system, it modulates gene, protein expression, and metabolite production in accordance with the level of nutrient it senses. As a result, different diets elicit different patterns of gene and protein expression and metabolite production. Nutrigenomics describes the patterns of these dietary signatures. This enables an understanding as to how nutrition influences homeostasis.

Maintenance of homeostasis is essential to the prolongation of good health and prevention or delay of disease. Although we have biomarkers for disease risk, biomarkers to quantify health are necessary. Quantifying homeostasis is a significant challenge. However, it has been suggested that measuring responses to a challenge to homeostasis may be more informative than a static measure [34]. Perturbation tests might use known detrimental nutritional challenges, such as high fat or high glucose, over a short time frame, then consider the ability of the body to restore itself to normal functioning. Comprehensive multidimensional, omics-based analyses provide a route to identifying key biomarkers, as well as leading to a greater understanding of health.

Metabolic flexibility is the capacity for an individual to adapt fuel oxidation to fuel availability. This concept is further developed as phenotypic flexibility, involving fundamental mechanisms essential for optimal metabolic health. The European FP7-funded NutriTech project will apply an integrated series of methods to assess the underlying and related cell biological and genetic mechanisms, and multiple physiological processes of adaptation when homeostasis is challenged in an integrated series of human intervention studies (http://www.nutritech.nl).

We have long considered most genetic states to be somewhat stable in the absence of the extreme physiological challenges described earlier. However, a recent study of a single individual over 14 months, using state of the art extremely high-coverage genomic analyses, described as an integrative personal omics profile, showed significant fluxing [35]. Extensive heteroallelic changes occurred, during both healthy and diseased states, as well as an unexpected RNA editing mechanism. The analysis combined genomic, transcriptomic, proteomic, metabolomic, and autoantibody profiles, revealing various medical risks, including a higher than normal susceptibility to type 2 diabetes. It also revealed extensive, dynamic changes in diverse molecular components and biological pathways.

NUTRIGENOMICS AND PREVENTIVE HEALTH

PC is the most common cancer in the Western world. After lung cancer, it is the second most important cancer causing male deaths in the United States and Britain. Dietary and lifestyle changes are recommended for men diagnosed with early-stage PC, but the evidence base for these has not been as strong as would be desirable. PC provides a good example on which gene-expression profiling, before and after dietary interventions, has led to a rationale for disease prevention.

Men with a diagnosis of high-grade prostatic intraepithelial neoplasia (HGPIN), the preinvasive in situ stage of prostatic adenocarcinoma, are known to be at increased risk of developing PC. Epidemiological studies have suggested that consumption of more than one portion of cruciferous vegetables (such as broccoli) per week may reduce both the incidence of PC and the risk of developing aggressive PC. Traka et al. [36] quantified and interpreted changes in global gene-expression patterns in the human prostate gland before, during, and after a 12 month broccoli-rich diet, as compared with a pea-rich diet. Volunteers with a diagnosis of HGPIN were randomly assigned to either of these two diets. Comparison of biopsies obtained pre- and postintervention revealed more changes in gene expression occurred in individuals on a broccoli-rich diet than in those on a pea-rich diet, and this stratified according to genotype. The authors suggested that regular consumption of broccoli interacts with GSTM1 genotype to result in complex changes to signaling pathways associated with inflammation and carcinogenesis in the prostate. That is, broccoli consumption shifted the gene-expression profile to a less cancer-prone state. This study, therefore, provides experimental evidence in humans to support observational studies that diets rich in cruciferous vegetables may reduce the risk of PC and other chronic disease.

NUTRIGENOMICS AND THE SLOWING OF DISEASE PROGRESSION

There are a number of examples whereby nutrigenomics technologies have given information relevant to the slowing of disease progression. PC again provides an exemplar.

In vitro studies, considering effects of nutrients on gene-expression profiles, may provide preliminary evidence for effective dietary intervention strategies. Friedrichs et al. [37] suggested that progression of PC to androgen independence is a key turning point in the progression of the disease. They had reason to believe that long-chain omega-3 polyunsaturated fatty acids (*n*-3 PUFA) could be effective at preventing and treating refractory PC. Thus, they used an in vitro model of androgen ablation to determine the effects of two *n*-3 PUFA, docosahexaenoic acid (DHA) and eicosapentaenoic acid (EPA), on progression of the LNCaP PC cell line to an androgen-independent state. Treatment with these PUFA was able to prevent progression of LNCaP cells, whereas the omega-6 PUFA, arachidonic acid (AA), promoted cell growth under conditions of hormone depletion. These results correlated with a decrease in the expression of the androgen receptor, as well as suppression of an important cancer-related signaling pathway.

In vivo studies are essential to confirm the efficacy of nutrient interventions. Thus, Magbanua et al. [38] considered the effects of supplementation with fish oil (which contains high levels of EPA and DHA) on prostate gene expression, in a double-blind placebo-controlled randomized clinical trial. They studied men with low-grade PC, stratified based on self-reported dietary consumption of fish, and then randomly assigned to a 3-month intervention of fish oil ($n = 27$) supplementation or placebo ($n = 28$). cDNA microarray analysis was used to study gene expression in morphologically normal prostate tissue at baseline and at 3 months. Differential gene expression and pathway analyses were then used to identify genes and pathways modulated by these dietary components. Pathway analyses of rank-ordered genes showed modulation of androgen and estrogen metabolism in men who routinely consumed more fish compared to men who ate less. In addition, modulation of AA metabolism and oxidative stress response was significantly different between the supplemented and nonsupplemented group.

cDNA microarray is the most powerful tool for studying gene expression

Metabolomics approaches have also been used in dietary intervention studies to slow cancer progression. For example, they have been used to study the mechanism by which a diet rich in WG rye reduces the progression of early-stage PC [39]. This study compared changes in the plasma metabolic signature of patients with early-stage PC, after a 6-week intervention with a diet rich in WG rye and rye bran product (RP), as compared with a similar intervention with a diet rich in a refined white wheat product (WP). Seventeen PC patients received 485 g RP or WP in a randomized, controlled, crossover design. At the end of each intervention period, fasting plasma samples were collected and studied using ^{1}H NMR-based metabolomics technologies. The data showed an increase in five metabolites, including 3-hydroxybutyric acid, acetone, betaine, *N*,*N*-dimethylglycine, and dimethyl sulfone, after the RP but not the WP intervention. The data suggested a shift in energy metabolism from an anabolic to a catabolic status, which could explain some of the beneficial health effects of WG rye. These would support the use of RP in dietary regimes for slowing cancer progression.

FUNCTIONAL FOODS

In the 1980s, Japan proposed the terminology and concepts of 'functional food', stimulating a considerable amount of basic and applied studies on food functionality across the globe. Although there are several definitions, an agreed working definition is "a food can be regarded as functional if it is satisfactorily demonstrated to affect beneficially one or more target functions in the body, beyond nutritional effects in a way which is relevant to either the state of health or well-being or the reduction of the risk of a disease." Functional foods are typically created to enhance the levels, bioavailability, or palatability of various nutrients and/or bioactive compounds.

How to Produce a Functional Food

Several methods can be used.

1. Eliminating or reducing the levels of a given food compound: This is appropriate to components known to cause a deleterious effect when consumed (e.g., an allergen).
2. Increasing the concentration of a component naturally present in food: For example, foods might be fortified with a micronutrient to reach a daily intake compatible with the dietary guidelines for reducing risk of disease.
3. Adding a novel component not normally present in most foods: Examples here would include probiotics or nonvitamin antioxidants.
4. Replacing a component whose intake may be at dietary excess levels: For example, starches may be replaced by dietary fibers in fiber-enhanced foods such as breads.
5. Increasing bioavailability or stability of a functional component: Examples here include studies on polyphenolic compounds.

Examples of typical ingredients added, and the claims associated with them, are provided in Table 1.2.

TABLE 1.2
Examples of Functional Food Ingredients, the Claims That Are Made or Implied, and the Evidence for the Efficacy of These Ingredients in Maintaining Health and/or Preventing Disease

Ingredient	Examples of Products	Claim	Strength of Evidence in Humans
		Macronutrients	
Carbohydrates as dietary fiber	Fiber-enhanced breads	Relieves constipation	++
Lipids as *n*-3 PUFA	Breads, eggs	Reduces risk of heart disease	++
Soy protein	Drinks, bars	Reduces cholesterol and risk of heart disease	+− For cholesterol lowering +− For reduction of heart disease
		Micronutrients	
Folic acid	Breakfast cereals	Protects against neural tube defects	++
Folic acid + vitamin B_6 (pyridoxine)	Breakfast cereals	Decreases homocysteine and risk of CVD	++ For homocysteine − For CVD
Vitamin D	Milk, breakfast cereals, and margarines	Immune function, bone health, and a decrease in mortality in elderly women	+ For all
Vitamin E	Supplements	Antioxidant, prevents CVD	− For CVD
Vitamin C	Drinks, sweets	Protects against CVD	+− In observational studies − In clinical trials
Calcium	Cereals, fruit juices, milk products, spreads	Protects against osteoporosis, helps maintain bone density	+ For consumers with a low calcium intake
Zinc	Sweets, lozenges	Prevention/cure of common cold	+−
		Novel functional food ingredients	
Plant stanols and sterols	Margarine, yogurt, cereal bars	Lower cholesterol and risk of coronary heart disease	++ For low-density lipoprotein cholesterol lowering +− For coronary heart disease No data on coronary heart disease
"Probiotic" live bacteria, plus fermentable sugars (prebiotics)	Yogurts	Enhance immunity	Some effects on biomarkers

(*Continued*)

TABLE 1.2 (*Continued*)
Examples of Functional Food Ingredients, the Claims That Are Made or Implied, and the Evidence for the Efficacy of These Ingredients in Maintaining Health and/or Preventing Disease

Ingredient	Examples of Products	Claim	Strength of Evidence in Humans
Isoflavones	Soy products	Reduce menopausal symptoms, osteoporosis, and CVD	– For hot flushes +– For osteoporosis and heart disease
Catechins	Tea	Reduce CVD	+– Some epidemiological evidence No trial data
Conjugated linoleic acid	Supplements (small amounts occur naturally in milk, beef, and lamb)	Anti-inflammatory effects reduce cancer and CVD risk	No data on cancer in humans – For blood lipids in humans

Whether the food itself will have a similar effect depends on the amounts and bioavailability of the claimed active ingredients.
++, Proven efficacy, consistent effect seen in multiple high-quality studies; +, reasonable evidence for efficacy, effect seen in a limited number of studies, or some inconsistency between studies; +–, evidence for no effect, absence of an effect evident from a limited number of studies; –, proven not to work, absence of an effect evident. More detailed references can be found in References [40–42].

Why might nutrigenomics be important for functional foods?

It is important to recognize that just adding a so-called functional ingredient to a food matrix does not prove that the food will benefit health. Theory does not always extrapolate to practice, and hitherto standard chemical, biochemical, or physiological methodologies may not be adequate to fully describe functional effects. Despite their increasing popularity, few functional foods are currently accompanied by scientifically supported health claims. The aims of nutrigenomics include being able to demonstrate the effect of known nutrients and bioactive food compounds and health foods on health, independent of the biological matrix which these are presented in. The technologies should lead to the development of functional foods that will keep people healthy according to their individual needs. Additional variables to be considered include the question as to whether the food is unprocessed and processed, the food matrix it is in, the amount that is actually eaten, and the eating-related behaviors of consumers. The studies are large and complex, and international cooperation in nutrigenomics research is highly desirable [43].

Functional foods are being designed for personalized nutrition, based on genetic information relevant to health risk profiles. An example might be functional food products designed to reduce the risk of CVDs. Despite excellent hypotheses for their design, effects induced by functional foods are hard to identify and prove, let alone to establish a recommended daily intake. Thus, defining the optimal intake and the upper limit of both functional foods and dietary supplements poses a technical challenge. Whole-genome transcriptome analysis can provide unbiased information on potentially affected biological processes, on a whole-genome level [40].

PERSONALIZED NUTRITION

A human phenotype is the composite of observable characteristics or traits, including appearance, behavior, development, and biochemical or physiological properties. Phenotypes result from the interaction between genes and environment, which ultimately determines the personalized nutritional requirements for an individual. As discussed earlier, there are a considerable number of genes that affect individual dietary requirements. However, we are not yet sufficiently in control of bioinformatics manipulation of that genetic information to understand how to optimally combine information on gene pathways and epistasis, thereby determining individual nutritional requirements. Alternative approaches (Figure 1.3) may provide answers to this dilemma. The identification of responders from nonresponders to diet must be a primary goal of personalizing nutrition, based on genetic and metabolic information.

The response of an individual to the combined effects of nutrient and caloric intake, genetic and epigenetic background, lifestyle choices, and environmental exposures, provides a sensitive indicator of nutritional and metabolic status, increasingly being measured as a metabolic phenotype [44]. Such information enables a rational basis for the selection of foods, including functional foods, and supplements,

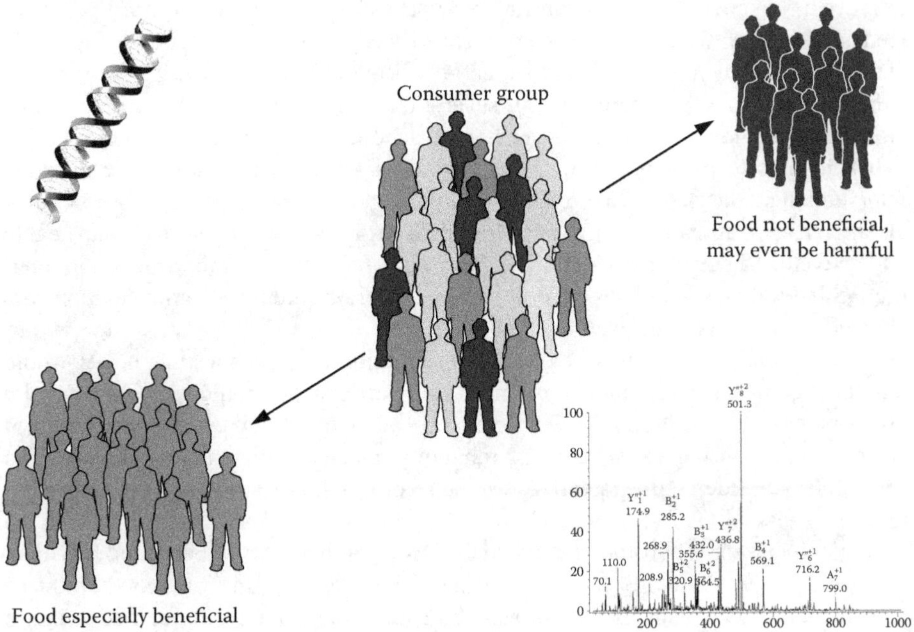

FIGURE 1.3 Both genetic and metabolomics methods may be appropriate for stratifying individuals for dietary benefits, in a comparable manner to pharmacogenomics.

along with lifestyle modification, to move an individual's health in a more personally beneficial direction. The ultimate goal is to develop a dietary pattern for each individual to maximize health and wellness, and prevent disease. This will also depend on age, activity level, and other lifestyle and environmental factors.

In addition to variations in the human genome, it is important to recognize the role of variation in the gut microbiota on human health [45]. These microbes and their by-products have been shown to alter the host genome, transcriptome, proteome, metabolome, and health status. Urinary metabolites reflect not only human metabolism, but also gut microflora metabolism. For example, distinctive urinary metabolites have been associated with the obesity phenotype [46]. Urinary metabolite profiling using ^{1}H NMR spectroscopy and pattern recognition methods has distinguished children with autism from closely related individuals without the disease [47]. The data suggest perturbations in sulfur and amino acid metabolism, as well as biochemical changes associated with an altered gut microbiota in the autistic children. Such distinctive metabolic profiles could be of potential value in monitoring the success of therapeutic interventions. This means that modulating the gut microbiota must be considered as an essential component of personalized nutrition. It becomes important to distinguish how different dietary components can enhance the selective growth of one microbial population over another. Metabolomics-based technologies have provided convincing evidence that regular consumption of synbiotics (a combination of probiotics and prebiotics) can lead to significant shifts in microbial flora [48].

TAKING PERSONALIZED NUTRITION TO THE PUBLIC

Surveys have generally shown consumers to have a positive attitude toward personalized foods. They would also be responsive to the use of their genetic profile, especially if guided by a dietician, and would be willing to buy the resulting product [49] (Chapter 18). However, there are still several challenges to targeted nutrition advice and functional food marketing according to genetic advice. Despite the promise of nutrigenomics to personalize diet, there have not yet been the large-scale nutrition intervention studies to prove the efficacy of the concept. The technology is now sufficiently sensitive and poised to make a significant difference to long-term human health.

Personalized nutrition uses familial, genetic, or metabolomics information to interpret an individual's health risk profile. The derived nutritional recommendations are claimed to help maintain wellness and/or reduce disease risk. Various Internet surveys have questioned consumers regarding their attitudes to such testing, if they would buy functional foods relevant to their individual nutrigenetic profile, or more generally use personalized nutrition. For example, such an Internet survey was conducted in December 2007 using a sample of 452 randomly selected adults in Germany [41]. The survey also considered the potential acceptance of functional food products claimed to reduce the risk of CVDs. In general, this group of consumers was positive toward the testing of their genetic profile, if it would lead to specific advice on beneficial nutrition. In addition, more than 40% would be willing to buy derived functional food products.

Ethical and practical considerations for various consumer groups can be found in Chapters 15 through 20.

REFERENCES

1. Ferguson, L.R. and Fenech, M.F. Vitamin and minerals that influence genome integrity, and exposure/intake levels associated with DNA damage prevention. *Mutation Research: Fundamental and Molecular Mechanisms of Mutagenesis* 733, 1–3 (2012).
2. Heyman, M.B. (for the Committee on Nutrition). From the American Academy of Pediatrics. Lactose intolerance in infants, children, and adolescents. *Pediatrics* 118, 1279–1286 (2006).
3. Fenech, M.F. Folate (vitamin B9) and vitamin B12 and their function in the maintenance of nuclear and mitochondrial genome integrity. *Mutation Research: Fundamental and Molecular Mechanisms of Mutagenesis* 733, 21–33 (2011).
4. Ferguson, L.R., Karunasinghe, N., Zhu, S. and Wang, A.H. Selenium and its role in the maintenance of genomic stability. *Mutation Research: Fundamental and Molecular Mechanisms of Mutagenesis* 733, 100–10 (2012).
5. Yamada, R. Primer: SNP-associated studies and what they can teach us. *Nature Clinical Practice Rheumatology* 4, 210–7 (2008).
6. van Binsbergen, E. Origins and breakpoint analyses of copy number variations: up close and personal. *Cytogenetic & Genome Research* 135, 271–6 (2011).
7. Johnson, L.J. and Tricker, P.J. Epigenomic plasticity within populations: its evolutionary significance and potential. *Heredity* 105, 113–21 (2010).
8. Gentshew, L. and Ferguson, L.R. Role of nutrition and microbiota in susceptibility to inflammatory bowel diseases. *Molecular Nutrition & Food Research* 56, 524–35 (2012).
9. Willett, C.W. The pursuit of optimal diets: a progress report. In *Nutritional genomics: discovering the path to personalized nutrition* (ed. Kaput, J.R. and Raymond L.) 37–56 (Wiley, New Jersey, 2006).
10. Willett, W.C., Skerrett, P.J., Giovannucci, E. and Callahan, M. *Eat, drink and be healthy: the Harvard Medical School guide to healthy eating* 299 (Simon & Schuster Source, New York, 2001).
11. Pan, A. et al. Red meat consumption and mortality: results from 2 prospective cohort studies. *Archives Internal Medicine* 172, 555–63 (2012).
12. Klein, E.A. et al. Vitamin E and the risk of prostate cancer: the Selenium and Vitamin E Cancer Prevention Trial (SELECT). *JAMA* 306, 1549–56 (2011).
13. Keys, A. et al. The seven countries study: 2,289 deaths in 15 years. *Preventive Medicine* 13, 141–54 (1984).
14. Razquin, C., Marti, A. and Martinez, J.A. Evidences on three relevant obesogenes: MC4R, FTO and PPARgamma. Approaches for personalized nutrition. *Molecular Nutrition & Food Research* 55, 136–49 (2011).
15. Scott, R.A. et al. FTO genotype and adiposity in children: physical activity levels influence the effect of the risk genotype in adolescent males. *European Journal of Human Genetics* 18, 1339–43 (2010).
16. Corella, D. et al. A high intake of saturated fatty acids strengthens the association between the fat mass and obesity-associated gene and BMI. *Journal of Nutrition* 141, 2219–25 (2011).
17. Alsaleh, A. et al. PPARgamma2 gene Pro12Ala and PPARalpha gene Leu162Val single nucleotide polymorphisms interact with dietary intake of fat in determination of plasma lipid concentrations. *Journal of Nutrigenetics & Nutrigenomics* 4, 354–66 (2011).
18. Varma, V., Wise, C. and Kaput, J. Carbohydrate metabolic pathway genes associated with quantitative trait loci (QTL) for obesity and type 2 diabetes: identification by data mining. *Biotechnology Journal* 5, 942–9 (2010).

19. Fisher, E. et al. Whole-grain consumption and transcription factor-7-like 2 (TCF7L2) rs7903146: gene-diet interaction in modulating type 2 diabetes risk. *British Journal of Nutrition* 101, 478–81 (2009).
20. Brauer, H.A. et al. Cruciferous vegetable supplementation in a controlled diet study alters the serum peptidome in a GSTM1-genotype dependent manner. *Nutrition Journal* 10, 11 (2011).
21. Ferrucci, L. et al. Common variation in the beta-carotene 15,15′-monooxygenase 1 gene affects circulating levels of carotenoids: a genome-wide association study. *American Journal of Human Genetics* 84, 123–33 (2009).
22. Phillips, C.M. et al. Dietary saturated fat, gender and genetic variation at the TCF7L2 locus predict the development of metabolic syndrome. *Journal of Nutritional Biochemistry* 23, 239–44 (2012).
23. Madden, J. et al. The impact of common gene variants on the response of biomarkers of cardiovascular disease (CVD) risk to increased fish oil fatty acids intakes. *Annual Review of Nutrition* 31, 203–34 (2011).
24. Laaksonen, M.M.L. et al. Associations of vitamin D receptor, calcium-sensing receptor and parathyroid hormone gene polymorphisms with calcium homeostasis and peripheral bone density in adult Finns. *Journal of Nutrigenetics & Nutrigenomics* 2, 55–63 (2009).
25. Reid, I.R., Bolland, M.J. and Grey, A. Calcium supplements and risk of myocardial infarction: a hypothesis twice tested. *American Journal of Medicine* 125, e15 (2012).
26. Poch, E. et al. Molecular basis of salt sensitivity in human hypertension. Evaluation of renin-angiotensin-aldosterone system gene polymorphisms. *Hypertension* 38, 1204–9 (2001).
27. van Ommen, B. et al. The micronutrient genomics project: a community-driven knowledge base for micronutrient research. *Genes & Nutrition* 5, 285–96 (2010).
28. Karunasinghe, N. et al. Serum selenium and single-nucleotide polymorphisms in genes for selenoproteins: relationship to markers of oxidative stress in men from Auckland, New Zealand. *Genes & Nutrition* 7, 179–90 (2012).
29. Kim, J. et al. Dietary intake of folate and alcohol, MTHFR C677T polymorphism, and colorectal cancer risk in Korea. *American Journal of Clinical Nutrition* 95, 405–12 (2012).
30. Kornman, K. et al. Interleukin-1 genotype-selective inhibition of inflammatory mediators by a botanical: a nutrigenetics proof of concept. *Nutrition* 23, 844–52 (2007).
31. Randolph, K. and Kornman, K. Award for nutrition and metabolism. A nutrigenetics proof-of-principle study: 12 years of molecular genetics meets 70 years of nutrition science. *Nutrition* 25, 258–60 (2009).
32. Otten, J.J., Hellwig, J.P. and Meyers, L.D. (eds.). *Dietary reference intakes: The essential guide to nutrient requirements* (The National Academies Press, Washington, DC, 2006).
33. Gentschew, L. and Ferguson, L.R. Role of nutrition and microbiota in susceptibility to inflammatory bowel diseases. *Molecular Nutrition & Food Research* 56, 524–35 (2012).
34. van Ommen, B., Keijer, J., Heil, S.G. and Kaput, J. Challenging homeostasis to define biomarkers for nutrition related health. *Molecular Nutrition & Food Research* 53, 795–804 (2009).
35. Chen, R. et al. Personal omics profiling reveals dynamic molecular and medical phenotypes. *Cell* 148, 1293–307 (2012).
36. Traka, M. et al. Broccoli consumption interacts with GSTM1 to perturb oncogenic signalling pathways in the prostate. *PLoS ONE [Electronic Resource]* 3, e2568 (2008).
37. Friedrichs, W., Ruparel, S.B., Marciniak, R.A. and deGraffenried, L. Omega-3 fatty acid inhibition of prostate cancer progression to hormone independence is associated with suppression of mTOR signaling and androgen receptor expression. *Nutrition & Cancer* 63, 771–7 (2011).

38. Magbanua, M.J.M. et al. Gene expression and biological pathways in tissue of men with prostate cancer in a randomized clinical trial of lycopene and fish oil supplementation. *PLoS ONE [Electronic Resource]* 6, e24004 (2011).
39. Moazzami, A.A. et al. Nuclear magnetic resonance-based metabolomics enable detection of the effects of a whole grain rye and rye bran diet on the metabolic profile of plasma in prostate cancer patients. *Journal of Nutrition* 141, 2126–32 (2011).
40. Keijer, J., van Helden, Y.G.J., Bunschoten, A. and van Schothorst, E.M. Transcriptome analysis in benefit-risk assessment of micronutrients and bioactive food components. *Molecular Nutrition & Food Research* 54, 240–8 (2010).
41. Roosen, J., Bruhn, M., Mecking, R.-A. and Drescher, L.S. Consumer demand for personalized nutrition and functional food. *International Journal for Vitamin & Nutrition Research* 78, 269–74 (2008).
42. O'Mahony, L., Stepien, M., Gibney, M.J., Nugent, A.P. and Brennan, L. The potential role of vitamin D enhanced foods in improving vitamin D status. *Nutrients* 3, 1023–41 (2011).
43. Kaput, J. et al. The case for strategic international alliances to harness nutritional genomics for public and personal health. *British Journal of Nutrition* 94, 623–32 (2005).
44. Zivkovic, A.M. and German, J.B. Metabolomics for assessment of nutritional status. *Current Opinion in Clinical Nutrition & Metabolic Care* 12, 501–7 (2009).
45. Turnbaugh, P.J. and Gordon, J.I. The core gut microbiome, energy balance and obesity. *Journal of Physiology* 587, 4153–8 (2009).
46. Calvani, R. et al. Gut microbiome-derived metabolites characterize a peculiar obese urinary metabotype. *International Journal of Obesity* 34, 1095–8 (2010).
47. Yap, I.K.S. et al. Urinary metabolic phenotyping differentiates children with autism from their unaffected siblings and age-matched controls. *Journal of Proteome Research* 9, 2996–3004 (2010).
48. Ndagijimana, M. et al. Effect of a synbiotic food consumption on human gut metabolic profiles evaluated by (1)H nuclear magnetic resonance spectroscopy. *International Journal of Food Microbiology* 134, 147–53 (2009).
49. DeBusk, R. The role of nutritional genomics in developing an optimal diet for humans. *Nutrition in Clinical Practice* 25, 627–33 (2010).

2 Variations in Solute Transporter Genes Affecting Micronutrient Solute Transport and Human Health

Peter Eck

CONTENTS

INTRODUCTION

Micronutrients are essential dietary compounds that are needed in small quantities to ensure normal metabolism. In regard to water-soluble compounds, often called solutes, micronutrients refer to water-soluble vitamins and mineral trace elements. Humans obtain these solutes through intestinal absorption from exogenous sources. After absorption, they will be distributed throughout the body. Solute carriers mediate the transport of water-soluble micronutrients across hydrophobic cell membranes. Therefore, external as well as genetic factors determine their intestinal absorption and systemic distribution, which can lead to pathophysiological consequences [1]. This chapter aims to demonstrate that genetic variations in micronutrients solute membrane carriers can profoundly influence health and disease states.

It has long been known that adequate dietary micronutrient supply is a determining factor for human health. Biochemical research determined how vitamins and trace elements serve as essential cofactors for enzymatic reactions in the biochemical machinery of the cell. Micronutrient deficiencies cause adverse health conditions, and dietary supplementation has proven highly beneficial in disease prevention, as illustrated by the decrease in neural tube birth defects after folate supplementation [2].

Adequate micronutrient status is determined by three main factors: (1) supply, (2) intrinsic utilization, and (3) metabolic capacity. Due to their essentiality, micronutrients are currently thought to represent a direct interface between nutrition and pathology, with the inferred prospect that therapeutic interventions may be achieved simply through altered nutrition or dietary supplementation. Expanding on this concept, this makes the genes in metabolic pathways candidates in increased disease susceptibilities through disturbance of the supply or utilization.

The recent advances in human and comparative genetics now make it possible to investigate intrinsic genetic variations contributing to disease susceptibility. Micronutrient solute carriers mediate transport processes across otherwise impenetrable cell membranes, hence regulating cellular supply. Disturbances in these transport processes lead to micronutrient imbalances and diseases. This chapter summarizes current knowledge about genetic variations in micronutrient solute carrier genes, impacting on their function to cause adverse health outcomes. Only transporters reasonably associated with a disease are discussed.

VITAMIN C (ASCORBIC ACID)

Vitamin C (L-ascorbic acid, ascorbate) is an essential cofactor for at least eight mammalian enzymatic reactions and functions as an intracellular and extracellular scavenger of free oxygen radicals. Humans rely on dietary intake of vitamin C because, unlike most mammals, humans do not synthesize vitamin C de novo [3].

SLC23A1

The human solute carrier family 23 member 1 gene *SLC23A1* on chromosome 5q31.2 contains 15 exons, and 2 alternatively spliced transcripts are listed in the NCBI database. The more predominant transcript variant encodes a shorter functional isoform a. Isoform b uses an alternative donor splice site to add 12 bases coding for 4 amino acids at the end of exon 5, which eliminates ascorbic acid transport by unknown mechanisms (Figure 2.1) [4,5]. UniGene cluster Hs.643467 identifies predominant expression in kidney, liver, and small intestine, with lower abundance in adipose tissue, blood, brain, lymph node, prostate, and spleen [6].

The SLC23A1 protein functions as a high-capacity, low-affinity ascorbic acid carrier in epithelial tissues. Cellular ascorbate enrichment against a gradient is based on sodium-coupled cotransport [5,7]. The renal reabsorption and in part intestinal absorption of ascorbate can be explained by the action of the SLC23A1 protein, which resides on the apical surface in polarized intestinal and renal epithelial cells to mediate cellular uptake from the lumen [3,8].

When *Slc23al* is globally deleted, as in *Slc23al*$^{-/-}$ mice, they lose the ability to reabsorb ascorbate in the proximal tubule of the kidney [3]. This results in up to 18-fold increased ascorbate loss into the urine, and as a consequence, the plasma ascorbate values are reduced up to 70%. The *Slc23al*$^{-/-}$ mice do not show decreases in intestinal ascorbic acid absorption, but very low hepatic levels, indicating the transporters' essential role in kidney and liver, but not small intestine. The low plasma ascorbic acid levels lead to five-fold elevated perinatal mortality, which could be eliminated after maternal oral ascorbate supplementation resulting in higher systemic concentrations. Therefore, the ascorbate provided by the dam is the key factor for perinatal survival of newborn pups. The findings in the *Slc23al*$^{-/-}$ mouse imply the possibility that human *SLC23A1* mutations and polymorphisms might reduce plasma ascorbate concentrations. This genetic phenomenon might be even more pronounced in susceptible individuals with insufficient intake.

Circulating ascorbate levels were reduced on average by 4.15 μmol/L in carriers of the single-nucleotide polymorphism (SNP) rs33972313-T genotype of *SLC23A1*

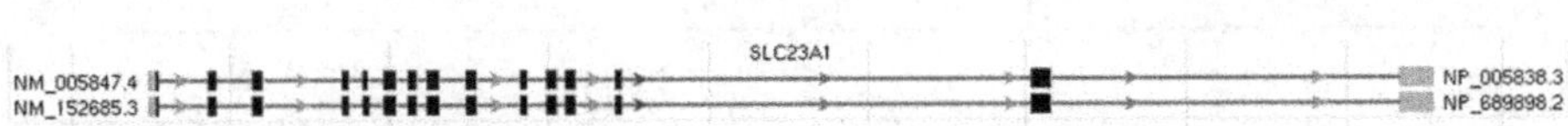

FIGURE 2.1 The two transcripts mapping to the *SLC23A1* locus on chromosome 5q31.2. Exon 5 is prolonged by 12 base pairs in NM 152685 (isoform b), adding 4 amino acids and rendering the protein nonfunctional for ascorbate transport. (From Wang, H. et al., *Biochim. Biophys. Acta*, 1461, 1–9, 1999.)

in a large European cohort (Figure 2.2) [9]. This nonsynonymous polymorphism causes a conversion of valine 264 to methionine (Val264Met). The methionine isoform, when expressed in *Xenopus laevis* oocytes, reduced the ascorbate uptake moderately compared to the common valine isoform [3]. The physiological implication of the moderate impact on function and plasma ascorbate levels needs further investigations to determine potential disease implications. Similarly, carriers of the intronic *SLC23A1* polymorphisms rs4257763-G showed reduced serum ascorbate levels compared to the rs4257763-A homozygotes, with 24.4 μmol/L compared to 29.7 μmol/L respectively [10]. It needs to be noted that these individuals show serum vitamin C levels comparable to those affecting perinatal mortality in the *Slc23a1*$^{-/-}$ pups [3]. This indicates that plasma ascorbate level in the low 20 μmol/L range might be common in humans, which could lead to pathological outcomes.

The two *SLC23A1* SNPs rs6596473 (IVS13+2515G>C) and rs11950646 (IVS9−110A>G) influence the risk of follicular lymphoma. The risk of follicular

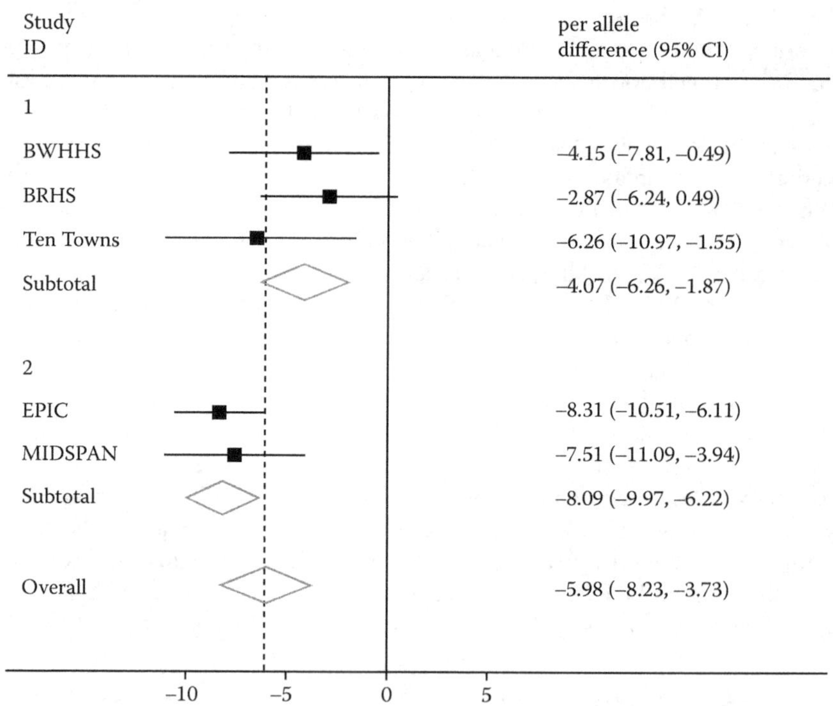

FIGURE 2.2 Meta-analysis summary of the association of *SLC23A1* polymorphisms rs33972313-T with circulating vitamin C from large European discovery and replication studies. Values represent a pooled estimate of per allele associations (random effects). The *x* axis represents the associated difference in L-ascorbic acid per rare allele at rs33972313 (μmol/L). Sections 1 and 2 show the results of the sub-analyses by L-ascorbic assay type. British Women's Heart and Health Study (BWHHS; $n = 3425$), British Regional Heart Study (BRHS; $n = 3740$), Ten Towns Study ($n = 1359$), European Prospective Investigation into Cancer and Nutrition (EPIC; $n = 4501$), and MIDSPAN ($n = 1814$). ID = identification.

lymphoma increases by 80% in homozygous carriers of the rs6596473-C and the rs11950646-G variants (Table 2.1). The mechanism behind this risk association remains to be explained, specifically since no correspondent ascorbic acid levels were reported and the association could not be replicated [11]. However, in the replication study, these genotypes were inversely and positively associated with diffuse large B-cell lymphoma and small lymphocytic lymphoma/chronic lymphocytic leukemia risk, respectively [11]. This warrants additional studies to conclude on the role of these variations in lymphomas.

The *SLC23A1* locus is also implicated in the predisposition to preterm birth. Individuals homozygous for *SLC23A1* haplotype 2 (AAGTAC) had the highest rate of spontaneous preterm birth in a Caucasian cohort. Heterozygosity for *SLC23A1* haplotype 1 (GAGCAG) resulted in 50% less preterm birth and homozygotes for the same haplotype 1 had 30% less preterm birth. These associations could not been confirmed for African-Americans [12], which warrant further functional and physiological studies.

SLC23A2

The human solute carrier family 23 member 2, *SLC23A2*, gene on chromosome 20p13 contains 17 exons; two alternatively spliced transcripts are listed in the NCBI database. The transcripts differ in the utilization of alternative 5′ exons and promoter regions, where the open reading frame is not altered (Figure 2.3) [4]. The *SLC23A2*

TABLE 2.1
Risks for Developing Follicular Lymphoma Expressed as Odds Ratios (OR) for Selected *slc23a1* Genotypes

SNP, Genotype	Controls ($N = 1049$)	Follicular Lymphoma ($N = 201$)	OR
SLC23A1			
rs6596473			
GG	496	82	1.0
CG	438	85	1.2
CC	110	33	1.8
CG/CC	548	118	1.3
p for trend			0.01
SLC23A1			
rs11950646			
AA	447	75	1.0
AG	460	84	1.1
GG	132	39	1.8
AG/GG	592	123	1.3
p for trend			0.02

Source: Data from the San Francisco Bay Area NHL Study. From Skibola, C.F., et al., *PLoS One*, 3, 7, e2816, 2008.

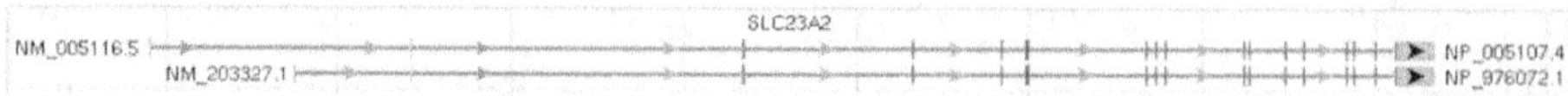

FIGURE 2.3 Transcripts mapped to the *SLC23A2* locus on chromosome 20p13. (http://www.ncbi.nlm.nih.gov/gene.)

transcript is found ubiquitously (Hs,516866 [6]), indicating its function as the main ascorbic acid solute carrier throughout the body. A *SLC23A2* variant resulting from a 345-bp deletion, which excludes the part of the predicted fourth as well as the fifth and sixth transmembrane domains, is reported. The truncated protein does not mediate ascorbate uptake [13]. The SLC23A2 protein is a high-affinity/low-capacity transporter concentrating ascorbate in the cells using a sodium gradient [7,14].

The global elimination of *Slc23a2* in mice is lethal in newborns, which suffer from respiratory failure and brain hemorrhage immediately after birth. *Slc23a2*'s role as the main placental ascorbate solute carrier is demonstrated by the failure to increase plasma ascorbate in the fetuses after supplementation to the pregnant dams. The uptake into tissues was severely decreased, as demonstrated in fibroblasts from *Slc23a2*$^{-/-}$ embryos, which had had only 5% of the expected ascorbic acid uptake [15].

Initial screening of the human *SLC23A2* gene did not detect any nonsynonymous SNPs, indicating a very low tolerance for genetic variations [16]. In studies of the general population, common genetic variations did not influence plasma ascorbate levels [10]. However, it was shown that *SLC23A2* rs1279386-G homozygote subjects had significantly lower plasma vitamin C concentrations in controls as well as primary open-angle glaucoma cases. Plasma ascorbic acid in primary open-angle glaucoma patients carrying the rs1279386-GG genotype was 51 μM, compared to 60 μM in carriers of the other genotypes. Similarly, control subjects of the rs1279386-GG genotype had plasma ascorbate of 62 μM compared to 69 μM determined for the other genotypes [17]. This indicates that SLC23A2 polymorphisms might affect open-angle glaucoma risk by influencing plasma vitamin C concentrations, since lower plasma ascorbate levels were associated with a 67% elevated risk of open-angle glaucoma [17]. However, the functional mechanism by which the intronic SNP rs1279386 modulates ascorbate levels need to be elucidated. Moreover, plasma ascorbate levels over 50 μM are considered to be sufficient for disease prevention, and it needs to be determined if a decrease from 60 μM in control subjects to 51 μM in primary open-angle glaucoma patients is truly contributing to disease development.

Genetic variations in the *SLC23A2* gene have been reported to impact cancer susceptibility. *SLC23A2* SNP rs12479919-AA homozygotes show 41% lower risk of gastric cancer when compared to rs12479919-GG carriers. A haplotype consisting of the alleles rs6139591-C, rs2681116-A, and rs14147458-T also protected from gastric malignancy [18].

Carriers of the *SLC23A2* rs4987219-GG/GC genotypes were found to have a twofold elevated risk of head and neck squamous cell carcinoma compared to rs4987219-CC individuals when they were infected with human papillomavirus 16 (HPV16) [19]. Remarkably, head and neck squamous cell carcinoma risk was more than sevenfold higher in SLC23A2 rs4987219-GG/GC individuals infected with HPV16 when they consumed high amounts of citrus fruits. Correspondingly, the risk was decreased for SLC23A2 rs4987219-CC carriers consuming little citrus fruit (Figure 2.4) [19].

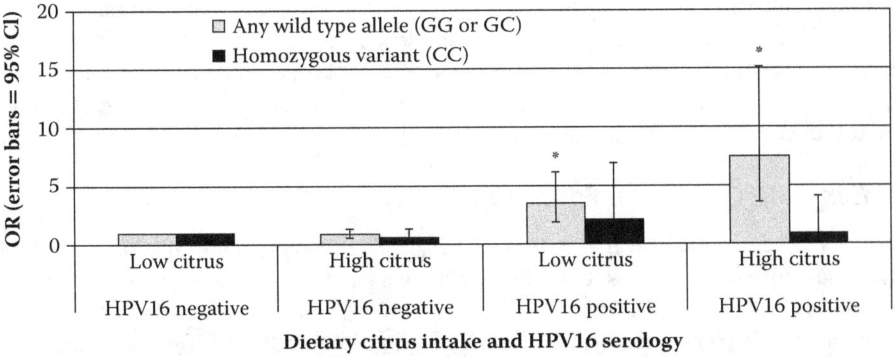

FIGURE 2.4 Risks for head and neck squamous cell carcinoma modulated by *SLC23A2* rs4987219 genotypes and human papillomavirus 16 (HPV16) infections. The risk is expressed as odds ratios (OR), low citrus intake is defined as <0.67 servings per day, high citrus intake is ≥0.67 servings per day. Number of cases = 319. Number of controls = 495. **P*-value < 0.0001 when compared with the low citrus, HPV-negative reference group for that genotype. (From Chen, A.A. et al., *Carcinogenesis*, 30, 977–981, 2009.)

A haplotype consistent of rs4987219-G and rs1110277-C lowered the risk of advanced colorectal carcinoma by 51% [20]. SNP rs4987219 resides in intron 8, rs1110277 in exon 8, and they are in strong linkage. The mechanism by which they mediate cancer susceptibility has not been determined. Overall, there is little knowledge of any biological mechanisms by which polymorphism in the *SLC23A2 gene* modulate cancer risk.

Caucasian individuals with the rs6139591-TT genotype showed a 70% elevated risk for preterm birth, and rs6139591-CT carriers had a 170% elevated risk. Similarly, a 190% higher risk was observed for rs2681116-G/A carriers, but not in subjects homozygous for the rs2681116-A allele. On the contrary, the rs1776964-TT genotype was associated with 70% decreased risk of spontaneous preterm birth [12].

Elevated risks for preterm birth as well as certain cancers have not been related to any physiologic mechanisms, highlighting the need to follow up association studies with functional experiments.

FOLATE

Folate, also called vitamin B_9, is an essential micronutrient with a central function in single-carbon transfer reactions, and folate status and metabolism are of significant interest to public health. Folate has proven highly successful in the prevention of neural tube defects, so much so that the United States prescribed a mandatory fortification of grain products with folate that began in 1998. This program led to a significantly reduced prevalence of birth defects such as spina bifida. Fortification with folate has been a clear public health success story and a victory for preventive medicine [2,21]. Beyond neural tube defects, such serious common diseases as colon cancer and other cancers are linked to low dietary folate intake [22]. For birth defects and cancers, folate is currently thought to represent a direct interface between nutrition and pathology, with the inferred prospect that therapeutic interventions may be achieved simply through altered nutrition or dietary supplementation. This certainly warrants investigations into the role of the genetic variations in metabolic folate pathways associated with increased disease susceptibilities through disturbance of the folate uptake or metabolism [21].

SLC19A1/RFC: Reduced Folate Carrier

Three transcripts map to the human *SLC19A1* gene locus on chromosome 21q22.3, two constituted of six exons, the third having five exons, all encoding different protein isoforms (Figure 2.5) [4]. Transcript 1 (NM 194255) is the longest mRNA translating into the longest protein isoform. Transcript variant 2 (NM 001205206) uses a different splicing in the 5′ region of the last exon, which results in a frameshift. This SLC19A1 protein isoform 2 therefore possesses a different shortened C-terminus. Transcript variant 3 utilizes an alternative exon containing some 5′ untranslated region (UTR) and the start codon. Therefore, protein isoform 3 possesses an alternative shorter N-terminus [4]. The gene is widely expressed (UniGene Hs.517356 and Hs.84190 [6]).

The 591–amino acid SLC19A1 protein is the major transporter that delivers folates to systemic tissues at their ambient neutral pH. It functions as an organic anion antiporter that utilizes the high transmembrane organic phosphate gradient to achieve uphill folate transport into cells at the optimum pH of 7.4 [23].

SLC19A1 accepts several alternative substrates, most notably methotrexate, the major antifolate anticancer agent in clinical use. For a further review on SLC19A1 and antifolate cancer therapy, see Zhao et al. [23].

Slc19a1 inactivation in the mouse is embryonically lethal under normal dietary conditions, but the phenotype can be rescued by sufficient folate supplementation during gestation. Even after gestational rescue, the surviving pups die within 2 weeks due to hematopoietic tissues failure [24]. *Slc19a1*$^{+/-}$ mice show increased susceptibility to colon adenocarcinoma [22], somewhat providing experimental evidence that the associations between low folate intake and carcinogenesis seen in human epidemiological studies might be valid.

Low *SLC19A1* expression or loss-of-function mutations in human or murine cancer cell lines confer resistance to methotrexate treatment due to impaired transport [23]. This observation indicates that variations and mutations in *SLC19A1* can cause impaired function or downregulation of the genes' expression, which both will contribute to resistance against anticancer treatments [25].

Various phenotypes have been associated with common nonsynonymous variants in *SLC19A1*. Genetic associations are seen for plasma or tissue folate concentrations, total homocysteine levels, birth defects (spina bifida and orofacial malformations), the risk to develop various cancers, the effect and toxicity of antifolate anticancer

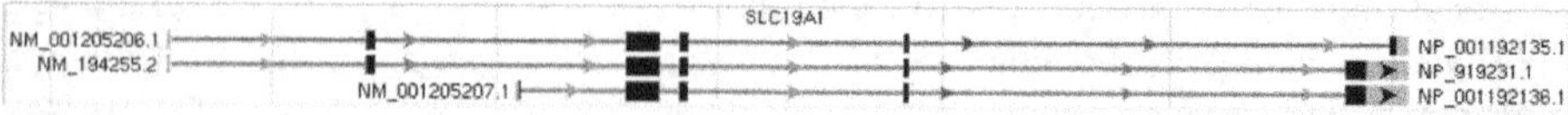

FIGURE 2.5 Three distinct transcripts mapping to the *SLC19A1* gene locus on chromosome 21q22.3. (http://www.ncbi.nlm.nih.gov/gene.)

agents, and infertility (see Table 2.2 for a list and the following paragraphs for details). Current evidence indicates complex gene–nutrient as well as gene–gene–nutrient interactions for the *SLC19A1* locus, which could explain significant inter-study variability and failures to replicate associations.

Reduced folate intake and subsequent reduced plasma and tissue levels are known to be initiating events in the development of such detrimental diseases as fetal neural tube defects. Consequently, if plasma and tissue folate levels are reduced due to a genetic defect, these individuals will have an elevated disease risk in spite of adequate intake. However, current studies demonstrating associations between folate levels and genetic variations in *SLC19A1* are inconsistent. This is highlighted by the fact that plasma folate levels are reported lower in carriers of the rs1051266-A allele, but higher in A-homozygotes when the *MTHFR* 677C/T is present [27]. In contrast, red blood cell folate levels are lower in rs1051266-G homozygotes [29]. These inconsistencies might be explained by complex gene–gene–nutrient interactions, which need to be confirmed in adequately designed epidemiological and biological functional studies.

Elevated plasma homocysteine levels elevate the risk for cardiovascular disease. In a genome-wide association studies (GWAS), the rs1051266-A, rs1131596-C, and the rs4819130-C alleles were each associated with 5.0% increased plasma homocysteine [31]. The three polymorphisms are in genetic linkage, but had previously not been associated with homocysteine levels [52,53]. rs1051266 is a nonsynonymous polymorphism, where rs1131596 falls into the 5′ region and rs4819130 in an intron of the gene. Functional studies will need to determine the SNP effects and role in disease susceptibility, where potential interactions with cobalamin have to be accounted for [31]. Reduced *SLC19A1* expression could play a significant role, since SNP rs1131596 seems to play a role in decreased SLC19A1 protein levels in cardiovascular disease patients [54,55].

Low folate intake causes birth defects in humans, and some emerging evidence seems to implicate *SLC19A1* polymorphism in disease etiology. The two alleles rs1888530-C and rs3788200-A were associated with the incidence of meningomyelocele, a lack of closure of the neural tube during embryologic development [46]. In a separate study, Bufalino et al. stated that they found gene–gene interactions between *MTHFR* rs2274976, *MTHFD1* rs2236225, and *SLC19A1* rs1051266, which defined the risk of nonsyndromic cleft lip and/or palate birth defects. However, they failed to mention the exact allelic combination and the impact [45]. Therefore, further evaluation or consideration of the validity of their findings is very difficult.

SLC19A1 polymorphisms are implicated in the risk of colorectal, esophageal and gastric, lung, head, and neck cancer, as well as lymphoblastic leukemia and leucopenia [32,33,35–38]. As seen before, results are inconsistent and often fail to be confirmed. For example, risks for colorectal cancer are reported to be elevated for rs1051266-A homozygotes [33] or carriers of the A-allele when the *MTHFR* 677-C is present, but seem to be decreased in carriers of the A-allele when they are *MTHFR* 677-T homozygotes [32]. On the contrary, the rs1051266-A homozygosity decreases the risk for leucopenia, and the rs1051266-G allele increases the risk for

TABLE 2.2
Polymorphisms and Mutations in the *SLC19A1* Gene Associated with Health-Related Phenotypes

Variations Identifier	Nucleotide/Amino Acid Change	Phenotype	Outcome
rs1051266	c.80A>G/p.His27Arg	Plasma folate levels	Lower in A-allele carriers [26]; however, higher in A-homozygotes when *MTHFR* 677C/T is present [27]
	–43T>C	Plasma folate levels	Lower in C-homozygotes [28]
rs1051266	c.80A>G/p.His27Arg	Red blood cell folate levels	Lower in G-homozygotes [29]
	–43T>C	Red blood cell folate levels	Lower in C-homozygotes [28]
rs1051266	c.80A>G/p.His27Arg	Total homocysteine in plasma	Increased in G-homozygotes combines when *MTHFR* 677T/T is present [27,30]
rs1051266, rs1131596, rs4819130		Total homocysteine in plasma	5.0% increased *for carriers of* rs1051266-*A*, rs1131596-*C*, rs4819130-*C* [31]
rs1051266	c.80A>G/p.His27Arg	Risk of distal colorectal adenoma	Elevated for carriers of the A-allele when *MTHFR* 677-C is present; however, decreased for A-allele in *MTHFR* 677-T homozygotes [32]
rs1051266	c.80A>G/p.His27Arg	Risk for colorectal cancer	Elevated for A-homozygotes [33]
rs1051266	c.80A>G/p.His27Arg	Risk for head and neck cancer	Increased in males over 50 years when G-allele carriers [34]
rs1051266	c.80A>G/p.His27Arg	Risk for leucopenia	Decreased in A-homozygotes [35]
rs1051266	c.80A>G/p.His27Arg	Risk for acute lymphoblastic leukemia	Reduced in heterozygosity and 3′-*TYMS*-6 bp/-6 bp homozygous deletion [36]
rs1051266	c.80A>G/p.His27Arg	Risk for oesophageal and gastric cancer	Increased in A-homozygotes [37]
rs1051266	c.80A>G/p.His27Arg	Risk for gastric cancer in subgroups	Elevated in female A-homozygotes over 60 years [37]

rs12659	c.696T>C/pPro232Pro	Risk of lung cancer	Increased for carriers of the C-allele risk [38]
rs1051266	c.80A>G/p.His27Arg	Survival after methotrexate treatment in childhood acute lymphoblastic leukemia	50% better chance of staying in remission for A-homozygotes [39]
rs1051266	c.80A>G/p.His27Arg	Bone marrow toxicity in methotrexate treatment	Higher in A-homozygotes [39].
rs1051266	c.80A>G/p.His27Arg	Liver toxicity in methotrexate treatment	Higher for G-homozygotes [39].
rs11702425, rs2838956, rs7499, rs2274808, rs9977268, rs7279445		Methotrexate efficacy in rheumatoid arthritis	Poor response for rs11702425-C, rs2838956-G, rs7499-A, rs2274808-T, rs9977268-T, rs7279445-T [40]
	IVS4(2117) C>T, IVS5(9148) C>A, exon 6 (2522) C>T	Overall survival at pemetrexed treatment	Improved in homozygotes [41]
–233T		Response after melphalan treatment and autologous stem cells transplantation in multiple myeloma	Improved for carriers of T-allele [42]
rs1051266	c.80A>G/p.His27Arg	Spina bifida birth defect	G-homozygotes show modest gene–nutrient interaction for spina bifida [43]
rs1051266	c.80A>G/p.His27Arg	Orofacial birth defects	G-allele increases risk in mothers not supplementing with folate [44]
rs1051266	c.80A>G/p.His27Arg	Maternal risk for nonsyndromic cleft lip and/or palate	A combination of *MTHFR* rs2274976, *MTHFD1* rs2236225, and *SLC19A1* rs1051266 increased maternal risk 5.3-fold [45]

(*Continued*)

TABLE 2.2 (*Continued*)
Polymorphisms and Mutations in the *SLC19A1* Gene Associated with Health-Related Phenotypes

Variations Identifier	Nucleotide/Amino Acid Change	Phenotype	Outcome
rs1888530		Risk for meningomyelocele	rs1888530-C overtransmitted in meningomyelocele cases [46]
rs3788200		Risk for meningomyelocele	rs3788200-A overtransmitted in meningomyelocele cases [46]
rs12659	c.696T>C/pPro232Pro	Risk of spontaneously aborted embryos	Elevated in C-homozygotes [47]
Haplotype –43T>C/80G>A/696C>T	43T>C/80G>A/696C>T	Idiopathic recurrent spontaneous abortion	–43C/80A/696 T and –43T/80G/696C elevate risk [48]
rs1051266	c.80A>G/p.His27Arg	Success of in vitro fertilization treatment (IVF)	G/A-heterozygotes had a decreased number of previously failed IVF and were more prevalent among fertile controls [49]
rs1051266	c.80A>G/p.His27Arg	Unexplained female infertility	G-allele is more prevalent in infertility [50]
Arg27His, Ser4 Pro, Ala7Val, Glu21Lys, Ser46Asn		Found in 162 osteosarcoma samples	Effect to be determined [51]

cancers of the head and neck in older males [34]. Future studies need to clarify exact mechanisms.

Murine and human cancer cells lines with low SLC19A1 levels or loss of function become resistant to methotrexate treatment [23]. This indicates a biological mechanism that provides the rationale for some genetic studies. Indeed, methotrexate treatment in acute lymphoblastic leukemia resulted in 50% elevated remission in rs1051266-A homozygote children, which correlated with higher bone marrow toxicity. In contrast, higher liver toxicity in GG homozygotes is reported [39].

Both cancer susceptibility and response to cancer treatment might be determined by mutations in *SLC19A1*, and sequencing of tumor specimens revealed several mutations in leukemia cells (Val29Leu, Glu45Lys, Ser46Ile Leu143Pro, Ala147Val, Arg148Gly, and Gln150Stop). Functional tests revealed that some of these mutations decreased SLC19A1 protein levels [25,56]. In three B-precursor specimens, the nonsynonymous variants, Asp56His and Asp522Asn, were found [57]. Methotrexate uptake is lower in the blast cells from B-precursor lymphoma patients with the Asp522Asn mutation as compared with cells from the wild-type carriers. *SLC19A1* re-sequencing in 162 osteosarcomas identified the new variants Ser46Asn, Glu21Lys, Ala7Val, and Ser4Pro, in addition to the common variant Arg27His [51]. Their functional and clinical significance terms of methotrexate transport and plasma level as well as therapy resistance have not been determined [25].

The link between dietary folate and birth defects connects systemic folate with early embryonic development and therefore fertility. It was reported that *SLC19A1* rs1051266-G/A heterozygotes had a decreased number of previously failed IVF treatments and were more prevalent among fertile controls [49]. Unexplained female infertility has been associated with the rs1051266-G allele [50].

SLC46A1/PCFT: Proton-Coupled Folate Transporter

The human *SLC46A1* gene on chromosome 17q11.2 is very compact, harboring a transcript of five exons (NM 542400) and encoding a protein of 459 amino acid residues. An alternative splice variant is mapped to the locus, lacking exon 3 (NM 001242366) (Figure 2.6) [4]. The gene is expressed in a wide variety of tissues (UniGene Hs.731770[6]), with high expression in the intestinal tract, kidney, liver, placenta, and spleen and low abundance in brain, testis, and lung [23].

FIGURE 2.6 Organization and alternative transcripts of the human *SLC46A1* gene on chromosome 17q11.2.

The human SLC46A1 protein mediates folate uptake and has a high affinity for folic acid, 5-methyltetrahydrofolate, and 5-formyltetrahydrofolate. It also has a high affinity for folate analogs, such as the anticancer agent pemetrexed [23]. The high electrogenic transport mechanism of this proton-coupled folate transporter is pH-dependent [58,59]. It also mediates heme uptake with significant lower affinity compared to folates [58,60].

Murine Slc46a1 protein is located on the apical brush-border membrane of proximal jejunum and duodenum. *Slc46a1*$^{-/-}$ mice develop severe macrocytic normochromic anemia and pancytopenia by 4 weeks of age. Erythroblasts do not develop to maturity and undergo premature apoptosis. Therefore, erythropoietin, soluble transferrin receptor (sCD71), and thrombopoietin are accumulated. Intestinal folate uptake is diminished causing systemic deficiency. The *Slc46a1*$^{-/-}$ mouse represents a model of human hereditary folate malabsorption [61].

Human hereditary intestinal folate malabsorption (OMIM 229050 [4]) is autosomal recessive, resulting in megaloblastic anemia, chronic infections, and persistent diarrhea. Neurological abnormalities such as delayed development, mental retardation, and seizures could be explained with diminished folate transport across the blood–brain barrier [62].

The mutations in the *SLC46A1* locus are summarized in Table 2.3. Several of these mutations locate to topologically important protein regions, where they have

TABLE 2.3
Mutations in the *SLC46A1* Gene Causing Human Hereditary Folate Malabsorption

Region	Nucleotide Change	Protein Change	Effect on Protein Structure or Function
Exon 1	c.17-18insC	p.Glu9Glyfs	Frameshift [65]
Exon 1	c.194delG	p.Gly65AlafsX25,	Frameshift abolishes transport [63]
Exon 1	c.194dupG	p.Cys66LeufsX99	Frameshift [66]
Exon 1	c.197_198 GC>AA	p.Cys66X	Nonsense [67]
Exon 1	c.204-205 delCC	p.Asn68Lysfs	Frameshift [65,68]
Exon 2	c.337C>A	p.Arg113Ser	Missense abolishes transport [63]
Exon 2	c.337 C>T	p.Arg113Cys	Missense [69]
Exon 2	c.439G>C	p.Gly147Arg	Missense decreases transport [63]
Exon 2	c.466G>T	p.Asp156Tyr	Missense [70]
Exon 2	c.954C>G	p.Ser318Arg	Missense abolishes transport [63]
Exon 2	c.1004C>A	p.Ala335Asp	Missense abolishes transport [65]
Exon 2	c.1012G>C	p.Gly338Arg	Missense abolishes transport [65]
Intron 2	c.1082-1G>A	Splice site deleted, p.Try362_Gly389del Exon 3 skipped	In-frame deletion of 28 amino acids causes intracellular trapping [58,71, 72]; note: transcript can be found in GeneBank (NM 001242366)
Exon 3	c.1126C>T	p.Arg376Trp	Missense abolishes transport [63]
Exon 3	c.1127G>A	p.Arg376Glu	Missense [72]
Exon 4	c.1274C>G	p.Pro425Arg	Missense decreases transport [63]

been shown to decrease or abolish folate transport at low pH in vitro (Figures 2.7 through 2.9) [58,63].

Human hereditary intestinal folate malabsorption is treated by parenteral administration [64].

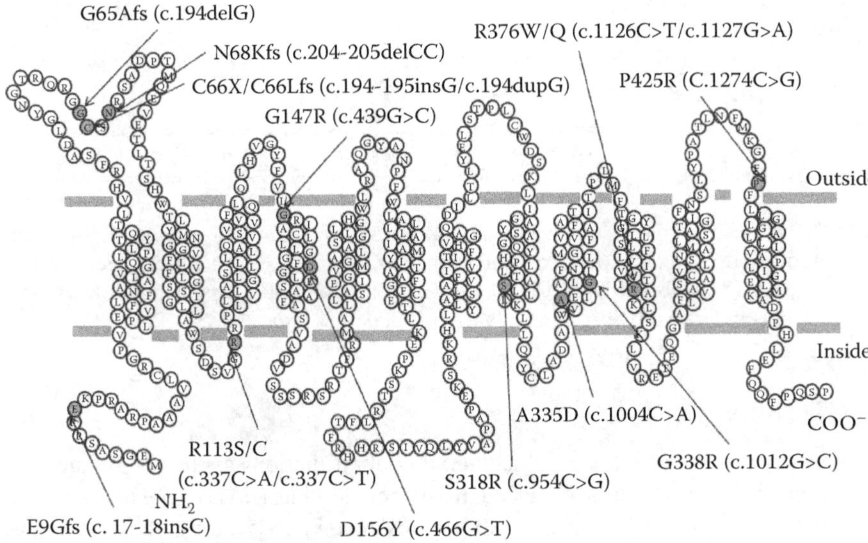

FIGURE 2.7 SLC46A1 topology and the location of some mutations associated with hereditary folate malabsorption. (http://omim.org/entry/201100.)

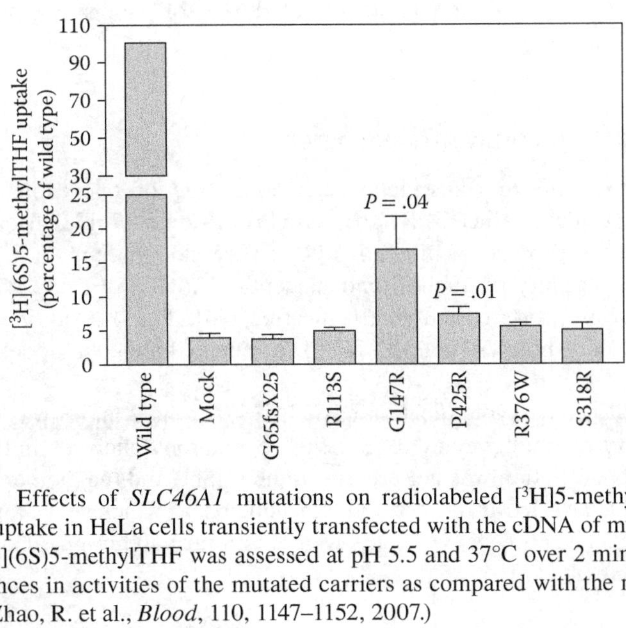

FIGURE 2.8 Effects of *SLC46A1* mutations on radiolabeled [^{3}H]5-methyl-tetra-hydrofolate (THF) uptake in HeLa cells transiently transfected with the cDNA of mutants. Uptake of 0.5 μM [^{3}H](6S)5-methylTHF was assessed at pH 5.5 and 37°C over 2 minutes; *P* values reflect differences in activities of the mutated carriers as compared with the mock transfectants. (From Zhao, R. et al., *Blood*, 110, 1147–1152, 2007.)

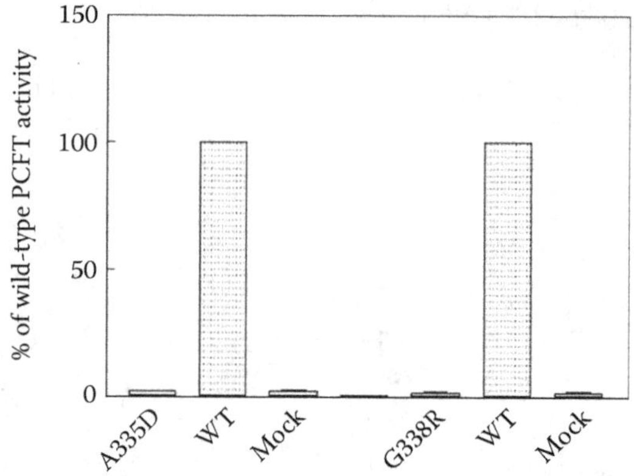

FIGURE 2.9 Functional assessment of SLC46A1 A335D and G338 mutants. Radiolabeled [3H]methotrexate influx was performed at a concentration of 0.5 μM at pH 5.5 over 1 minutes with R1-11 cells transfected with A335D and G338R mutant plasmids along with wild-type and mock plasmids. (From Shin, D.S. et al., *Mol. Genet. Metab.*, 103, 33–37, 2011.)

RIBOFLAVIN

Riboflavin, alias vitamin B_2, exhibits its metabolic functions as the coenzyme flavin mononucleotide (FMN) and flavin adenine dinucleotide (FAD). These coenzymes mediate the activation of folic acid and pyridoxine and are therefore central to pathways in carbohydrate, amino acid, and lipid metabolism.

Riboflavin deficiency is characterized by endocrine dysfunction leading to anemia and skin lesions. Degeneration of the nervous system could also be observed. Suboptimal levels are linked to an elevated risk of esophageal squamous cell carcinoma [73].

SLC52A1/RFT1 Riboflavin Transporter 1

Two alternative spliced transcripts, each consisting of five exons, map to the *SLC52A1* gene locus (alias GPR172B) on chromosome 17p13.2. Both transcripts encode the same protein (Figure 2.10) [4]. Expression in humans is restricted to embryonic tissue, larynx, mouth, and placenta (UniGene Hs.632247[6]), as well as kidney, colon, prostate, and small intestine [74]. The 448–amino acid protein mediates cellular riboflavin uptake [74,75]. A murine knockout model has not been described.

A maternal heterozygote deletion of *SLC52A1* exons 2 and 3 was postulated to be the cause of the multiple acyl-CoA dehydrogenation deficiency in the infant offspring [75]. The deletion was not present in the infant, and the mother's haploinsufficiency might have led to mild riboflavin deficiency, which was amplified in the nursing infant. The clinical symptoms were temporary and might also be related to low maternal intake [75].

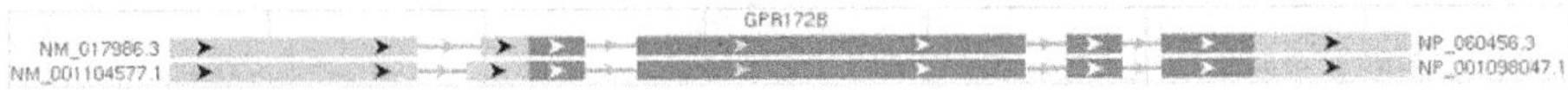

FIGURE 2.10 Alternative transcripts mapping to the *SLC52A1* gene locus (alias GPR172B) on chromosome 17p13.2.

SLC52A2/RFT3 Riboflavin Transporter 3

Five exons are transcribed from the *SLC52A2* gene locus on chromosome 8q24.3, with almost ubiquitous expression (UniGene Hs.6459 [6]) [4]. Very high abundance is demonstrated within the brain and the salivary gland [76]. The 445–amino acid SLC52A2 protein mediates cellular uptake of riboflavin [76].

The rare autosomal recessive Brown–Vialetto–Van Laere syndrome is in part attributed to the mutation c.916G>A (p.G306R) in *SLC52A2*, which is found in cases, but not in healthy controls [77]. The syndrome presents in the second decade of life with severe neurological defects of the spinal motor nerves and upper motor neurons, causing cranial nerve palsies as well as hearing loss. Typically hearing loss is the first symptom, and later muscle degeneration might lead to respiratory failure. Atypical cases might not develop hearing loss, but bulbar palsy [78]. This presentation is referred to as Fazio–Londe syndrome, which involves the same *SLC52A2* c.916G>A mutation [79].

Due to these findings, it is speculated that riboflavin might be an option as a therapy for these *SLC52A2* mutation-positive patients. Riboflavin treatment of one of these patients showed a positive response [77].

SLC52A3/RFT2: Riboflavin Transporter 2

The *SLC52A3* gene on chromosome 20p13 contains five exons and encodes a 469–amino acid protein functioning as a riboflavin transporter [4,80]. Its transcripts can be found in various tissues, including brain, heart, intestine, kidney, mammary gland, pancreas, placenta, prostate, and testis (UniGene Hs.283865 [6]).

SLC52A3 mediates Na^+-independent high-affinity riboflavin, lumiflavin, FMN, and FAD transport [81,82]. No knockout of the gene in an animal model is described.

Mutations in the human *SLC52A3* gene contribute to the Brown–Vialetto–Van Laere syndrome (OMIM 211530) and the Fazio–Londe disease (OMIM 211500). These diseases are sometimes considered to be the same disease entity and are related to mutations in riboflavin transporter genes [83].

Fourteen mutations segregate with the disease in individuals with Brown–Vialetto–Van Laere syndrome (Table 2.4) and seem to be causative by virtue of their exclusive presence in homozygote or compound heterozygote patients [78]. In fact, the majority of the mutations map to conserved regions (Figure 2.11) and affect membrane targeting as well as transporter functions (Figures 2.12 and 2.13, Table 2.4). It has been shown that the Pro28Thr, Glu36Lys, Glu71K, and Arg132Try mutants are retained within the endoplasmic reticulum, while the Trp17Arg and Leu350Met mutants are targeted to the cell membrane (Figure 2.13) [84].

TABLE 2.4
Mutations in the *SLC52A3* Gene Causing Brown–Vialetto–Van Laere Syndrome and Fazio–Londe Disease

Region	Nucleotide Change	Effect	Effect on Protein Structure or Function
Exon 1	c.49T>C	p.Trp17Arg	Missense, transport abrogated [79,84]
Exon 2	c.82C>A	p.Pro28Thr	Missense, retained within the endoplasmic reticulum [85,84]
Exon 2	c.106G>A	p.Glu36Lys	Missense, retained within the endoplasmic reticulum [78,84]
Exon 2	c.160G>A	p.Gly54Arg	Missense [77]
Exon 2	c.211G>T	p.Glu71X	Nonsense, retained within the endoplasmic reticulum [85,78,84]
Exon 2	c.394C>T	p.Arg132Try	Missense, retained within the endoplasmic reticulum [78,84]
Exon 2	c.224T>C	p.Iso75Thr	Missense [77]
Exon 3	c.639C>G	p.Tyr213X	Nonsense [78]
Exon 3	c.670T>C	p.Phe224Leu	Missense [78]
Exon 3	c.989G>T>C	p.Gly330Val	Missense [86]
Exon 3	c.1048T>A	p.Leu350Met	Missense, no change in transport [78,84]
Exon 5	c.1237T>C	p.Val413Ala	Missense [78]
Exon 5	c.1325_1326 delTG	p.L442RfsX35	Frameshift, 35 amino acids longer protein than the wild-type [78]
Exon 5	c.1371C>G	p.Phe457Leu	Missense [78]

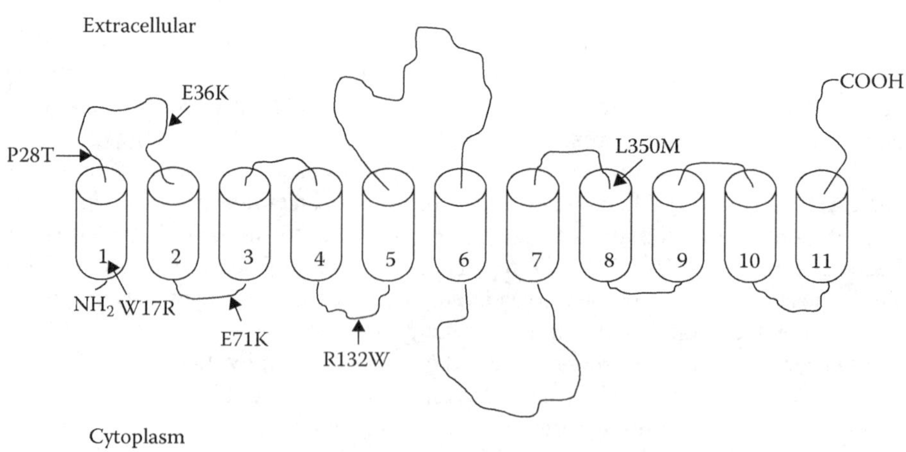

FIGURE 2.11 Hypothetical membrane topology of hSLC52A3 protein and location of selected Brown–Vialetto–Van Laere syndrome missense mutations. Human SLC52A3 is predicted to have 11 potential transmembrane domains and an extracellular oriented COOH-terminus. Arrows indicate the location of Brown–Vialetto–Van Laere syndrome missense mutations. (From Nabokina, S.M. et al., *Mol. Genet. Metab.*, 105, 652–657, 2012.)

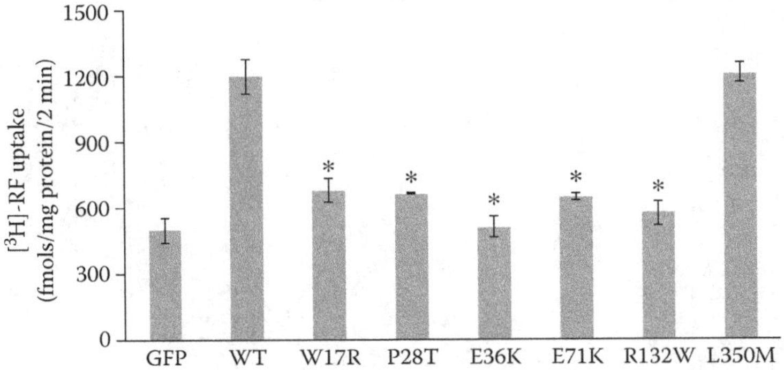

FIGURE 2.12 Effect of Brown–Vialetto–Van Laere syndrome missense mutations on riboflavin uptake. Radiolabeled ^{3}H-riboflavin (RF) uptake by human intestinal epithelial CaCo-2 cells transiently transfected with wild-type (WT) and mutated hSLC52A3, matched to green fluorescent protein controls. *Note*: *Significance level $p \geq 0.05$. (From Nabokina, S.M. et al., *Mol. Genet. Metab.*, 105, 652–657, 2012.)

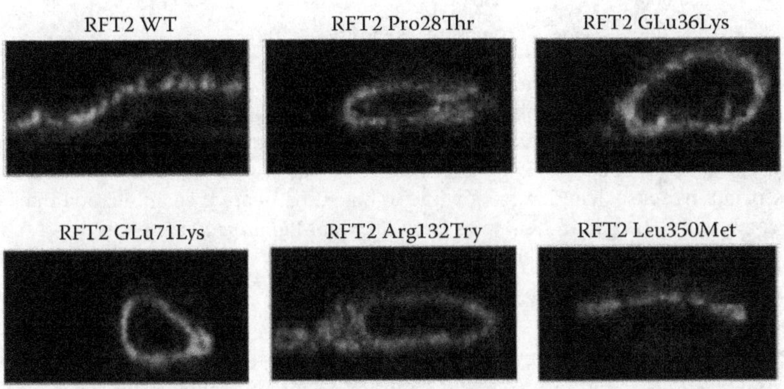

FIGURE 2.13 Cellular location of different hSLC52A3 mutants in polarized CaCo-2 cells. Confocal fluorescent images show the *x-z* axis with the apical pole on top. Green fluorescent protein–tagged human RFT2 wild-type (RFT2 WT) shows an exclusive apical localization, while several mutations cause the protein to be retained in the endoplasmic reticulum. (www.healthcare.uiowa.edu/labs/pendredandbor/slcMutations.htm.)

Supplementation with riboflavin can improve the clinical symptoms in some cases, demonstrating that high-dose riboflavin is a potential treatment for the Brown–Vialetto–Van Laere syndrome as well as for the Fazio–Londe disease [79].

On a genome-wide scale, the *SLC52A3 (C20orf54)* gene locus on chromosome 20p13 has also been associated with the susceptibility of esophageal squamous cell carcinoma and gastric cardia adenocarcinoma in Chinese populations (Figure 2.14). The T allele of rs13042395 decreases the risk [73,87]. This corresponds to the evidence of increased risk of esophageal squamous cell carcinoma and gastric cardia

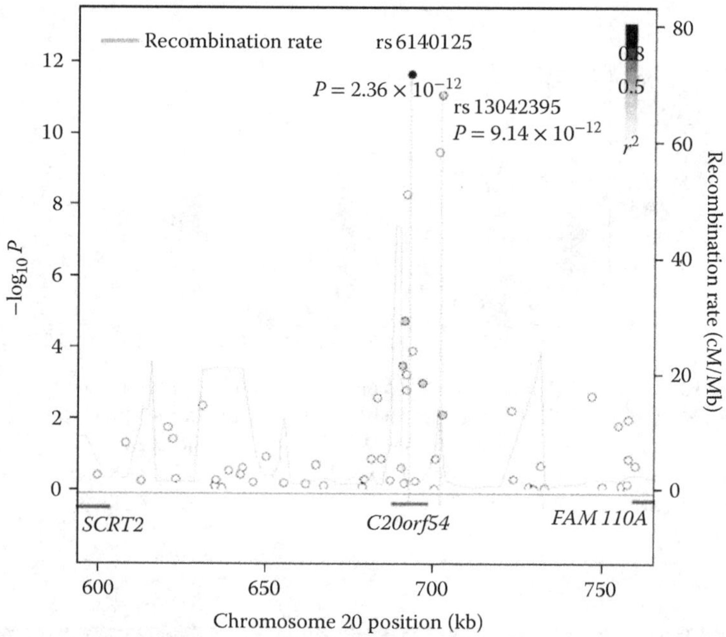

FIGURE 2.14 Scatterplot of the association within 20p13 (*C20orf54*) for esophageal squamous cell carcinoma. The *P* values of SNPs (shown as −log10 values in *y* axis, from the genome-wide single-marker association analysis) are plotted against their map positions (*x* axis). The shading of each SNP spot reflects its r^2 with the top SNP (darkest circle) within each association locus, changing from white to black. Estimated recombination rates (based on the combined CHB and JPT samples from the HapMap project) are plotted as a light line. (From Wang, L.D. et al., *Nat. Genet.*, 42, 759–763, 2010.)

adenocarcinoma in riboflavin deficiency. It is reported that riboflavin supplementation reduces the risk of esophageal squamous cell carcinoma and gastric cardia adenocarcinoma. The exact nature of the functional changes caused by these *SLC52A3* polymorphisms remains to be determined.

THIAMINE

Thiamin (vitamin B_1) as a coenzyme has a ubiquitous presence in all cells, and thiamine-dependent enzymes are found in key pathways of the energy metabolism. The heart and the nervous system are the first organs to be negatively affected in thiamine deficiency, most likely due to their high-energy metabolism. Therefore, the thiamine deficiency beriberi is characterized by neurological and cardiovascular symptoms [1].

SLC19A2

The *SLC19A2* gene located on human chromosome 1q23.3 contains six exons and is expressed in a wide variety of tissues (UniGen Hs.30246 [6]) [88,89]. The 497–amino acid SLC19A2 protein mediates cellular thiamine uptake independent of sodium, at an optimum pH of 8 [89,90].

Disruption of the *Slc19a2* gene in mice eliminates the high-affinity thiamine transport component of erythrocytes, but intestinal uptake is not altered [91,92]. *Slc19a2*$^{-/-}$ mice develop diabetes mellitus only when they are on a thiamine-free diet, and the phenotype is reversed after 6 weeks of thiamine repletion. In addition, neurological responses are altered in the *Slc19a2*$^{-/-}$ mice when they are on a thiamine depletion diet. Hearing loss due to selective loss of inner hair cells in the cochlea is one of the more dramatic phenotypes [93]. Defective formation of erythrocyte, myeloid, and megakaryocyte cells results in megaloblastosis [91].

Various mutations in the human *SLC19A2* gene cause the recessive thiamine-responsive megaloblastic anemia syndrome (OMIM 249270) (Table 2.5, Figure 2.15). Onset is typically between infancy and adolescence, and symptoms include megaloblastic anemia, diabetes mellitus, and sensorineural deafness. Symptoms such as anemia and sometimes diabetes improve with high doses of thiamine. Other more variable features include optic atrophy, congenital heart defects, short stature, and stroke [94]. Table 2.5 lists mutations reported to segregate with disease patients. However, the impacts of most listed mutations on the transporters' functions still remain to be determined. The mutation location within the gene might indicate the degree of impact on the function and therefore disease development (Figure 2.15).

SLC19A3

The human *SLC19A3* gene (alias ThTr2) on chromosome 2q37 is expressed in a wide variety of tissues, showing specifically high presence in placenta and liver (UniGene

TABLE 2.5
Mutations in the *SLC19A2* Gene Segregating with Megaloblastic Anemia Syndrome

Region	Nucleotide Change	Protein Change	Effect on Protein Structure or Function
Exon 1	c.121G>C	p.G41R	Missense [94–96]
Exon 1	c.152C>T	p.P51L	Missense [97]
Exon 1	c.196G>T	p.E66X	Nonsense [95]
Exon 2	c.242insA	p.Ins81fs/ter97	Frameshift [95,98,99]
Exon 2	c.277G>C	p.D93H	Missense [95]
Exon 2	c.287delG	p.Del96fs/ter117	Frameshift [99]
Exon 2	c.413G>A	p.E138K	Missense [94]
Exon 2	c.428C>T	p.S143F	Missense [100,95]
Exon 2	c.429delTT	p.Del143fs/ter239	Frameshift [99]
Exon 2	c.473C>G	p.T158R	Missense [101]
Exon 2	c.454_458del GGCATinsTA	p.G152X	Nonsense [94]
Exon 2	c.484 C > T, rs74315373	p.Arg162X	Nonsense [88,102,95]

(Continued)

TABLE 2.5 (*Continued*)
Mutations in the *SLC19A2* Gene Segregating with Megaloblastic Anemia Syndrome

Region	Nucleotide Change	Protein Change	Effect on Protein Structure or Function
Exon 2	c.515 G>A	p.G172D	Missense [94,88]
Exon 2	c.566_567 delGC insTCT	p.Insdel189fs/ter239	Frameshift [103]
Exon 2	c.602C>T	p.A201V	Missense [94]
Exon 2	c.688A>T	p.I230F	Missense [94]
Exon 2	c.697C>T	p.Q233X	Nonsense [104]
Exon 2	c724 Cdel	p.Del242fs/ter259	Frameshift [88]
Exon 2	c.750G>A	p.W250X	Nonsense [88]
Exon 2	c.758delT	p.Del253fs/ter260	Frameshift [94]
Exon 2	c.760insT	p.E254X	Nonsense [94]
Exon 3	c.885delT	p.Del295fs/ter313	Frameshift [105,90]
Exon 3	c.1001 G>A	p.G334D	Missense [102]
Exon 3	c.1002G>A	p.G335D	Missense [94]
Exon 4	c.1074G>A	p.W358X	Nonsense [106]
Exon 4	c.1105delTT	p.Del369fs/ter385	Frameshift [107]
Exon 4	c.1147delGT	p.Del383fs/ter385	Frameshift [108,90]
Exon 4	c.1172insCAT	p.Ins393S	Insertion [94]
Intron 4	c.1223+1G>A	p.408+1splice	Splice site deleted [95]

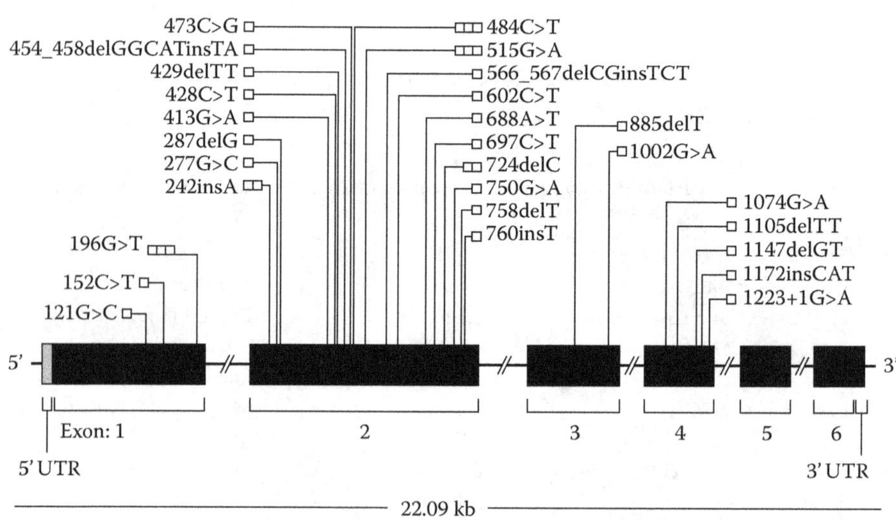

FIGURE 2.15 Known mutations in *hSLC19A2* gene segregating with patients of the thiamine-responsive megaloblastic anemia syndrome (OMIM 249270). All mutations are presented according to their location in the thiamine transporter gene *SLC19A2*. (From O'Brien, B.A. et al., *J. Autoimmun.*, 31, 42–51, 2008.)

Hs.221597 [6,4]). The 496–amino acid SLC19A3 protein mediates thiamin uptake and locates to the apical side in polarized cells [109].

Slc19a3-deficient mice have reduced intestinal thiamin uptake with a significant decrease in blood thiamin levels. *Slc19a3*$^{-/-}$ mice die prematurely at 1 year of age after showing lethargic behavior and progressive wasting starting approximately 3 months before death. The hepatic parenchyma is inflamed and necrotic; the renal cortex is also inflamed with signs of proximal convoluted tubular degeneration and nephrosclerosis [92].

The autosomal recessive thiamine metabolism dysfunction syndrome seems to be caused by mutations in the human *SLC19A3* gene. Within this syndrome, two phenotypes are observed, the biotin-responsive basal ganglia disease (BBGD) (MIM 607483) and Wernicke's-like encephalopathy (MIM 606152) [110]. Table 2.6 represents a list of mutations in the *SLC19A3* gene found in thiamine metabolism dysfunction syndrome patients. The disease is generally characterized by episodic encephalopathy, febrile illness, presenting as confusion, seizures, external ophthalmoplegia, dysphagia, and sometimes coma and death. Either partial or complete improvement of early symptoms is achieved by high-dose biotin or thiamine treatment. If untreated, encephalopathies can result in permanent dystonia, with lesions of the basal ganglia. It is not known why biotin administration results in clinical improvement, as mutations in the thiamine transporter *SLC19A3* seem to be causative in the disorder (Table 2.6) [110] (Figure 2.16).

TABLE 2.6
Mutations in the *SLC19A3* Gene Found in Patients with Biotin-Responsive Basal Ganglia Disease and Wernicke's-Like Encephalopathy

Region	Nucleotide Change	Protein Change	Effect on Protein Structure or Function/Syndrome
Exon 1	c.68G>T	p.Gly23Val	Missense [111] abolishes transport function [112]/basal ganglia disease
Exon 2	c.74dupT	p.Ser26LeufsX19	Frameshift/basal ganglia disease [113]
Exon 2	c.218A>G	p.Lys44Glu	Missense causes retention in the endoplasmic reticulum/Wernicke's encephalopathy [114]
Exon 3	c.1047G>C	p.Glu320Gln	Missense causing reduced transporter activity/Wernicke's encephalopathy [114]
Exon 3	c.958G>C	p.E320Q	Missense causing reduced transporter activity [110]/Wernicke's encephalopathy[114]
Intron 3	980-14A-G	Splice alteration, exon 4 skipped (r.980_1172del) resulting in p.Gly327AspfsX8	Exon 4 skipped, frameshift results in nonsense-mediated RNA decay/basal ganglia disease [113]
Exon 5	c.1264A>G	p.Thr422Ala	Missense [111] abolishes transport function [112]/basal ganglia disease

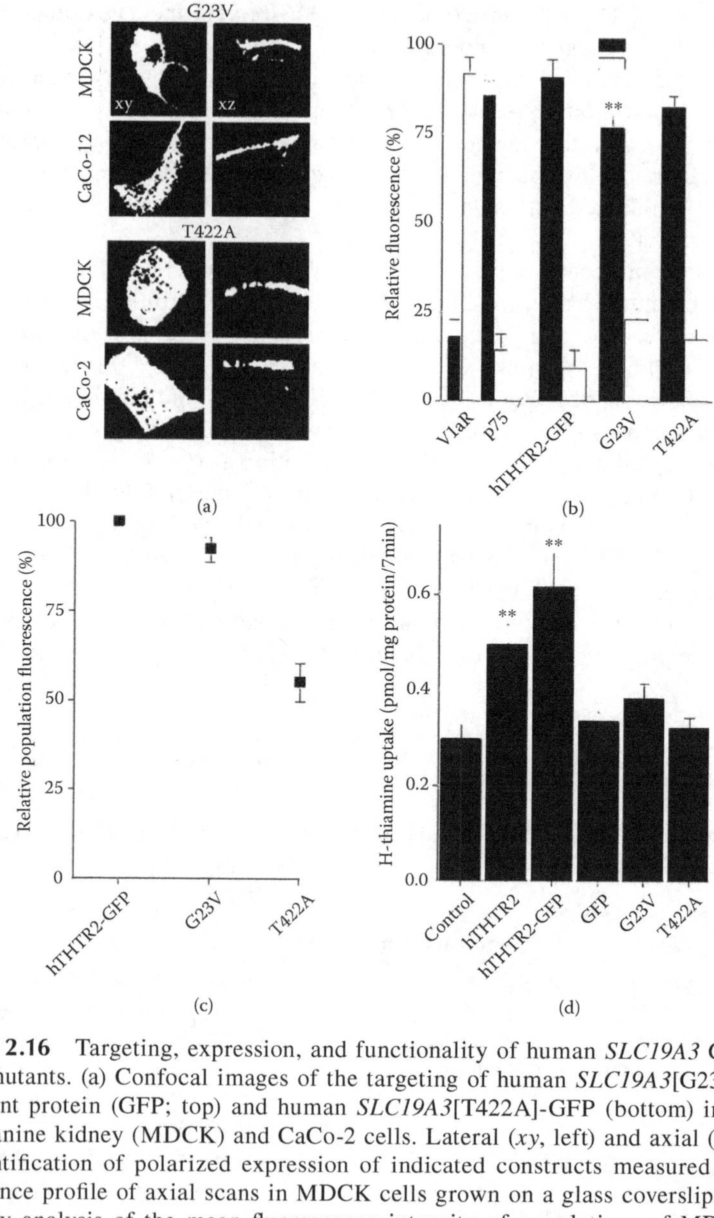

FIGURE 2.16 Targeting, expression, and functionality of human *SLC19A3* G23V and T422A mutants. (a) Confocal images of the targeting of human *SLC19A3*[G23V]-green fluorescent protein (GFP; top) and human *SLC19A3*[T422A]-GFP (bottom) in Madin–Darby canine kidney (MDCK) and CaCo-2 cells. Lateral (*xy*, left) and axial (*xz*, right). (b) Quantification of polarized expression of indicated constructs measured from the fluorescence profile of axial scans in MDCK cells grown on a glass coverslip. (c) Flow cytometry analysis of the mean fluorescence intensity of populations of MDCK cells transfected with the clinical mutant constructs. (d) Measurements of radiolabeled [^{3}H] thiamine uptake by stable MDCK cell lines expressing the indicated constructs. *Note*: *Significance level $p \geq 0.01$. (From Subramanian, V.S. et al., *Am. J. Physiol. Cell Physiol.*, 291, C851–C859, 2006.)

The common intronic *SLC19A3* polymorphism rs13007334 is associated with plasma total homocysteine on a genome-wide level [31]. A 6.9% elevation of total homocysteine in plasma was reported for the rs13007334-C/T heterozygotes. This seems to indicate a novel and uncharacterized biological phenomenon, since SLC19A3 is not known to transport either folate or vitamins B_6/B_{12}, which are known to impact plasma total homocysteine.

IODINE (I^-)

The chemical element iodine (I^-) is incorporated into the thyroid hormones triiodothyronine (T_3) and thyroxine (T_4), which regulate metabolic pathways in the skeletal muscle, central nervous system, and the lungs. Iodine deficiencies lead to a swelling of the thyroid gland called goiter as well as developmental delays and mental retardation [115].

SLC5A5

Iodine uptake into the thyroid is mediated by the Na^+/I^- symporter SLC5A5 (alias NIS). The *SLC5A5* gene on human chromosome 19p13.2-p12 contains 15 exons [4]. The UniGene database (Hs584804 [6]) identifies expression in the brain, eye, and muscle. However, UniGene does not include the thyroid, where it is highly expressed, and expression has also been characterized in the additional extrathyroidal tissues, such as the lactating mammary, the salivary gland, and stomach as well as small intestinal epithelia. The functions for iodine in extrathyroidal tissues have not been determined [116].

The SLC5A5 transcript encodes for a 643–amino acid protein [117], which in the thyroid follicular cell is found on the basolateral pole [115]. The iodine transport is sodium dependent, concentrating it in the thyroid cell. The SLC5A5-mediated I^- transport is electrogenic: two Na^+ ions are transported with each I^- [115,116]. Circulating iodide and thyroid-stimulating hormone regulate SLC5A5's activity and therefore intrathyroidal iodide concentrations, which are 20–50-fold higher than plasma levels [116].

Mutations in *SLC5A5* cause various iodine transport defects leading to congenital hypothyroidism (OMIM 274400) [118]. Most known *SLC5A5* mutations change the amino acid sequence and therefore substrate kinetics; however, some frameshift mutations and truncated proteins have been reported (Table 2.7), which severely compromise the proteins' cellular location and function.

Figure 2.17 depicts the secondary structure model of the SLC5A5 protein and shows the locations of some known mutations. The locations of specific mutations influence the clinical presentations, where onset of hypothyroidism and goiter varies widely (Table 2.7). For example, homozygotes for p.Thr354Pro developed hypothyroidism during infancy, childhood, or not at all [118], indicating a significant influence of the individual genetic background. In contrast, high penetrance is observed for the p.Gly395Arg mutation, where disease is seen within the first month of life.

TABLE 2.7
Mutations of the *SLC5A5* Gene and Their Impact on the Sodium Iodide Symporter's Function as Well as Onset of Hypothyroidism

Mutation	Functional Impact	Onset of Hypothyroidism
p.Val59Glu (V59E)	Nonfunctional protein	Childhood
p.Gly93Arg (G93R), dbSNP rs121909178	Nonfunctional protein due to altered Na^+/I^-coupling stoichiometry	Childhood
p.Arg124His (R124H)	Nonfunctional protein	Neonatal
p.Met143_Gln323del (DelM143-Q323)	Nonfunctional protein due to impaired membrane trafficking	Neonatal
p.Gln267Glu (Q267E), dbSNP rs121909176	Proper membrane targeting but nonfunctional protein marked by decreased turnover	Neonatal
p.Cys272X (C272X), dbSNP rs121909175	Premature stop, truncated protein	Infancy
p.Thr354Pro (T354P), dbSNP rs121909174	Proper membrane targeting but nonfunctional protein due to impaired Na^+ binding	Infancy, childhood, or normal thyroid function
p.Gly395Arg (G395R), dbSNP rs121909180	Proper membrane targeting but nonfunctional protein due to impaired Na^+/I^-coupling	Neonatal
p.Ala439_Pro443del (DelA439-P443)	Nonfunctional protein	Infancy
p.Tyr531X (Y531X), dbSNP rs121909177 p.Ser509ArgfsX7 (FS515X)	67 nt. deletion, frameshift, premature stop, truncated protein	Neonatal
p.Gly543Glu (G543E), dbSNP rs121909179	Nonfunctional protein due to defective maturation and membrane trafficking	Childhood

Source: Adapted from Spitzweg, C. and J.C. Morris, *Mol. Cell. Endocrinol.*, 322, 56–63, 2010.

Residual iodine transporter function, as measured by uptake into the thyroid gland, is markedly lower in neonatal compared to later onset. However, not all patients develop developmental delays [118].

SLC26A4

The *SLC26A4* gene located on human chromosome 7q31 is constituted of 21 exons [4], and its expression is limited to thyroid, vascular, uterus, trachea, testis, prostate, muscle, lung, kidney, and brain (Hs571246 [6]). Expression is also found in inner ear cells [116]. SLC26A4 encodes a multifunctional anion exchanger called pendrin, which transports chloride, bicarbonate, and iodide. In the thyrocytes, the SLC26A4 protein locates to the apical pole, where it contributes to iodide release from the cell into the follicular lumen [119].

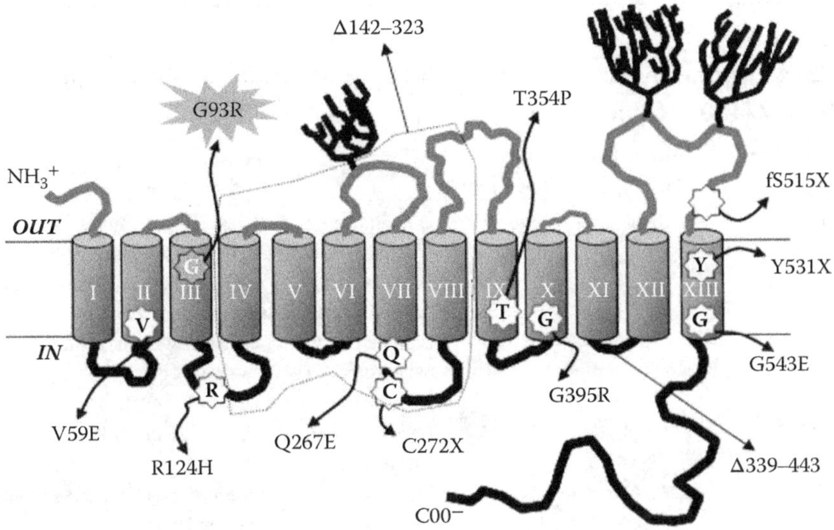

FIGURE 2.17 Secondary structure model of the SLC5A5 protein and the location of selected mutations segregating with congenital hypothyroidism patients. Orange cylinders represent transmembrane segments (TMS); gray lines, extracellular segments; black lines, intracellular segments; branches, N-linked glycosylation sites (N225, 485, 497). Mutations are indicated. (From Paroder-Belenitsky, M. et al., *Proc. Natl. Acad. Sci. USA*, 108, 17933–17938, 2011.)

Slc26a4 knockout mice have no apparent thyroid abnormalities but are completely deaf and display signs of vestibular dysfunction. The vestibular system is constituted of part of the inner ear and the brain that process information to control balance. In *Slc26a4*$^{-/-}$ mice, inner ears show severe endolymphatic dilatation, destruction of sensory cells, and malformation of otoconia and otoconial membranes [120].

In a recessive mouse mutant termed "loop," a homozygous Ser408Phe substitution within the ninth transmembrane domain of Slc26a4 was found. Homozygous Ser408Phe mice are deaf and unable to completely control their body. Slc26a4-Ser408Phe-mediated anion efflux is severely decreased, which seems to cause a change in mineral composition of the inner ear demonstrated by the presence of ectopic stones. This compromises proper hair cell stimulation and vestibular functions [121].

The autosomal recessive Pendred syndrome (OMIM 274600) is caused by bi-allelic mutations in the *SLC26A4* gene. The syndrome develops in early infants and presents with deafness, goiter, and hypothyroidism [116,119]. To date, at least 175 mutations have been reported for the *SLC26A4* gene; however, most of them have not been related to a specific phenotype yet [122]. Table 2.8 lists *SLC26A4* associated with a known disease phenotype.

SLC26A4's role in extrathyroid tissues such as lung, endometrium, prostate, testis, and the lactating mammary gland is not known [123].

TABLE 2.8
***SLC26A4* Mutations Associated with a Pendred Syndrome Phenotype (OMIM 274600) Gene**

Nucleotide Change	Amino Acid Change	Gene Location	Phenotype
84C>A	S28R	Exon 2	Bilateral severe sensorineural hearing loss, subclinical hypothyroidism, language disturbance
398T>A	S133T	Exon 4	Bilateral severe sensorineural hearing loss, subclinical hypothyroidism, language disturbance
626G>T	G209V	Exon 6	Enlarged vestibular aqueduct without Pendred syndrome
707T>C	L236P	Exon 6	Recessive locus for deafness (DFNB4)
917delT	X308	Exon 7	Enlarged vestibular aqueduct without Pendred syndrome
1115C>T	A372V	Exon 9	Enlarged vestibular aqueduct without Pendred syndrome
1334T>G	L445W	Exon 11	Hearing loss, goiter, vestibular aqueduct
1468A>C	I490L	Exon 13	Recessive locus for deafness (DFNB4)
1489G>A	G497S	Exon 13	Recessive locus for deafness (DFNB4)
2000T>G	F667C	Exon 17	Sensorineural hearing loss, goiter
2111insGCTGG	X722	Exon 19	Enlarged vestibular aqueduct without Pendred syndrome
2162C>T	T721M	Exon 19	Enlarged vestibular aqueduct without Pendred syndrome
2168A>G	H723R	Exon 19	Enlarged vestibular aqueduct without Pendred syndrome, Mondini dysplasia, vertigo spells
2182-2183insG	Y728X	Exon 19	Enlarged vestibular aqueduct, sensorineural hearing loss, goiter

Source: www.healthcare.uiowa.edu/labs/pendredandbor/slcMutations.htm.

IRON

The trace metal iron participates in cellular functions as a redox cofactor in oxygen and electron transport. Iron helps to control the cellular redox potential, maintenance of energy metabolism, oxidative stress, and DNA synthesis [124]. Systemic iron abundance and location is tightly controlled through storage in the liver and macrophages. However, the kidneys have no excretion function, and iron is lost only through bleeding and sloughing of cells. Excessive amounts of iron cannot be bound to its designated binding proteins, and will catalyze the formation of highly reactive oxygen radicals, and therefore damage hepatic, cardiac, and endocrine tissues. Iron transport can be mediated through solute carriers, or when bound to proteins like transferrin, through receptor-mediated endocytosis [125].

Transporters of the SLC11A family mediate iron transport across cell membranes. However, they are multispecific, also accepting other divalent metal ions such as manganese (Mn^{2+}), cobalt (Co^{2+}), or cadmium (Cd^{2+}) as substrates [126].

SLC11A1

The *SLC11A1* gene, containing 15 exons, is located on human chromosome 2q35 and encodes the natural resistance-associated macrophage protein 1 (NRAMP1) [4,127]. The UniGene database shows almost ubiquitous expression, with high abundance in spleen, placenta, lung, larynx, and blood (Hs.591607 [6]). The 550–amino acid SLC11A1 protein releases divalent cations from the phagosome of macrophages, aiding the defense against microbes [124,128]. The removal of iron and other metals from the phagolysosome is thought to deplete the trapped bacteria of essential trace elements [128].

Slc11a1$^{-/-}$ mice exhibit disturbed systemic iron distribution, with higher transferrin saturation and elevated concentrations in the spleen, while dietary absorption is increased. However, the transferrin saturation is reduced when the mice are under stress, and non-heme iron in the liver and spleen and macrophages increases. The chronic iron overload observed in these mice indicates the existence of a similar phenotype when the human transporter is affected [128].

A role for *Slc11a1* as a modifying gene in the susceptibility to type 1 diabetes has been proposed based on a naturally occurring protective mutation in the so-called Idd5.2 *Slc11a1* haplotype. In these mice, Slc11a1 does not function, which protects the nonobese diabetic mouse from type 1 diabetes [129].

Various studies in different human cohorts report increased risks for tuberculosis associated with *SLC11A1* polymorphisms [130]. Two recent meta-analysis of case–control studies confirmed associations of the coding polymorphism rs17235409 (G>A, D543N), the 3′ UTR rs17235416 (1729+55del4TGTG), the intronic rs3731865 (c.469 +14G>C, INT4), and the 5′ promoter rs34448891 ([GT]n repeat) [130,131] to tuberculosis. The following modulations in tuberculosis risks were demonstrated:

- Carriers of rs34448891 allele 3 have a 35% [131] or 31% [130] reduced risk.
- Carriers of the rs3731865-C allele have a 27% [131] or 23% [130] elevated risk.
- Carriers of the rs17235409-A allele have a 31% [131] or 24% [130] elevated risk.
- Carriers of the rs17235416-TGTG deletion have a 45% [131] or 35% [130] elevated risk.

The association between *SLC11A1* polymorphisms and tuberculosis susceptibility observed in these analyses supports the hypothesis that the protein might play an important role in the host defense [130,131]. However, disease mechanisms and possible gene–gene–nutrient interaction remain to be determined.

SLC11A1 polymorphisms are implicated in autoimmune diseases, such as systemic lupus erythematosus, Crohn's disease, ulcerative colitis, type 1 diabetes, and sarcoidosis (Table 2.9) [132–137].

Specifically, the *SLC11A1* 5′ promoter rs34448891 $(GT)_n$ polymorphisms (Table 2.9) has been investigated due to its proposed effect on gene expression. The so-called allele 3 mediates high while allele 2 mediates decreased expression. Therefore, it is speculated that the high expression provoked by allele 3 will lead to increased macrophage

TABLE 2.9
Details of Individual Association Studies of *SLC11A1* 5′ Promoter rs34448891 $(GT)_n$ Polymorphisms, and Autoimmune or Inflammatory Disease

Study	Disease	Population	rs34448891 Allele Elevating Risk
Graham et al. (2000)	Primary biliary cirrhosis	English	Allele 5[a]
Maliarik et al. (2000)	Sarcoidosis	African-Americans	Allele 3 (allele 2 protective)[a]
Sanjeevi et al. (2000)	Juvenile rheumatoid arthritis	Latvian/Russian	Allele 3 (allele 2 protective)[a]
Yang et al. (2000)	Rheumatoid arthritis	Korean	No association
Kojima et al. (2001)	Inflammatory bowel disease	Japanese	Allele 7[a]
Kotze et al. (2001)	Multiple sclerosis	South African	Allele 5[a]
Bassuny et al. (2002)	Type 1 diabetes	Japanese	Allele 2 protective[b]
Rodriguez et al. (2002)	Rheumatoid arthritis	Spanish	Allele 2 protective[c]
Comabella et al. (2004)	Multiple sclerosis	Spanish	No association
Takahashi et al. (2004)	Type 1 diabetes	Japanese	Allele 7 (allele 2 protective)[d]
Crawford et al. (2005)	Inflammatory bowel disease	Caucasian	No association
Dubaniewicz et al. (2005)	Sarcoidosis	Polish	Allele 3[a]
Nishino et al. (2005)	Type 1 diabetes	Japanese	Allele 2 protective[e]
Zaahl et al. (2005b)	Inflammatory bowel disease	South African (mixed)	Allele 3[f]

Source: O'Brien, B.A. et al., *J. Autoimmun.*, 31, 42–51, 2008.

[a] The specified allele was positively associated with the incidence of disease.

[b] Frequency of allele 2 slightly lower, albeit not significantly, in the early onset (2–10 years) cohort than in controls.

[c] Only when patients and controls stratified according to MHC risk alleles. An increase in 2/2 genotype frequency among patients carrying MHC risk alleles compared to controls. Frequency of patients with allele 3 significantly decreased among patients without MHC risk alleles compared to controls also not carrying MHC risk.

[d] Allele 2 significantly lower when data analyzed using χ^2 test, but not after Bonferroni multiple adjustment.

[e] In all diabetic patients, allele 2 was less frequent and allele 3 was more frequent, albeit not significantly, than in controls. Decreased frequency of allele 2 only among patients with early-onset (<11 years) compared to late onset (>11 years) patients and control subjects.

[f] No statistically significant differences when comparing $(GT)^n$ promoter alleles in patients and controls, except when data stratified according to the presence of the –237C/T polymorphism in association with allele 3.

activation resulting in higher risk for autoimmune diseases. A variety of associations are reported, although results are inconsistent (Table 2.9). All of the published association studies for the rs34448891 $(GT)_n$ polymorphisms had small sample sizes, which warrant caution in extrapolating results to the general population. A recent meta-analysis of these studies found that rs34448891 allele 3 does not confer an increased risk for autoimmune and inflammatory diseases [132]. This controversy demonstrates the need for adequately powered experimental design in genetic association studies as well as the need to validate findings in biological experiments and specific human trials.

SLC11A2/NRAMP2

Nine differentially spliced transcripts are mapped to the human *SLC11A2* locus on chromosome 12q13, illustrating complex splicing with four protein isoforms reported in the NCBI database (Figure 2.18) [4].

Expression can be found in almost all tissues (UniGene Hs.505545), and four different protein isoforms have been characterized [138, 139]. In one isoform, an alternative upstream 5′ exon, termed exon 1A, adds an in-frame translation initiation codon and extends the open reading frame of the protein by 31 amino acids. SLC11A2 expression levels are in part regulated by an iron-responsive element in the 3′ UTR [138, 139].

Solute carrier family 11 member 2, SLC11A2, alias divalent metal ion transporter 1 DMT1, NRAMP2, and DCT1, mediates iron (Fe^{2+}) transport into cells using a proton-dependent mechanism. Alternative substrates are the divalent metal cations Mn^{2+}, Co^{2+}, Cu^{2+}, and Zn^{2+}.

SLC11A2 is involved in non-transferrin-bound iron uptake on the apical side of the enterocyte, into the hepatocyte, erythroid precursors, and placental cells. Therefore, it plays a major role in iron absorption, storage, and distribution, including maternal transfer into the fetus [125].

Murine autosomal recessive microcytic anemia (mk) is caused by the Arg182Gly missense mutation in *Slc11a2*, resulting in decreased intestinal iron absorption as well as altered utilization in the red blood cell. The same Arg185Gly substitution causes a similar phenotype in the Belgrade (b) rat [140]. This specific mutation alters iron transport functions and introduces a calcium channel–like activity [125]. Subcellular targeting is also altered.

Slc11a2 inactivation in the mouse results in decreased postnatal non-heme iron absorption and disturbed hemoglobin formation in the erythroid precursor, but transfer to the fetus was not altered. Despite the fact that iron overload in a mouse with

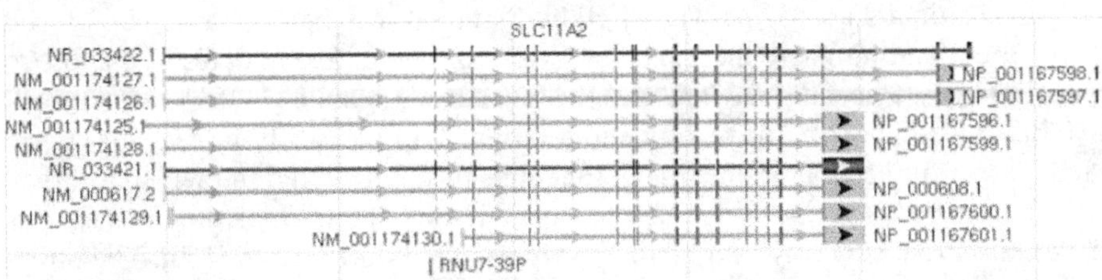

FIGURE 2.18 Transcripts mapped to the SLC11A2 locus.

hereditary hemochromatosis seems to be mediated by Slc11a2, its loss conferred enhanced tolerance to the disease [125].

Human recessive autosomal hypochromic microcytic anemia and iron overload (OMIM 206100) is caused by missense mutations in the *SLC11A2* gene, which lead to decreased erythroid iron utilization [141,142]. Alternatively, the syndrome can be caused by abnormalities in globin or heme synthesis, as well as unknown alterations diminishing availability or acquisition of iron. The following *SLC11A2* mutations have been found in hypochromic microcytic anemia patients:

- A homozygous c.1197G>C (p.GLU399Asp) substitution [143]
- Compound heterozygous c.310-3_5delCTT deletion and c.1246C>T (p.Arg416Cys) substitution [144]
- Compound heterozygous c.340_342delGTG deletion and c.635G>T (p.Gly212Val) substitution [142]
- A homozygous c.223G>A (p.Gly75Arg) substitution [145,146]
- Compound heterozygous c.1472A>G (p.Asn491Ser) and c.635G>T (p.Gly212Val) substitutions [147]

The c.1197G>C mutation alters splicing of exon 12 as well as changing glutamic acid in position 399 to aspartic acid in the remaining properly spliced transcript. The improper splicing seems to reduce mRNA levels and protein abundance resulting in reduced functionality [148].

The c.310-3_5delCTT deletion modifies the splice acceptor for intron 4, and as a consequence, exon 5 is partially spliced out. The resulting SLC11A2 protein misses 40 amino acids, abolishing transport activity [148].

The c.1246C>T transition causes a substitution of the evolutionary conserved arginine at position 416 to cysteine. The resulting protein is retained in the endoplasmic reticulum and cannot fulfill its transport functions [148]

SLC40A1/Ferroportin-1

The human *SLC40A1* gene containing eight exons is located on chromosome 2q32; the transcript shows a pattern of ubiquitous expression. The 5′ UTR contains an iron response element modulating gene expression. Human SLC40A1 (alias ferroportin-1) is a 571–amino acid protein, which represents the sole known iron exporter in mammals. It mediates release across basolateral membranes of intestinal enterocytes and the hepatocytes as well as out of macrophages [149].

The global *Slc40a1* knockout in mice results in embryonic lethality, while heterozygous animals are viable with slightly disrupted iron homeostasis. High levels of iron are found in macrophages, enterocytes, as well as hepatocytes of *Slc40a1*$^{-/-}$ mice. Enterocyte-specific *Slc40a1* inactivation causes anemia [149].

In the flatiron mouse, the histidine in position 32 of the Slc40a1 protein is substituted with arginine, compromising its functions through altered intracellular targeting and transport activity. As a consequence, ferritin contains high amounts of iron, while transferrin is poorly saturated, and Kupffer cells overloaded [150]. The observations in mice define the physiologic implications of Slc40a1 activity and serve as a basic model for hemochromatosis and a syndrome called ferroportin disease.

Human hereditary hemochromatosis is an iron homeostasis disorder caused by homozygous mutations in the hemochromatosis 1, transferrin receptor 2, *hepcidin*, and hemochromatosis 2 genes [149]. Patients have pathological iron deposition in parenchymal cells of the liver, heart, pancreas, and other tissues. Paradoxically, macrophages retain less iron than in normal individuals. The peptide hepcidin binds to ferroportin and targets it for destruction. One form of hemochromatosis results from nonfunctional hepcidin causing unimpeded iron transport through SLC40A1/ferroportin. Clinical findings are explained by a greater transfer of iron from absorptive intestinal epithelial cells to the bloodstream and accelerated macrophage iron release.

Impairment or loss of SLC40A1 functions results in a syndrome called ferroportin disease [151]. The syndrome presents itself in the classical, the nonclassical, or a variable phenotype (Figure 2.19) with significant biochemical heterogeneity and the following diagnostic parameters [152]:

- Classical: normal transferrin saturation, hyperferritinemia, and iron overload in macrophages.
- Nonclassical: high transferrin saturation, hyperferritinemia, and iron overload in macrophages and hepatocytes.

In a recent meta-analysis, 176 ferroportin cases and the underlying 31 genetic mutations were analyzed [152]. The following mutations were found to correlate with the classical disease presentation [152]:

1. Glycine at position 80 changed to valine (Gly80Val, G80V)
2. Aspartic acid at position 157 changed to asparagine (Asp157Asn, D157N)
3. Valine at position 162 deleted (Val 162del)
4. Aspartic acid at position 181 changed to valine (Asp181Val, D181V)
5. Glutamine at position 182 changed to histidine (Gln182His, Q182H)
6. Arginine at position 489 changed to lysine (Arg489Lys, R489K)

The following mutations have been correlated to the nonclassical presentation [152]:

1. Tyrosine at position 64 changed to asparagine (Tyr64Asn, Y64N)
2. Valine at position 72 changed to phenylalanine (Val72Phe, V72F)
3. Asparagine at position 144 changed to histidine (Asn144His, N144H)
4. Cysteine at position 326 changed to either tyrosine or serine (Cys326Tyr/Ser, C326Y/S)
5. Serine at position 338 changed to arginine (Ser338Arg, S338R)
6. Tyrosine at position 501 changed to cysteine (Tyr501Cys, Y501C)

The following mutations resulted in a variable phenotype [152]:

1. Alanine at position 77 changed to aspartic acid (Ala77Asp, A77D)
2. Asparagine at position 144 changed to histidine (Asn144His, N144H)
3. Asparagine at position 185 changed to aspartic acid (Asn185Asp, N185D)
4. Arginine at position 88 changed to threonine (Arg88Thr, R88T)

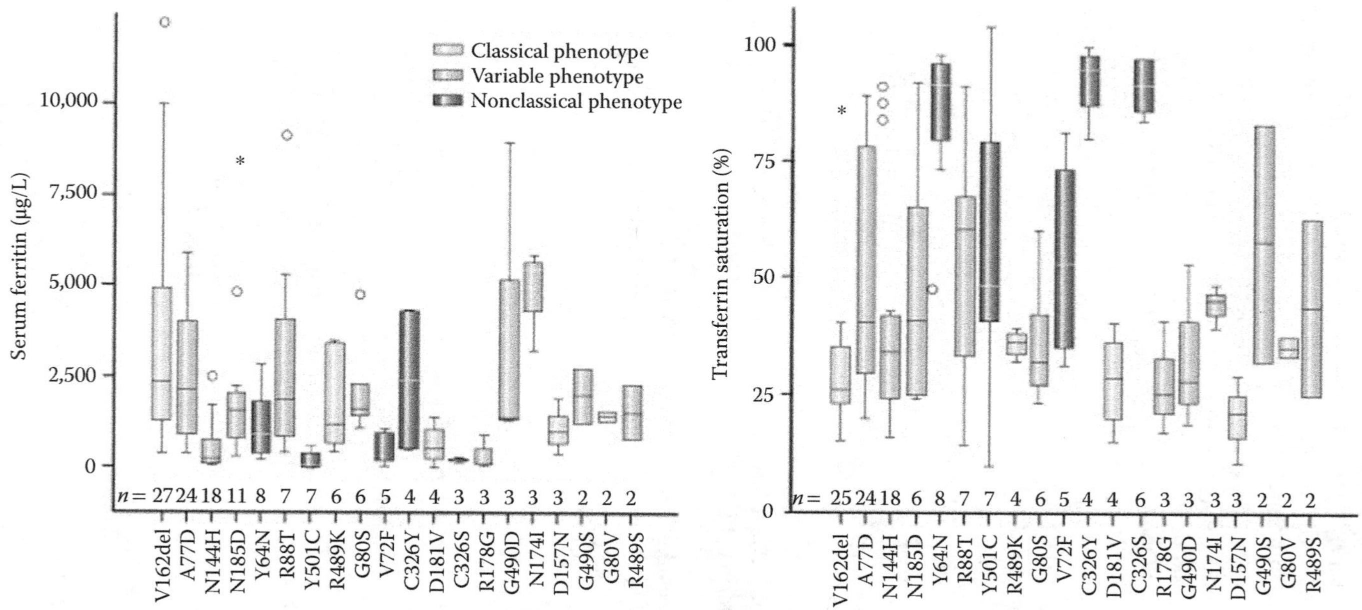

(a) (b)

FIGURE 2.19 Genotype to phenotype correlation of ferroportin disease: patients with ferroportin disease identified from the systematic meta-analysis were grouped according to the *SLC40A1* mutation. Box–Whisker plots of (a) serum ferritin and (b) transferrin saturation in mutations reported in more than five patients are shown. Boxes represent 25th and 75th percentile. Whiskers range and horizontal lines represent the median. Outliers are shown as circles. Light gray, gray, and black boxes indicate that all patients reported with the respective mutation were classified as *classical*, *nonclassical*, or variable biochemical phenotype, respectively, that is, all patients had low or normal transferrin saturation (gray), increased transferrin saturation (black), or different patients with the same mutation had variable transferrin saturation (light gray). Any outliers are marked with a circle and extreme cases with an asterisk. (From Mayr, R. et al., *J. Hepatol.*, 55, 734–736, 2011.)

5. Glycine at position 80 changed to serine (Gly80Ser, G80S)
6. Arginine at position 178 changed to glycine (Arg178Gly, R178G)
7. Glycine at position 490 changed to aspartic acid (Gly490 Asp, G490D)
8. Asparagine at position 174 changed to isoleucine (Asn174Ile, N174I)
9. Glycine at position 490 changed to serine (Gly490Ser, G490S)
10. Arginine at position 489 changed to serine (Arg489Ser, R489S)

The presence of the variable phenotype and its clinical presentation shows that ferroportin disease is multifactorial and that modifying genetic factors play a significant role. Functional biological experiments need to clarify the exact impacts of individual genetic variations.

ZINC

The essential trace metal zinc interacts as a catalytic element or as a structural stabilizer with hundreds of different proteins or peptides. Zinc deficiency has a range of symptoms including embryonic malformations, growth retardation, skin abnormalities with delayed wound healing, compromised immunity, hypogonadism, and lack of appetite [153]. On the contrary, zinc can be toxic when overdosed, and therefore uptake and systemic levels are tightly regulated by various different solute carriers [154]. Zinc uptake and efflux is mediated by solute carriers encoded by members of the *SLC30A* and the *SLC39A* gene groups (Figure 2.20) (Suzuki et al., 2005a,b) [154].

SLC30A1/ZnT1

The *SLC30A1* gene, located on chromosome 1q32.2, is constituted of only two exons [4] and has a broad tissue distribution (UniGene Hs.519469 [6]). SLC30A1 is involved in cellular zinc efflux and can therefore confers resistance to zinc toxicity. The protein is located on the basolateral pole of the enterocytes indicating a major role in zinc release into the circulation [155,156].

SLC30A1 knockout in mice is lethal to the developing embryos, which cannot be rescued by excess maternal zinc supplementation. Heterozygote *SLC30A1* knockout mice develop normally but are three times more likely to have abnormal embryos under dietary zinc deficiency. The abnormal embryos are smaller, have a curled tail, and no digits, which are due to the maternal but not embryonic heterozygosity [157].

Mutations in human *SLC30A1* have been linked to a rare genetic disease, epidermodysplasia verruciformis, in which patients have an unusual sensitivity to cutaneous papillomavirus (epidermodysplasia verruciformis human papillomavirus [EV-HPV]) infections. It is speculated that the disease results from a disturbance of zinc homeostasis by disruptions in SLC30A1's interaction with the products of the *EVER1* or *EVER2* genes, both encoding transmembrane channel–like proteins [158].

SLC30A2/ZnT2

The *SLC30A2* gene is located on chromosome 1p35.3, where a shorter transcript is derived from seven exons, and a longer one constituted of eight exons (Figure 2.21) [4]. *SLC30A2* shows restricted expression in tissues with unique zinc requirements,

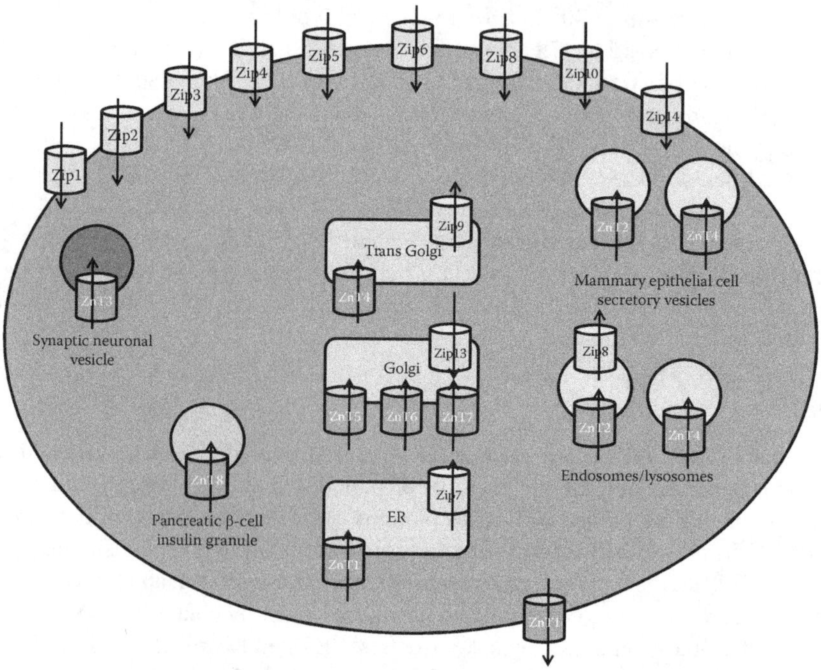

FIGURE 2.20 Solute carrier proteins of the SLC30A (ZnT) and the SLC39A (Zip) families mediate zinc and divalent cation uptake and cellular distribution. A hypothetical example cell representing different tissues is shown.

FIGURE 2.21 Two alternative transcripts map to the *SLC30A2* locus on chromosome 1p35.3. Exon 3 is skipped in reference sequence NM032513.3.

such as the cervix, eye, kidney, lung, ovary, placenta, thyroid, uterus (UniGene Hs.143545 [6]), and prostate gland [159].

In its most notable function, SLC30A2 is involved in zinc export from the mammary gland by transporting zinc from the cytosol into excretory vesicles in epithelial cells (Figure 2.20) [159,160]. Remarkably, the longer protein isoform localizes primarily to the endosomal/secretory compartments, whereas the shorter isoform is associated with the plasma membrane [159].

Women having SLC30A2's arginine 54 substituted by histidine (Arg54His) secreted less zinc into the milk, which caused temporary zinc deficiencies in newborns [161]. Various SNPs in *SLC30A2* have been shown to alter subcellular location. Specifically, the leucine to proline substitution in position 23 (Leu23Pro, SNP rs35235055) results in the protein's mislocalization to lysosomes. Similarly, the arginine to cysteine substitution at amino acid 340 (Arg340Cys, SNP rs35623192) causes a faulty targeting to the Golgi apparatus instead of the endosomal compartments [160]. The physiological consequences of these polymorphisms remain to be determined.

The nonsynonymous polymorphism 1031A>G and the promoter variation −697G>T (rs117153535) were associated with low zinc concentrations in breast milk. However, the reported decrease of zinc in the breast milk appears small and physiologic consequences need to be investigated further. On contrast, extremely low zinc levels are reported in carriers of the rare variation 68T>C (Leu23Pro, rs35235055), which could lead to zinc deficiency in the exclusively breast-fed infant [162].

SLC30A3/ZnT3

The *SLC30A3* gene located on chromosome 2p23.3 is constituted of eight exons [4]. The transcript has a discrete expression pattern in blood, bone, brain, mouth, and testis (UniGene Hs.467981 [6]). In adipose tissue, SLC30A3 has a lower abundance in visceral as compared to subcutaneous areas of lean subjects; however, the reverse is observed for obese individuals [163]. In mice, Slc30a3 is found in the intestine, kidney, liver, spleen, seminal vesicles, testis, submaxillary glands, tongue, brain and epithelial cells of the choroid plexus, the Bergmann glial cells of cerebellar cortex, the postganglionic neurons of superior cervical ganglia, and pancreatic islet [163]. The transport mechanism is driven by an electrogenic antiport of a proton with zinc [163].

Slc30a3 knockout in the mouse decreases hippocampal and cortical zinc content, while pancreatic β-cells or testicular seminiferous tubular cells maintain normal levels [163]. The lower zinc level in the brain resulted in impaired cognitive functions during maturation, eventually resembling Alzheimer's disease symptoms [164]. The *Slc30a3*$^{-/-}$ mice had normal fear behavior, but trace fear conditioning and fear extinction was altered [165].

In spite of unaltered zinc concentrations in the pancreatic islet β-cells, *Slc30a3*$^{-/-}$ mice could not maintain normal glucose metabolism, most likely due to reduced insulin secretion or stability [163]. Although 17 nonsynonymous mutations in human *SLC30A3* are reported to date in dbSNP [166], none have been linked to a disease phenotype. However, potential functional impacts of mutations have been shown in regard to impaired dimerization [167].

SLC30A8/ZnT8

SLC30A8 is located on human chromosome 8q24.11, with five differentially spliced transcripts mapped to the locus (Figure 2.22) [4]. The primary site of expression in humans is the pancreas, with minor expression in kidney, liver, lung, mammary gland, placenta, testis (UniGene Hs.532270 [6]), and amygdala [168]. In addition to pancreatic β-cells, *SLC30A8* is confirmed for adipose tissue, lymphocytes, thyroid follicles, adrenal cortex, α- and pancreatic polypeptide islet cells [169]. The

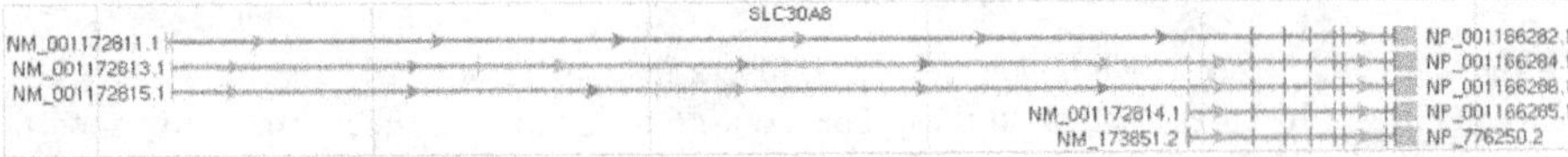

FIGURE 2.22 Differentially spliced transcripts aligning to the *SLC30A8* locus on human chromosome 8q24.11.

369–amino acid protein locates to intracellular membranes where it is responsible for zinc transfer into subcellular compartments [170].

Slc30a8 knockout mice are predisposed to diet-induced obesity and consequent insulin resistance [169–171]. The Slc30a8 protein is an essential component of the membrane of pancreatic β-cell insulin granules, representing the main zinc carrier for the structure. Diminished transport in the *Slc30a8*$^{-/-}$ mice leads to reduced granular zinc levels and incomplete crystallization of insulin [169]. As a result, fasting glucose is increased, while glucose tolerance is compromised in female *Slc30a8*$^{-/-}$ mice [169–171].

The *SLC30A8* rs13266634-C allele is consistently associated with an elevated risk of type 2 diabetes mellitus in individuals of Caucasian, Asian, and African backgrounds [172–175,169,176–179]. Three recent meta-analysis estimated the overall risk of type 2 diabetes for carriers of the *SLC30A8* rs13266634-C allele elevated by 14%–16% (Figure 2.23) [180–182]. Similarly, the risk for impaired glucose tolerance was 15% higher for individuals carrying the *SLC30A8* rs13266634-C allele (Figure 2.24) [181].

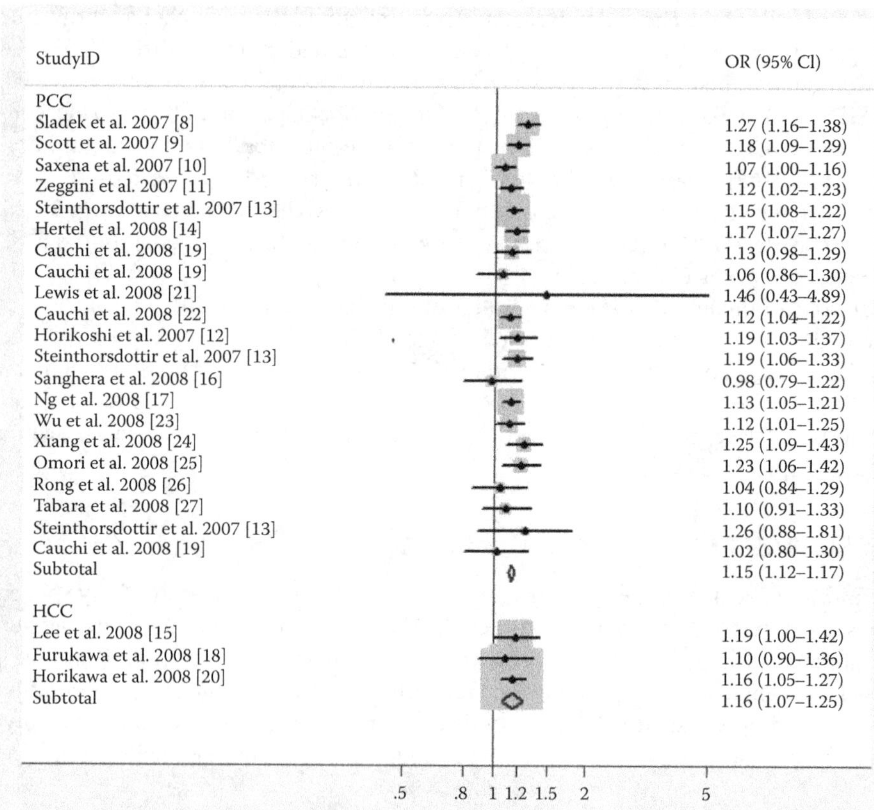

FIGURE 2.23 Stratified analysis pooled odds ratios, expressing the risk of type 2 diabetes mellitus, in case–control studies. The area of the squares reflects the study-specific weight (i.e., inverse of the variance). Diamonds represent the pooled odds ratios and the solid lines the 95% confidence interval of every subgroup. (From Jing, Y.L. et al., *Nutr. Metab. Cardiovasc. Dis.*, 21, 398–405, 2011.)

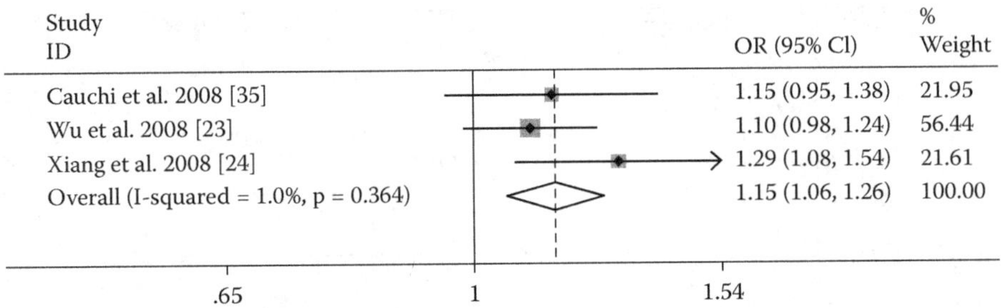

FIGURE 2.24 Pooled odds ratios for the association between rs13266634 C/T polymorphism of *SLC30A8* and susceptibility to impaired glucose tolerance (IGT). The area of the squares reflects the study-specific weight. The diamond shows the summary fixed-effects odds ratio estimate from three studies. (From Xu, K. et al., *Diabetes Res. Clin. Pract.*, 91, 195–202, 2011.)

The nonsynonymous rs13266634-C→T nucleotide change results in an arginine 325 to tryptophane substitution (Arg325Trp, R325W). The disease-associated arginine 325 protein has a reduced zinc transport activity as compared to the tryptophan 325 isoform [171]. However, insulin release from isolated human islets did not differ for the two genotypes, but higher *SLC30A8* expression elevated the insulin and glucagon levels [182]. Overall, the epidemiological evidence is compelling, but further functional studies are needed to elucidate the disease mechanism.

SLC30A10/ZnT10

SLC30A10 resides on human chromosome 1q41 and is constituted of four exons [4]. UniGene mRNA expression profiles indicate very selected expression in brain, liver, and testis [6], and restricted expression in fetal liver and fetal brain is also reported [168]. The 485–amino acid SLC30A10 protein encodes a magnesium membrane carrier, which seems to play a key role in release from the liver [183].

Manganese is an essential trace element that acts as a cofactor in a multitude of enzymatic reactions to mediate oxidative events, transfers, hydrolysis, ligations, and more. It has a very prominent role in the manganese-containing superoxide dismutase, which detoxifies harmful superoxide species [184]. Exposure to high levels of manganese can be toxic, with symptoms manifesting through behavioral mood changes, leading to Parkinson's disease–like presentation.

A variety of autosomal recessive homozygous *SLC30A10* mutations are found in patients with hypermagnesemia, higher red blood cell volume, hepatic cirrhosis, and neurological movement disorder (Figure 2.25). The mutations segregate with the disease in affected families, suggesting that they are causative. Functional studies revealed that the missense mutation c.266T>C, changing leucine 89 to proline (Leu89Pro), and the nonsense mutation c.585del, causing a frameshift (Thr196Profs17), do abolish magnesium transport. It is therefore deduced that defective SLC30A10 leads to magnesium accumulation in the liver and brain [183].

Family	Exon	Mutation	
A	1-2	g.1qdel218.057.426_218.158.564bp	
B	1	c.266T>C,	p.Leu89Pro
C	1	c.292_402del,	p.Val98_Phe134del
D	1	c.314_322del	p.Ala105_Pro107del
E	1	c.585del	p.Thr196Profs*17
F	3	c.765_767del	p.Val256del
G	3	c.922C>T	p.Gln308*
H	4	c.1046T>C	p.Leu349Pro

(a)

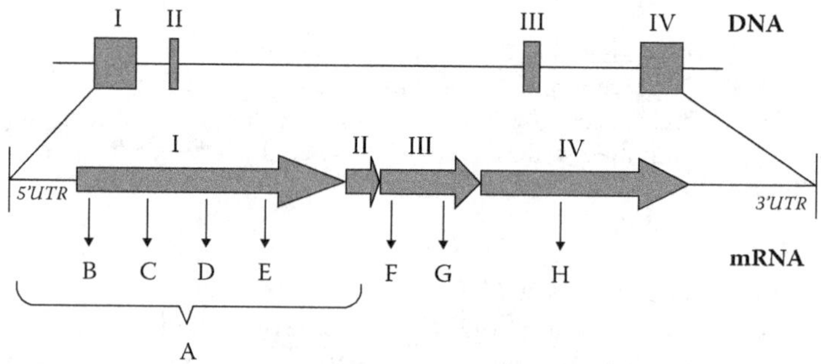

(b)

FIGURE 2.25 *SLC30A10* mutations in affected families with a syndrome of hepatic cirrhosis, dystonia, polycythemia, and hypermagnesemia. (a) Mutations in *SLC30A10* as identified by DNA sequencing. (For families D and G, no DNA was available for analysis of deceased siblings D-II-3 and G-II-1). (b) Genomic structure of the exons encoding SLC30A10 and positions of identified mutations. The large deletion spanning exon 1 and 2 in family A is indicated by a bracket [183]. In addition to the mutations listed in Figure 2.25, a case of c.1235delA deletion in exon 4 has been described. This causes a frameshift for 25 amino acids leading to a stop codon. (From Quadri, M. et al., *Am. J. Hum. Genet.*, 90, 467–477, 2012.)

SLC39A2/Zip2

The *SLC39A2* gene locus on human chromosome 14q11.2 accommodates five exons, and two alternative splice variants are listed in the NCBI database. Variant isoform A represents a longer transcript (NM014579) and protein, whereas isoform B (NM001256588) uses an alternate splice site that results in a frameshift in the 3′ coding region creating a distinct and significantly shorter C-terminus of the full-length 309–amino acid protein (Figure 2.26) [4]. Expression maps to brain, mammary gland, pharynx, placenta, prostate, and uterus indicate a very restricted abundance in specific tissues (UniGene Hs.175783 [6]).

The SLC39A2 protein exclusively locates to the plasma membrane, increases cellular zinc uptake, concentration-, time-, temperature-, pH-dependent, but energy independent. The other transition metals, cadmium, copper, and manganese, might be alternative substrates. It is proposed that SLC39A2 is a Zn^{2+}/HCO_3^- symporter [186].

Slc39a2$^{-/-}$ mice exhibit no obvious adverse phenotype, but are more sensitive to dietary zinc deficiency during pregnancy [154].

The *SLC39A2* rs2234632-G/G genotype is overrepresented in individuals with carotid stenosis. This genotype encodes an arginine at position 43 in the amino

FIGURE 2.26 The *SLC39A2* gene locus on human chromosome 14q11.2 and its two alternative transcripts. (http://www.ncbi.nlm.nih.gov/gene.)

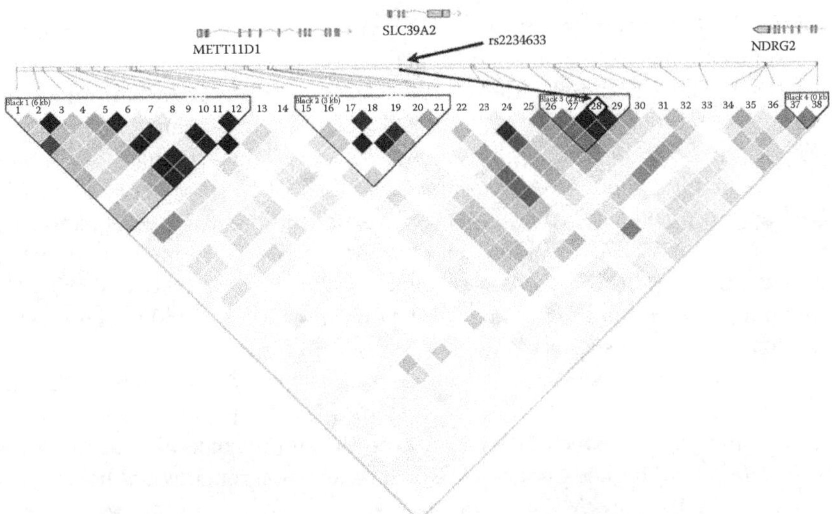

FIGURE 2.27 Linkage disequilibrium (LD) between pairs of SNPs around rs2234633 as determined by Haploview. Relative distances between SNPs in the region are marked as *vertical hash marks* in the *white bar* above the LD plot. The relative positions of the genes in the region are shown in the *top level*. *Gray boxes* in the genes represent exons, while *gray lines* represent introns. The name of each gene is written below its graphical representation. *Black triangular outlines* in the LD plot mark areas of high LD. The *borders* of these LD blocks were determined by Haploview. The position of rs2234633 is marked by *black arrows* below the gene in which it is located (SLC39A2) and by a *black diamond* in the LD plot (SNP 27). *Darker areas* in the LD plot indicate higher levels of LD. (From Karagas, M.R. et al., *Hum. Genet.*, 131, 453–461, 2012.)

acid sequence. Two other alleles exist, the rs2234632-T encoding a leucine, and the rs2234632-A encoding a glutamine [187]. Functional differences were not investigated and disease mechanisms need to be determined.

In individuals with high arsenic exposure, the risk of bladder cancer is elevated for carriers of the *SLC39A2* SNP rs2234636-TC or -CC genotypes by 96% or 91%, respectively. This association was not found in individuals with low arsenic exposure [188]. The effect of a zinc transporter on an arsenic disease is hard to explain, specifically since the SLC39A2 protein is not known to bind arsenic. However, rs2234636 is a nonsynonymous SNP causing a Phe115Leu conversion. It is not in linkage with other SNPs and might therefore be the causative variation (Figure 2.27) [188].

SLC39A3/Zip3

Three exons constitute the *SLC39A3* gene on human chromosome 19p13.3, where two alternative splice variants align (Figure 2.28) [4]. Expression is almost ubiquitous (UniGene Hs.515046 [6]).

FIGURE 2.28 Alternative transcripts mapping to the human *SLC39A3* locus on chromosome 19p13.3. (http://www.ncbi.nlm.nih.gov/gene.)

The SLC39A3 protein is present on intracellular organelles in zinc deprivation and recruited to the cell surface under normal conditions, where it mediates zinc uptake [189]. The zinc uptake can be inhibited by copper, cadmium, manganese, cobalt, silver, and nickel, indicating alternative substrate acceptance [190].

Mice lacking *Slc39a3* are slightly more sensitive to dietary zinc restriction, but have no detrimental phenotype in normal conditions [191]. However, if *Slc39a3* and *Slc39a1* are eliminated together, embryonic abnormalities become apparent [191]. Triple knockout of *Slc39a1*, *Slc39a2*, and *Slc39a3* does not adversely affect the mice in adequate zinc supply, but show embryonic abnormalities in zinc deficiency [192]. The findings in mice imply redundancy of *SLC39A3*, which could explain a lack of association to human diseases.

The *SLC39A3* SNP rs4806874-G allele is consistently associated with bipolar disorder in a meta-analysis of two GWAS studies [193]. This association was replicated in an independent study [194]. However, the significance of the intronic SNP rs4806874 in regard to disease mechanism and causation remains unknown.

SLC39A4/ZIP4

The *SLC39A4* gene locus on human chromosome 8q24.3 harbors 12 exons; two alternative spliced transcripts are aligned in the NCBI database. Variant isoform 1 (NM 017767) contains a distinct 5' UTR and 5' coding region, resulting in a distinct N-terminus compared to isoform 2 (NM 130849), which represents the shorter transcript but encodes the longer isoform (Figure 2.29) [4].

The site of expression indicates SLC39A4's key role in intestinal zinc absorption or renal reabsorption [195]. The transcripts can also be found in uterus, trachea, skin, salivary gland, prostate, placenta, pancreas, ovary, mammary gland, liver, lung, heart, eye, blood, and ascites (UniGene Hs.521934 [6]). These two transcripts encode proteins of 647 and 622 amino acids where they share the last 583 residues [196]. Zinc, copper, and nickel are substrates for the human SLC39A4. [197]. The SLC39A4 protein is found in endosomes when extracellular zinc is sufficient, but relocates to the apical pole of the enterocyte in zinc deficiency [198].

Slc39a4 knockout mouse embryos die in the early postimplantation period [199]. *Slc39a4*$^{+/-}$ littermates are found in low numbers (compared to wild-types) and show significant growth retardation. *Slc39a4*$^{+/-}$ have severe malformation of the skull, exposed brains, might lack one or both eyes, and accumulate fluid in the cerebral ventricles.

An autosomal recessive hereditary zinc deficiency is reported in cattle, with symptoms of diarrhea and skin lesions, as well as high susceptibility to infections. When calves receive supplemental zinc, all symptoms are alleviated. A single nucleotide G to A change alters the bovine *Slc39a4* gene splice donor site for intron 10. The altered splicing eliminates coding regions for transmembrane domain 4 and most of transmembrane domain 5. This change is predicted to abolish transporter functions and therefore causes the bovine hereditary zinc deficiency with a phenotype resembling human acrodermatitis enteropathica (AE) [200].

Human autosomal recessive AE appears in early infancy with growth retardation, diarrhea, and behavioral and neurological abnormalities. It is attributed to zinc malabsorption and is reversed with a dietary zinc supplementation of 1–3 mg/kg/day (Figure 2.30) (OMIM 201100 [83]). Plasma zinc concentrations are under 50 mg/dL, while normal values are between 60 and 120 mg/dL. Severe disease ends in organ failure and death [198].

Over 30 mutations in the human *SLC39A4* gene have been determined in cases of AE (Table 2.10). Affected individuals are mostly homozygotes or compound heterozygotes, but five heterozygote cases are reported [198].

The functional implications of six human mutations introduced into the mouse Slc23a4 cDNA have been tested in vitro. The amino acids altered are conserved between human and mouse and are mainly located in transmembrane domains [215]. All mutations decreased zinc uptake activity of SLC39A4 (Figure 2.31). Slc23a4 proteins with the amino acid changes, Gly340Asp (human Gly330Asp), Leu382Pro

FIGURE 2.29 Alternative transcripts mapped to the human *SLC39A4* locus on chromosome 8q24.3. (http://www.ncbi.nlm.nih.gov/gene.)

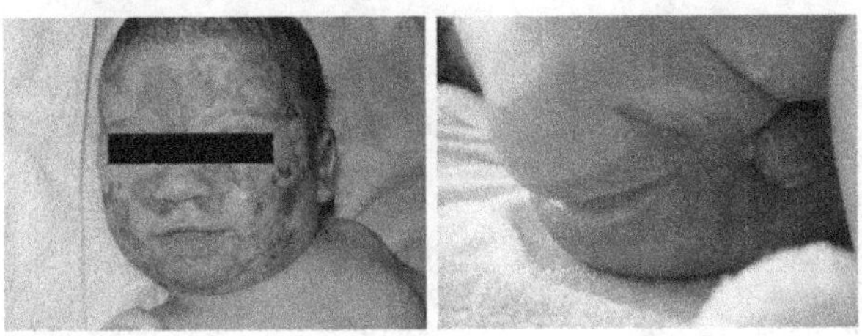

(a) (b)

FIGURE 2.30 Acrodermatitis enteropathica erythematous erosive lesions on the face (a) and involvement of the anogenital area (b). (From Santiago, F. et al., *Pediatr. Dermatol.*, 28, 735–736, 2011.)

TABLE 2.10
Mutations in the *SLC39A4* Gene of Acrodermatitis Enteropathica Cases

Region	Nucleotide Change	Effect on Amino Acid	Effect on Protein Structure or Function
Exon 1	c.184T>C [202]	p.Cys62Arg	Missense
Exon 1	c.143T>G [203, 204, 202]	p.Leu48X	Nonsense
Intron 1	c.192119G>A [196]	Possible donor splice site error	ND
Exon 2	c.283C>T [205]	p.Arg95Cys	Missense
Exon 2	c.318C>A [206]	p.Asn106Lys	Missense
Intron 2	c.475-2>4 [202]	Possible acceptor splice site error	

(*Continued*)

TABLE 2.10 (*Continued*)
Mutations in the SLC39A4 Gene of Acrodermatitis Enteropathica Cases

Region	Nucleotide Change	Effect on Amino Acid	Effect on Protein Structure or Function
Exon 2	c.251C>T [195]	p.Pro84Leu	Missense
Exon 3	c.511G>T [198]	p.Val171Leu	Missense
Exon 3	c.599C>T [196]	p.Pro200Leu	Missense decreases V_{max}
Exon 3	c.631C>T [207]	p.Gln211X	Nonsense
Exon 3	c.641_642ins10 [201]	p.Ser214ArgfsX30	Frameshift
Exon 4	c.766delC [208]	p.Leu256SerfsX16	Frameshift
Exon 4	c.751C>T [195]	p.Arg251Trp	Missense
Exon 5	c.850G4A (dbSNP rs7823979) [202]	p.Glu284Lys	Missense
Exon 5	c.909G>C [204]	p.Gln303His	Missense
Exon 5	c.926G>A [206]	p.Cys309Tyr	Missense
Exon 5	c.968_971delAGTC [196]	p.Ser324ArgfsX24	Frameshift
Exon 6	c.989G>A [206]	p.Gly330Asp	Missense causes cellular mislocalization
Exon 6	c.1016_1017ins53 [204]	p.Thr357AlafsX10	Frameshift
Exon 6	c.1115T>C [206]	p.Leu372Pro	Missense with reduced protein levels
Exon 6	c.1120G>A [196]	p.Gly374Arg	Missense with reduced protein levels
Exon 6	c.1191insC [209]	p.Gln398fsX18	Frameshift
Exon 6	c.1141A>G [208]	p.Thr381Ala	Missense
Exon 6	c.1115T>G [210]	p.Leu372Arg	Missense
Intron 6	c.1150-2A>G [195]	Possible acceptor splice site error	
Exon 7	c.1203G>A [202]	p.Trp401X	Nonsense
Exon 7	c1223delC [211]	p.Ala408fsX481	Frameshift
Exon 7	c.1223_1227delCCGGG [196]	p.Trp411ArgfsX7	Frameshift
Exon 7	c.1229T>C [195]	p.Leu410Pro	Missense
Intron 7	c.1287+2T>C [205]	Possible acceptor splice site error	
Exon 9	c.1438G>T[212]	p.Glu480Sto	Stop
Exon 9	c.1462_147411+delAGACTGA GCCCAGG [213]	p.Arg488SerfsX2	Frameshift
Exon 10	c.1534G>T [208]	p.Gly512Trp	Missense
Exon 10	c.1576G>A [196]	p.Gly526Arg	Missense decreases V_{max}
Exon 11	c.1784G>T [214]	p.Gly595Val	Missense
Exon 11	c.1646_1648delTGC [208]	p.549delLeu	Deletion
Exon 12	c.1888G>C [206]	p.Gly630Arg	Missense with reduced protein levels

Source: Modified and expanded from Schmitt, S. et al., *Hum. Mutat.*, 30, 926–933, 2009.
The numbering for the nucleotide changes are based on cDNA sequence in accordance with the GenBank entry NM_130849.2. Position +1 corresponds to the A of the ATG translation initiation codon in the reference sequence.

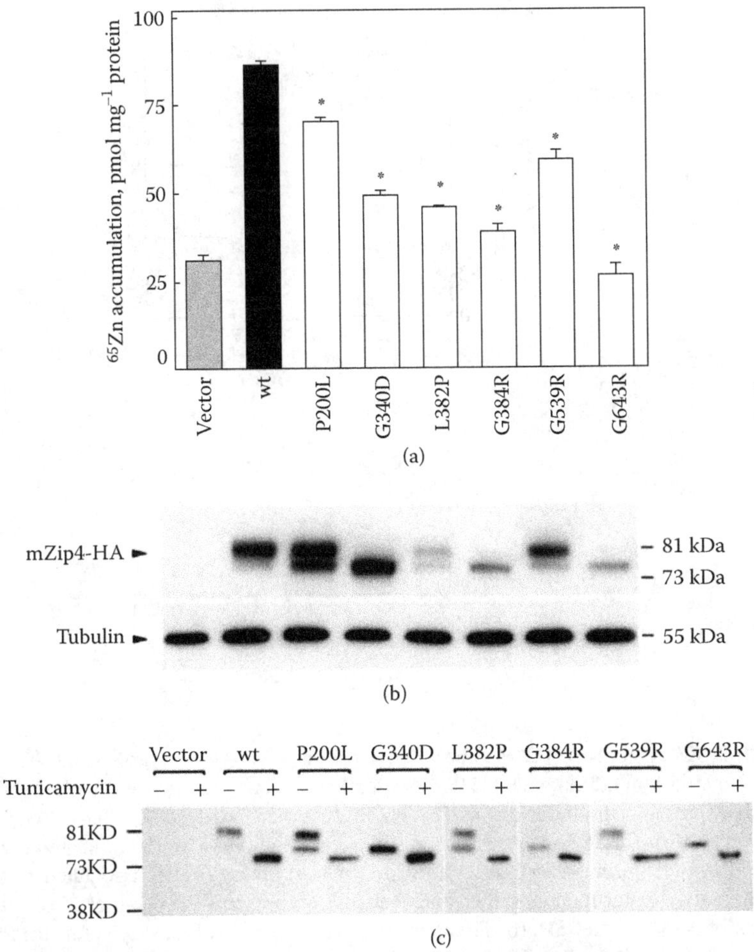

FIGURE 2.31 SLC39A4 mutant proteins have reduced radiolabeled ^{65}Zn uptake activity. Human embryonic kidney 293 (HEK293) cells were transiently transfected with the vector or the indicated mZip4-HA allele, grown for 36–48 hours and then assayed for (a) ^{65}Zn uptake activity or (b) mZip4-HA expression by immunoblotting. ^{65}Zn uptake was assayed with 2 μM $^{65}ZnCl_2$ for 15 minutes. Previous studies showed that zinc accumulation is linear over this time period for the wild-type protein. The cells were then washed and cell-associated ^{65}Zn was measured. The figure shows a representative experiment ($n = 3$) and the asterisks indicate significant differences ($P < 0.01$) from wild-type. In (b), total protein extracts were prepared from transfected cells and analyzed by immunoblotting. Tubulin was used as a loading control and the positions of molecular weight markers are shown. (c) Effects of AE mutations on mZip4-HA N-glycosylation. Stably transfected carbohydrate (CHO) cells bearing the vector or expressing the indicated mZip4-HA allele were treated with tunicamycin (5 μg/mL) for 16 hours. Treated and untreated control cells were harvested and lysed and protein extracts were prepared and analyzed by immunoblotting using anti-HA antibody. L382P was loaded at a higher protein level/lane to compensate for its lower accumulation. (From Wang, F. et al., *Hum. Mol. Genet.*, 13, 563–571, 2004.)

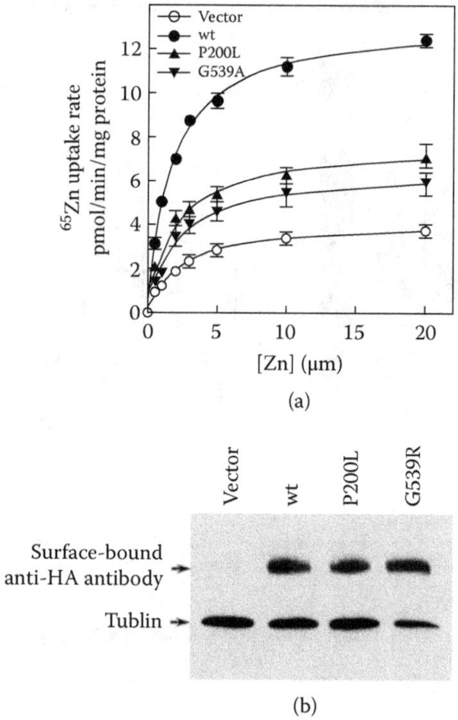

FIGURE 2.32 Effects of P200L and G539R on the kinetics of radiolabeled ^{65}Zn uptake. (a) Human embryonic kidney 293 (HEK293) cells transiently transfected with the vector or plasmids expressing the indicated mZip4-HA alleles were assayed for ^{65}Zn uptake activity over a range of substrate concentrations. Cells were incubated with the indicated concentration of ^{65}Zn for 15 minutes before washing and measurement of cell-associated zinc levels. A representative experiment is shown and each point represents the mean of three replicates. The error bars indicate ±1 SD. (b) The same cells as in (a) were also assayed for surface levels of mZip4-HA protein as described in Figure 2.31.

(human Gly372Asp), Gly384Arg (human Gly374Asp), and Gly643Arg (human Gly630Arg), did not get targeted to the plasma membrane (Figure 2.31).

The two protein alterations, Pro200Leu (same in humans) and Gly539Arg (human Gly526Arg), were targeted correctly to the plasma membrane, but maximal zinc uptake was decreased by 30% (Figure 2.32). In addition, they did not undergo endocytosis in conditions of adequate zinc supply, as seen for the wild-type [215].

CONCLUSIONS

In past decades, the discovery of a variety of monogenic disorders has clearly demonstrated that disruptions of micronutrient transporter genes lead to severe syndromes. With the development of transgenic animal models, especially knockout mice, we now have a tool to study each solute carrier's biology and disease impact in model systems, which will lead to the discovery of further disease phenotypes.

The current development of GWAS enables us to determine gene–gene and gene–diet interactions beyond the scope of a single gene. Future applications of adequately powered design in GWAS will permit the discovery of genetic associations of micronutrient imbalances leading to common and complex diseases, such as cancers and cardiovascular diseases. The major challenge will be the translation of the association into clinical or population health. Each putative risk genotype needs to be validated using biological systems, such as model animals or affected human individuals.

This chapter demonstrates our ability to determine disease-causing rare mutations, but at the same time, there is still an apparent lack of identification and validation of disease-causing polymorphisms in common and complex diseases. We should take that as a motivation for further research into the biology and genetics of micronutrients and their solute carriers. If successful, this research could lead to significant early diagnostics and prevention of some of the most detrimental common and complex diseases, such as cancer, metabolic syndrome, type 2 diabetes, and cardiovascular disease.

REFERENCES

1. Said, H.M., Intestinal absorption of water-soluble vitamins in health and disease. *Biochemical Journal*, 2011. **437**(3): pp. 357–372.
2. Običan, S.G. et al., Folic acid in early pregnancy: a public health success story. *The FASEB Journal*, 2010. **24**(11): pp. 4167–4174.
3. Corpe, C.P. et al., Vitamin C transporter Slc23a1 links renal reabsorption, vitamin C tissue accumulation, and perinatal survival in mice. *Journal of Clinical Investigation*, 2010. **120**(4): pp. 1069–1083.
4. http://www.ncbi.nlm.nih.gov/gene.
5. Wang, H. et al., Human Na+-dependent vitamin C transporter 1 (hSVCT1): primary structure, functional characteristics and evidence for a non-functional splice variant. *Biochimica et Biophysica Acta*, 1999. **1461**(1): pp. 1–9.
6. http://www.ncbi.nlm.nih.gov/unigene.
7. Tsukaguchi, H. et al., A family of mammalian Na+-dependent L-ascorbic acid transporters. *Nature*, 1999. **399**(6731): pp. 70–75.
8. Varma, S. et al., Hierarchal contribution of N- and C-terminal sequences to the differential localization of homologous sodium-dependent vitamin C transporters, SVCT1 and SVCT2, in epithelial cells. *Biochemistry*, 2009. **48**(13): pp. 2969–2980.
9. Timpson, N.J. et al., Genetic variation at the SLC23A1 locus is associated with circulating concentrations of L-ascorbic acid (vitamin C): evidence from 5 independent studies with >15,000 participants. *American Journal of Clinical Nutrition*, 2010. **92**(2): pp. 375–382.
10. Cahill, L.E. and A. El-Sohemy, Vitamin C transporter gene polymorphisms, dietary vitamin C and serum ascorbic acid. *Journal of Nutrigenetics and Nutrigenomics*, 2010. **2**(6): pp. 292–301.
11. Skibola, C.F. et al., Polymorphisms in the estrogen receptor 1 and vitamin C and matrix metalloproteinase gene families are associated with susceptibility to lymphoma. *PLoS One*, 2008. **3**(7): p. e2816.
12. Erichsen, H.C. et al., Genetic variation in the sodium-dependent vitamin C transporters, SLC23A1, and SLC23A2 and risk for preterm delivery. *American Journal of Epidemiology*, 2006. **163**(3): pp. 245–254.

13. Lutsenko, E.A., J.M. Carcamo, and D.W. Golde, A human sodium-dependent vitamin C transporter 2 isoform acts as a dominant-negative inhibitor of ascorbic acid transport. *Molecular and Cellular Biology*, 2004. **24**(8): pp. 3150–3156.
14. Daruwala, R. et al., Cloning and functional characterization of the human sodium-dependent vitamin C transporters hSVCT1 and hSVCT2. *FEBS Letters*, 1999. **460**(3): pp. 480–484.
15. Sotiriou, S. et al., Ascorbic-acid transporter Slc23a1 is essential for vitamin C transport into the brain and for perinatal survival. *Nature Medicine*, 2002. **8**(5): pp. 514–517.
16. Eck, P. et al., Comparison of the genomic structure and variation in the two human sodium-dependent vitamin C transporters, SLC23A1 and SLC23A2. *Human Genetics*, 2004. **115**(4): pp. 285–294.
17. Zanon-Moreno, V. et al., Association between a SLC23A2 gene variation, plasma vitamin C levels, and risk of glaucoma in a Mediterranean population. *Molecular Vision*, 2011. **17**: pp. 2997–3004.
18. Wright, M.E. et al., Genetic variation in sodium-dependent ascorbic acid transporters and risk of gastric cancer in Poland. *European Journal of Cancer*, 2009. **45**(10): pp. 1824–1830.
19. Chen, A.A. et al., Genetic variation in the vitamin C transporter, SLC23A2, modifies the risk of HPV16-associated head and neck cancer. *Carcinogenesis*, 2009. **30**(6): pp. 977–981.
20. Erichsen, H.C. et al., Genetic variation in sodium-dependent vitamin C transporters SLC23A1 and SLC23A2 and risk of advanced colorectal adenoma. *Nutrition and Cancer*, 2008. **60**(5): pp. 652–659.
21. Salbaum, J.M. and C. Kappen, Genetic and epigenomic footprints of folate. *Progress in Molecular Biology and Translational Science*, 2012. **108**: pp. 129–158.
22. Ma, D.W.L. et al., Folate transport gene inactivation in mice increases sensitivity to colon carcinogenesis. *Cancer Research*, 2005. **65**(3): pp. 887–897.
23. Zhao, R. et al., Mechanisms of membrane transport of folates into cells and across Epithelia. *Annual Review of Nutrition*, 2011. **31**(1): pp. 177–201.
24. Zhao, R.B. et al., Rescue of embryonic lethality in reduced folate carrier-deficient mice by maternal folic acid supplementation reveals early neonatal failure of hematopoietic organs. *Journal of Biological Chemistry*, 2001. **276**(13): pp. 10224–10228.
25. Yee, S.W. et al., SLC19A1 pharmacogenomics summary. *Pharmacogenetics and Genomics*, 2010. **20**(11): pp. 708–715.
26. Eklof, V. et al., The reduced folate carrier (RFC1) 80G>A and folate hydrolase 1 (FOLH1) 1561C>T polymorphisms and the risk of colorectal cancer: a nested case-referent study. *Scandinavian Journal of Clinical & Laboratory Investigation*, 2008. **68**(5): pp. 393–401.
27. Chango, A. et al., A polymorphism (80G>A) in the reduced folate carrier gene and its associations with folate status and homocysteinemia. *Molecular Genetics and Metabolism*, 2000. **70**(4): pp. 310–315.
28. Chatzikyriakidou, A. et al., Distinct association of SLC19A1 polymorphism -43T>C with red cell folate levels and of MTHFR polymorphism 677C>T with plasma folate levels. *Clinical Biochemistry*, 2008. **41**(3): pp. 174–176.
29. Stanisławska-Sachadyn, A. et al., The reduced folate carrier (SLC19A1) c.80G>a polymorphism is associated with red cell folate concentrations among women. *Annals of Human Genetics*, 2009. **73**(5): pp. 484–491.
30. Devlin, A.M. et al., Interactions among polymorphisms in folate-metabolizing genes and serum total homocysteine concentrations in a healthy elderly population. *American Journal of Clinical Nutrition*, 2006. **83**(3): pp. 708–713.

31. Wernimont, S.M. et al., Folate network genetic variation, plasma homocysteine, and global genomic methylation content: a genetic association study. *BMC Medical Genetics*, 2011. **12**: p. 150.
32. Levine, A.J. et al., Variation in folate pathway genes and distal colorectal adenoma risk: a sigmoidoscopy-based case-control study. *Cancer Causes & Control*, 2011. **22**(4): pp. 541–552.
33. Eussen, S.J.P.M. et al., Plasma folate, related genetic variants, and colorectal cancer risk in EPIC. *Cancer Epidemiology Biomarkers and Prevention*, 2010. **19**(5): pp. 1328–1340.
34. Galbiatti, A.L.S. et al., A80G polymorphism of reduced folate carrier 1 (RFC1) gene and head and neck squamous cell carcinoma etiology in Brazilian population. *Molecular Biology Reports*, 2011. **38**(2): pp. 1071–1078.
35. Faganel Kotnik, B. et al., Association of genetic polymorphism in the folate metabolic pathway with methotrexate pharmacokinetics and toxicity in childhood acute lymphoblastic leukaemia and malignant lymphoma. *European Journal of Clinical Pharmacology*, 2011. **67**(10): pp. 993–1006.
36. Yeoh, A.E.J. et al., Genetic susceptibility to childhood acute lymphoblastic leukemia shows protection in Malay boys: results from the Malaysia-Singapore ALL study group. *Leukemia Research*, 2010. **34**(3): pp. 276–283.
37. Wang, L.N. et al., Reduced folate carrier gene G80A polymorphism is associated with an increased risk of gastroesophageal cancers in a Chinese population. *European Journal of Cancer*, 2006. **42**(18): pp. 3206–3211.
38. Shen, M. et al., Polymorphisms in folate metabolic genes and lung cancer risk in Xuan Wei, China. *Lung Cancer*, 2005. **49**(3): pp. 299–309.
39. Gregers, J. et al., The association of reduced folate carrier 80G>A polymorphism to outcome in childhood acute lymphoblastic leukemia interacts with chromosome 21 copy number. *Blood*, 2010. **115**(23): pp. 4671–4677.
40. Owen, S.A. et al., Genetic polymorphisms in key methotrexate pathway genes are associated with response to treatment in rheumatoid arthritis patients. *The Pharmacogenomics Journal*, 2012. DOI:10.1038/tpj.2012.7.
41. Adjei, A.A. et al., Correlation between polymorphisms of the reduced folate carrier gene (SLC19A1) and survival after pemetrexed-based therapy in non-small cell lung cancer: a north central cancer treatment group-based exploratory study. *Journal of Thoracic Oncology*, 2010. **5**(9): pp. 1346–1353.
42. Maggini, V. et al., Association of folate transporter SLC19A1 polymorphisms with the outcome of multiple myeloma after chemotherapy and tandem autologous transplantation. *Leukemia*, 2006. **21**(1): pp. 176–178.
43. Shaw, G.M. et al., Maternal periconceptional vitamin use, genetic variation of infant reduced folate carrier (A80G), and risk of spina bifida. *American Journal of Medical Genetics*, 2002. **108**(1): pp. 1–6.
44. Pei, L. et al., Genetic variation of infant reduced folate carrier (A80G) and risk of orofacial defects and congenital heart defects in China. *Annals of Epidemiology*, 2006. **16**(5): pp. 352–356.
45. Bufalino, A. et al., Maternal polymorphisms in folic acid metabolic genes are associated with nonsyndromic cleft lip and/or palate in the Brazilian population. *Birth Defects Research Part A: Clinical and Molecular Teratology*, 2010. **88**(11): pp. 980–986.
46. O'Byrne, M.R. et al., Association of folate receptor (FOLR1, FOLR2, FOLR3) and reduced folate carrier (SLC19A1) genes with meningomyelocele. *Birth Defects Research. Part A, Clinical and Molecular Teratology*, 2010. **88**(8): pp. 689–694.
47. Jeon, Y.J. et al., The reduced folate carrier-1 (RFC1 696T>C) polymorphism is associated with spontaneously aborted embryos in Koreans. *Genes and Genomics*, 2011. **33**(3): pp. 223–228.

48. Rah, H. et al., Solute carrier family 19, member 1 (SLC19A1) polymorphisms (-43T>C, 80G>A, and 696C>T), and haplotypes in idiopathic recurrent spontaneous abortion in a Korean population. *Reproductive Sciences*, 2012. **19**(5): pp. 513–519.
49. Laanpere, M. et al., Folate-metabolizing gene variants and pregnancy outcome of IVF. *Reproductive BioMedicine Online*, 2011. **22**(6): pp. 603–614.
50. Altmae, S. et al., Variations in folate pathway genes are associated with unexplained female infertility. *Fertility and Sterility*, 2010. **94**(1): pp. 130–137.
51. Yang, R. et al., Sequence alterations in the reduced folate carrier are observed in osteosarcoma tumor samples. *Clinical Cancer Research*, 2003. **9**(2): pp. 837–844.
52. Fredriksen, Å. et al., Large-scale population-based metabolic phenotyping of thirteen genetic polymorphisms related to one-carbon metabolism. *Human Mutation*, 2007. **28**(9): pp. 856–865.
53. Giusti, B. et al., Genetic analysis of 56 polymorphisms in 17 genes involved in methionine metabolism in patients with abdominal aortic aneurysm. *Journal of Medical Genetics*, 2008. **45**(11): pp. 721–730.
54. Chatzikyriakidou, A. et al., Transcription regulatory polymorphism-43T>C in the 5'-flanking region of SLC19A1 gene could affect rheumatoid arthritis patient response to methotrexate therapy. *Rheumatology International*, 2007. **27**(11): pp. 1057–1061.
55. Hilton, J.E. et al., The molecular basis of glutamate formiminotransferase deficiency. *Human Mutation*, 2003. **22**(5): pp. 416–416.
56. Drori, S. et al., Clustering of mutations in the first transmembrane domain of the human reduced folate carrier in GW1843U89-resistant leukemia cells with impaired antifolate transport and augmented folate uptake. *Journal of Biological Chemistry*, 2000. **275**(40): pp. 30855–30863.
57. Kaufman, Y. et al., Reduced folate carrier mutations are not the mechanism underlying methotrexate resistance in childhood acute lymphoblastic leukemia. *Cancer*, 2004. **100**(4): pp. 773–782.
58. Qiu, A. et al., Identification of an intestinal folate transporter and the molecular basis for hereditary folate malabsorption. *Cell*, 2006. **127**(5): pp. 917–928.
59. Thwaites, D.T. and C.M.H. Anderson, H+-coupled nutrient, micronutrient and drug transporters in the mammalian small intestine. *Experimental Physiology*, 2007. **92**(4): pp. 603–619.
60. Shayeghi, M. et al., Identification of an intestinal heme transporter. *Cell*, 2005. **122**(5): pp. 789–801.
61. Salojin, K.V. et al., A mouse model of hereditary folate malabsorption: deletion of the PCFT gene leads to systemic folate deficiency. *Blood*, 2011. **117**(18): pp. 4895–4904.
62. Geller, J. et al., Hereditary folate malabsorption: family report and review of the literature. *Medicine*, 2002. **81**(1): pp. 51–68.
63. Zhao, R. et al., The spectrum of mutations in the PCFT gene, coding for an intestinal folate transporter, that are the basis for hereditary folate malabsorption. *Blood*, 2007. **110**(4): pp. 1147–1152.
64. Watkins, D. and D.S. Rosenblatt, Update and new concepts in vitamin responsive disorders of folate transport and metabolism. *Journal of Inherited Metabolic Disease*, 2011. **35**(4): 665–670.
65. Shin, D.S. et al., Identification of novel mutations in the proton-coupled folate transporter (PCFT-SLC46A1) associated with hereditary folate malabsorption. *Molecular Genetics and Metabolism*, 2011. **103**(1): pp. 33–37.
66. Meyer, E. et al., A novel PCFT gene mutation (p.Cys66LeufsX99) causing hereditary folate malabsorption. *Molecular Genetics and Metabolism*, 2010. **99**(3): pp. 325–328.
67. Min, S.H. et al., The clinical course and genetic defect in the PCFT gene in a 27-year-old woman with hereditary folate malabsorption. *Journal of Pediatrics*, 2008. **153**(3): pp. 435–437.

68. Atabay, B. et al., Mutation of the proton-coupled folate transporter gene (PCFT-SLC46A1) in Turkish siblings with hereditary folate malabsorption. *Pediatric Hematology and Oncology*, 2010. **27**(8): pp. 614–619.
69. Lasry, I. et al., A novel loss-of-function mutation in the proton-coupled folate transporter from a patient with hereditary folate malabsorption reveals that Arg 113 is crucial for function. *Blood*, 2008. **112**(5): pp. 2055–2061.
70. Shin, D.S. et al., Functional roles of aspartate residues of the proton-coupled folate transporter (PCFT-SLC46A1); a D156Y mutation causing hereditary folate malabsorption. *Blood*, 2010. **116**(24): pp. 5162–5169.
71. Borzutzky, A. et al., Reversible severe combined immunodeficiency phenotype secondary to a mutation of the proton-coupled folate transporter. *Journal of Allergy and Clinical Immunology*, 2009. **133**(3): pp. 287–294.
72. Mahadeo, K.M. et al., Prevalence of a loss-of-function mutation in the proton-coupled folate transporter gene (PCFT-SLC46A1) causing hereditary folate malabsorption in Puerto Rico. *Journal of Pediatrics*, 2011. **159**(4): pp. 623–627.e1.
73. Wang, L.D. et al., Genome-wide association study of esophageal squamous cell carcinoma in Chinese subjects identifies susceptibility loci at PLCE1 and C20orf54. *Nature Genetics*, 2010. **42**(9): pp. 759–763.
74. Yonezawa, A. et al., Identification and functional characterization of a novel human and rat riboflavin transporter, RFT1. *American Journal of Physiology. Cell Physiology*, 2008. **295**(3): pp. C632–C641.
75. Ho, G. et al., Maternal riboflavin deficiency, resulting in transient neonatal-onset glutaric aciduria type 2, is caused by a microdeletion in the riboflavin transporter gene GPR172B. *Human Mutation*, 2011. **32**(1): pp. E1976–E1984.
76. Yao, Y. et al., Identification and comparative functional characterization of a new human riboflavin transporter hRFT3 expressed in the brain. *Journal of Nutrition*, 2010. **140**(7): pp. 1220–1226.
77. Johnson, J.O. et al., Exome sequencing reveals riboflavin transporter mutations as a cause of motor neuron disease. *Brain*, 2012. **135**(Pt 9): pp. 2875–2882.
78. Green, P. et al., Brown-Vialetto-Van Laere syndrome, a ponto-bulbar palsy with deafness, is caused by mutations in C20orf54. *American Journal of Human Genetics*, 2010. **86**(3): pp. 485–489.
79. Bosch, A.M. et al., Brown-Vialetto-Van Laere and Fazio Londe syndrome is associated with a riboflavin transporter defect mimicking mild MADD: a new inborn error of metabolism with potential treatment. *Journal of Inherited Metabolic Disease*, 2011. **34**(1): pp. 159–164.
80. Moriyama, Y. Riboflavin transporter is finally identified. *Journal of Biochemistry*, 2011. **150**(4): pp. 341–343.
81. Yamamoto, S. et al., Identification and functional characterization of rat riboflavin transporter 2. *Journal of Biochemistry*, 2009. **145**(4): pp. 437–443.
82. Fujimura, M. et al., Functional characteristics of the human ortholog of riboflavin transporter 2 and riboflavin-responsive expression of its rat ortholog in the small intestine indicate its involvement in riboflavin absorption. *The Journal of Nutrition*, 2010. **140**(10): pp. 1722–1727.
83. http://omim.org/entry/201100.
84. Nabokina, S.M., V.S. Subramanian, and H.M. Said, Effect of clinical mutations on functionality of the human riboflavin transporter-2 (hRFT-2). *Molecular Genetics and Metabolism*, 2012. **105**(4): pp. 652–657.
85. Johnson, J.O. et al., Exome sequencing in Brown-Vialetto-Van Laere syndrome. *American Journal of Human Genetics*, 2010. **87**(4): pp. 567–569.
86. Koy, A. et al., Brown-Vialetto-Van Laere syndrome: a riboflavin-unresponsive patient with a novel mutation in the C20orf54 gene. *Pediatric Neurology*, 2012. **46**(6): pp. 407–409.

87. Wei, W. et al., Functional single nucleotide polymorphism in C20orf54 modifies susceptibility to esophageal squamous cell carcinoma. *Diseases of the Esophagus*, 2012. **26**(1): pp. 97–103.
88. Labay, V. et al., Mutations in SLC19A2 cause thiamine-responsive megaloblastic anaemia associated with diabetes mellitus and deafness. *Nature Genetics*, 1999. **22**(3): pp. 300–304.
89. Dutta, B. et al., Cloning of the human thiamine transporter, a member of the folate transporter family. *Journal of Biological Chemistry*, 1999. **274**(45): pp. 31925–31929.
90. Fleming, J.C. et al., The gene mutated in thiamine-responsive anaemia with diabetes and deafness (TRMA) encodes a functional thiamine transporter. *Nature Genetics*, 1999. **22**(3): pp. 305–308.
91. Oishi, K. et al., Targeted disruption of Slc19a2, the gene encoding the high-affinity thiamin transporter Thtr-1, causes diabetes mellitus, sensorineural deafness and megaloblastosis in mice. *Human Molecular Genetics*, 2002. **11**(23): pp. 2951–2960.
92. Reidling, J.C. et al., Impaired intestinal vitamin B-1 (Thiamin) uptake in thiamin transporter-2-deficient mice. *Gastroenterology*, 2010. **138**(5): pp. 1802–1809.
93. Liberman, M.C. et al., Deletion of SLC19A2, the high affinity thiamine transporter, causes selective inner hair cell loss and an auditory neuropathy phenotype. *Journal of the Association for Research in Otolaryngology: JARO*, 2006. **7**(3): pp. 211–217.
94. Bergmann, A.K. et al., Thiamine-responsive megaloblastic anemia: identification of novel compound heterozygotes and mutation update. *Journal of Pediatrics*, 2009. **155**(6): pp. 888–892.e1.
95. Raz, T. et al., The spectrum of mutations, including four novel ones, in the thiamine-responsive megaloblastic anemia gene SLC19A2 of eight families. *Human Mutation*, 2000. **16**(1): pp. 37–42.
96. Olsen, B.S. et al., Thiamine-responsive megaloblastic anaemia: a cause of syndromic diabetes in childhood. *Pediatric Diabetes*, 2007. **8**(4): pp. 239–241.
97. Lagarde, W.H. et al., Novel mutation in the SLC19A2 gene in an African-American female with thiamine-responsive megaloblastic anemia syndrome. *American Journal of Medical Genetics Part A*, 2004. **125A**(3): pp. 299–305.
98. Bay, A. et al., Thiamine-responsive megaloblastic anemia syndrome. *International Journal of Hematology*, 2010. **92**(3): pp. 524–526.
99. Diaz, G.A. et al., Mutations in a new gene encoding a thiamine transporter cause thiamine- responsive megaloblastic anaemia syndrome. *Nature Genetics*, 1999. **22**(3): pp. 309–312.
100. Habeb, A.M. et al., Incidence, genetics, and clinical phenotype of permanent neonatal diabetes mellitus in northwest Saudi Arabia. *Pediatric Diabetes*, 2011. **13**(6): pp. 499–505.
101. Ricketts, C.J. et al., Thiamine-responsive megaloblastic anaemia syndrome: long-term follow-up and mutation analysis of seven families. *Acta Paediatrica, International Journal of Paediatrics*, 2006. **95**(1): pp. 99–104.
102. Pichler, H. et al., Thiamine-responsive megaloblastic anemia (TRMA) in an Austrian boy with compound heterozygous SLC19A2 mutations. *European Journal of Pediatrics*, 2012. **171**(11): pp. 1711–1715.
103. Yesilkaya, E. et al., A novel mutation in the SLC19A2 gene in a Turkish female with thiamine-responsive megaloblastic anemia syndrome. *Journal of Tropical Pediatrics*, 2009. **55**(4): pp. 265–267.
104. Ozdemir, M.A. et al., TRMA syndrome (thiamine-responsive megaloblastic anemia): a case report and review of the literature. *Pediatric Diabetes*, 2002. **3**(4): pp. 205–209.
105. Mathews, L., K. Narayanadas, and G. Sunil, Thiamine responsive megaloblastic anemia. *Indian Pediatrics*, 2009. **46**(2): pp. 172–174.

106. Scharfe, C. et al., A novel mutation in the thiamine responsive megaloblastic anaemia gene SLC19A2 in a patient with deficiency of respiratory chain complex I. *Journal of Medical Genetics*, 2000. **37**(9): pp. 669–673.
107. Kurtoglu, S. et al., Thiamine withdrawal can lead to diabetic ketoacidosis in thiamine responsive megaloblastic anemia: report of two siblings. *Journal of Pediatric Endocrinology and Metabolism*, 2008. **21**(4): pp. 393–397.
108. Aycan, Z. et al., Thiamine-responsive megaloblastic anemia syndrome with atrial standstill: a case report. *Journal of Pediatric Hematology Oncology*, 2011. **33**(2): pp. 144–147.
109. Rajgopal, A. et al., SLC19A3 encodes a second thiamine transporter ThTr2. *Biochimica et Biophysica Acta*, 2001. **1537**(3): pp. 175–178.
110. Yamada, K. et al., A wide spectrum of clinical and brain MRI findings in patients with SLC19A3 mutations. *BMC Medical Genetics*, 2010. **11**(1): p. 171.
111. Zeng, W.-Q. et al., Biotin-responsive basal ganglia disease maps to 2q36.3 and is due to mutations in SLC19A3. *The American Journal of Human Genetics*, 2005. **77**(1): pp. 16–26.
112. Subramanian, V.S., J.S. Marchant, and H.M. Said, Biotin-responsive basal ganglia disease-linked mutations inhibit thiamine transport via hTHTR2: biotin is not a substrate for hTHTR2. *American Journal of Physiology. Cell Physiology*, 2006. **291**(5): pp. C851–C859.
113. Debs, R. et al., Biotin-responsive basal ganglia disease in ethnic Europeans with novel SLC19A3 mutations. *Archives of Neurology*, 2010. **67**(1): pp. 126–130.
114. Kono, S. et al., Mutations in a thiamine-transporter gene and Wernicke's-like encephalopathy. *New England Journal of Medicine*, 2009. **360**(17): pp. 1792–1794.
115. Paroder-Belenitsky, M. et al., Mechanism of anion selectivity and stoichiometry of the Na+/I- symporter (NIS). *Proceedings of the National Academy of Sciences of the United States of America*, 2011. **108**(44): pp. 17933–17938.
116. Leung, A. E.N. Pearce, and L.E. Braverman, Role of iodine in thyroid physiology. *Expert Review of Endocrinology and Metabolism*, 2010. **5**(4): pp. 593–602.
117. Smanik, P.A. et al., Expression, exon-intron organization, and chromosome mapping of the human sodium iodide symporter. *Endocrinology*, 1997. **138**(8): pp. 3555–3558.
118. Spitzweg, C. and J.C. Morris, Genetics and phenomics of hypothyroidism and goiter due to NIS mutations. *Molecular and Cellular Endocrinology*, 2010. **322**(1–2): pp. 56–63.
119. Bizhanova, A. and P. Kopp, Genetics and phenomics of Pendred syndrome. *Molecular and Cellular Endocrinology*, 2010. **322**(1–2): pp. 83–90.
120. Everett, L.A. et al., Pendred syndrome is caused by mutations in a putative sulphate transporter gene (PDS). *Nature Genetics*, 1997. **17**(4): pp. 411–422.
121. Dror, A.A. et al., Calcium oxalate stone formation in the inner ear as a result of an Slc26a4 mutation. *Journal of Biological Chemistry*, 2010. **285**(28): pp. 21724–21735.
122. www.healthcare.uiowa.edu/labs/pendredandbor/slcMutations.htm.
123. Kopp, P. L. Pesce, and J.C. Solis-S, Pendred syndrome and iodide transport in the thyroid. *Trends in Endocrinology and Metabolism*, 2008. **19**(7): pp. 260–268.
124. Courville, P. R. Chaloupka, and M.F.M. Cellier, Recent progress in structure–function analyses of Nramp proton-dependent metal-ion transporters. *Biochemistry and Cell Biology*, 2006. **84**(6): pp. 960–978.
125. Gunshin, H. et al., Slc11a2 is required for intestinal iron absorption and erythropoiesis but dispensable in placenta and liver. *Journal of Clinical Investigation*, 2005. **115**(5): pp. 1258–1266.
126. Neves, J.V. et al., Natural history of SLC11 genes in vertebrates: tales from the fish world. *BMC Evolutionary Biology*, 2011. **11**: p. 106.
127. Blackwell, J.M. et al., Genomic organization and sequence of the human NRAMP gene: identification and mapping of a promoter region polymorphism. *Molecular Medicine*, 1995. **1**(2): pp. 194–205.

128. Soe-Lin, S. et al., Nramp1 promotes efficient macrophage recycling of iron following erythrophagocytosis in vivo. *Proceedings of the National Academy of Sciences of the United States of America*, 2009. **106**(14): pp. 5960–5965.
129. Wicker, L.S. et al., Fine mapping, gene content, comparative sequencing, and expression analyses support Ctla4 and Nramp1 as candidates for Idd5.1 and Idd5.2 in the nonobese diabetic mouse. *The Journal of Immunology*, 2004. **173**(1): pp. 164–173.
130. Li, X.W. et al., SLC11A1 (NRAMP1) polymorphisms and tuberculosis susceptibility: updated systematic review and meta-analysis. *PLoS One*, 2011. **6**(1): p. e15831.
131. Meilang, Q. et al., Polymorphisms in the SLC11A1 gene and tuberculosis risk: a meta-analysis update [Review article]. *The International Journal of Tuberculosis and Lung Disease*, 2012. **16**(4): pp. 437–446.
132. O'Brien, B.A. et al., Association of SLC11A1 promoter polymorphisms with the incidence of autoimmune and inflammatory diseases: a meta-analysis. *Journal of Autoimmunity*, 2008. **31**(1): pp. 42–51.
133. Akcakaya, P. et al., The functional SLC11A1 gene polymorphisms are associated with sarcoidosis in Turkish population. *Molecular Biology Reports*, 2012. **39**(4): pp. 5009–5016.
134. Yang, J.H.M. et al., Evidence of association with type 1 diabetes in the SLC11A1 gene region. *BMC Medical Genetics*, 2011. **12**: p. 59.
135. Pedroza, L.S.R.A. et al., Systemic lupus erythematosus: association with KIR and SLC11A1 polymorphisms, ethnic predisposition and influence in clinical manifestations at onset revealed by ancestry genetic markers in an urban Brazilian population. *Lupus*, 2011. **20**(3): pp. 265–273.
136. Stewart, L.C. et al., SLC11A1 polymorphisms in inflammatory bowel disease and *Mycobacterium avium* subspecies paratuberculosis status. *World Journal of Gastroenterology*, 2010. **16**(45): pp. 5727–5731.
137. Gazouli, M. et al., Role of functional polymorphisms of NRAMP1 gene for the development of Crohn's disease. *Inflammatory Bowel Diseases*, 2008. **14**(10): pp. 1323–1330.
138. Hubert, N. and M.W. Hentze, Previously uncharacterized isoforms of divalent metal transporter (DMT)-1: implications for regulation and cellular function. *Proceedings of the National Academy of Sciences of the United States of America*, 2002. **99**(19): pp. 12345–12350.
139. Ludwiczek, S. et al., Ca^{2+} channel blockers reverse iron overload by a new mechanism via divalent metal transporter-1. *Nature Medicine*, 2007. **13**(4): pp. 448–454.
140. Fleming, R.E. et al., Mechanism of increased iron absorption in murine model of hereditary hemochromatosis: increased duodenal expression of the iron transporter DMT1. *Proceedings of the National Academy of Sciences of the United States of America*, 1999. **96**(6): pp. 3143–3148.
141. Iolascon, A. and L. De Falco, Mutations in the gene encoding DMT1: clinical presentation and treatment. *Seminars in Hematology*, 2009. **46**(4): pp. 358–370.
142. Iolascon, A. et al., Microcytic anemia and hepatic iron overload in a child with compound heterozygous mutations in DMT1 (SCL11A2). *Blood*, 2006. **107**(1): pp. 349–354.
143. Mims, M.P. et al., Identification of a human mutation of DMT1 in a patient with microcytic anemia and iron overload. *Blood*, 2005. **105**(3): pp. 1337–1342.
144. Beaumont, C. et al., Two new human DMT1 gene mutations in a patient with microcytic anemia, low ferritinemia, and liver iron overload. *Blood*, 2006. **107**(10): pp. 4168–4170.
145. Blanco, E. et al., Not all DMT1 mutations lead to iron overload. *Blood Cells, Molecules, and Diseases*, 2009. **43**(2): pp. 199–201.
146. Barrios, M. et al., The homozygous mutation G75R in the human SLC11A2 gene leads to microcytic anaemia and iron overload. *British Journal of Haematology*, 2012. **157**(4): pp. 514–516.

147. Bardou-Jacquet, E. et al., A novel N491S mutation in the human SLC11A2 gene impairs protein trafficking and in association with the G212V mutation leads to microcytic anemia and liver iron overload. *Blood Cells Molecules and Diseases*, 2011. **47**(4): pp. 243–248.
148. Lam-Yuk-Tseung, S. V. Picard, and P. Gros, Identification of a tyrosine-based motif (YGSI) in the amino terminus of Nramp1 (Slc11a1) that is important for lysosomal targeting. *Journal of Biological Chemistry*, 2006. **281**(42): pp. 31677–31688.
149. Donovan, A. et al., The iron exporter ferroportin/Slc40a1 is essential for iron homeostasis. *Cell Metabolism*, 2005. **1**(3): pp. 191–200.
150. Zohn, I.E. et al., The flatiron mutation in mouse ferroportin acts as a dominant negative to cause ferroportin disease. *Blood*, 2007. **109**(10): pp. 4174–4180.
151. Schimanski, L.M. et al., In vitro functional analysis of human ferroportin (FPN) and hemochromatosis-associated FPN mutations. *Blood*, 2005. **105**(10): pp. 4096–4102.
152. Mayr, R. et al., Ferroportin disease: a systematic meta-analysis of clinical and molecular findings. *Journal of Hepatology*, 2010. **53**: pp. 941–949.
153. Stathopoulou, M.G. et al., Mineral intake. *Progress in Molecular Biology and Translational Science*, 2012. **108**, pp. 201–236.
154. Peters, J.L. et al., Targeting of the mouse Slc39a2 (Zip2) gene reveals highly cell-specific patterns of expression, and unique functions in zinc, iron, and calcium homeostasis. *Genesis*, 2007. **45**(6): pp. 339–352.
155. Palmiter, R.D. and S.D. Findley, Cloning and functional characterization of a mammalian zinc transporter that confers resistance to zinc. *The EMBO Journal*, 1995. **14**(4): pp. 639–649.
156. Wang, X. and B. Zhou, Dietary zinc absorption: a play of Zips and ZnTs in the gut. *IUBMB Life*, 2010. **62**(3): pp. 176–182.
157. Andrews, G.K. et al., Mouse zinc transporter 1 gene provides an essential function during early embryonic development. *Genesis*, 2004. **40**(2): pp. 74–81.
158. Lazarczyk, M. et al., Regulation of cellular zinc balance as a potential mechanism of EVER-mediated protection against pathogenesis by cutaneous oncogenic human papillomaviruses. *Journal of Experimental Medicine*, 2008. **205**(1): pp. 35–42.
159. Lopez, V. and S.L. Kelleher, Zinc transporter-2 (ZnT2) variants are localized to distinct subcellular compartments and functionally transport zinc. *Biochemical Journal*, 2009. **422**(1): pp. 43–52.
160. Seo, Y.A. and S.L. Kelleher, Functional analysis of two single nucleotide polymorphisms in SLC30A2 (ZnT2): implications for mammary gland function and breast disease in women. *Physiological Genomics*, 2010. **42A**(4): pp. 219–227.
161. Chowanadisai, W. B. Lonnerdal, and S.L. Kelleher, Identification of a mutation in SLC30A2 (ZnT-2) in women with low milk zinc concentration that results in transient neonatal zinc deficiency. *Journal of Biological Chemistry*, 2006. **281**(51): pp. 39699–39707.
162. Qian, L. et al., Polymorphisms of SLC30A2 and selected perinatal factors associated with low milk zinc in Chinese breastfeeding women. *Early Human Development*, 2012. **88**(8): pp. 663–668.
163. Smidt, K. and J. Rungby, ZnT3: a zinc transporter active in several organs. *Biometals: An International Journal on the Role of Metal Ions in Biology, Biochemistry, and Medicine*, 2012. **25**(1): pp. 1–8.
164. Adlard, P.A. et al., Cognitive loss in zinc transporter-3 knock-out mice: a phenocopy for the synaptic and memory deficits of Alzheimer's disease? *Journal of Neuroscience*, 2010. **30**(5): pp. 1631–1636.
165. Martel, G. et al., Zinc transporter 3 is involved in learned fear and extinction, but not in innate fear. *Learning and Memory*, 2010. **17**(11): pp. 582–590.
166. http://www.ncbi.nlm.nih.gov/projects/SNP/.

167. Salazar, G. et al., SLC30A3 (ZnT3) oligomerization by dityrosine bonds regulates its subcellular localization and metal transport capacity. *PLoS One*, 2009. **4**(6): p. e5896.
168. Seve, M. et al., In silico identification and expression of SLC30 family genes: an expressed sequence tag data mining strategy for the characterization of zinc transporters' tissue expression. *BMC Genomics*, 2004. **5**(1): p. 32.
169. Hardy, A.B. et al., Effects of high-fat diet feeding on Znt8-null mice: differences between β-cell and global knockout of Znt8. *American Journal of Physiology. Endocrinology and Metabolism*, 2012. **302**(9): pp. E1084–E1096.
170. Lemaire, K. et al., Insulin crystallization depends on zinc transporter ZnT8 expression, but is not required for normal glucose homeostasis in mice. *Proceedings of the National Academy of Sciences of the United States of America*, 2009. **106**(35): pp. 14872–14877.
171. Nicolson, T.J. et al., Insulin storage and glucose homeostasis in mice null for the granule zinc transporter ZnT8 and studies of the type 2 diabetes–associated variants. *Diabetes*, 2009. **58**(9): pp. 2070–2083.
172. Sladek, R. et al., A genome-wide association study identifies novel risk loci for type 2 diabetes. *Nature*, 2007. **445**(7130): pp. 881–885.
173. Saxena, R. et al., Genome-wide association analysis identifies loci for type 2 diabetes and triglyceride levels. *Science*, 2007. **316**(5829): pp. 1331–1336.
174. Zeggini, E. et al., Replication of genome-wide association signals in UK samples reveals risk loci for type 2 diabetes. *Science*, 2007. **316**(5829): pp. 1336–1341.
175. Scott, L.J. et al., A genome-wide association study of type 2 diabetes in Finns detects multiple susceptibility variants. *Science*, 2007. **316**(5829): pp. 1341–1345.
176. Steinthorsdottir, V. et al., A variant in CDKAL1 influences insulin response and risk of type 2 diabetes. *Nature Genetics*, 2007. **39**(6): pp. 770–775.
177. Cauchi, S. et al., The genetic susceptibility to type 2 diabetes may be modulated by obesity status: implications for association studies. *BMC Medical Genetics*, 2008. **9**: p. 45.
178. Wu, Y. et al., Common variants in CDKAL1, CDKN2A/B, IGF2BP2, SLC30A8, and HHEX/IDE genes are associated with type 2 diabetes and impaired fasting glucose in a Chinese Han population. *Diabetes*, 2008. **57**(10): pp. 2834–2842.
179. Mtiraoui, N. et al., Contribution of common variants of ENPP1, IGF2BP2, KCNJ11, MLXIPL, PPARγ, SLC30A8 and TCF7L2 to the risk of type 2 diabetes in Lebanese and Tunisian Arabs. *Diabetes and Metabolism*, 2012. **38**(5): pp. 444–449.
180. Jing, Y.L. et al., SLC30A8 polymorphism and type 2 diabetes risk: evidence from 27 study groups. *Nutrition, Metabolism and Cardiovascular Diseases*, 2011. **21**(6): pp. 398–405.
181. Xu, K. et al., Association between rs13266634 C/T polymorphisms of solute carrier family 30 member 8 (SLC30A8) and type 2 diabetes, impaired glucose tolerance, type 1 diabetes—A meta-analysis. *Diabetes Research and Clinical Practice*, 2011. **91**(2): pp. 195–202.
182. Cauchi, S. et al., Meta-analysis and functional effects of the SLC30A8 rs13266634 polymorphism on isolated human pancreatic islets. *Molecular Genetics and Metabolism*, 2010. **100**(1): pp. 77–82.
183. Tuschl, K. et al., Syndrome of hepatic cirrhosis, dystonia, polycythemia, and hypermanganesemia caused by mutations in SLC30A10, a manganese transporter in man. *American Journal of Human Genetics*, 2012. **90**(3): pp. 457–466.
184. Law, N.A. M.T. Caudle, and V.L. Pecoraro, Manganese redox enzymes and model systems: properties, structures, and reactivity. *Advances in Inorganic Chemistry*, 1999. **46**: pp. 305–440.
185. Quadri, M. et al., Mutations in SLC30A10 cause parkinsonism and dystonia with hypermanganesemia, polycythemia, and chronic liver disease. *American Journal of Human Genetics*, 2012. **90**(3): pp. 467–477.

186. Gaither, L.A. and D.J. Eide, Functional expression of the human hZIP2 zinc transporter. *Journal of Biological Chemistry*, 2000. **275**(8): pp. 5560–5564.
187. Giacconi, R. et al., A novel Zip2 Gln/Arg/Leu codon 2 polymorphism is associated with carotid artery disease in aging. *Rejuvenation Research*, 2008. **11**(2): pp. 297–300.
188. Karagas, M.R. et al., SLC39A2 and FSIP1 polymorphisms as potential modifiers of arsenic-related bladder cancer. *Human Genetics*, 2012. **131**(3): pp. 453–461.
189. Wang, F. et al., Zinc-stimulated endocytosis controls activity of the mouse ZIP1 and ZIP3 zinc uptake transporters. *Journal of Biological Chemistry*, 2004. **279**(23): pp. 24631–24639.
190. Dufner-Beattie, J. et al., Structure, function, and regulation of a subfamily of mouse zinc transporter genes. *Journal of Biological Chemistry*, 2003. **278**(50): pp. 50142–50150.
191. Dufner-Beattie, J. et al., Mouse ZIP1 and ZIP3 genes together are essential for adaptation to dietary zinc deficiency during pregnancy. *Genesis*, 2006. **44**(5): pp. 239–251.
192. Kambe, T. et al., Slc39a1 to 3 (subfamily II) Zip genes in mice have unique cell-specific functions during adaptation to zinc deficiency. *American Journal of Physiology. Regulatory, Integrative and Comparative Physiology*, 2008. **294**(5): pp. R1474–R1481.
193. Baum, A.E. et al., Meta-analysis of two genome-wide association studies of bipolar disorder reveals important points of agreement. *Molecular Psychiatry*, 2008. **13**(5): pp. 466–467.
194. Ollila, H.M. et al., Findings from bipolar disorder genome-wide association studies replicate in a Finnish bipolar family-cohort. *Molecular Psychiatry*, 2009. **14**(4): pp. 351–353.
195. Wang, K. et al., A novel member of a zinc transporter family is defective in acrodermatitis enteropathica. *The American Journal of Human Genetics*, 2002. **71**(1): pp. 66–73.
196. Kury, S. et al., Identification of SLC39A4, a gene involved in acrodermatitis enteropathica. *Nature Genetics*, 2002. **31**(3): pp. 239–240.
197. Antala, S. and R.E. Dempski, The human ZIP4 transporter has two distinct binding affinities and mediates transport of multiple transition metals. *Biochemistry*, 2012. **51**(5): pp. 963–973.
198. Schmitt, S. et al., An update on mutations of the SLC39A4 gene in acrodermatitis enteropathica. *Human Mutation*, 2009. **30**(6): pp. 926–933.
199. Dufner-Beattie, J. et al., The mouse acrodermatitis enteropathica gene Slc39a4 (Zip4) is essential for early development and heterozygosity causes hypersensitivity to zinc deficiency. *Human Molecular Genetics*, 2007. **16**(12): pp. 1391–1399.
200. Yuzbasiyan-Gurkan, V. and E. Bartlett, Identification of a unique splice site variant in SLC39A4 in bovine hereditary zinc deficiency, lethal trait A46: an animal model of acrodermatitis enteropathica. *Genomics*, 2006. **88**(4): pp. 521–526.
201. Santiago, F. et al., Acrodermatitis enteropathica: a novel SLC39A4 gene mutation found in a patient with an early-onset. *Pediatric Dermatology*, 2011. **28**(6): pp. 735–736.
202. Küry, S. et al., Mutation spectrum of human SLC39A4 in a panel of patients with acrodermatitis enteropathica. *Human Mutation*, 2003. **22**(4): pp. 337–338.
203. Kharfi, M. et al., Acrodermatite entéropathique chez un nourrisson né à terme nourri exclusivement au sein. *Annales de Dermatologie et de Vénéréologie*, 2005. **132**(3): pp. 246–248.
204. Nakano, A. et al., Novel SLC39A4 mutations in acrodermatitis enteropathica. *Journal of Investigative Dermatology*, 2003. **120**(6): pp. 963–966.
205. Park, C.-H. et al., Congenital zinc deficiency from mutations of the SLC39A4 gene as the genetic background of acrodermatitis enteropathica. *Journal of Korean Medical Science*, 2010. **25**(12): pp. 1818–1820.
206. Wang, K. et al., A novel member of a zinc transporter family is defective in acrodermatitis enteropathica. *American Journal of Human Genetics*, 2002. **71**(1): pp. 66–73.

207. Meftah, S.P. et al., A new mutation in exon 3 of the SCL39A4 gene in a Tunisian family with severe acrodermatitis enteropathica. *Nutrition*, 2006. **22**(10): pp. 1067–1070.
208. Schmitt, S. et al., An update on mutations of the SLC39A4 gene in acrodermatitis enteropathica. *Human Mutation*, 2009. **30**(6): pp. 926–933.
209. Coromilas, A. et al., Novel SLC39A4 mutation in acrodermatitis enteropathica. *Pediatric Dermatology*, 2011. **28**(6): pp. 697–700.
210. Li, C.-R. et al., One novel homozygous mutation of SLC39A4 gene in a Chinese patient with acrodermatitis enteropathica. *Archives of Dermatological Research*, 2010. **302**(4): pp. 315–317.
211. Vardi, A. et al., A new genetic isolate of acrodermatitis enteropathica with a novel mutation. *British Journal of Dermatology*, 2009. **160**(6): pp. 1346–1348.
212. Nakano, H. et al., Novel and recurrent nonsense mutation of the SLC39A4 gene in Japanese patients with acrodermatitis enteropathica. *British Journal of Dermatology*, 2009. **161**(1): pp. 184–186.
213. Wang, S. et al., A novel SLC39A4 gene mutation in the family of an acrodermatitis enteropathica patient with an unusual presentation. *British Journal of Dermatology*, 2008. **159**(4): pp. 976–978.
214. Kilic, S.S. et al., A novel mutation of the SLC39A4 gene causing acrodermatitis enteropathica. *British Journal of Dermatology*, 2007. **157**(2): pp. 386–387.
215. Wang, F. et al., Acrodermatitis enteropathica mutations affect transport activity, localization and zinc-responsive trafficking of the mouse ZIP4 zinc transporter. *Human Molecular Genetics*, 2004. **13**(5): pp. 563–571.

3 Genetic Variants in the Omega-6 and Omega-3 Fatty Acid Metabolic Pathways

Their Role in the Determination of Nutritional Requirements and Chronic Disease Risk

Artemis P. Simopoulos

CONTENTS

INTRODUCTION

A fundamental aspect of the genetic approach to disease is an appreciation of human variation: its nature and extent, origin and maintenance, distribution in families and populations, interactions with environment, especially diet and exercise, and consequences for normal development and homeostasis [1–3]. Some of the earliest studies of human biochemical genetics showed considerable variability within and between populations, which is highly relevant for nutrition [3]. Variation in nutritional requirements and interaction of certain nutrients with genetically determined biochemical and metabolic factors suggest different requirements for individuals [4,5]. This variation (such as sex differences) is inborn and needs to be differentiated from variations caused by the life cycle (growth, pregnancy, and old age). Research is defining the mechanisms by which genes influence nutrient absorption, metabolism and excretion, taste perception, and degree of satiation and the mechanisms by which nutrients influence gene expression [6]. Genetic variation and gene–nutrient interactions are also important in drug metabolism and adverse reactions to drugs.

During the past few years, genome-wide association studies (GWASs) have revealed genomic variants (alleles) predisposing to diabetes [7], prostate cancer [8], lupus [9], age-related macular degeneration [10], Crohn's disease [11], and other diseases. For coronary heart disease (CHD), a major locus has been identified on chromosome 9p21 [12]. The locus is heterozygous in 50% of Caucasians with an increased risk of 15%–20% and homozygous in 25% of Caucasians with an increased risk of 30%–40%. This variation has been confirmed in Icelandic, British, German, and Central European populations for 60,000 Caucasians and in Korean, Japanese, Chinese, and East Asians. Preliminary evidence suggests 9p21 is not a risk factor for African-Americans. The 9p21 variant is a novel risk factor for CHD and cerebral vascular disease, independent of known risk factors such as diabetes, hypertension, cholesterol, and obesity. This information implies a new mechanism for CHD with respect to vascular pathology, perhaps separate from the lipid hypothesis [13].

The interaction of genetics and environment, nature and nurture, is the foundation for all health and disease [3,14,15]. Genes define susceptibility to a disease or condition, and environmental factors such as diet and exercise determine who among the susceptibles will develop the disease or condition (Figure 3.1).

Nutrition is an environmental factor of major importance. Methodological advances in molecular biology and genetics have facilitated the study of inherited

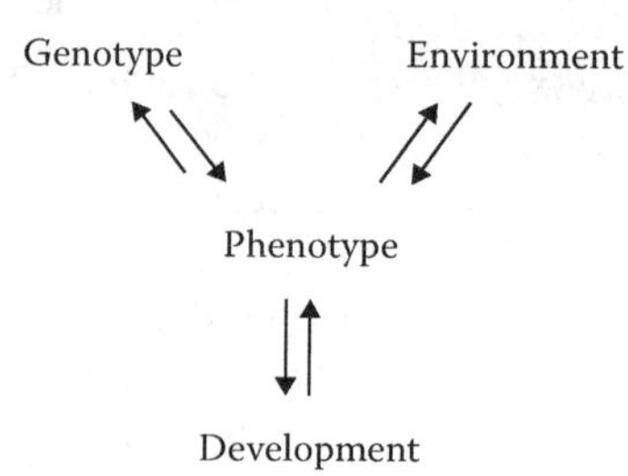

FIGURE 3.1 Relationships between genes, environment, and development are dynamic. (From Childs, B., *Genetic Variation and Nutrition*, World Rev Nutr Diet, Basel, Karger, 63, 14–24, 1990.)

disease at the DNA level and of nutrients at the molecular level. This research has led to (1) the development of concepts and research on genetic variation and dietary response, known as nutrigenetics (e.g., individuals responding differently to the same diet by attaining different levels of serum cholesterol and blood pressure because of genetic variation) and (2) the studies on the evolutionary aspects of diet and the role of nutrients in gene expression, known as nutrigenomics (e.g., polyunsaturated fatty acids [PUFAs] suppress fatty acid synthase [mRNA] gene expression). The term nutrigenetics was introduced by Brennan in 1977 in *Nutrigenetics: New Concepts for Relieving Hypoglycemia* [16]. Nutrigenetics/nutrigenomics could provide a framework for development of genotype-dependent novel foods for health promotion and for prevention and management of chronic diseases. National general dietary guidelines have been issued for the prevention of chronic diseases without considering the effects of genetic variation on dietary responses, despite such evidence [4,5].

Heritability is the proportion of the total variance that can be explained by genes and gene–environment interactions [17]. For example, 50% of the variance in plasma cholesterol concentration is genetically determined [18,19]; 30%–60% for blood pressure [20]; 15% in the United Kingdom [21] to 50% in Sweden [22] for fibrinogen, an independent risk factor for CHD; and 75% in Australia for bone density [23]. Calculations of heritability are tied to the specific population and environment studied and vary if populations differ in the prevalence of the relevant genetic alleles. Population subgroups may need to have specific dietary recommendations for the prevention of CHD or certain cancers or other diseases. CHD, high blood pressure, diabetes, cancers, and other chronic diseases tend to aggregate in families; risk among relatives is higher than in the general population [24]. Families share both genes and environment; similarity may result from either. In families with CHD onset before age 46, heritability was estimated to be 92%–100%; within families with older index cases, the heritability ranges from 15% to 30%.

On the basis of estimates from studies in paleolithic nutrition and modern-day, hunter-gatherer populations, humans evolved on a diet that was much lower in saturated fatty acids than is today's diet. Furthermore, the diet contained small but roughly equal amounts of omega-6 and omega-3 PUFAs (Figure 3.2) [25–27].

Humans and animals can convert linoleic acid (LA) to arachidonic acid (AA) and α-linolenic acid (α-LNA) to eicosapentaenoic acid (EPA) and docosahexaenoic acid (DHA) [28] (Figure 3.3). This conversion was shown by using deuterated LNA [29]. There is competition between omega-3 and omega-6 fatty acids for the desaturation enzymes fatty acid desaturase 1 (*FADS1*) and fatty acid desaturase 2 (*FADS2*). However, both Delta-5 and Delta-6 desaturases prefer omega-3 to omega-6 fatty acids [28,30,31]. There is some evidence that Delta-6 desaturase decreases with age [28]. Premature infants [32], hypertensive individuals [33], and some diabetics [34] are limited in their ability to make EPA and DHA from LNA. These findings are important and need to be considered when making dietary recommendations. EPA and DHA are found in the oils of fish, particularly fatty fish (Table 3.1) [35]. AA is found predominantly in the phospholipids of grain-fed animals.

LA, LNA, and their long-chain derivatives are important components of animal and plant cell membranes. In mammals and birds, the omega-3 fatty acids are distributed selectively among lipid classes. LNA is found in triglycerides, in cholesteryl

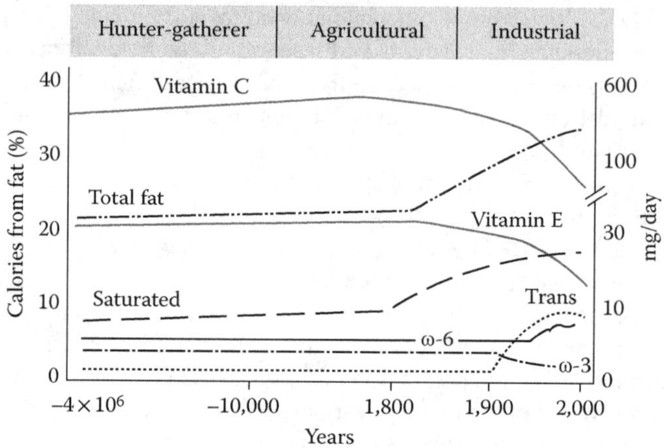

FIGURE 3.2 Hypothetical scheme of fat, fatty acid (ω-6, ω-3, trans, and total) intake (as percent of calories from fat) and intake of vitamins E and C (mg/day). (From Simopoulos, A.P., *Antioxidant Status, Diet, Nutrition and Health*, CRC Press, Boca Raton, 65–88, 1999.)

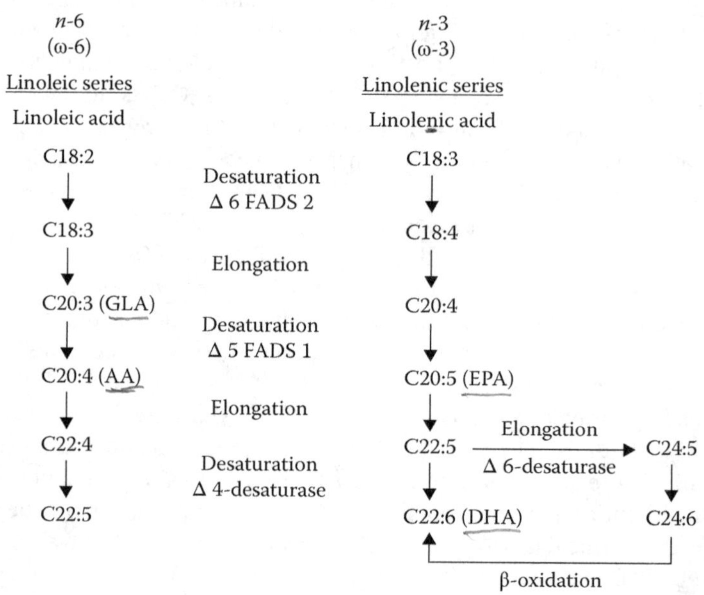

FIGURE 3.3 Desaturation and elongation of omega-3 and omega-6 fatty acids. The enzymes Delta-6 and Delta-5 desaturases are encoded by *FADS2* and *FADS1*, respectively.

esters, and in very small amounts in phospholipids. EPA is found in cholesteryl esters, triglycerides, and phospholipids. DHA is found mostly in phospholipids. In mammals, including humans, the cerebral cortex [36], retina [37], and testis and sperm [38] are particularly rich in DHA. DHA is one of the most abundant components of the brain's structural lipids. DHA, like EPA, can be derived only from direct ingestion or by synthesis from dietary EPA or LNA.

TABLE 3.1
Content of ω-3 Fatty Acids and Other Fat Components in Selected Fish[a]

			Fatty Acids					
Fish	**Total Fat**	**Total Saturated**	**Total Monounsaturated g/100 g**	**Total Polyunsaturated g/100 g**	**18:3**	**20:5**	**22:6**	**Cholesterol mg/100 g**
Anchovy, European	2.3	0.5	0.7	0.8	Tr	0.2	0.6	80
Bass, striped	6.5	1.4	2.9	1.6	—	0.4	0.8	59
Bluefish	5.6	1.1	2.3	1.4	0.3	0.2	0.1	67
Carp	2.7	0.6	1.0	0.8	0.1	0.2	0.2	75
Catfish, brown bullhead	4.3	1.0	1.6	1.0	Tr	0.1	0.2	58
Catfish, channel	0.7	0.1	0.1	0.3	Tr	0.1	0.2	43
Cod, Atlantic	3.2	1.1	1.2	0.5	Tr	0.1	0.1	61
Flounder, unspecified	1.0	0.2	0.3	0.3	Tr	0.1	0.1	46
Grouper, red	0.8	0.2	0.1	0.2	—	Tr	0.2	—
Haddock	0.7	0.1	0.1	0.2	Tr	0.1	0.1	63
Halibut, Greenland	13.8	2.4	8.4	1.4	Tr	0.5	0.4	46
Halibut, Pacific	2.3	0.3	0.8	0.7	0.1	0.1	0.3	32
Herring, Pacific	13.9	3.3	6.9	2.4	0.1	1.0	0.7	77
Herring, round	4.4	1.3	0.8	1.5	0.1	0.4	0.8	28
Mackerel, king	13.0	2.5	5.9	3.2	—	1.0	1.2	53
Mullet, striped	3.7	1.2	1.1	1.1	0.1	0.3	0.2	49
Ocean perch	1.6	0.3	0.6	0.5	Tr	0.1	0.1	42
Plaice, European	1.5	0.3	0.5	0.4	Tr	0.1	0.1	70
Pollock	1.0	0.1	0.1	0.5	—	0.1	0.4	71
Pompano, Florida	9.5	3.5	2.6	1.1	—	0.2	0.4	50

(Continued)

TABLE 3.1 (*Continued*)
Content of ω-3 Fatty Acids and Other Fat Components in Selected Fish[a]

	Fatty Acids							
Fish	Total Fat	Total Saturated	Total Monounsaturated g/100 g	Total Polyunsaturated g/100 g	18:3	20:5	22:6	Cholesterol mg/100 g
Salmon, Chinook	10.4	2.5	4.5	2.1	0.1	0.8	0.6	—
Salmon, pink	3.4	0.6	0.9	1.4	Tr	0.4	0.6	—
Snapper, red	1.2	0.2	0.2	0.4	Tr	Tr	0.2	—
Sole, European	1.2	0.3	0.4	0.2	Tr	Tr	0.1	50
Swordfish	2.1	0.6	0.8	0.2	—	Tr	0.1	39
Trout, rainbow	3.4	0.6	1.0	1.2	0.1	0.1	0.4	57
Tuna, albacore	4.9	1.2	1.2	1.8	0.2	0.1	1.0	54
Tuna, unspecified	2.5	0.9	0.6	0.5	—	0.1	0.4	—

Source: Adapted from the United States Department of Agriculture Provisional Table on the Content of Omega-3 Fatty Acids and Other Fat Components in Seafoods as presented by Simopoulos et al. (*Health Effects of Polyunsaturated Fatty Acids in Seafoods*, Academic Press, Orlando, FL, 1986).

[a] Per 100 g edible portion, raw.

- denotes lack of reliable data for nutrient known to be present; Tr, trace (<0.05 g/100 g food).

BIOLOGICAL ASPECTS OF OMEGA-6 AND OMEGA-3 FATTY ACIDS

About 80 years ago (1929–1930), Burr and Burr [39] were the first to discover the importance of LA 18:2ω-6 and ALA 18:3ω-3 in restoring the effects caused by the fat-free diet in deprived animals. They coined the term "essential fatty acids" (EFAs). Whereas healthy skin and successful growth, reproduction, and lactation were obtained in mammals fed LA as the only source of EFA, linolenic acid was found to permit growth but was unable to prevent the skin lesions of EFA deficiency or support reproduction [39].

Today, we know that LA and ALA are essential for normal growth and development of human beings. The two families of omega-6 (LA) and omega-3 (ALA) fatty acids are physiologically and metabolically distinct, cannot be synthesized in the human body, and must be obtained from the diet. Figure 3.3 shows the metabolism of LA and ALA into very long-chain polyunsaturated fatty acids (LC-PUFAs) through a series of desaturases and elongases. Both LA and ALA use the same enzymes and compete with each other for enzyme availability. During evolution, there was a balance in the intake of LA and ALA with a ratio of ω-6: ω-3 = 1, whereas today in Western societies, the ratio is about 16/1 ω-6: ω-3 because of the high intake of vegetable oils—soybean, corn oil, sunflower, safflower, and linseed oil—which are high in 18:2ω-6 [40]. LA is found in high amounts in grains with the exception of flaxseed, chia, perilla, rapeseed, and walnuts that are rich in ALA. The green leaves of plants, particularly wild plants, are higher in ALA than in LA [40–43].

The capacity for desaturation and chain elongation of PUFAs appears to be limited and variable. From isotope-labeled ALA feeding studies, the range of conversion of ALA to EPA has been estimated between 0.2% and 21% [44]. The PUFA composition of red blood cell (RBC) membrane phospholipids has been shown to be associated with normal growth and development, as well as in the outcome of chronic diseases such as CHD, hypertension, cancer, arthritis, allergies and other autoimmune diseases, since both omega-6 and omega-3 PUFAs are processed in the human body to powerful promoters of eicosanoids such as prostaglandins and leukotrienes (Figure 3.4) [40–42]. Plasma levels of LC-PUFAs are determined by both dietary intake and endogenous metabolism. Desaturases and elongases catalyze the conversion of PUFAs in humans. Figure 3.3 shows the metabolic pathway of omega-6 and omega-3 fatty acids. The key enzymes in this pathway are the Delta-5 and Delta-6 desaturases, which are encoded by *FADS1* and *FADS2*, respectively [45,46]. They are the rate-limiting enzymes in the synthesis of LC-PUFA, AA, EPA, and DHA from their dietary precursors LA and ALA. AA and EPA are the parent fatty acids for the formation of eicosanoids and DHA for docosanoids.

Competition between the omega-6 and omega-3 fatty acids occurs in prostaglandin formation. EPA competes with AA for prostaglandin and leukotriene synthesis at the cyclooxygenase and lipoxygenase (LO) level (Figure 3.4). When humans ingest fish or fish oil, the EPA and DHA from fish or fish oil lead to (1) a decreased production of prostaglandin E_2 (PGE_2) metabolites; (2) a decrease in thromboxane A_2, a potent platelet aggregator and vasoconstrictor; (3) a decrease in leukotriene B_4 formation, an inducer of inflammation and a powerful inducer of leukocyte chemotaxis and adherence; (4) an increase in thromboxane A_3, a weak platelet aggregator and

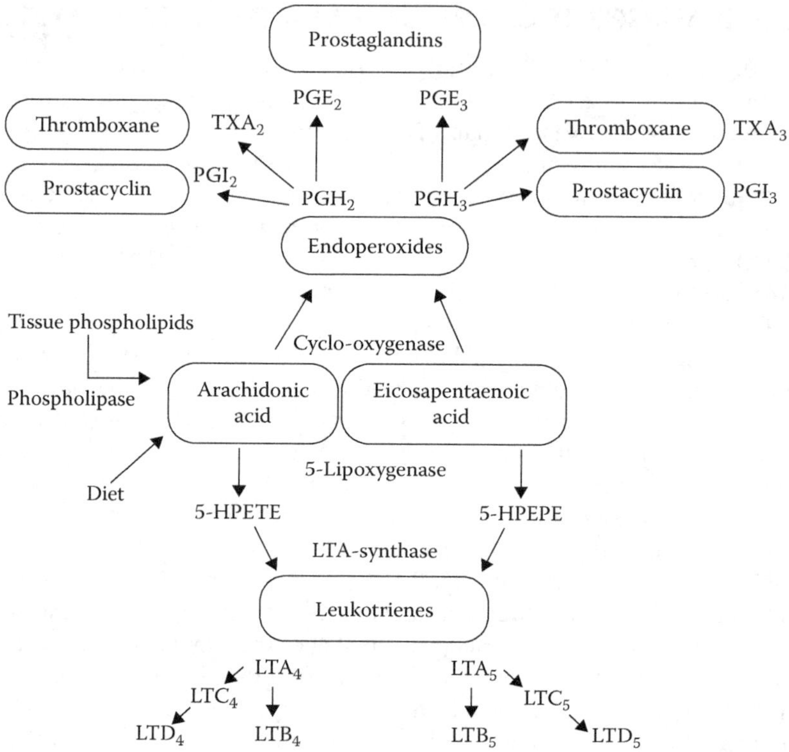

FIGURE 3.4 Oxidative metabolism of arachidonic acid and eicosapentaenoic acid by the cyclooxygenase and 5-lipoxygenase pathways. 5-HPETE, 5-hydroperoxyeicosatetranoic acid; 5-HPEPE, 5-hydroxyeicosapentaenoic acid.

a weak vasoconstrictor; (5) an increase in prostacyclin PGI_3, leading to an overall increase in total prostacyclin by increasing PGI_3 without a decrease in PGI_2 (both PGI_2 and PGI_3 are active vasodilators and inhibitors of platelet aggregation); and (6) an increase in leukotriene B_5, a weak inducer of inflammation and a weak chemotactic agent [47,48]. Omega-3 fatty acids modulate prostaglandin metabolism and decrease triglycerides, and in high doses, lower cholesterol and have antithrombotic and anti-inflammatory properties. These studies have been extensively reviewed [35,49–53]. In the early phase of inflammation, excessive amounts of interleukins (ILs) and lipid mediators are released and play a crucial role. Proinflammatory eicosanoids of AA metabolism are released from membrane phospholipids in the course of inflammatory activation. EPA is released to compete with AA for enzymatic metabolism inducing the production of less inflammatory and chemotactic derivatives. Recent studies using lipidomic approaches have discovered the production of novel lipid mediators termed resolvins E1 and protectins D1 from EPA and DHA and lipoxins from AA that are involved in the resolution of inflammation and in the return to homeostasis [54].

AA is involved in growth and produces PGE_2, which is important for the normal development of many organs and cells including the central nervous system [55–60].

DHA is found in high amounts in the membranes of brain and retina and is critical for proper neurogenesis, neurotransmitter metabolism, neuroprotection, and vision [61,62].

The *FADS1* and *FADS2* gene cluster involved in the metabolic pathway of LA and ALA and the enzymes involved in the production of eicosanoids, 5-LO and cyclo-oxygenase from the AA and EPA, are polymorphic. Recent studies on their polymorphisms indicate that the minor alleles of the genetic variants in *FADS1* and *FADS2* are associated with higher LA and lower AA levels in RBC membrane and plasma phospholipids those may influence the estimation of dietary requirements [63,64], particularly during pregnancy and lactation [65], as well as the infant's intelligence quotient (IQ), [66] whereas an increase in the activity of the desaturase increases the AA-to-LA ratio and the risk for CHD [67]. Furthermore, genetic variants in the *5-LO* and cyclooxygenase-2 (*COX-2*) genes have been associated with increased risk for CHD [68] and cancer, respectively [69].

GENETIC VARIANTS, *FADS1*, AND *FADS2* IN ESTIMATING NUTRITIONAL REQUIREMENTS OF OMEGA-3 AND OMEGA-6 FATTY ACIDS

Omega-6 fatty acids account for the majority of PUFAs in the U.S. food supply [70,71]. They are the predominant PUFA in all diets, especially Western diets. The major omega-6 fatty acid in Western diets is LA, representing about 90% of all the PUFA in North American diets.

The levels of LC-PUFA in plasma serum or RBC membrane phospholipids depend on dietary intake and endogenous metabolism. (Figure 3.3) There have been many indications for considerable interindividual variation in the capacity for endogenous formation of LC-PUFAs. For example, over 20 years ago, Koletzko et al. [72] showed a rather close correlation of omega-6 and omega-3 fatty acid content in mature milk in human beings even though the main dietary sources were different. Thus, it appears that some women have a higher ability to synthesize and secrete milk LC-PUFAs of both the omega-6 and omega-3 series than others. Further, Guerra et al. [73] showed that there was a tracking of plasma LC-PUFA levels in the absence of tracking of dietary intake patterns, suggesting that there is interindividual variation in the ability to endogenously synthesize LC-PUFAs among children, which persists over time and could most likely be due to genetically determined differences in metabolic turnover. Changes in PUFA conversion have been shown with stable isotope studies [74,75].

The key enzymes in omega-6 and omega-3 fatty acid metabolism are the Delta-5 and Delta-6 desaturases, which are encoded by the *FADS1* and *FADS2* genes, respectively [45–46,76]. *FADS1* and *FADS2* are located on the desaturase gene cluster on chromosome 11 (11q12-13.1). This cluster also includes a *FADS3* gene that shares 52% and 62% sequence identity with *FADS1* and *FADS2* genes, as well as a cytochrome b5 domain and a multiple membrane spanning desaturase region.

Schaeffer et al. [64] first reported the association of *FADS1* and *FADS2* polymorphisms with the levels of omega-6 and omega-3 fatty acids in serum phospholipids.

In 2006, Schaeffer et al. [64] showed that common genetic variants of the *FADS1* and *FADS2* gene cluster and their reconstructed haplotypes are associated with the fatty acid composition in serum phospholipids (p values $<1.0 \times 10^{-13}$). Subjects carrying the minor alleles of the single nucleotide polymorphisms (SNPs), rs174544, rs174553, rs174566, rs174561, rs174568, rs968567, rs99780, rs174570, rs2072114, rs174583, and rs174589, were associated with increased levels of 18:2ω-6, 20:2ω-6, 20:3ω-6, and 18:3ω-3 and decreased levels of 20:4ω-6, 22:4ω-6, 20:5ω-3, and 22:5ω-3. Oleic acid 18:1ω-9 and 22:6ω-3 did not show statistically significant associations with the genetic variants. A significant decrease of AA and EPA and dihomo-γ-linolenic acid is associated with decreased production of strong inflammatory mediators. Schaeffer et al. [64] found associations of the *FADS1* and *FADS2* gene cluster with allergic rhinitis and atopic eczema. Various genome-wide scans suggest linkage of the chromosomal region 11q12-13.1, where the *FADS1* and *FADS2* gene cluster is located, with atopy and asthma [77]. However, Schaeffer et al. did not find a statistical significance between *FADS1* and *FADS2* cluster and atopic diseases, and a larger study will be needed. Schaeffer et al. unequivocally showed that the fatty acid composition of serum phospholipids is genetically controlled by the *FADS1* and *FADS2* gene cluster [64].The investigated SNPs in this cluster explained 28% of the variance of AA and up to 12% of its precursor fatty acids. The frequency of the minor alleles was about 26%. It can be concluded that the genetic variants indicate a difference in the conversion of omega-6 and omega-3 fatty acids catalyzed by the delta-5 and delta-6 desaturase, which suggests that individuals may require different amounts of dietary PUFAs or LC-PUFAs to achieve comparable biological effects. Therefore, further studies addressing the biological effects of PUFAs and LC-PUFAs should include genotyping for *FADS1* and *FADS2* polymorphisms.

GENETIC VARIANTS IN OMEGA-6 AND OMEGA-3 FATTY ACID METABOLISM AND IQ

Children's intellectual development is influenced by both genetic and environmental experiences. In general, breast-fed children attain higher IQ scores than children not fed breast milk. Breast-feeding is thought to influence brain development through nutritional processes involving fatty acids [78]. The predominant LC-PUFAs present in human milk, but not in cow's milk, are AA and DHA. Substantial amounts of AA and DHA accumulate in the human brain during the first postnatal months [79] and infants who are breast-fed have higher concentrations of AA and DHA than infants fed unsupplemented formulas [80, 81]. Randomized controlled clinical trials comparing the neurodevelopment of infants fed DHA-supplemented versus unsupplemented formula have produced inconsistent results [82]. Caspi et al. [66] searched the Kyoto Encyclopedia of Genes and Genomes database [83] for genes involved in LC-PUFA metabolism that might moderate the effect of breast-feeding on IQ. The search led them to *FADS2*. *FADS2* gene expression is regulated through end product inhibition and dietary LC-PUFA such as those available in breast milk [84]. The authors selected two SNPs (rs174575 and rs1535) as candidate biomarkers and tested the hypothesis that the cognitive advantage associated with breast-feeding in human beings is related to genetic differences in LC-PUFA metabolism, which they replicated in two birth cohorts. The authors found the difference in IQ test scores between breast-fed and not breast-fed to be 5.6 in one birth cohort and 6.3 IQ points in the other cohort. Analyses revealed that the rs174575 interacted with breast-feeding to influence IQ in both cohorts. There was a dominant effect of the C allele in response to breast-feeding, with those carrying the C allele having a 6.4-IQ-point advantage relative to children not breast-fed (± = 6.35, $p < .001$). In contrast, GG homozygous neither gained an advantage from breast-feeding nor suffered a disadvantage from not being breast-fed ($t = 0.50$, $p = .02$). The interaction between children's rs174575 genotype and breast-feeding suggests that C carrying children benefit from breast milk more than do GG homozygotes. There were not significant IQ differences among children fed breast milk as a function of maternal genotypes. Therefore, these results suggest that the rs174575 influence of breast-feeding effects on IQ involves genetic differences in children's LC-PUFA metabolism rather than rs174575 differences among lactating women in their milk composition. The difference in IQ was 6.8 IQ points with C carriers having the advantage of 0.48 standard deviation units in the general population. This advantage corresponds to a moderate effect size that is associated with many important life outcomes [85,86]. This finding needs to be replicated in much larger cohorts and populations. The molecular mechanism by which rs174575 may influence cognitive development is not known. The rs174575 C allele is linked with the major alleles of *FADS1* and *FADS2* SNPs which are associated with more efficient fatty acid processing, possibly because of increased transcriptomal activity or a more active protein.

Caspi et al. [66] point out that "Comparative genomics shows that rs174575 is in a sequence conserved between human (hg17), chimpanzee (panTro1), dog (canFAm1), rat (rn3), and mouse (mm5) having regulatory potential [87], and there are nonhuman animal models for dietary deprivation/supplementation [88] and for the study of intelligence" [89]. This study represents an excellent example of how a genetic variant can enhance a favorable response (increased IQ) to an environmental exposure (breast-feeding) that was present throughout evolution when our genes were programmed to respond to a balanced omega-6/omega-3 ratio. It also points to the need that GWAS must include environmental exposures especially diet in the interaction between genetic variation and disease associations.

GENETIC VARIANTS OF THE *FADS1* AND *FADS2* GENE CLUSTER INFLUENCE OMEGA-6 AND OMEGA-3 FATTY ACID COMPOSITION IN BOTH PLASMA AND RED CELL MEMBRANE PHOSPHOLIPIDS DURING PREGNANCY AND LACTATION

AA, EPA, and DHA play central roles in infant growth, neural development, and immune function. The maternal status of AA, EPA, and DHA during gestation influences maternal to infant transfer via the placenta, and breast milk provides fatty acids to infants after birth. Xie and Innis [65] determined that *FADS1* and *FADS2* SNPs influence plasma phospholipid and erythrocyte ethanolamine phosphoglyceride (EPG) omega-6 and omega-3 fatty acids during pregnancy and their breast milk during lactation. The authors genotyped rs174553, rs99780, rs174575, and rs174583 in the *FADS1* and *FADS2* gene cluster and analyzed plasma and erythrocyte fatty acid and dietary intake for 69 pregnant women and breast milk for a subset of 54 women exclusively breast-feeding at 1 month postpartum. Minor allele homozygotes of rs174553 (GG), rs99780 (TT), and rs174583 (TT) had lower AA but higher LA in plasma phospholipids and erythrocyte EPG and decreased omega-6 and omega-3 fatty acid product to precursor ratio at 16 and 36 week gestation, $p < .001$. Breast milk fatty acids were influenced by genotype, with significantly lower 14.0, AA and EPA, but higher 20:2ω-6 in the minor allele homozygotes of rs174553 (GG), rs99780 (TT), and rs174583 (TT) and lower AA EPA 22:5ω-3 and DHA in the minor allele homozygotes GG of rs174575. The results indicate a robust association between minor alleles of the four SNPs and lower AA and other omega-6 fatty acids relative to precursor LA. Similar results were found for the omega-3 series. Genetic variation in the *FADS1* and *FADS2* gene cluster is important to the composition of fatty acids provided to breast-fed infants in mother's milk.

Similar results were obtained in a recent study by Koletzko et al. [90] who investigated the relation between *FADS* gene cluster polymorphisms and RBC Fatty acid concentrations in over 4000 pregnant women participating in the Avon Longitudinal Study of Parents and Children. These are important findings indicating that FADS genotypes influence the amount of DHA that might affect the supply of DHA during pregnancy affecting brain and retina development.

GENETIC VARIANTS IN *FADS1* AND *FADS2* AND CORONARY HEART DISEASE RISK AND THE METABOLIC SYNDROME

Desaturase activity is assayed in vitro or in animals by measurement of the rate of conversion of radiolabeled precursor fatty acids to their respective products [91], but ethical and practical reasons prevent this possibility in humans. Instead, a product to precursor ratio (e.g., AA/LA or EPA/ALA) as a surrogate measure to estimate desaturase activity is well established.

Malerba et al. [92] genotyped 13 SNPs located on the *FADS1–FADS2–FADS3* cluster in 658 Italian adults (78% males; mean age 59.7 ± 11.1 years) participating in the Verona Heart Project. Polymorphisms and statistically inferred haplotypes showed a strong association with AA levels in serum phospholipids and in erythrocyte cell membranes (rs174545 adjusted p value for multiple tests, $p < .0001$ and $p < .0001$, respectively). Other significant associations were observed for LA, ALA, and eicosadienoic acid (EDA). Minor allele homozygotes and heterozygotes were associated with higher levels of LA and ALA and lower levels of AA. No significant associations were observed with EPA and DHA. All genotyped SNPs were found to be polymorphic. The minor allele frequency ranged from 9% to 41%. The frequency of most SNPs ranged between 20% and 30%, with only one SNP (rs 2524299) showing a minor allele frequency of <10% (9.1%). Carriers of the minor variants showed significantly lower levels of AA. In RBC membrane phospholipids, some of the minor variants showed higher levels of LA. Similar significant results were also observed in the subgroup of individuals without CHD. The authors concluded "The observed strong association of *FADS* gene polymorphisms with the levels of AA which is a precursor of molecules involved in inflammation and immunity processes, suggests that SNPs of the *FADS1* and *FADS2* gene region are worth studying in diseases related to inflammatory conditions or alterations in the concentration of omega-6 and omega-3 fatty acids."

In a recent GWAS to identify genetic contributors of plasma omega-6 and omega-3 fatty acid concentrations in 1075 participants in the InCHIANTI Study on aging, Tanaka et al. [93] noted that the strongest evidence was in the region of chromosome 11 that encodes *FADS1*, *FADS2*, and *FADS3*. The SNP with the most significant association was rs174537 near *FADS1* in the analysis of AA ($p = 5.95 \times 10^{-46}$). Minor allele homozygotes had lower AA compared to the major allele homozygotes and rs174537 accounted for 18.6% of the additive variance in AA concentrations. Participants carrying the allele associated with higher AA, EDA ($p = 6.78 \times 10^{-9}$), and EPA ($p = 1.07 \times 10^{-14}$) also had higher low-density lipoprotein (LDL) and total cholesterol levels. These results show that SNPs of genes encoding enzymes in the metabolism of PUFA contribute to plasma concentrations of fatty acids, especially AA and higher LDL and total cholesterol levels.

Martinelli et al. [67] analyzed RBC membrane fatty acids, genotyped 13 SNPs in the FADS region, and estimated the ratio of RBC-AA to RBC-LA, C-reactive protein (CRP) in an ongoing case–control study with or without angiographic evidence of coronary artery disease (CAD). Both AA/LA and the ratio of EPA to LNA were higher in participants with CAD than in those without CAD, but in a multiple logistic regression model, only a higher AA/LA resulted as an independent risk factor for CAD (odds ratio: 2.55; 95% CI:1.61, 4.05 for higher) compared with lower ratio tertile; p for trend <.001. Concentrations of high-sensitivity C-reactive protein (hs-CRP) increased progressively across tertiles of AA/LA. Graded increases in hs-CRC concentrations and CAD risk were related to the carriership of FADS haplotypes, including the alleles associated with a higher ratio.

Studies by Kark et al. [94] and Baylin and Campos [95] have shown that higher amounts of AA in adipose tissue are associated with higher risk of acute myocardial infarction. In populations eating a Western diet rich in omega-6 PUFA, a high desaturase activity may promote an increased bioavailability of AA with prevailing synthesis of AA-derived proinflammatory eicosanoids leading to atherosclerosis and vascular damage. On the other hand, high desaturase activity in subjects on a diet rich in omega-3 fatty acids or receiving EPA and DHA supplementation could result in an opposite situation with a preferential synthesis of anti-inflammatory eicosanoids.

African-Americans in the United States [96] have a higher proportion of chronic inflammatory diseases such as CHD, diabetes, and the metabolic syndrome than Africans in the African continent. Type 2 diabetes occurs in only 1%–2% of Africans, whereas the incidence in African-Americans is 11%–13% [97, 98]. Could diet and specifically the high intakes of LA and genetic variants might be the culprit? In a study carried out by Sergeant et al. [99], it was shown that high LA in the diet, in the presence of *FADS1* polymorphisms with high desaturase activity, African-Americans had higher AA than European Americans and a much higher prevalence of diabetes and metabolic syndrome. About 81% of African-Americans and 46% European Americans had the GG allele associated with high AA levels.

Analysis of allele frequencies at rs174537 in HapMap populations around the world shows major differences in allele frequencies among populations suggesting that the efficiency of LA to AA conversion is probably population dependent. Furthermore, haplotypes of the *FADS* gene cluster including variants associated with an elevated AA:LA ratio are related to both a higher systemic inflammation and greater risk of CHD [67].

GENETIC VARIANTS IN THE 5-LIPOXYGENASE AND THE ROLE OF OMEGA-6 AND OMEGA-3 FATTY ACIDS IN CORONARY HEART DISEASE

Since atherosclerosis involves arterial inflammation, Dwyer et al. [100] hypothesized that a polymorphism in the *5-LO* gene promoter could relate to atherosclerosis in humans and that this effect could interact with the dietary intake of competing 5-LO substrates. The study consisted of 470 healthy middle-aged women and men from the Los Angeles Atherosclerosis study, randomly sampled. The investigators determined 5-LO genotypes, carotid-artery intima-media thickness, markers of inflammation, CRP, IL-6, dietary AA, EPA, DHA, LA, and ALA with the use of six 24-hour recalls of food intake. The results showed that 5-LO variant genotypes were found in 6.0% of the cohort. Mean intima-media thickness adjusted for age, sex, height, and racial or ethnic group was increased by $80 \pm 19\ \mu m^{-1}$ from among the carriers of two variant alleles as compared with the carrier of the common (wild-type) allele. In multivariate analysis, the increase in intima-media thickness among carriers of two variant alleles (62 μm, $p < .001$) was similar in this cohort to that associated with diabetes (64 μm, $p < .001$), the strongest common cardiovascular risk factor. Increased dietary AA significantly enhanced the apparent atherogenic effect of genotype, whereas increased dietary intake of omega-3 fatty acids EPA and DHA blunted this effect. Furthermore, the plasma level of CRP of two variant alleles was increased by a factor of two, as compared with that among carriers of the common allele. Thus, genetic variation of *5-LO* identifies a subpopulation with increased risk for atherosclerosis. The diet–gene interaction further suggests that dietary omega-6 fatty acids promote, whereas marine omega-3 fatty acids EPA and DHA inhibit leukotriene-mediated inflammation that leads to atherosclerosis in this subpopulation.

The prevalence of variant genotypes did differ across racial and ethnic groups with higher prevalence among blacks (24.0%), Asians or Pacific Islanders (19.4%), and other racial or ethnic groups (18.2%) than among Hispanic subjects (3.6%) and non-Hispanic whites (3.1%). The study constitutes evidence that genetic variation in an inflammatory pathway—in this case the leukotriene pathway—can trigger atherogenesis in humans. These findings could lead to new dietary and targeted molecular approaches for the prevention and treatment of cardiovascular disease according to genotype, particularly in the populations of non-European descent [101].

GENETIC VARIANTS IN THE 5-LIPOXYGENASE, OMEGA-6 FATTY ACIDS AND BREAST CANCER

Several epidemiologic studies and animal experiments suggest that omega-6 fatty acids increase the risk of cancer whereas omega-3s decrease the risk. However, not all studies have produced consistent results. The 5-LO pathway has been implicated in carcinogenesis and tumor progression in many types of cancer: lung [102], colon [103,104], prostate [105,106], kidney [107], and bladder [108]. Earlier epidemiologic studies on dietary fat intake and breast cancer did not find positive association between omega-6 and breast cancer risk. Those studies, however, did not take into account genetic predisposition related to omega-6 fatty acid metabolism. Wang et al. [109] determined genetic variants in the 5-LO gene (*ALOX5*) and 5-lipoxygenase-activating protein gene (*ALOX5AP*) in combination with dietary LA intake in a population-based multiethnic case–control study on breast cancer in Latin-American, African-American, and White women in the San Francisco area. The authors did not find significant main effects of *ALOX5* and *ALOX5AP* genotypes on breast cancer risk that were consistent across race or ethnicity. There was, though, a significant interaction between the *ALOX5AP*-4900 A> G polymorphisms and dietary LA intake ($p = .03$) among women consuming a diet high in LA (top quartile of intake > 17.4 g/day), carrying the AA genotype. The AA genotype was associated with higher breast cancer risk, compared to genotype AG or GG, whereas in women consuming ≤ 17.4 g/day of LA, the *ALOX5AP*-4900 genotype was not associated with breast cancer risk. These findings indicate that studies on dietary fat intake and cancer should take into consideration type of fat, quantity of fat, and genetic variants. Furthermore in the United States, 17.4 g/day is the intake that a significant portion of the population ingests. It is unfortunate that the American Heart Association recommended a LA intake up to 10% of calories, that is, 22 g/day on a 2000 cal/day, thus putting a significant number of women at risk.

GENETIC VARIANTS OF CYCLOOXYGENASE-2 AND THE PROTECTIVE EFFECT OF LONG-CHAIN OMEGA-3 FATTY ACIDS IN PROSTATE CANCER

Prostate cancer is one of the most common cancers in men. Increasing evidence points to chronic inflammation as one of the factors leading to cancer. Inflammation may result from bacterial or viral infections, intraprostatic urine reflux, or diet. Dietary components that are potent anti-inflammatory agents are the omega-3 PUFAs. Studies have shown that genetic variants at the *COX-2* gene modify prostate inflammation through the COX-2 enzymatic pathway. As discussed previously, COX-2 is a key enzyme in fatty acid metabolism and inflammation. In a case–control study of 466 men diagnosed with aggressive prostate cancer and 478 age- and ethnicity-matched controls, Fradet et al. [69] genotyped nine COX-2 tag SNPs. Dietary history was assessed with a semiquantitatively food frequency questionnaire. Increasing omega-3 intake was associated with a decreased risk of aggressive prostate cancer (p trend $\leq .0001$), and this inverse association was even stronger among men with genetic variants rs4648310 (+ 8897 A/G) flanking the three region of COX-2 (p interaction $= .02$). The patients with the lowest intake of omega-3s and the genetic variant had the most aggressive tumor, whereas the omega-3 PUFAs were protective and this effect was modified by the genetic variant. This gene by diet (omega-3s) interaction clearly shows that the main dietary effect was modified by the genetic variant, whereas men with the variant genotype AG or GG and low intake of omega-3s had much higher risk than men with the variant genotype and high intake of omega-3s.

Another study [110] of Swedish men found that frequent consumption of fatty fish (rich in omega-3s) was inversely associated with prostate cancer risk, and this effect was modified by rs5275 (+ 6364 A>G) SNP in COX-2 where only men carrying the variant allele maintained a strong inverse association between fatty fish intake and prostate cancer, suggesting that the protective effect of omega-3s on prostate cancer may be modified by COX-2 variants.

The interaction between dietary factors and genetic variants could explain the differences noted in association and epidemiological studies. Considering that a low omega-3 intake in the presence of certain genetic variants leads to a more aggressive disease, an increase in omega-3 intake and a decrease in omega-6 leading to a balanced omega-6/omega-3 ratio, as it was during evolution, when our genes were programmed to respond to a balanced ratio, is the recommendation most appropriate to improve public health.

CONCLUSIONS AND RECOMMENDATIONS

The fatty acid composition of RBC membranes and serum phospholipids plays an important role in cellular processes, and is associated with normal growth and development and with the etiology of several complex chronic diseases in humans. The metabolism of EFAs, linoleic and alpha-linolenic, and their metabolic derivatives are controlled by enzymes encoded by polymorphic genes. Therefore, the availability of PUFAs to various tissues is of major importance to health and depends on both dietary intake and endogenous production or metabolic turnover.

Variants in the human genes of Delta-5 and Delta-6 desaturase *FADS1* and *FADS2* that influence both serum and red cell membrane phospholipid levels of PUFA, have a frequency of 26%. The minor alleles are associated with lower AA and higher LA and account for 28% of the variation in serum phospholipid AA and up to 12% of its precursor fatty acids. Smaller percentage values were found for omega-3 fatty acids. These findings suggest that individuals may require different amounts of dietary LA, ALA or AA, EPA, and DHA, for both normal development and in the prevention and management of chronic diseases.

As shown by the studies included in this review, the interaction of *FADS1* and *FADS2* gene cluster with breast-feeding influences IQ in children as well as the levels of LA, ALA, and LC-PUFA in pregnancy and lactation and CHD risk. Similarly, polymorphisms at 5-LO increase the risk for CHD and cancer of the breast, whereas polymorphisms at the cyclooxygenase-2 increase the risk of cancer of the prostate. The risk for CHD and cancer of the prostate is decreased by higher EPA and DHA intake. EPA and DHA downregulate the expression of genes involved in inflammation, oxidative stress, and atherosclerosis and upregulate the nitric oxide synthase gene and genes involved in apoptosis, regulation of cell cycle, mRNA-processing Reactome, RNA binding, and DNA replication Reactome, in peripheral blood mononuclear cells and in adipose tissue cells.

Of interest is the fact that weight loss or caloric restriction has similar effects on gene expression as those obtained by EPA and DHA supplementation. Considering that today's Western societies are characterized by high amounts of omega-6 and low amounts of omega-3 fatty acids, are sedentary with high prevalence of obesity, and that obesity is associated with low omega-3 fatty acids in adipose tissue and muscle, it becomes evident that there is a need to precisely define the nutritional requirements for omega-6 and omega-3 fatty acids taking into consideration *FADS1* and *FADS2* polymorphisms, dietary intake, and endogenous production.

There are important differences in the capacity of different populations to synthesize long-chain PUFA. These differences suggest genetic variants are important factors that may contribute to health disparities between and among populations.

Nutrigenetics/Nutrigenomics will continue to provide data on the importance of genetic variants and on the mechanisms of nutrients and gene interactions in both health and disease. It is necessary to bridge successfully the rapidly widening gap between gene nutrient disease association research and the critical investigations needed to be carried out to improve clinical management and public health.

REFERENCES

1. Bonne-Tamir B, Adam A. *Genetic Diversity among Jews: Diseases and Markers at the DNA Level.* New York: Oxford University Press, 1992.
2. Bowman JE, Murray RF. *Genetic Variation and Disorders in Peoples of African Origin.* Baltimore, MD: Johns Hopkins University Press, 1990.
3. Simopoulos AP, Childs B, eds. Genetic variation and nutrition. *World Rev Nutr Diet* 1990;63:1–300.
4. Molloy AM, Daly S, Mills JL, Kirke PN, Whitehead AS, Ramsbottom D, Conley MR, Weir DG, Scott JM. Thermolabile variant of 5, 10-methylenetetrahydrofolate reductase associated with low red-cell folates: implications for folate intake recommendations. *Lancet* 1997;349:1591–93.
5. Zeisel SH. Genetic polymorphisms in methyl-group metabolism and epigenetics: lessons from humans and mouse models. *Brain Res* 2008;1237:5–11.
6. Ordovas JM. Genetic influences on blood lipids and cardiovascular disease risk: tools for primary prevention. *Am J Clin Nutr* 2009;89(suppl):S1509–17.
7. Sladek R, Rocheleau G, Rung J, Dina C, Shen L et al. A genome-wide association study identifies novel risk loci for type 2 diabetes. *Nature* 2007;445:881–85.
8. Amundadottir LT, Sulem P, Gudmundsson J, Helgason A, Baker A et al. A common variant associated with prostate cancer in European and African populations. *Nat Genet* 2006;38:652–58.
9. Graham RR, Kozyrev SV, Baechler EC, Reddy MV, Plenge RM et al. A common haplotype of interferon regulatory factor 5 (IRF5) regulates splicing and expression and is associated with increased risk of systemic lupus erythematosus. *Nat Genet* 2006;38:550–55.
10. Klein RJ, Zeiss C, Chew EY, Tsai JY, Sackler RS et al. Complement factor H polymorphism in age-related macular degeneration. *Science* 2005;308:385–89.
11. Zhang HF, Qiu LX, Chen Y, Zhu WL, Mao C, Zhu LG, Zheng MH, Wang Y, Lei L, Shi J. ATG16L1 T300A polymorphism and Crohn's disease susceptibility: evidence from 13022 cases and 17,532 controls. *Hum Genet* 2009;125(5–6):627–31.
12. McPherson R, Pertsemlidis A, Kavaslar N, Stewart A, Roberts R et al. A common allele on chromosome 9 associated with coronary heart disease. *Science* 2007;316:1488–91.
13. Roberts R. A customized genetic approach to the number one killer: coronary artery disease. *Curr Opin Cardiol* 2008;23(6):629–33.

14. Simopoulos AP, Nestel P, eds. Genetic variation and dietary response. *World Rev Nutr Diet* 1997;80:1–170.
15. Simopoulos AP, Ordovas JM, eds. Nutrigenetics and nutrigenomics. *World Rev Nutr Diet* 2004;93.
16. Brennan RO. *Nutrigenetics: New Concepts for Relieving Hypoglycemia.* New York: Signet, 1977.
17. Suzuki DT, Griffiths AJF, Miller JH, Lewontin RC. *An Introduction to Genetic Analysis.* New York: Freeman, 1989.
18. National Heart, Lung and Blood Institute. *Report of the Task Force on Research in Atherosclerosis.* Washington, DC: U.S. Department of Health Human Services, 1991.
19. Williams RR. Nature, nurture, and family predisposition. *N Engl J Med* 1988;318:769–71.
20. Mongeau J-G. Heredity and blood pressure. *Semin Nephrol* 1989;9:208–16.
21. Humphries SE, Cook M, Dubowitz M, Stirling Y, Meade TW. Role of genetic variation at the fibrinogen locus in determination of plasma fibrinogen concentrations. *Lancet* 1987;1:1452–55.
22. Hamsten A, Iselius L, de Faire U, Blomback M. Genetic and cultural inheritance of plasma fibrinogen concentration. *Lancet* 1987;1:988–91.
23. Morrison NA, Qi JC, Tokita A, Kelly PJ, Crofts L, Nguyen TV, Sambrook PN, Eisman JA. Prediction of bone density from vitamin D receptor alleles. *Nature* 1994;367:284–87.
24. Scott J. Molecular genetics of common diseases. *Br Med J* 1987;295:769–71.
25. Leaf A, Weber PC. A new era for science in nutrition. *Am J Clin Nutr* 1987;45 (suppl):1048–53.
26. Eaton SB, Konner M. Paleolithic nutrition. A consideration of its nature and current implications. *N Engl J Med* 1985;312:283–9.
27. Simopoulos AP. Genetics and nutrition: or what your genes can tell you about nutrition. In: Simopoulos AP, Childs B, eds. Genetic variation and nutrition. *World Rev Nutr Diet*, Vol. 63. Basel: Karger, 1990:25–34.
28. de Gomez Dumm INT, Brenner RR. Oxidative desaturation of alpha-linolenic, linoleic, and stearic acids by human liver microsomes. *Lipids* 1975;10:315–7.
29. Emken EA, Adlof RO, Rakoff H, Rohwedder WK. Metabolism of deuterium-labeled linolenic, linoleic, oleic, stearic and palmitic acid in human subjects. In: Baillie TA, Jones JR, eds. *Synthesis and Applications of Isotopically Labelled Compounds 1988.* Amsterdam: Elsevier Science Publishers, 1989:713–6.
30. Hague TA, Christofferson BO. Effect of dietary fats on arachidonic acid and eicosapentaenoic acid biosynthesis and conversion to C22 fatty acids in isolated liver cells. *Biochim Biophys Acta* 1984;796:205–17.
31. Hague TA, Christofferson BO. Evidence for peroxisomal retroconversion of adrenic acid (22:4n6) and docosahexanoic acid (22:6n3) in isolated liver cells. *Biochim Biophys Acta* 1986;875:165–73.
32. Carlson SE, Rhodes PG, Ferguson MG. Docosahexaenoic acid status of preterm infants at birth and following feeding with human milk or formula. *Am J Clin Nutr* 1986;44:798–804.
33. Singer P, Kaeger W, Voigt S, Thiel H. Defective desaturation and elongation of n-6 and n-3 fatty acids in hypertensive patients. *Prostaglandins Leukot Med* 1984; 15:159–65.
34. Honigmann G, Schimke E, Beitz J, Mest HJ, Schliack V. Influence of a diet rich in linolenic acid on lipids, thrombocyte aggregation and prostaglandins in type I (insulin-dependent) diabetes. *Diabetologia* 1982;23:175 (abstr).
35. Simopoulos AP, Kifer RR, Martin RE, eds. *Health Effects of Polyunsaturated Fatty Acids in Seafoods.* Orlando, FL: Academic Press, 1986.
36. O'Brien JS, Sampson EL. Fatty acid and aldehyde composition of the major brain lipids in normal gray matter, white matter and myelin. *J Lipid Res* 1965;6:545–51.

37. Anderson RE. Lipids of ocular tissues. IV. A comparison of the phospholipids from the retina of six mammalian species. *Exp Eye Res* 1970;10:339–44.
38. Poulos A, Darin-Bennett A, White IG. The phospholipid bound fatty acids and aldehydes of mammalian spermatozoa. *Comp Biochem Physiol* 1975;46B:541–9.
39. Burr GO, Burr MM. On the nature and role of fatty acids essential in nutrition. *J Biol Chem* 1930;86:587–622.
40. Simopoulos AP. The importance of the omega-6/omega-3 fatty acid ratio in cardiovascular disease and other chronic diseases. *Exp Biol Med (Maywood)* 2008;233:674–88.
41. Simopoulos AP. Omega-3 fatty acids in health and disease and in growth and development. *Am J Clin Nutr* 1991;54:438–63.
42. Simopoulos AP, Norman HA, Gillaspy JE, Duke JA. Common purslane: a source of omega-3 fatty acids and antioxidants. *J Am Coll Nutr* 1992;11:374–82.
43. Simopoulos AP. Omega-6/omega-3 essential fatty acids: biological effects. In: Simopoulos AP, Bazan NG, eds. Omega-3 Fatty Acids, the Brain and Retina. *World Rev Nutr Diet*, Vol. 99. Basel: Karger, 2009:1–16.
44. Burdge G. Alpha-linolenic acid metabolism in men and women: nutritional and biological implications. *Curr Opin Clin Nutri Metab Care* 2004;7:137–44.
45. Cho HP, Nakamura MT, Clarke SD. Cloning, expression, and nutritional regulation of the mammalian delta-6 desaturase. *J Biol Chem* 1999;274:471–7.
46. Cho HP, Nakamura M, Clarke SD. Cloning, expression, and fatty acid regulation of the human delta-5 desaturase. *J Biol Chem* 1999;274:37335–9.
47. Weber PC, Fischer S, von Schacky C, Lorenz R, Strasser T. Dietary omega-3 polyunsaturated fatty acids and eicosanoid formation in man. In: Simopoulos AP, Kifer RR, Martin RE, eds. *Health Effects of Polyunsaturated Fatty Acids in Seafoods*. Orlando, FL: Academic Press, 1986:49–60.
48. Lewis RA, Lee TH, Austen KF. Effects of omega-3 fatty acids on the generation of products of the 5-lipoxygenase pathway. In: Simopoulos AP, Kifer RR, Martin RE, eds. *Health Effects of Polyunsaturated Fatty Acids in Seafoods*. Orlando, FL: Academic Press, 1986:227–38.
49. Burr ML, Fehily AM, Gilbert JF, Rogers S, Holliday RM, Sweetnam PM, Elwood PC, Deadman NM. Effects of changes in fat, fish, and fibre intakes on death and myocardial reinfarction: diet and reinfarction trial (DART). *Lancet* 1989;2:757–61.
50. Leaf A. Cardiovascular effects of fish oils. Beyond the platelet. *Circulation* 1990; 82:624–8.
51. Leaf A, Weber PC. Cardiovascular effects of n-3 fatty acids. *N Engl J Med* 1988; 318:549–57.
52. Simopoulos AP, Kifer RR, Martin RE, Barlow SM, eds. *Health Effects of w3 Polyunsaturated Fatty Acids in Seafoods*. World Rev Nutr Diet, Vol. 66. Basel: Karger, 1991.
53. Von Schacky C. Prophylaxis of atherosclerosis with marine omega-3 fatty acids: a comprehensive strategy. *Ann Intern Med* 1988;107:890–9.
54. Spite M, Serhan CN. Novel lipid mediators promote resolution of acute inflammation: impact of aspirin and statins. *Circ Res* 2010;107(10):1170–84.
55. Innis SM. Essential fatty acids in growth and development. *Prog Lipid Res* 1991; 30:39–103.
56. Cha YI, Solnica-Krezel L, DuBois RN. Fishing for prostanoids: deciphering the developmental functions of cyclooxygenase-derived prostaglandins. *Dev Biol* 2006;289:263–72.
57. Harizi H, Gualde N. The impact of eicosanoids on the crosstalk between innate and adaptive immunity: the key role of dendritic cells. *Tissue Antigens* 2005;65:507–14.
58. Leu BH, Schmidt JT. Arachidonic acid as a retrograde signal controlling growth and dynamics of retinotectal arbors. *Dev Neurobiol* 2008;68:18–30.

59. Khanapure SP, Garvey DS, Janero DR, Letts LG. Eicosanoids in inflammation: biosynthesis, pharmacology and therapeutic frontiers. *Curr Top Med Chem* 2007;7:311–40.
60. Peskar BM, Sawka N, Ehrlich K, Peskar BA. Role of cyclooxygenase-1 and -2, phospholipase C, and protein kinase C in prostaglandin mediated gastroprotection. *J Pharmacol Exp Ther* 2003;305:1233–8.
61. Simopoulos AP, Bazan NG, eds. *Omega-3 Fatty Acids, the Brain and Retina.* World Rev Nutr Diet, Vol. 99. Basel: Karger, 2009.
62. Serhan CN, Chiang N, Van Dyke TE. Resolving inflammation: dual anti-inflammatory and pro-resolution lipid mediators. *Nat Rev Immunol* 2008;8:349–61.
63. Koletzko B, Demmelmair H, Schaeffer L, Illig T, Heinrich J. Genetically determined variation in polyunsaturated fatty acid metabolism may result in different dietary requirements. *Nestle Nutr Workshop Ser Pediatr Program* 2008;62:35–44; discussion 44–9.
64. Schaeffer L, Gohlke H, Muller M, Heid IM, Palmer LJ, Kompauer I, Demmelmair H, Illig T, Koletzko B, Heinrich J. Common genetic variants of the FADS1 FADS2 gene cluster and their reconstructed haplotypes are associated with the fatty acid composition in phospholipids. *Hum Mol Genet* 2006;15:1745–56.
65. Xie L, Innis SM. Genetic variants of the FADS1 FADS2 gene cluster are associated with altered (n-6) and (n-3) essential fatty acids in plasma and erythrocyte phospholipids in women during pregnancy and in breast milk during lactation. *J Nutr* 2008;138:2222–8.
66. Caspi A, Williams B, Kim-Cohen J, Craig IW, Milne BJ, Poulton R, Schalkwyk LC, Taylor A, Werts H, Moffitt TE. Moderation of breastfeeding effects on the IQ by genetic variation in fatty acid metabolism. *Proc Natl Acad Sci USA* 2007;104:18860–5.
67. Martinelli N, Girelli D, Malerba G, Guarini P, Illig T et al. FADS genotypes and desaturase activity estimated by the ratio of arachidonic acid to linoleic acid are associated with inflammation and coronary artery disease. *Am J Clin Nutr* 2008;88:941–9.
68. Allayee H, Baylin A, Hartiala J, Wijesuriya H, Mehrabian M, Lusis AJ, Campos H. Nutrigenetic association of the 5-lipoxygenase gene with myocardial infarction. *Am J Clin Nutr* 2008;88:934–40.
69. Fradet V, Cheng I, Casey G, Witte JS. Dietary omega-3 fatty acids, cyclooxygenase-2 genetic variation, and aggressive prostate cancer risk. *Clin Cancer Res* 2009;15:2559–66.
70. Simopoulos AP, Herbert V, Jacobson B. *The Healing Diet.* New York: Macmillan, 1995.
71. Simopoulos AP. Nutrition policies for the prevention of atherosclerosis in industrialized societies. In: Moyal MF, ed. *Diet and Life Style: New Technology.* Paris: Libby, 1988:373–80.
72. Koletzko B, Mrotzek M, Bremer HJ. Fatty acid composition of mature human milk in Germany. *Am J Clin Nutr* 1988;47:954–9.
73. Guerra A, Demmelmair H, Toschke AM, Koletzko B. Three-year tracking of fatty acid composition of plasma phospholipids in healthy children. *Ann Nutr Metab* 2007;51:433–8.
74. Del Prado M, Villalpando S, Elizondo A, Rodríguez M, Demmelmair H, Koletzko B. Contribution of dietary and newly formed arachidonic acid to human milk lipids in women eating a low fat diet. *Am J Clin Nutr* 2001;74:242–7.
75. Demmelmair H, von Schenck U, Behrendt E, Sauerwald T, Koletzko B. Estimation of arachidonic acid synthesis in full term neonates using natural variation of 13C content. *J Pediatr Gastroenterol Nutr* 1995;21:31–6.
76. Marquardt A, Stohr H, White K, Weber BH. Cdna cloning, genomic structure, and chromosomal localization of three, members of the human fatty acid desaturase family. *Genomics* 2000;66:175–83.
77. Daniels SE, Bhattacharrya S, James A, Leaves NI, Young A et al. A genome-wide search for quantitative trait loci underlying asthma. *Nature* 1996;383:247–50.

78. Institute of Medicine. *Infant Formula: Evaluating the Safety of New Ingredients.* Washington, DC: National Academies of Press, 2004.
79. Heird WC, Lapillonne A. The role of essential fatty acids in development. *Annu Rev Nutr* 2005;25:549–71.
80. Farquharson J, Cockburn F, Patrick WA, Jamieson EC, Logan RW. The role of essential fatty acids in development. *Lancet* 1992;340:810–3.
81. Makrides M, Neumann MA, Byard RW, Simmer K, Gibson RA. Fatty acid composition of brain, retina, and erythrocytes in breast- and formula-fed infants. *Am J Clin Nutr* 1994;60:189–94.
82. McCann JC, Ames BN. Is docosahexaenoic acid, an n-3 long-chain polyunsaturated fatty acid, required for development of normal brain function? An overview of evidence from cognitive and behavioral tests in humans and animals. *Am J Clin Nutr* 2005;82:281–95.
83. Kanehisa M, Goto S, Hattori M, Aoki-Kinoshita KF, Itoh M, Kawashima S, Katayama T, Araki M, Hirakawa M. From genomics to chemical genomics: new developments in KEGG. *Nucleic Acids Res* 2006;34:D354–7.
84. Nakamura MT, Nara TY. Structure, function, and dietary regulation of delta6, delta5, and delta9 desaturases. *Annu Rev Nutr* 2004;24:345–76.
85. Cohen J. *Statistical Power Analysis for the Behavioral Sciences.* Hillsdale, NJ: Lawrence Erlbaum Associates, 1988.
86. Gottfredson LS. Why g matters: the complexity of everyday life. *Intelligence* 1997;24:79–132.
87. Karolchik D, Baertsch R, Diekhans M, Furey TS, Hinrichs A et al. The UCSC Genome Browser Database. *Nucleic Acids Res* 2003;31:51–4.
88. Fedorova I, Salem N Jr. Omega-3 fatty acids and rodent behavior. *Prostaglandins Leukot Essen Fatty Acids* 2006;75:271–89.
89. Plomin R. The genetics of G in human and mouse. *Nat Rev Neurosci* 2001;2:136–41.
90. Koletzko B, Lattka E, Zeilinger S, Illig T, Steer C. Genetic variants of the fatty acid desaturase gene cluster predict amounts of red blood cell docosahexaenoic and other polyunsaturated fatty acids in pregnant women: findings from the Avon Longitudinal study of parents and children. *Am J Clin Nutr* 2011;93(1):211–9.
91. Narce M, Asdrubal P, Delachambre MC, Véricel E, Lagarde M, Poisson JP. Age-related changes in linoleic acid bioconversion by isolated hepatocytes from spontaneously hypertensive and normotensive rats. *Mol Cell Biochem* 1994;141(1):9–13.
92. Malerba G, Schaeffer L, Xumerle L, Klopp N, Trabetti E et al. SNPs of the FADS gene cluster are associated with polyunsaturated fatty acids in a cohort of patients with cardiovascular disease. *Lipids* 2008;43(4):289–99.
93. Tanaka T, Shen J, Abecasis GR, Kisialiou A, Ordovas JM et al. Genome-wide association study of plasma polyunsaturated fatty acids in the InCHIANTI Study. *PLoS Genet* 2009;5(1):e1000338.
94. Kark JD, Kaufmann NA, Binka F, Goldberger N, Berry EM. Adipose tissue n-6 fatty acids and acute myocardial infarction in a population consuming a diet high in polyunsaturated fatty acids. *Am J Clin Nutr* 2003;77(4):796–802.
95. Baylin A, Campos H. Arachidonic acid in adipose tissue is associated with nonfatal acute myocardial infarction in the central valley of Costa Rica. *J Nutr* 2004;134(11):3095–9.
96. American Heart Association (2009) Heart Disease and Stroke Statistics—2008 Update. http://www.americanheart.org/downloadable/heart/1200082005246HS_Stats%202008.final.pdf (accessed November 2009).
97. World Health Organization (2009) Diabetes Programme: Facts and Figures. http://www.who.int/diabetes/facts/en/index.html (accessed November 2009).
98. American Diabetes Association (2009) Diabetes Statistics—2007. http://www.diabetes.org/diabetes-basics/diabetes-statistics/ (accessed November 2009).

99. Sergeant S, Hugenschmidt CE, Rudock ME, Ziegler JT, Ivester P et al. Differences in arachidonic acid levels and fatty acid desaturase (FADS) gene variants in African Americans and European Americans with diabetes or the metabolic syndrome. *Br J Nutr* 2012;107(4):547–55.
100. Dwyer JH, Allayee H, Dwyer KM, Fan J, Wu H, Mar R, Lusis AJ, Mehrabian M. Arachidonate 5-lipoxygenase promoter genotype, dietary arachidonic acid, and atherosclerosis. *N Engl J Med* 2004;350(1):29–37.
101. Simopoulos AP. Genetic variation and dietary response: nutrigenetics/nutrigenomics. *Asia Pacific J Clin Nutr* 2002;11(S6):S117–28.
102. Avis IM, Jett M, Boyle T, Vos MD, Moody T, Treston AM, Martínez A, Mulshine JL. Growth control of lung cancer by interruption of 5-lipoxygenase-mediated growth factor signaling. *J Clin Invest* 1996;97:806–13.
103. Soumaoro LT, Iida S, Uetake H, Ishiguro M, Takagi Y, Higuchi T, Yasuno M, Enomoto M, Sugihara K. Expression of 5-lipoxygenase in human colorectal cancer. *World J Gastroenterol* 2006;12:6355–60.
104. Ye YN, Wu WK, Shin VY, Bruce IC, Wong BC, Cho CH. Dual inhibition of 5-LOX and COX-2 suppresses colon cancer formation promoted by cigarette smoke. *Carcinogenesis* 2005;26:827–34.
105. Ghosh J, Myers CE. Arachidonic acid stimulates prostate cancer cell growth: critical role of 5-lipoxygenase. *Biochem Biophys Res Commun* 1997;235:418–23.
106. Sundaram S, Ghosh J. Expression of 5-oxoETE receptor in prostate cancer cells: critical role in survival. *Biochem Biophys Res Commun* 2006;339:93–8.
107. Faronato M, Muzzonigro G, Milanese G, Menna C, Bonfigli AR, Catalano A, Procopio A. Increased expression of 5-lipoxygenase is common in clear cell renal cell carcinoma. *Histol Histopathol* 2007;22:1109–18.
108. Hayashi T, Nishiyama K, Shirahama T. Inhibition of 5-lipoxygenase pathway suppresses the growth of bladder cancer cells. *Int J Urol* 2006;13:1086–91.
109. Wang J, John EM, Ingles SA. 5-Lipoxygenase and 5-lipoxygenaseactivating protein gene polymorphisms, dietary linoleic acid, and risk for breast cancer. *Cancer Epidemiol Biomarkers Prev* 2008;17:2748–54.
110. Hedelin M, Chang ET, Wiklund F, Bellocco R, Klint A et al. Association of frequent consumption of fatty fish with prostate cancer risk is modified by COX-2 polymorphism. *Int J Cancer* 2007;120:398–405.

4 Nutrigenomic Approaches to Unraveling the Physiological Effects of Complex Foods

Peter J. Gillies and John P. Vanden Heuvel

CONTENTS

INTRODUCTION

Although much has been written on the promise and practice of nutrigenomics [1–3], far less has been written on the prospective application of nutrigenomics to product development. In this chapter, a novel omega-3 fatty acid-enriched oil is discussed as an example of how nutrigenomics can be leveraged as part of the product life-cycle management process (Figure 4.1). As will become evident, the various technologies in the nutrigenomic tool kit have different values at different times in the process.

PRODUCT BACKGROUND: THE UNMET NEED

Evidence-based reviews and population-based risk assessment models underscore the need to increase the consumption of long-chain omega-3 fatty acids [4,5]. The estimated dietary intake of eicosapentaenoic acid (EPA) and docosahexaenoic

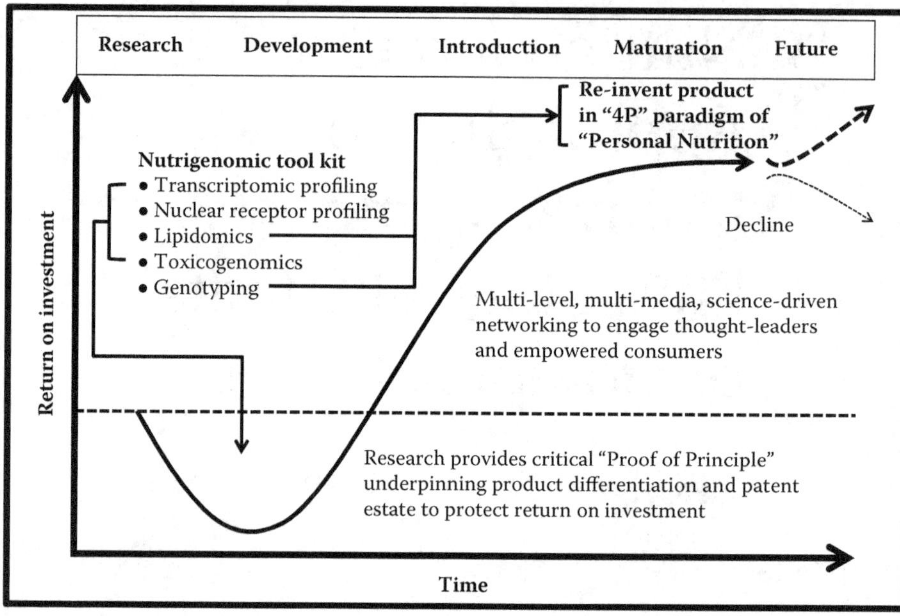

FIGURE 4.1 A nutrigenomic view of the product life cycle.

acid (DHA) hovers around 138 mg/day. In contrast, the recommended intake of these long-chain omega-3 fatty acids is between 250 and 500 mg/day, depending on whether one adopts an international or U.S. centric view of the data [6]. The proposal to increase intake by two- to fourfold comes at a time when the sustainability of fish has been called into question and the amount and ratio of EPA and DHA in fish is highly variable [7,8]. Thus, from both health and product perspective, there is a need to find new and sustainable sources of long-chain omega-3 fatty acids of consistent composition and content. In this regard, advances in agricultural and fermentation biotechnology have enabled the development of high-quality, sustainable sources of omega-3-enriched oils for use in foods and dietary supplements [9]. Two recent commercial examples of such oils include stearidonic acid–enriched oil from soybeans (Soymega™) and EPA-enriched oil from yeast (NewHarvest™ [NH]).

The commercialization of a novel oil carries with it the responsibility to validate and, if necessary, redefine the nutritional pharmacology of the oil. This is much more than "best practice," given that the scientific literature teaches that fatty acids are major modulators of gene expression and the molecular signatures of structurally similar fatty acids, for example, EPA and DHA, can be more different than the same depending on the ontological pathways of interest [10,11]. In this regard, it is unlikely that the nutritional pharmacology of a novel oil is the simple sum of parts and that its health benefit profile while guided cannot be defined by the literature on other related oils. Herein, the critical questions become the following: (1) When in the new product life cycle should one consider the realities of molecular nutrition? (2) Which nutrigenomic tools enable a useful understanding of the oil?

NUTRIGENOMIC TOOL KIT

Nutrition science has been one of the many beneficiaries of the human genome project, particularly in terms of new technologies. Indeed, the "-omic" revolution has provided the field of nutrition with a remarkable set of molecular tools, a "nutrigenomic tool kit," which enables not only basic research but also product development. The development of NH provides an example of how various nutrigenomic tools can be used, or not used as the case may be, in the research and development phase of a novel oil. NH is an EPA-enriched oil, produced in a genetically modified yeast (*Yarrowia lipolytica*), which contains approximately 35% EPA, 18% linoleic acid, 5% oleic acid (OA), and a small percentage of other well-known fatty acids, none of which exceed 5% on an individual basis [12].

TRANSCRIPTOMIC PROFILING

The transcriptomic profiling of the EPA-enriched oil (NH) was undertaken with three basic premises in mind: (1) the transcriptomic profile of a related series of fatty acids will show a degree of similarity, but discrete patterns of gene expression will exist within the profile for a given fatty acid or mixtures thereof; (2) the genes being regulated will provide key insights into the defining nutritional pharmacology of a fatty acid or mixtures thereof; and (3) a deeper understanding of the molecular nutrition of fatty acids will enable more specific and efficacious health claims to be made around novel oil products. The profiling studies were conducted using a human monocyte cell line (THP-1) that when differentiated and challenged with lipopolysaccharides (LPSs) offers a useful model in which to examine the anti-inflammatory effects of fatty acids or extracts of foods or dietary supplements [13,14]. As shown in Figure 4.2a, LPS-challenged THP-1 cells treated with 100 μM α-linolenic acid (ALA), DHA, EPA, OA, or NH resulted in distinct gene expression signatures for each fatty acid. When a list of 180 genes that were significantly regulated by the fatty acids was examined, it became obvious that the predominant mode of regulation was a repression in mRNA levels (shown as light grey bars), an observation that is consistent with the ability of certain fatty acids to decrease inflammatory signaling. NH resulted in a response that was more similar to that of purified EPA and OA than that of DHA. Pathway analysis of the genes regulated by NH, ALA, DHA, and EPA indicated that the primary biological impact of these fatty acids fell into three main ontological categories, lipid/cholesterol metabolism, inflammation, and cell differentiation/cancer (Figure 4.2b), and that the NH expression profile was driven by members of the nuclear receptor superfamily (Figure 4.2c). In summary, the transcriptomic profiling study provides support for the differential molecular pharmacology of omega-3 fatty acids in general and NH in particular. Furthermore, the profiling studies suggest that a major underlying mechanism of action for NH resides in the oil's ability to activate specific nuclear receptors, a hypothesis worthy of more detailed examination.

(a)

Function	p-value	#
Diseases and disorders		
Cancer	3E-14	59
Organismal injury	3E-9	24
Inflammatory response	1E-9	31
Molecular and cellular function		
Cell growth and proliferation	2E-12	53
Lipid metabolism	4E-12	33
Small molecule biochemistry	4E-12	41

(b)

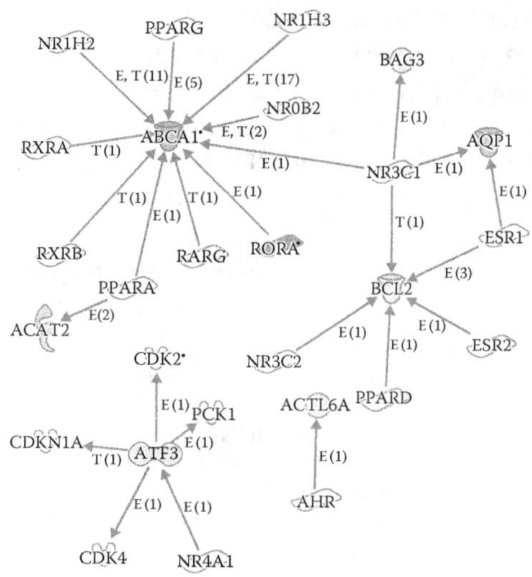

(c)

FIGURE 4.2 Transcriptomic profiling of fatty acids. THP-1 cells were grown under standard conditions and treated with fatty acids, an extract of the NewHarvest product (100 μM, as a BSA conjugate), or control (BSA) for 24 hours. RNA was extracted using Qiagen RNeasy and quality assessed by RNA Nano Chips on the Agilent Bioanalyzer. Each sample was labeled using the Affymetrix IVT Express Kit according to the manufacturer's protocol. The GeneChip Human Genome U133A 2.0 (Affymetrix), representing 14,500 well-characterized genes, was hybridized with the labeled RNA using GeneChip Hybridization Wash and Stain Kit (#702232) in the Affymetrix GeneChip Hybridization Oven 640, according to the manufacturer's instructions. Following hybridization, the arrays were washed and stained using the Affymetrix GeneChip Fluidics Station 450 according to the manufacturer's protocol and scanned using the GeneChip Scanner 3000 7G. The scanned image file (DAT) and the intensity data (CEL) were imported into GeneSpring 10.0 (Agilent Technologies). One-way analysis of variance with asymptotic p-value and Benjamini–Hochberg multiple corrections was performed. In a separate analysis, unpaired t-tests were used to find genes that were significantly regulated by the fatty acid relative to vehicle control (volcano plots, $p < .05$ with 2.5-fold differences). (a) Gene expression patterns for the significantly regulated genes is depicted (dark grey is shown an increased whereas light grey is shown as decreased, expression relative to control). Hierarchical analysis was performed by JMP (SAS Institute, Cary, NC). (b) Ontological analysis was performed using Ingenuity Pathway Analysis (IPA) (Ingenuity Systems Inc., Redwood City, CA). (c) Pathway analysis was performed by IPA. Shown is a network that is involved in lipid metabolism that contains a preponderance of nuclear receptors.

Nuclear Receptor Profiling

Ligand-activated nuclear receptors are intracellular transcription factors that directly regulate gene expression in response to a broad spectrum of lipophilic molecules ranging from fatty acids to drugs [15–17]. The nuclear receptors that may be responsive to individual omega-3 fatty acids and NH were identified from pathway mapping of the transcriptomic profiles; however, the candidate receptors needed to be confirmed in specific gene reporter assays as shown in Figure 4.3. Of the nuclear receptors examined, the proliferator-activated receptor (PPAR) isoforms, retinoid X receptor α (RXRα), retinoic acid receptor (RAR)γ and farnesoid X receptor (FXR) were affected by treatment with the various fatty acids and NH. PPARα was activated by all fatty acids, whereas the other receptors showed varying degrees of selectivity. Of particular note is the extent of PPARβ/δ activation observed with EPA as well as the relatively high amount of activation of PPARγ with DHA. The NH oil had a transcription factor activation profile similar to SDA, ALA, and EPA. When NH was examined in more detail (Figure 4.3b and c), the two predominant targets were PPARα and PPARβ/δ with lesser effects seen with the other receptors. In summary,

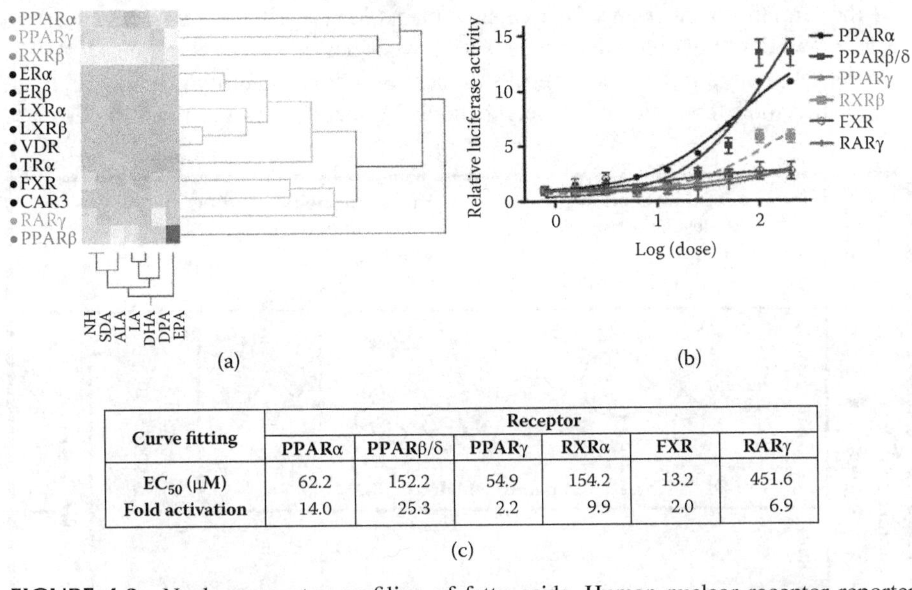

Curve fitting	Receptor					
	PPARα	PPARβ/δ	PPARγ	RXRα	FXR	RARγ
EC_{50} (μM)	62.2	152.2	54.9	154.2	13.2	451.6
Fold activation	14.0	25.3	2.2	9.9	2.0	6.9

(c)

FIGURE 4.3 Nuclear receptor profiling of fatty acids. Human nuclear receptor reporter assay systems were purchased from INDIGO Biosciences Inc. (State College, PA). Assays were performed according to the manufacturer's instructions. (a) The activation of the NRs by 100 μM of the indicated fatty acids is shown, relative to vehicle control (DMSO, dark grey is shown an increased, whereas light grey is shown as decreased). Hierarchical analysis was performed by JMP (SAS Institute, Cary, NC). (b) A select group of NRs were examined with a dose–response of the NewHarvest extract. (c) Nonlinear regression analysis of the data shown in panel b (Prism 5.01, GraphPad Software Inc., San Diego, CA).

the nuclear receptor profiling data suggested that the NH oil may have beneficial effects on lipid metabolism and inflammatory process through PPARα and PPARβ/γ activation; furthermore, the robust activation of PPARβ/γ by EPA relative to DHA suggests research aimed at this receptor may differentiate EPA-enriched oils from DHA-enriched oils.

Metabolomic Profiling

In the evaluation of a novel oil, lipidomics is the metabolomic platform of choice [18]. Herein, there are several technical platforms from which to choose, examples of which are presented in Figure 4.4. Of these, fatty acid profiling by gas–liquid chromatography [19] was extensively used to characterize both the fatty acid composition of the EPA-enriched oil and the human response to the oil in the clinical studies. With regard to the latter, 600 mg/day of the EPA-rich oil for 6 weeks increased serum EPA and the Omega Score™ by 200% and 124%, respectively [20]. Comprehensive lipoprotein analysis was done through a combination of clinical analyzer and enzyme-linked immunosorbent assays (*vide infra*) to anchor the biological activity of the oil in the reported literature. Advanced lipid species profiling by mass spectrometry has not been undertaken to date; however, it would be interesting to quantitate both the oil and the human serum from EPA-treated subjects looking at EPA-enrichment of the various acyl lipid fractions with a focus on triglycerides, given the emerging story that EPA-enrichment of triglycerides results in increased bioavailability [21,22]. Although technically more complicated, a search for EPA metabolites such as 18S E-series

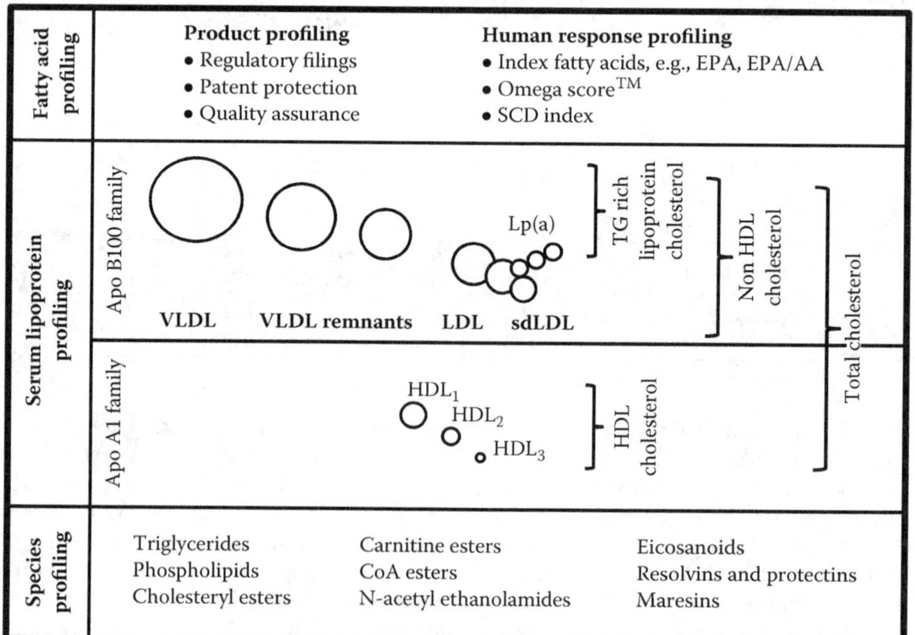

FIGURE 4.4 Overview of lipidomic analyses of oil products and product responses.

resolvins, metabolites which may be the ultimate effector molecules of EPA's biological activity, could prove to be germane in understanding and expanding the biology of an EPA-rich oil [23]. In summary, the value capture of lipidomics is that it provided quantitative data on the absorption and distribution of the novel oil and created a physiological context for the nutrient–gene interactions identified by transcriptomic and nuclear receptor profiling. Advanced species profiling could offer future opportunities to promote product differentiation in the market place as new science unfolds.

Toxicogenomic Profiling

Toxicogenomics is a powerful safety assessment tool, particularly for a new chemical entity about which little is known [24–26]; however, its utility in the primary safety assessment of mixtures or complex matrices such as food or supplements is less certain, if not potentially problematic from a regulatory perspective. For NH, a product that is a simpler compositional form of fish oil, the classical approach of comparing a commercially representative sample of the EPA-enriched oil head-to-head with a "generally recognized as safe" fish oil was considered to be the best strategy. The only toxicologically remarkable findings surfaced in the formal safety assessment studies were a gender-specific (male) thyroid follicular cell hypertrophy in 28, but not 90 day rat studies, and decreased serum cholesterol in both the high-density lipoprotein (HDL) and the non-HDL fractions [27,28]. The thyroid effect represents a classic example of a gender-specific "metabolic food reaction," and the cholesterol-lowering effect in the HDL fraction is a well-documented rodent-specific difference in the transcriptional regulation of apoA-1 [29]. The non-HDL lowering may reflect a down regulation of the cholesterol biosynthetic pathway secondary to posttranscriptional suppression of SREBP-2 [30]. However, the clinical meaning of this observation in rodents is unclear, given that omega-3 fatty acids in food and drugs are used to lower serum triglycerides, not serum cholesterol, in humans [31]. Herein, the decision to forego a toxicogenomics approach to the safety evaluation of the EPA-enriched oil appears to have been well considered.

Nutrigenetics

Nutrigenetics, the tailoring of nutritional products to the genetic makeup of a consumer analogous to that of pharmacogenetics, can be a double-edged sword. On the one hand, nutrigenetics can open the door to personal nutrition, increase product efficacy, and create avenues for product reinvention; on the other hand, it leads to segmentation of the consumer population and niche product development, events that run contrary to the mass marketing model of the food industry. With respect to personal nutrition, two trends may be germane. First, consumer surveys suggest that 78% of Americans are favorably disposed to using genetic information to optimize their personal nutrition [32]. Second, the discovery of genetic polymorphisms in the omega-3 biosynthetic pathway, notably in fatty acid desaturase 1 and fatty acid desaturase 2 [33], and in the nuclear receptors that are activated by omega-3 fatty acids such as PPARα [34] all foretell of an era of genetic testing and nutrigenomic counseling. In a paradigm similar to "4P" medicine [35,36], the future of nutrition and health can be framed as "4P" nutrition that is "predictive, preemptive, personal, and participatory." The 4P paradigm may be attractive to empowered consumers looking to proactively manage their health or to physicians whose clinical assessment of a patient may suggest that more aggressive dietary management is in order. The success of the 4P paradigm may be enabled by single cell oil biotechnology that produces defined oils of novel and defined composition that can be leveraged with a deeper understanding of an individual's omega-3 fatty acid genetic response profile. Although the science underpinning the 4P paradigm continues to move ahead, regulatory hurdles such as direct to consumer marketing of genetic tests and ethical considerations are problematic at the moment, but likely resolvable in time.

NUTRIGENOMICS AND THE EVIDENTIARY HIERARCHY

Prospective transcriptomic profiling can set up an exciting array of molecular hypotheses, but only studies in humans can prove them. In this regard, nutrigenomic data sit at the bottom of the evidentiary hierarchy. The practical corollary of this statement is that as one moves from discovery science in the laboratory to reduction science in the clinic, specific hypotheses start to drive study design and the selection outcome variables. With regard to the EPA-enriched oil, the primary focus of the first study in humans was safety and product compliance, with a secondary focus on lipid and lipoprotein metabolism in an effort to tether the nutritional pharmacology of the product to the omega-3 literature. With regard to the first objective, there were no untoward or clinically meaningful safety issues identified in the study with capsule compliance exceeding 85% [37]. With regard to the second objective, the EPA-rich oil at 1800 mg/day lowered triglyceride-rich lipoprotein cholesterol ~12%, small dense low-density lipoprotein (sdLDL) ~9%, and Lp-PLA2 (a vascular specific biomarker of inflammation) ~6%. At 600 mg/day, it was notable that EPA was without effect on LDL cholesterol, whereas DHA raised LDL cholesterol ~14%. An objective assessment of the clinical data was that the effects of EPA and the differential effects of EPA versus DHA were neither unexpected based on the literature [38] nor predicted by the prospective transcriptomic profiling of the product. In this regard, one is left to speculate that the differential nutritional pharmacology of the EPA-rich oil that is so evident in the molecular profiling resides largely outside of known or traditional endpoints. On the one hand, this is intriguing in terms of opportunities to reinvent the health benefit story of a novel EPA-enriched oil; however, the exploration of the hypothesis is not without considerable R&D expense and likely falls outside of the "return on investment" model for a food ingredient.

CONCLUSIONS

The nutrigenomic tool kit offers an impressive array of technologies that can be used to define the nutritional pharmacology of complex nutritional bioactives and food. At different points in the product life cycle, these tools can frame new opportunities, enable product characterization, and allow sophisticated insight into the human response to the product. There is, however, a practical and resource-driven tension between discovery science and reduction science that needs to be managed with the recognition that both have value although perhaps not at the same time.

P.J. Gillies holds patents on the use of omega-3 fatty acids derived from yeast, which he invented while an employee of the E.I. DuPont Company. Portions of this work were conducted under a contract between E.I. Du Pont Company and INDIGO Biosciences Inc. J.P. Vanden Heuvel is an employee of Penn State University and has a financial stake with INDIGO Biosciences Inc.

REFERENCES

1. Wittwer J, Rubio-Aliaga I, Hoeft B et al. Nutrigenomics in human intervention studies: Current status, lesson learned and future perspectives. *Molecular Nutrition and Food Research* 2011; 55:341–358.
2. German JB, Zivkovic AM, Dallas DC et al. Nutrigenomics and personalized diets: What will they mean for food? *Annual Reviews in Food Science Technology* 2011; 2:97–123.
3. Fenech M, El-Sohemy A, Cahill L et al. Nutrigenetics and nutrigenomics: Viewpoints on the current status and applications in nutrition research and practice. *Journal of Nutrigenetics and Nutrigenomics* 2011; 4:69–89.
4. Balk EM, Horsley TA, Newberry SJ et al. A collaborative effort to apply the evidence-based review process to the field of nutrition: Challenges, benefits, and lessons learned. *American Journal of Clinical Nutrition* 2007; 85:1448–1456.
5. Danaei G, Ding EL, Mozaffarian D et al. The preventable causes of death in the United States: Comparative risk assessment of dietary, lifestyle, and metabolic risk factors. *PLoS Medicine* 2009; 6:e1000058. doi:10.1371/journal.pmed.1000058.
6. Harris WS, Mozaffarian D, Lefevre M et al. Towards establishing dietary reference intakes for eicosapentaenoic and docosahexaenoic acids. *Journal of Nutrition* 2009; 139:804S–819S.
7. Jenkins DJA, Sievenpiper JL, Pauly D et al. Are dietary recommendations for the use of fish oils sustainable? *Canadian Medical Association Journal* 2009; 180:633–637.
8. Harris K, Fleming J, and Kris-Etherton P. Challenges in estimating omega-3 fatty acid content of seafood from US nutrient databases: A salmon case study. *Journal of Food Composition and Analysis* 2011; 24:1168–1173.
9. Gillies PJ, Harris WS, and Kris-Etherton PM. Omega-3 fatty acids in food and pharma: The enabling role of biotechnology. *Current Atherosclerosis Reports* 2011; 13(6):463–473. doi:10.1007/s11883-011-0206-z.
10. Bouwens M, van de Rest O, Dellschaft N et al. Fish-oil supplementation induces anti-inflammatory gene expression profiles in human blood mononuclear cells. *American Journal of Clinical Chemistry* 2009; 90:415–424.
11. Gorjao R, Azevedo-Martins AK, Rodrigues HG et al. Comparative effects of DHA and EPA on cell function. *Pharmacology and Therapeutics* 2009; 122:56–64.
12. MacKenzie SA, Belcher LA, Sykes GP et al. Safety assessment of EPA-rich oil produced from yeast: Results of a 90-day subchronic toxicity study. *Regulatory Toxicology and Pharmacology* 2010; 58:490–500.
13. Zhao G, Etherton TD, Martin KR et al. Anti-inflammatory effects of polyunsaturated fatty acids in THP-1 cells. *Biochemical and Biophysical Research Communications* 2005; 336:909–917.
14. Zhang J, Grieger JA, Kris-Etherton PM et al. Walnut oil increases cholesterol efflux through inhibition of stearoyl CoA desaturase 1 in THP-1 macrophage-derived foam cells. *Nutrition and Metabolism* 2011; 8:61–74.

15. Francis GA, Fayard E, Picard F et al. Nuclear receptors and the control of metabolism. *Annual Review of Physiology* 2003; 65:261–311.
16. Sampath H, and Ntambi JM. Polyunsaturated fatty acid regulation of genes of lipid metabolism. *Annual Review of Nutrition* 2005; 25:317–340.
17. Schulman IG. Nuclear receptors as drug targets for metabolic disease. *Advance Drug Delivery Reviews* 2010; 62(13):1307–1315.
18. Quehenberger O, and Dennis EA. The human plasma lipidome. *New England Journal of Medicine* 2011; 365:1812–1823.
19. Holub BJ, Wlodek M, Rowe W et al. Correlation of omega-3 levels in serum phospholipids from 2053 human blood samples with key fatty acid ratios. *Nutrition Journal* 2009; 8:58. doi:10.1186/1475-2891-8-58.
20. Gillies PJ. Effect of a novel eicosapentaenoic acid-rich oil on serum cholesterol in man: Comparison to docosahexaenoic acid. *Presented at the 37th Annual Texas Human Nutrition Conference*, February 5, 2010, Texas A&M University, College Station, TX.
21. Dyerberg J, Madsen P, Moller JM et al. Bioavailability of marine n-3 fatty acids formulations. *Prostaglandins, Leukotrienes and Essential Fatty Acids* 2010; 83:137–141.
22. Neubronner J, Schuchardt JP, Kressel G et al. Enhanced increase of omega-3 index in response to long-term n-3 fatty acid supplementation from triacylglycerides versus ethyl esters. *European Journal of Clinical Nutrition* 2010; 65:247–254.
23. Oh SF, Pillai PS, Recchiuti A et al. Pro-resolving actions and stereoselective biosynthesis of 18S E-series resolvins in human leukocytes and murine inflammation. *Journal of Clinical Investigation* 2011; 121:569–581.
24. Boverhof DR, and Zacharewski TR. Toxicogenomics in risk assessment: Applications and needs. *Toxicological Sciences* 2006; 89:352–360.
25. Foster WR, Chen SJ, He A et al. A retrospective analysis of toxicogenomics in the safety assessment of drug candidates. *Toxicologic Pathology* 2007; 35:621–635.
26. Thompson K. Toxicogenomics and studies of genomic effects of dietary components. *World Review of Nutrition and Dietetics* 2010; 101:115–122.
27. MacKenzie SA, Belcher LA, Sykes GP et al. Safety assessment of EPA-rich oil produced from yeast: Results of a 90-day subchronic toxicity study. *Regulatory Toxicology and Pharmacology* 2010; 58:490–500.
28. Belcher LA, MacKenzie SA, Donner M et al. Safety assessment of EPA-rich triglyceride oil produced from yeast: Genotoxicity and 28-day oral toxicity in rats. *Regulatory Toxicology and Pharmacology* 2011; 59:53–63.
29. Vu-Dac N, Chopin-Delannoy S, Gervois P et al. The nuclear receptors peroxisome proliferator-activated receptor-α and rev-erbα mediate the species-specific regulation of apoliporotein A-1 expression by fibrates. *Journal of Biological Chemistry* 1998; 273:25713–25720.
30. Sugiyama E, Ishikawa Y, Li Y et al. Eicosapentaenoic acid lowers plasma and liver cholesterol levels in the presence of peroxisome proliferators-activated receptor alpha. *Life Sciences* 2008; 83:19–28.
31. Davidson MH. Mechanisms for the hypotriglyceridemic effect of marine omega-3 fatty acids. *American Journal of Cardiology* 2006; 98(suppl):27i–33i.
32. International Food Information Council Foundation. Functional Foods/Foods for Health Consumer Trending Survey Food and Health. 2009. Available at: http://www.foodinsight.org/Resources/Detail.aspx?topic=2009_Functional_Foods_For_Health_Consumer_Trending_Survey_executive_Summary (accessed May 22, 2011).
33. Glaser C, Heinrich J, and Koletzko B. Role of FADS1 and FADS2 polymorphisms in polyunsaturated fatty acid metabolism. *Metabolism* 2010; 59:993–999.
34. Rudkowska I, Caron-Dorval D, Verreault M et al. PPARalpha L162Vpolymorphism alters the potential of n-3 fatty acids to increase lipoprotein lipase activity. *Molecular Nutrition and Food Research* 2010; 54:543–550.

35. Zerhouni EA. Understanding the NIH "4P's of Medicine" Excerpt from FY2009 Director's Budget Request Statement, U.S. Department of Health and Human Services, National Institutes of Health. March 5, 2008.
36. Barker R. *2030 The Future of Medicine, Avoiding a Medical Meltdown.* Oxford University Press, Oxford, 2011.
37. Schaefer EJ, Asztalos IB, Gleason JA et al. Effects of eicosapentaenoic acid, docosahexaenoic acid, and olive oil on cardiovascular disease risk factors. *Circulation* 2010; 122:A20007.
38. Jacobson TA, Glickstein SB, Rowe JD et al. Effects of eicosapentaenoic acid and docosahexaenoic acid on low-density lipoprotein cholesterol and other lipids: A review. *Journal of Clinical Lipidology* 2012; 6:5–18.

Section II

Modifying Disease Risk through Nutrigenetics and Nutrigenomics

5 Modulating the Risk of Cardiovascular Disease through Nutrigenetics

Antonio Garcia-Rios, Javier Delgado-Lista, Pablo Perez-Martinez, Francisco Pérez-Jimenez, and Jose Lopez-Miranda

CONTENTS

INTRODUCTION

Cardiovascular diseases (CVDs) continue to be the major cause of morbidity and mortality in developed countries [1–3], and so our future understanding of their homeostasis and pathogenesis is an important factor when considering therapy and prevention targets. In this regard, it is well known that CVDs are a paradigm of multifactorial disorders related to genetic and modifiable risk factors (Figure 5.1). The influence of modifiable risk factors, such as smoking status, physical activity, and dietary intake, has been clearly established and nowadays, nobody questions the negative effect of tobacco, a sedentary lifestyle, or high-saturated fat diets. However, in clinical practice, it is not uncommon to find patients with premature CVD without any of these conventional risk factors. These situations are probably because of the influence of genetic factors, which could lead toward a susceptibility to atherosclerosis. Indeed, it is well known that genetic variations lead to phenotypic variations and that these variations on the key players involved in the process of atherosclerosis lead to changes in cellular response that accelerate, or predispose someone to, the development of CVD. Nowadays, the subject of genetic markers is one of the areas in which our understanding of the development and progression of CVD has been studied in greater depth over the past 10 years [4–6]. However, it is important to note that in our current knowledge about CVD, the role of genetic factors needs to be clarified and strengthened, so that they acquire the status they deserve inside of the cardiovascular risk factors.

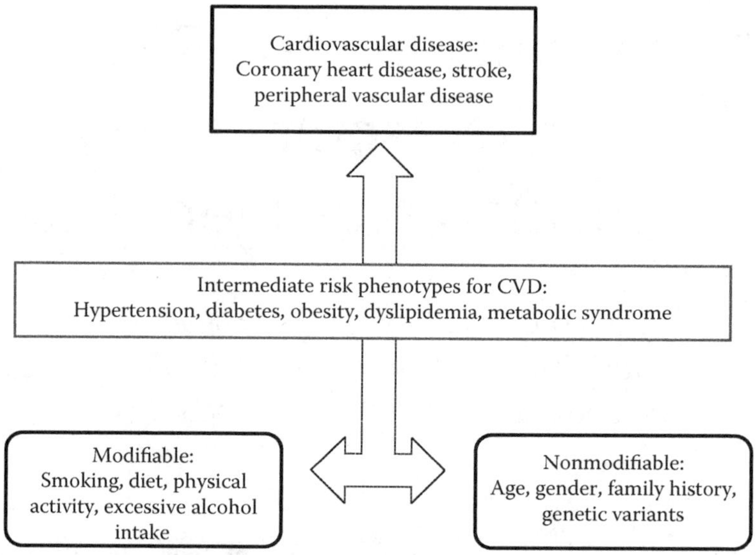

FIGURE 5.1 Cardiovascular risk factors.

In addition to their complex pathogenesis, enormous interindividual variability has been observed in both CVD and its intermediate risk factors. In this regard, it is very important to take into account another clue observed in the development of CVD—the interaction between genes and environmental factors, which influences the final clinical phenotype of this disease or some of its intermediate risk factors, such as lipid metabolism, hypertension (HTA), or glucose metabolism. Indeed, it has been shown that the interaction between genes and smoking can affect final plasma lipid concentrations in patients with familial hypercholesterolemia [7,8], and these findings could help to explain the differences in the susceptibility to coronary heart disease observed in these patients. In addition, findings of this kind may support the notion that interaction between genes and environment could explain the enormous variability in intermediate phenotypes linked to cardiovascular disorders, such as lipoprotein metabolism, plasma glucose, blood pressure (BP), or markers of inflammation and endothelial damage. Among environmental factors, diet and dietary fat can be considered to be the most important factors that can influence CVD [9]. Indeed, dietary modification continues to be a cornerstone in the prevention of metabolic disorders. However, it is well known that although general recommendations can explain general changes for a group of people, it is not possible to predict individual variations and that the effect of dietary changes on plasma marker concentrations differs significantly among individuals. Thus, the concept is being established that this variability in response is an intrinsic characteristic of the individual, rather than being the result of differing dietary compliance with experimental protocols. In this regard, the growing evidence derived from the study of gene–diet interactions has helped us to understand this variability over the past few years. Thus, nutrigenetics has emerged in the past decade to help us understand individual differences in the dietary response that may be related to the presence of individual genetic markers, such as single nucleotide polymorphisms (SNPs), or through the interaction between these genetic markers and dietary components. This knowledge could help in the prevention and treatment of metabolic diseases in high-risk population across of personalized nutrition [10–12].

In summary, the development of CVD is influenced not only by both environmental and genetic factors but also by the interaction between genes and environment, which can determine the intermediate risk phenotype for CVD or the presence of CVD itself and, at the same time, these interactions can provide the key to explaining the wide variability among individuals regarding CVD or intermediate risk phenotypes. Given that diet can be considered one of the most influential factors in the maintenance of homeostasis and a cornerstone in both prevention and therapy for CVD, this chapter discusses some evidence derived from the role of gene–nutrient interactions and how these interactions can modify the intermediate risk factors for CVDs, such as lipid metabolism and HTA. It also explores how this interaction can explain the variability observed in the development of those risk factors or CVD. The importance of nutrigenetics in obesity and diabetes will be discussed in other chapters of this book. All this knowledge together could help to pave the way for prevention of CVD as well as to develop personalized nutrition and individual therapy.

NUTRIGENETICS AND LIPID METABOLISM

Lipid metabolism is one of the most important determining factors in the development of chronic diseases worldwide, such as obesity, CVD, or metabolic syndrome (MetS). In this regard, lipid and lipoprotein metabolism is one of the areas in which more studies have been carried out to further our understanding of the development and progression of CVD disorders. Thus, growing evidence has shown that although universal recommendations about the control of lipid metabolism could be appropriate for the general population, there is wide variability in this area among individuals, related to a combination of environmental and genetic factors, as well as interaction between genes and environment (and, in particular, diet). Indeed, it has been shown that the presence of specific genetic variants or SNPs in key enzymes for lipid homeostasis can affect final concentrations in the main players of lipid metabolism, such as low-density cholesterol, high-density cholesterol, or triglycerides (TGs), and how their phenotypic manifestations may be modified by dietary intake.

In this regard, it has been clearly established that low-density lipoprotein cholesterol (LDL-C) concentrations are directly related to the development of CVD and subsequent death from this cause. Therefore, LDL-C remains a cornerstone in the treatment of dyslipidemia and the prevention of CVD [13]. However, it is well known that there is considerable heterogeneity in LDL-C levels among groups, probably as a result of a combination of genetic factors and gene–diet interaction (Table 5.1). A good example of this has been shown with apolipoprotein E (apoE), in which its role in lipid metabolism and cholesterol transport is well established. apoE presents three major isoforms (*APOE2*, *APOE3*, and *APOE4*) that differ in their affinity for binding to apoE and low-density lipoprotein receptors and thus their ability to influence lipid metabolism [14]. In this regard, a recent

TABLE 5.1
Evidence of Genetic Factors or Gene–Diet Interaction on Lipid Metabolism

Lipid Metabolism	Genes/Proteins [References]	Results
LDL-C	*APOE*/apoE [15–17]	Compared with *E3/E3* genotype, *E2* carriers had a 20% lower risk of coronary heart disease and *E4* carriers had a slightly higher risk. In addition, subjects with the *E2/E2* genotype had 31% lower mean of LDL-C concentrations than those with the *E4/E4* genotype [15]
		Carriers of the T allele for rs405509 SNP showed higher concentrations of apoB and LDL-C after a saturated diet compared with *GG* subjects [16]
		APOE genotypes could modulate the effect of habitual saturated fat on lipid metabolism in a population with an average habitual total fat intake of less than 30% [17]
HDL-C	LIPC/HL [20]	The-*514C/T* SNP interacts with dietary fat and determines HDL-C levels and subclasses of HDL-C, in which the T allele is associated with significantly greater HDL-C concentrations and large HDL-C size only in subjects consuming <30% of energy from fat
TG	LPL/LPL [24,25]	rs328 and rs1059611 SNPs have been related with changes in plasma lipid concentrations, mainly TRL, and interact with plasma *n*-6 polyunsaturated to modulate lipid metabolism [24]
		Carriers of the H1 allele (H1S447 and H1X447 genotypes) on rs320 SNP presented a lower postprandial lipemic response compared with H2S447 subjects [25]

meta-analysis that included 82 studies of lipid levels with 86,067 healthy participants and 121 studies of coronary outcomes with 37,850 cases and 82,727 controls found a very consistent relationship between *APOE* genotypes and LDL-C in coronary risk [15]. Compared with individuals with the most common *E3/E3* genotype, *E2* carriers had a 20% lower risk of coronary heart disease and *E4* carriers had a higher risk. Indeed, subjects with the *E2/E2* genotype had about 31% lower mean LDL-C concentrations than those with the *E4/E4* genotype, which could explain the differences in coronary risk. In short, carriers of the *APOE4* allele had a higher total and LDL-C plasma concentration and a greater coronary risk of myocardial infarction. However, it has been observed in clinical practice that not everyone with the *E4* allele develops CVD, and this fact suggests that other genetic or environmental factors must be involved, or that the interaction between them determines the final phenotype. In this context, it has been shown that the *APOE* gene promoter–*219G/T* SNP increases LDL-C levels and susceptibility to oxidation in response to a saturated fatty acid (SFA)-rich diet [16]. In this study, this particular SNP was genotyped in 55 healthy men with the *APOE3/E3* genotype who completed three dietary periods, each lasting 4 weeks. The first was a SFA-rich diet (38% fat-20% SFA and 12% monounsaturated fatty acid [MUFA] and 47% carbohydrates [CHO]), which was followed by a CHO-rich diet (30% fat-<10% SFA and 12% MUFA and 55% CHO) or a MUFA-rich diet (38% fat-<10% SFA and 22% MUFA and 47% CHO) in a randomized crossover design, in which all subjects followed each of the three diets. In this study, carriers of the T allele showed higher concentrations of apoB and LDL-C after the SFA diet compared with *GG* subjects. However, in carriers of the T allele, the decrease in concentrations of LDL-C and apoB was significantly greater when they changed from the saturated to the high-CHO diet, compared with *GG* subjects. Therefore, this particular SNP in the *APOE* gene could explain the differences in response to a diet among individuals. In addition, it has been shown that saturated fat intake can interact with *APOE* genotypes and modulate the final concentrations of lipoproteins. Ordovás and coworkers [17] studied these interactions in a population with 420 subjects. The *APOE* genotype was determined and the median saturated fat intake was used to divide the population into two groups: low saturated fat intake (mean intake 8.6% energy), and high saturated fat intake (mean intake 13.5%). They showed that although higher saturated fat intake was associated with higher very-low-density lipoprotein cholesterol (+29%) and lower high-density lipoprotein cholesterol (HDL-C) (−22%) in *APOE2* carriers, the opposite effect was observed in subjects with the *APOE4* genotype. They suggest that the *APOE* genotypes could modulate the effect of habitual saturated fat on lipid metabolism in a population with an average habitual total fat intake of less than 30%. This interaction between *APOE* genotypes and fat intake has been replicated later in a different population in which differences were found not only in lipid metabolism, but also in the risk of myocardial infarction [18]. Therefore, based on findings from different studies, there is clear evidence supporting the notion that the *APOE* locus could interact with dietary saturated fat, modifying plasma lipid concentrations, and also modifying CVD risk, which appears more evident in *E4* carriers.

Following on with independent risk factors for CVD in lipid metabolism, the inverse relation between HDL-C and the presence of CVD has been clearly established. HDL-C molecules serve to transport excess cholesterol to the liver and thus prevent CVD through their implication in reverse cholesterol transport (RCT) [19]. Therefore, the presence of genetic variations in the key players of the RCT pathway, as well as producing important gene–diet interactions, also contributes greatly to phenotypic variation in humans. A good example is the effect shown for the hepatic lipase (*LIPC*) gene on HDL-C concentrations. This gene encodes a key enzyme involved in RCT, and variability in the *LIPC* gene interacts with the intake of fat in diet and determines final HDL-C concentrations. Thus, it has been shown that the presence of the-*514C/T* SNP in the *LIPC* gene interacts with dietary fat and determines HDL-C levels and subclasses of HDL-C [20], in which the T allele is associated with significantly greater HDL-C concentrations and large HDL-C size only in subjects consuming <30% of energy from fat. This gene–nutrient interaction confirms previous findings in other populations [21] and could explain some of the findings that show no association between this particular SNP and HDL-C.

Finally, accumulated evidence suggests that TGs, in both fasting and postprandial states, are an independent risk factor for CVD [22,23]. However, it is well known that TG concentrations can vary among individuals, whether by a different response to diet, by the presence of genetic variations in key enzymes, or by the interaction between these genetic markers and diet. This fact has been shown for lipoprotein lipase (LPL), a key enzyme in the metabolism of triacylglycerol-rich lipoproteins (TRLs). Thus, two genetic variations at the *LPL* gene (rs328 and rs1059611) have been related with changes in plasma lipid concentrations, mainly TRL, and interact with plasma *n*-6 PUFA to modulate lipid metabolism [24]. In this study, plasma lipid concentrations and *LPL* SNPs were determined in 452 subjects with MetS in the European LIPGENE human study and were replicated in 1754 subjects from the LIPGENE-SU.VI.MAX study. Subject carriers for the minor allele for both SNPs were associated with lower TG and higher HDL-C concentrations. In addition, an interaction between genes and fatty acids was observed, in which carriers of the minor allele for both SNPs displayed a lower fasting TG and TRL concentrations only when they had *n*-6 polyunsaturated fatty acids. These results, provided from two independent studies, show that genetic variations at the *LPL* gene influence plasma TG concentrations and that this association may be influenced by the plasma fatty acid pattern. The importance of genetic variants at the *LPL* gene has also been studied during the postprandial state. Here, we investigated whether the association of *LPL Hin*dIII (H1/H2) and serine447-Stop (S447X) SNPs explained the interindividual variability observed during the postprandial state [25]. To do this, 51 healthy *APOE3/E3* male volunteers underwent a vitamin A fat-load test consisting of 1 g of fat/kg body weight and 60,000 IU of vitamin A. The meal provided 1 g fat and 7 mg cholesterol/kg body weight and contained 60% fat, 15% protein, and 25% CHO. After the meal, subjects were not allowed to consume any calorie-containing food for 11 h. Blood samples were taken before the meal, every hour until the sixth hour, and every second hour and 30 minutes until the eleventh hour. We found that carriers of the H1 allele (H1S447 and H1X447 genotypes) presented a lower postprandial lipemia response than subjects with the H2S447 genotype (homozygotes for the H2 allele of the *LPL Hin*dIII SNP and S447 allele). This is extremely significant, since the modifications observed in postprandial lipoprotein metabolism might be involved in the increased prevalence of coronary artery disease observed in subjects homozygous for the H2 allele of the *Hin*dIII SNP [26,27] and the lower risk of myocardial infarction associated with the H1X447 genotype [28].

In conclusion, it has been shown that the presence of genetic variations in the main key enzymes of lipid metabolism modifies final plasma lipid concentrations. In addition, the interaction between these genetic variants and dietary nutrients modifies final phenotypes and may explain the interindividual differences observed as regards diet. All these findings are of great importance, given that it has been clearly established that final concentrations of LDL-C, HDL-C, and TGs are independent risk factors for CVD.

NUTRIGENETICS AND HYPERTENSION

HTA is a major cardiovascular risk factor directly associated with the development of CVD. As we have explained previously for lipid metabolism, it is necessary to understand the complex mechanisms responsible for the control of BP to find the main factors involved in this control. Thus, it has been clearly established that environmental factors participate in the control of BP, of which diet is probably the key factor in the control and treatment of HTA. Indeed, alterations in diet are the first step and the most important changes in lifestyle recommended in the treatment. In addition, over the past 10 years we have learned more about the influence of genetic factors in the control of BP. Thus, an important locus has been discovered that can influence the control of BP and can predispose us to developing or becoming susceptible to HTA [29,30]. This is of major importance because it provides new insights in the control of BP and may help to develop new targets for the treatment of HTA. However, as the focus of the current chapter is CVD and lipid metabolism, it is important to note that the control of BP is influenced not only by genetic variants but also by the interaction between those genetic markers and environmental factors, mainly gene–diet interactions, which can influence the final clinical phenotype of this disease.

In this regard, it has been shown that some specific genetic variations known to affect metabolic disorders can influence the control of BP and how their final phenotype may be modified by dietary intake (Table 5.2). One example is the *TCF7L2* gene, a subgroup of T-cell-specific transcription factors, as major genetic predictors for the development of type 2 diabetes mellitus [31,32] but with other implications discovered in metabolic disorders such as HTA [33]. Thus, Delgado-Lista et al. have shown that the presence of determined genetic variants at *TCF7L2* gene (rs7903146 and rs17685538 SNPs) can influence BP. Thus, homozygotes for the major allele of rs7903146 showed higher diastolic BP than heterozygotes and minor allele homozygotes and showed a similar trend for systolic BP. In addition, homozygotes for the major allele of rs17685538 showed lower diastolic BP than heterozygotes. This last SNP, the rs17685538, had a low frequency for minor allele homozygotes and this could imply that the increased BP observed in the minor allele carriers may

TABLE 5.2
Evidence of Genetic Factors or Gene–Diet Interactions on HTA

Genes [Reference]	Results
TCF7L2 [33]	rs7903146 and rs17685538 SNPs can influence BP. Homozygotes for the major allele of rs7903146 showed higher diastolic BP than heterozygotes and minor allele homozygotes and showed a similar trend for systolic BP. In addition, homozygotes for the major allele of rs17685538 showed lower diastolic BP than heterozygotes. However, the higher diastolic BP found in carriers of the minor allele of rs17685538 was limited to those with higher plasma SFA concentrations
β2-AR [34]	β2-AR G46A polymorphism is associated with increased BP responsiveness to the DASH diet and altered activation of the RAAS

be responsible for an evolutionary disadvantage that may be greater in homozygotes. Moreover, this study showed an interesting interaction between this SNP and dietary SFAs, in which the higher diastolic BP found in carriers of the minor allele of rs17685538 was limited to those with higher plasma SFA concentrations [33].

Another specific locus for HTA has been studied. Here, genetic variations of the β2-adrenergic receptor (β2-AR) gene have been linked to salt sensitivity and low plasma renin activity. In addition, specific gene–diet interactions have been shown for this locus, such as that observed between the dietary approaches to stop hypertension (DASH) dietary pattern and genotype status at β2-AR G46A SNP [34]. This study showed significant gene–diet interactions for changes in systolic BP and an association between the A allele of βAR G46A and greater BP reduction and plasma renin activity responses to the DASH diet. With this study, the authors have shown that β2-AR G46A polymorphism is associated with increased BP responsiveness to the DASH diet and altered activation of the renin–angiotensin–aldosterone system (RAAS), which suggests that there is an interaction of this genotype with renin release. These findings are greatly significant, given that β2-AR could be considered as a genetic modifier of diet response.

In conclusion, the information we know about the importance of diet in the control of BP, together with the recent findings of a new genetic locus that influences BP and our understanding of the interactions between these loci and diet, may help to further our knowledge of the pathogenesis of HTA and thus help to develop new therapeutic strategies.

FUTURE DIRECTIONS AND CONCLUSIONS

The main objective of cardiovascular risk modification is to avoid the presence of coronary artery disease, stroke, or peripheral vascular disease, as well as to maintain good health and increase life expectancy. To achieve this, first, it is important to recognize the key players that influence the development of CVD and, second, to try to control them. It is well known that CVDs are a paradigm of multifactorial disorders related to genetic and modifiable risk factors as well as the interaction between both factors. With genetic factors, nowadays, we are discovering more and more loci with potential influence on CVD or intermediate risk phenotypes, but these new targets need to be clarified in the future. However, with respect to modifiable risk factors, everyone recognizes, and no one questions, the importance of smoking, physical activity, or diet as determinant risk factors for CVD, as well as intermediate risk factors such as HTA, blood lipid profile, glucose metabolism, or obesity. However, it is also known that although general recommendations about those factors, mainly diet, can help a group of people, it is not possible to predict individual responses or interindividual differences with respect to the same pattern of diet to prevent or treat CVD. In this regard, we have found great support in nutrigenetics, as we have learned more about how specific genetic variations and the interaction between these genetic modifications and the environment (in particular dietary intake) influence overall CVD risk factors, as well as the final phenotype of the manifestations of CVD. Therefore, it is important to recognize this new approach, in which certain genetic polymorphisms affect CVD risk factors and how their phenotypic manifestations may be modified by dietary intake. Taking into account this new knowledge may help us to understand the interindividual variability observed in intermediate risk factors, such as lipid metabolism or HTA, and in the development of CVD. However, the most important point is that with this new knowledge, it could be possible to provide individuals with dietary guidance specifically tailored to their genetic map.

However, we need to be cautious before drawing general conclusions, since the current evidence about new genetic markers or gene–diet interactions is extracted from studies with a wide heterogeneity in number of subjects, diet composition, duration of dietary intervention, and statistical methods of analysis. Therefore, although the basis of this complex knowledge has been clearly established by current evidence, it is time to build strong, well-established foundations. To achieve this, replication studies are urgently required to achieve greater consistency in the conclusions drawn from the results, mainly in the study of the interaction between nutritional and genetic factors in dietary intervention studies. In this context, it is important to use large sample sizes and a range of ethnicities and to standardize the design of future studies, for which it is necessary to homogenize nutritional information and the measure of potential confounding factors that could have some influence, such as gender, age, body mass index, smoking, or physical activity. In addition, there are numerous studies about intermediate risk factors, such as lipid metabolism and HTA, as final outcomes and it is necessary to carry out more studies with specific outcomes in cardiovascular end points (coronary heart disease, stroke, or peripheral vascular disease) [35]. Finally, it will be necessary to know more about the influence of epigenetics, since the final assembly of the coded proteins and their functionality, as well as the post-transcriptional changes applied to them, may exert a great influence on their final effects.

In conclusion, over the past few years we have advanced in our knowledge of the pathogenesis of CVDs. We already know a lot about the influence of modifiable risk factors such as diet, but this is not enough in clinical practice. Nowadays, we must venture beyond that point. Advances in the understanding of new genetic markers, as well as the interaction between these genetic factors and diet, are helping us to predict individual responses and to clarify the differences in response among individuals. It is still in the early days, but we are progressing toward what in the future will become personalized strategies in the prevention and treatment of CVDs.

REFERENCES

1. Allender S, Peto V, Scarborough P, Boxer A, Rayner M. *Coronary Heart Disease Statistics*. 2007. London: British Heart Foundation.
2. O'Flaherty M, Ford E, Allender S, Scarborough P, Capewell S. Coronary heart disease trends in England and Wales from 1984 to 2004: Concealed levelling of mortality rates among young adults. *Heart*. 2008;94:178–181.
3. Lloyd-Jones DM, Hong Y, Labarthe D, Mozaffarian D, Appel LJ, VanHorn L, Greenlund K et al. Defining and setting national goals for cardiovascular health promotion and disease reduction: The American Heart Association's strategic impact goal through 2020 and beyond. *Circulation*. 2010;121(4):586–613.
4. Ioannidis JP. Prediction of cardiovascular disease outcomes and established cardiovascular risk factors by genome-wide association markers. *Circ. Cardiovasc. Genet.* 2009;2(1):7–15.

5. Ding K, Kullo IJ. Genome-wide association studies for atherosclerotic vascular disease and its risk factors. *Circ. Cardiovasc. Genet.* 2009;2(1):63–72.
6. Govindaraju DR, Cupples LA, Kannel WB, O'Donnell CJ, Atwood LD, D'Agostino RB Sr, Fox CS et al. Genetics of the Framingham Heart Study population. *Adv. Genet.* 2008;62:33–65.
7. Garcia-Rios A, Perez-Martinez P, Mata P, Fuentes F, Lopez-Miranda J, Alonso R, Caballero J, Mata N, Perez-Jimenez F, Ordovas JM. Polymorphism at the TRIB1 gene modulates plasma lipid levels: Insight from the Spanish familial hypercholesterolemia cohort study. *Nutr. Metab. Cardiovasc. Dis.* 2011;21(12):957–63.
8. Garcia-Rios A, Perez-Martinez P, Fuentes F, Mata P, Lopez-Miranda J, Alonso R, Rodriguez F et al. Genetic variations at ABCG5/G8 genes modulate plasma lipid concentrations in patients with familial hypercholesterolemia. *Atherosclerosis.* 2010;210(2):486–92.
9. Phillips CM, Goumidi L, Bertrais S, Field MR, Ordovas JM, Cupples LA, Defoort C et al. Leptin receptor polymorphisms interact with polyunsaturated fatty acids to augment risk of insulin resistance and metabolic syndrome in adults. *J. Nutr.* 2010;140(2):238–44.
10. Perez-Martinez P, Delgado-Lista J, Garcia-Rios A, Ferguson JF, Gulseth HL, Williams CM, Karlström B et al. Calpain-10 interacts with plasma saturated fatty acid concentrations to influence insulin resistance in individuals with the metabolic syndrome. *Am. J. Clin. Nutr.* 2011;93(5):1136–41.
11. Smith CE, Ordovás JM. Fatty acid interactions with genetic polymorphisms for cardiovascular disease. *Curr. Opin. Clin. Nutr. Metab. Care.* 2010;13(2):139–44.
12. Ordovas JM, Shen J. Gene-environment interactions and susceptibility to metabolic syndrome and other chronic diseases. *J. Periodontol.* 2008;79(8 Suppl):1508–13.
13. Expert Panel on Detection, Evaluation, and Treatment of High Blood Cholesterol in Adults. Executive summary of the third report of the National Cholesterol Education Program (NCEP) expert panel on detection, evaluation, and treatment of high blood cholesterol in adults (Adult treatment panel III). *JAMA.* 2001;285:2486–97.
14. Anoop S, Misra A, Meena K, Luthra K. Apolipoprotein E polymorphism in cerebrovascular & coronary heart diseases. *Indian J. Med. Res.* 2010;132:363–78.
15. Bennet AM, DiAngelantonio E, Ye Z, Wensley F, Dahlin A, Ahlbom A, Keavney B et al. Association of apolipoprotein E genotypes with lipid levels and coronary risk. *JAMA.* 200719;298(11):1300–11.
16. Moreno JA, Pérez-Jiménez F, Marín C, Gómez P, Pérez-Martínez P, Moreno R, Bellido C, Fuentes F, López-Miranda J. Apolipoprotein E gene promoter -219G->T polymorphism increases LDL-cholesterol concentrations and susceptibility to oxidation in response to a diet rich in saturated fat. *Am. J. Clin. Nutr.* 2004;80(5):1404–9.
17. Campos H, D'Agostino M, Ordovás JM. Gene-diet interactions and plasma lipoproteins: Role of apolipoprotein E and habitual saturated fat intake. *Genet. Epidemiol.* 2001;20(1):117–28.
18. Yang Y, Ruiz-Narvaez E, Kraft P, Campos H. Effect of apolipoprotein E genotype and saturated fat intake on plasma lipids and myocardial infarction in the Central Valley of Costa Rica. *Hum. Biol.* 2007;79(6):637–47.
19. Miller G, Miller N. Plasma high density lipoprotein concentration and development of ischaemic heart disease. *Lancet* 1975;1(7897):16.
20. Ordovas JM, Corella D, Demissie S, Cupples LA, Couture P, Coltell O, Wilson PW, Schaefer EJ, Tucker KL. Dietary fat intake determines the effect of a common polymorphism in the hepatic lipase gene promoter on high-density lipoprotein metabolism: Evidence of a strong dose effect in this gene-nutrient interaction in the Framingham Study. *Circulation.* 2002;106(18):2315–21.

21. Couture P, Otvos JD, Cupples LA, Lahoz C, Wilson PW, Schaefer EJ, Ordovas JM. Association of the C-514T polymorphism in the hepatic lipase gene with variations in lipoproteins subclass profiles: The Framingham Offspring Study. *Arterioscler. Thromb. Vasc. Biol.* 2000;20(3):815–22.
22. Le NA, Walter MF. The role of hypertriglyceridemia in atherosclerosis. *Curr. Atheroscler. Rep.* 2007;9:110–5.
23. Perez-Martinez P, Garcia-Rios A, Delgado-Lista J, Perez-Jimenez F, Lopez-Miranda J. Nutrigenetics of the postprandial lipoprotein metabolism: Evidences from human intervention studies. *Curr. Vasc. Pharmacol.* 2011;9(3):287–91.
24. Garcia-Rios A, Delgado-Lista J, Perez-Martinez P, Phillips CM, Ferguson JF, Gjelstad IMF, Williams CM et al. Genetic variations at the lipoprotein lipase gene influence plasma lipid concentrations and interact with plasma n-6 polyunsaturated fatty acids to modulate lipid metabolism. *Atherosclerosis.* 2011;218(2):416–22.
25. López-Miranda J, Cruz G, Gómez P, Marín C, Paz E, Pérez-Martínez P, Fuentes FJ, Ordovas JM, Pérez-Jiménez F. The influence of lipoprotein lipase gene variation on postprandial lipoprotein metabolism. *J. Clin. Endocrinol. Metab.* 2004;89(9):4721–8.
26. Mattu RK, Needham EW, Morgan R, Rees A, Hackshaw AK, Stocks J, Elwood PC, Galton DJ. DNA variants at the LPL gene locus associate with angiographically defined severity of atherosclerosis and serum lipoprotein levels in a Welsh population. *Arterioscler. Thromb.* 1994;14(7):1090–7.
27. Thorn JA, Chamberlain JC, Alcolado JC, Oka K, Chan L, Stocks J, Galton DJ. Lipoprotein and hepatic lipase gene variants in coronary atherosclerosis. *Atherosclerosis.* 1990;85(1):55–60.
28. Humphries SE, Nicaud V, Margalef J, Tiret L, Talmud PJ. Lipoprotein lipase gene variation is associated with a paternal history of premature coronary artery disease and fasting and postprandial plasma triglycerides: The European Atherosclerosis Research Study (EARS). *Arterioscler. Thromb. Vasc. Biol.* 1998;18(4):526–34.
29. International Consortium for Blood Pressure Genome-Wide Association Studies, Ehret GB, Munroe PB, Rice KM, Bochud M, Johnson AD, Chasman DI et al. Genetic variants in novel pathways influence blood pressure and cardiovascular disease risk. *Nature.* 2011;478(7367):103–9.
30. Kato N, Takeuchi F, Tabara Y, Kelly TN, Go MJ, Sim X, Tay WT et al. Meta-analysis of genome-wide association studies identifies common variants associated with blood pressure variation in East Asians. *Nat. Genet.* 2011;43(6):531–8.
31. Grant SF, Thorleifsson G, Reynisdottir I, Benediktsson R, Manolescu A, Sainz J, Helgason A et al. Variant of transcription factor 7-like 2 (TCF7L2) gene confers risk of type 2 diabetes. *Nat. Genet.* 2006;38(3):320–3.
32. Tabara Y, Osawa H, Kawamoto R, Onuma H, Shimizu I, Miki T, Kohara K, Makino H. Replication study of candidate genes associated with type 2 diabetes based on genome-widescreening. *Diabetes.* 2009;58(2):493–8.
33. Delgado-Lista J, Perez-Martinez P, García-Rios A, Phillips CM, Williams CM, Gulseth HL, Helal O et al. Pleiotropic effects of TCF7L2 gene variants and its modulation in the metabolic syndrome: From the LIPGENE study. *Atherosclerosis.* 2011;214(1):110–6.
34. Sun B, Williams JS, Svetkey LP, Kolatkar NS, Conlin PR. Beta2-adrenergic receptor genotype affects the renin-angiotensin-aldosterone system response to the dietary approaches to stop hypertension (DASH) dietary pattern. *Am. J. Clin. Nutr.* 2010; 92(2):444–9.
35. Do R, Xie C, Zhang X, Männistö S, Harald K, Islam S, Bailey SD et al. The effect of chromosome 9p21 variants on cardiovascular disease may be modified by dietary intake: Evidence from a case/control and a prospective study. *PLoS Med.* 2011;9(10):e1001106.

6 Modulating the Risk of Obesity and Diabetes through Nutrigenetics

Helen M. Roche and Catherine Phillips

CONTENTS

INTRODUCTION

The increasing incidence of obesity is the single most important determinant of the global pandemic of metabolic syndrome (MetS) and type 2 diabetes mellitus (T2DM), the combination of which is often referred to as diabesity. Nutrition and physical activity are key environmental factors, which potentially interact with genetic predisposition to promote the progression and pathogenesis of these combined environmental and polygenic, diet-related diseases. Excessive caloric intake and sedentary lifestyle promote the obese phenotype. More than half of adults in Europe and the United States are overweight or obese, leading to MetS, which in turn greatly enhances subsequent risk of T2DM and cardiovascular disease (CVD) [1].

It is estimated that 60%–90% of diabetes is directly related to obesity or weight gain [2]. There is no doubt that a genetic component can also impact on the risk of insulin resistance and type 2 diabetes, sensitivity to which may be further amplified by poor diet. Conversely, if we have a greater understanding of potential gene–nutrient interactions, then it may be possible to manipulate diet in such a way to minimize the metabolic risk of obesity, to attenuate insulin resistance and T2DM. Figure 6.1 illustrates that the pathway between obesity and insulin resistance, toward MetS and T2DM, represents a progressive phenotype. Some individuals may have a greater genetic sensitivity or predisposition toward obesity and diabetes, as reviewed later. But the combination of metabolic stress (including excessive energy intake, low physical activity, saturated fatty acids [SFAs], etc.) and a heightened inflammatory state accelerates the progression toward insulin resistance and diabetes.

With increasing obesity, adipose tissue loses optimal functionality. The exact molecular mechanisms that lead to loss of optimal adipose tissue function in obesity

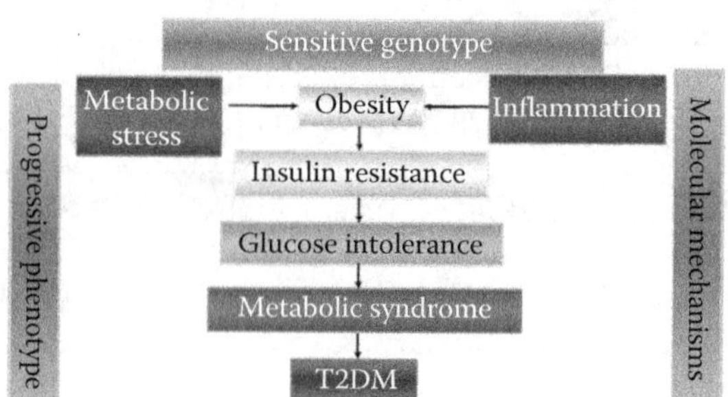

FIGURE 6.1 Development and progression of diabesity, link between obesity, MetS, and diabetes. (Adapted from Roche, H.M., *Proc Nut Soc*, 64, 23, 2005. With permission.)

promoting diabetes are not fully elucidated. Substantial evidence points toward adipose tissue inflammation as a key etiological factor in the development of insulin resistance and T2DM. Immune cell recruitment into adipose tissue begins with infiltration with T cells [3,4] followed by recruitment of proinflammatory macrophages [5,6]. Adipose-derived cytokines including tumor necrosis factor alpha (TNF-α), interleukin-6 (IL-6), and interleukin-1β (IL-1β) are well-characterized insulin desensitizing agents [7–9], and lack of key inflammatory molecules/receptors including TNF-α, IκB kinase, toll-like receptor-4 (TLR4), and IL-1 receptor 1 [10–13] protect against obesity-induced insulin resistance. Other important processes relate to a combination of (1) lipotoxicity associated with ectopic fat deposition, (2) endoplasmic reticulum stress, (3) oxidative stress and altered reactive oxygen species production, and (4) mitochondrial dysfunction [14,15]. The culmination of all these results in peripheral insulin resistance, wherein insulin-responsive tissues such as skeletal muscle and liver lose optimal functionality, followed by suboptimal pancreatic function that leads to glucose intolerance that precedes MetS and overt diabetes [16].

There are some individuals who seem exceptionally resilient to the adverse effects of obesity, who despite being overweight are "inappropriately" healthy for their degree of obesity. Indeed, it has been shown that obese but metabolically healthy individuals lack the enhanced inflammatory response associated with obesity [17], mediated via cytokines including IL-1β, IL-6, and TNF-α, promoted by transcription factors including extracellular signal-regulated kinase and nuclear factor kappa-light-chain-enhancer of activated B cells, which are important effectors that promote insulin resistance. The challenge for nutrigenomics is to understand the molecular mechanisms that explain the differences between equally obese but insulin-resistant versus insulin-sensitive individuals, which may be ascribed to differences in genetic susceptibility and/or differences in sensitivity versus resilience against the metabolic and inflammatory stressors that coexist with obesity. This, in turn, could provide important insights into the mechanistic link between adipose tissue expansion and risk of diabetes. From the dietary advice perspective, a deeper understanding of the underlying nutrient-sensitive molecular mechanisms to aid understanding of the link between nutrition and health will provide the platform to defining whether more targeted nutritional advice is an appropriate public health approach.

GENETIC PREDISPOSITION TO OBESITY, DIABETES, AND THE METABOLIC SYNDROME

Although the current global diabesity pandemic is being driven by an obesogenic environment created through industrialization and modernization, which in turn has resulted in more sedentary lifestyles and freely available caloric abundance, it is also clear that this trend is facilitated by an individuals' genetic predisposition to excessive weight gain. Obesity and diabetes are common, complex multifactorial conditions with high heritability. The familial clustering associated with obesity is not just because of common environmental factors. Studies of twins, adoptees, and families indicate that up to 80% of the variance in body mass index (BMI) is attributable to genetic factors. High relative risk ratios [18] and concordance rates for monozygotic twins compared to dizygotic twins have also been estimated for obesity

[19]. Interestingly, adoption studies revealed that adoptees' weight is more similar to that of the biological parents than the adoptive parents [20]. Heritability rates of 25%–40% for BMI and body fat [20–22] and 10%–30% for MetS have been estimated [23,24], indicating that these conditions are partly heritable. Genetic factors are estimated to contribute approximately 50% toward T2DM risk. Family studies have shown that first-degree relatives of individuals with T2DM are approximately three times more likely to develop the disease than individuals without a positive family history of the disease [25,26]. Furthermore, twin studies have shown that concordance rates for monozygotic twins, ranging from 60% to 90%, are significantly higher than those for dizygotic twins. Thus, it is clear that obesity, MetS, and diabetes have a strong genetic component. However, the genetics of these conditions have been difficult to study owing to their wide phenotypic variability. For example, obese phenotypes range from overweight to morbid obesity, with and without insulin resistance and other metabolic perturbations, and include differences in body fat distribution. Depending on the MetS criteria used to define the condition, MetS individuals may have at least 3–5 or 6 metabolic abnormalities, and the age of onset of these conditions varies among individuals.

Monogenic and Polygenic Forms of Obesity and Diabetes

Animal models and family studies have been useful in identifying rare monogenic forms of obesity and diabetes and thus important pathways and candidate genes. Six genes account for the majority of the monogenic forms of diabetes: hepatic nuclear factor 4α (*HNF-4α*), glucokinase (*GCK*), *HNF-1α*, insulin promoter factor-1 (*IPF-1*), *HNF-1β*, and neuroD1 transcription factor (*NEUROD1*) [26]. Over the past 15–20 years, mutations in a number of genes including leptin (*LEP*), leptin receptor (*LEPR*), pro-opiomelanocortin (*POMC*), and melanocortin-4 receptor (*MC4R*) have been associated with monogenic obesity [27]. However for most individuals, genetic predisposition to obesity, MetS, and T2DM has a polygenic basis. The absence of large single-gene effects and the detection of multiple small effects support this notion, which suggests that only in combination with other predisposing variants does a sizeable phenotypic effect arise. In addition, this implies that certain sets of polygenic variants relevant to these conditions in one individual may not be the same in another individual.

Approaches to Identify Genetic Determinants of Disease

Identifying genes associated with any complex trait involves a range of experimental strategies, including positional cloning using genome-wide linkage analysis, candidate gene association, and more recently, genome-wide association analysis. With the advent of high-throughput genetic analysis and the completion of the Human Genome Project, our understanding of the genetic architecture and biology of common diet-related polygenic disorders including obesity and T2DM is improving. Genome-wide association studies (GWAS) represent a powerful approach to the identification of genes involved in common polygenic diseases such as obesity and T2DM. This analysis is performed without any prior knowledge regarding the nature or location of the causative gene(s). Typically, these studies analyze hundreds of thousands of single nucleotide polymorphisms (SNPs) across the entire genome and involve very large subject numbers. Patterns of association between genotypes and disease status are then identified and evaluated statistically. In the past 5 years, GWAS have identified a number of novel loci relevant to obesity and diabetes. Prior to high-throughput, large-scale, whole-genome-wide studies, genome scanning by positional cloning and the candidate gene approach have been the traditional techniques for identification of genes associated with obesity, T2DM, and MetS. The positional cloning approach allows identification of genes without any previous knowledge of biological function or the disease mechanism. This method involves mapping the susceptibility or causative loci purely on their chromosomal location using multigenerational pedigrees and/or a large number of sibling pairs. In contrast, the hypothesis-driven candidate gene approach identifies genes according to biological function and/or linkage studies and association tests for significant differences in their allele frequencies between a patient group and a control population. In terms of obesity, MetS, and diabetes, given the different physiologies and metabolic pathways involved that produce the same apparent disease, it is immediately obvious that the number of potential candidate genes is very large. Varying degrees of success have been achieved for each approach in terms of defining genetic determinants of diabesity. Some of the most pertinent findings are presented.

Transcription Factor 7-Like 2

The year 2006 heralded the identification of the most important T2DM susceptibility gene known so far, transcription factor 7-like 2 (*TCF7L2*). Two novel SNPs in the Wnt signaling regulated *TCF7L2* gene were associated with increased T2DM risk [28,29], most likely through defective β-cell function and impaired insulin secretion [28]. Several large studies subsequently replicated and confirmed the association with T2DM risk in various populations and the *TCF7L2* rs7903146 SNP has emerged as one of the most important T2DM susceptibility gene variants known to date [30–35]. TCF7L2 polymorphisms have also been associated with the MetS components such as dyslipidemia and waist circumference [36,37]. However, prospective and population-based MetS association studies have produced conflicting results, with some reporting an association with MetS, hyperglycemia, impaired insulin secretion, and hypertriglyceridemia [37,38] while others found no association with MetS or insulin resistance [39,40]. More recently, *TCF7L2* rs7903146 was associated with increased MetS risk, arising from their impaired insulin sensitivity, greater insulin resistance, and increased abdominal obesity and hypertension [41]. This association has also been confirmed in a recent systematic review [42].

Fat Mass and Obesity-Associated Gene

Following the identification of TCF7L2, previously unknown genetic variants in the fat mass and obesity-associated (*FTO*) gene on chromosome 16 were also linked to T2DM risk through an effect on BMI [43], such that the 16% of adults homozygous for the rs9939609 "risk" A allele were 3 kg heavier and had 1.7-fold increased risk of obesity relative to the homozygous nonrisk allele carriers. It has been suggested that the impaired satiety, greater food intake, and more frequent loss of eating control reported by individuals with at least one risk allele may account for the observed increased obesity risk [44–46]. Importantly, researchers have shown increased obesity risk associated with this polymorphism from childhood into old age [43]. A number of large studies replicated and confirmed the association with obesity risk in European populations [47–49] and the *FTO* rs9939609 SNP is now recognized as one of the most important gene variants predisposing to obesity. Furthermore, a recent systematic review on the genetics of MetS confirmed increased MetS risk with *FTO* [42].

Calpain 10

Genome scanning in several different ethnic groups has identified a number of chromosome regions harboring T2DM and obesity susceptibility genes. Calpain 10 (*CAPN10*), which encodes the cysteine protease calpain 10, was the first T2DM susceptibility gene identified through a genome-wide scan followed by positional cloning [50]. Genetic and functional data indicate that *CAPN10* plays an important role in insulin resistance and intermediate phenotypes [51]. *CAPN10* variants have been linked with several MetS phenotypes including hypertriglyceridemia, BMI, and hypertension [52–54].

Proinflammatory Cytokines

Obesity is a chronic low-grade inflammatory state that is associated with increased risk for MetS, diabetes, and CVD. Promoter region genetic variants of the proinflammatory cytokines *TNF-α* (rs1800629) and *IL-6* (rs1800795 and rs1800797) have also been linked to increased risk of diabetes and MetS phenotypes [55–59], although results have been inconsistent [60,61]. Such inconsistencies may be, in part, explained by the fact that as cytokines act in a complex network, single-gene activity may not provide full insight into the role of cytokine genes in MetS. In a recent MetS case–control study, *TNF-α* rs1800629 major G allele homozygotes and lymphotoxin α (LTA) rs915654 minor A allele carriers had 20%–40% higher risk of MetS [62]. The combined effect of carrying both risk genotypes, which represent half of this population, further increased MetS risk probably attributable to their greater risk of abdominal obesity. Interestingly, this additive effect was further influenced by the presence of *IL-6* rs1800797 G allele. Risk genotype carriers who were also homozygous for the *IL-6* rs1800797 G allele were most at risk of developing MetS (odds ratio [OR] 2.10), fasting hyperglycemia (OR 2.65), and abdominal obesity (OR 1.52).

Signal Transducer and Activator of Transcription 3

Signal transducer and activator of transcription 3 (STAT3) is a transcription factor released during the acute-phase response wherein it is activated by cytokines, such as IL-6 [63]. Animal studies initially highlighted the importance of STAT3 in body weight regulation and normal glucose homeostasis [64–69]. However, few human studies have been performed to examine genetic associations and results have been inconsistent [70,71], perhaps because of gender differences, sample size, and genetic heterogeneity of the populations studied. Common genetic variants at the *STAT3* locus have recently been associated with increased risk of abdominal obesity [72]. As individual genetic variants generally confer only a moderate risk to a trait, analyzing multiple risk alleles simultaneously can be more informative and enhance predictive power [73], particularly in polygenic conditions. A significant genotype effect between the number of risk alleles and risk of abdominal obesity was identified, with approximately a 2.5-fold increased risk in individuals carrying more than two risk alleles compared to individuals carrying one or fewer risk alleles [73].

Adiponectin

Adiponectin (*ADIPOQ*) is an adipokine that is abundantly expressed in adipose tissue and sensitizes the body to insulin, thus it is a good candidate gene for obesity, MetS, and T2DM. Levels of circulating adiponectin are reduced in obese and T2DM subjects [74]. Associations have been found between a number of polymorphisms in *ADIPOQ* and its receptors *ADIPOR1* and *ADIPOR2* with adiponectin levels, insulin resistance, and MetS phenotypes [75,76].

Complement Component 3

Complement component 3 (*C3*) is another potential candidate gene with respect to inflammation and diabesity. Elevated concentrations of C3, a protein with a central role in the innate immune system, have been associated with insulin resistance, obesity, MetS, and diabetes [77–80]. In keeping with previous findings, a dose-dependent relationship between C3 concentrations and the number of MetS components were identified in the LIPGENE-SU.VI.MAX study, indicating that elevated proinflammatory status is associated with increased MetS risk [81]. Furthermore, examination of associations between *C3* polymorphisms and MetS risk showed that common genetic variants at the *C3* locus were associated with risk of MetS and its phenotypes, including dyslipidemia, abdominal obesity, and insulin sensitivity [81].

Peroxisome Proliferator-Activated Receptor-γ

Dyslipidemia is one of the very early features of an obese or MetS phenotype and frequently precedes metabolic disturbances in insulin and glucose homeostasis. A number of lipid-sensitive transcription factors, including peroxisome proliferator-activated receptor-γ (PPARγ), have been implicated in the development of these conditions. *PPARγ* is a good candidate gene for obesity, MetS, and T2DM because of its multiple roles in adipocyte differentiation, fatty acid metabolism, insulin sensitivity, and glucose homeostasis. Prior to the GWAS era, the *PPARγ* Pro12Ala polymorphism had been identified as the most widely reproduced genetic variation for the risk of T2DM [25]. The original study investigating the polymorphism in T2DM showed that the alanine allele of the Pro12Ala polymorphism was associated with lower BMI, improved insulin sensitivity, and thus reduced diabetes risk by 75% [82]. Inconsistent results from subsequent association studies prompted a meta-analysis that confirmed a modest (1.25-fold) but significant increase in diabetes risk for the Pro12Pro genotype [83]. The Pro12Pro genotype also predicts conversion from impaired glucose tolerance to T2DM with a threefold increased risk of developing diabetes in the Pro12 homozygotes compared to 12Ala carriers [84]. In obese subjects, diabetes risk is almost doubled among the Pro12 allele carriers. Interestingly, the obese phenotype seems to exacerbate the detrimental effect of the PPARγ Pro12 allele on insulin sensitivity [85]. Perhaps, more importantly is that this variant is very common in most populations. Approximately 98% of Europeans carry at least one copy of the Pro allele, so it is reasonable to speculate that this SNP contributes to a considerable proportion of T2DM risk.

GENETIC DETERMINANTS OF DIABESITY: CONCLUDING THOUGHTS

A major role for genetic susceptibility to obesity, T2DM, and MetS has been identified. However, regardless of the approach used, gene–disease association studies are fraught with difficulties including lack of replication, inadequate statistical power, multiple hypothesis testing, population stratification, publication bias, and phenotypic differences. It is becoming increasingly evident that the identification of true genetic associations in common multifactorial conditions, such as these diet-related conditions, requires large studies consisting of thousands rather than hundreds of subjects. Also, the absence of large single-gene effects and the detection of multiple small effects accentuate the need for the study of larger populations to reliably identify the size of the effect now expected for complex diseases. There is no doubt that development of high-density arrays that permit the genotyping of hundreds of thousands of polymorphisms in very large populations will rapidly advance our understanding of the genetic basis of T2DM, MetS, and obesity. Indeed, the discovery of associated variants in unsuspected genes and outside coding regions illustrates the ability of GWAS to provide potentially important clues into the pathogenesis of these common conditions. However, considering the limited success in confirming polygenic variants for diabesity to date, it is obvious that more polygenic variants await discovery. Furthermore, to further improve our understanding of how these genetic variants interact with environmental factors to modulate disease risk, more extensive phenotypic data are required, especially in relation to diet and lifestyle factors.

DIETARY ENVIRONMENT: POTENTIAL ROLE OF DIFFERENT NUTRIENTS

The primary strategy to alleviate insulin resistance in obese individuals is to promote weight loss through a combination of diet and physical activity, the combination of which is as effective as pharmacological agents [86]. The increasing incidence of type 2 diabetes worldwide is a major challenge, as 60%–90% of cases appear to be directly related to obesity or weight gain [2]. Given the dramatic rise in obesity rates worldwide [87,88], future health is extremely worrisome. Since public health approaches have limited success in impeding weight gain, alternative strategies to attenuate the metabolic risk factors associated with obesity need to be explored. Within this context, several groups have sought to determine whether manipulating the composition of the diet, within an isocaloric context, can improve the metabolic phenotype despite obesity. The role of specific dietary macronutrients in development and/or treatment of insulin resistance is controversial, nevertheless there is some evidence to suggest that individual manipulations targeting different fatty acids, glycemic index, and/or protein levels may be of value.

Dietary Fatty Acids

We recently reviewed the literature that suggests that dietary fats may be particularly detrimental, not only because of their greater calorific value but also because lipids can directly impede insulin signaling [89]. Briefly, epidemiological and cohort studies show the detrimental effects of total fat on insulin resistance and the development of T2DM [90–92]. SFAs seem to be particularly potent at promoting insulin resistance [93–95]. However, the optimal amount and type of dietary fat for the prevention and/or treatment of insulin resistance remains unclear. Some studies have shown that diets rich in monounsaturated fatty acids (MUFAs) improved insulin sensitivity in healthy subjects [96]. The MUFA in Obesity (MUFObes) study determined the effect of MUFA on insulin sensitivity and weight maintenance. It showed that MUFA diets produced less body fat regain with improved insulin and glucose levels [97,98]. The KANWU study showed that a high-SFA diet reduced insulin sensitivity in overweight subjects, and post hoc analysis indicated that isoenergetic substitution of SFAs for MUFA improved insulin sensitivity but only in subjects whose habitual preintervention dietary fat intake was below the median [99]. In subjects with MetS, LIPGENE, a large pan-European isocaloric dietary intervention study, showed that substitution of SFAs with either MUFA or as part of a low-fat, high-complex carbohydrate improved insulin sensitivity in only those subjects whose preintervention dietary fat intake was less than the median [100]. Clearly, the effects of fatty acid interventions are variable. Important determinants such as the prediet environment may affect outcome. In addition we need to take account of the genetic background as discussed in more detail later.

Dietary Carbohydrate

Manipulating dietary carbohydrates quality also needs to be considered within the context of obesity and insulin resistance. In 1981, Jenkins introduced the concept of the glycemic index (GI) [101], which classifies carbohydrates according to their postprandial effects on blood glucose level. The Nurse's Health Study showed that high-GI foods were strongly associated with an increased T2DM [102]. Substituting whole-grain foods, such as brown rice, for white rice can reduce the risk of T2DM [103,104]. But other studies have shown inconsistent effects of manipulating GI and glycemic load on metabolic health. For example, the RISCK (Reading, Imperial,

Surrey, Cambridge and Kings) study, a multicentre, parallel design, randomized control trial, investigated whether replacement of SFAs in the diet with MUFA or carbohydrates, and modifying GI intake, could improve insulin sensitivity in subjects with MetS. However, there was no overall effect of GI on insulin sensitivity. Nevertheless, post hoc analysis did suggest an improvement in insulin sensitivity of the low-GI diet when in combination with a low SFA [105].

Dietary Protein

In the case of optimal protein intake, the Diet, Obesity, and Genes (Diogenes) study, a pan-European, multicenter, randomized, dietary intervention study was designed to assess the efficacy of moderate-fat diets that vary in protein content and GI for preventing weight regain and insulin sensitivity after weight loss. Weight regain was significantly less following a high-protein diet and a low-GI diet [106]. Also importantly, the low-GI diet continued to reduce plasma C-reactive protein concentrations [107], which is indicative of low-grade inflammation that is fundamental to insulin resistance in overweight/obese adults.

Other Dietary Components

Overwhelming evidence points to localized adipose tissue inflammation and dysfunction during the development of insulin resistance, which is a prerequisite to the development of type 2 diabetes. Within this context, it may be possible to attenuate the impact of adipose tissue inflammation with a view to improving insulin sensitivity despite obesity. Anti-inflammatory pharmacological agents, including aspirin (sodium salicylate) or salsalate, improve glycemic control including HbA1c, fasting blood glucose, and adiponectin concentration in patients with T2DM [108]. Several nutrient and nonnutrient food components have anti-inflammatory and antioxidant properties, including polyphenols, resveratrol, catechins, vitamin E, long-chain (LC) *n*-3 polyunsaturated fatty acids (PUFAs), and conjugated linoleic acid [109–111]. In vitro and animal studies show proof of concept that these anti-inflammatory food components can attenuate inflammation and improve insulin sensitivity [111,112]. However, translating this effect into humans has proven more difficult; for example, low doses of LC *n*-3 PUFA do not improve insulin sensitivity [99,100]. Nevertheless, this may reflect dose or the need for a combination of anti-inflammatory agents to maximize effects. Bakker et al. [110] showed that a combination of anti-inflammatory nutrients, including resveratrol, green tea extract, α-tocopherol, vitamin C, and LC *n*-3 PUFA, did improve adiponectin concentrations in healthy, overweight, and obese men. Nevertheless the concept of whether anti-inflammatory nutrients/food components have the potential to attenuate adipose tissue inflammation and insulin resistance needs to be clarified.

PERSPECTIVES FOR FUTURE DIETARY INTERVENTION SUCCESS

Although all of the above provide some insight that macronutrient manipulations may improve the metabolic phenotype despite overweight and obesity, it must be acknowledged that variable response is an important factor. This factor goes beyond poor compliance, wherein typically up to 30% of subjects do not respond to interventions. The major challenge for nutrigenomics is to define indicators of potential efficacy of dietary interventions. The reasons for variable response are many including genetic background, the preintervention dietary environment [99,100], or indeed metabolic phenotypes (or metabotypes) that reflect both genetic and dietary components may determine response. Metabolic phenotyping promises to be a useful tool in human intervention studies in terms of identifying responders versus nonresponders to preempt dietary efficacy. For example, O'Sullivan et al. [113] used a combination of biochemical markers, inflammatory indices, H-NMR metabolomic analysis, and k-means clustering to identify responsive phenotypes. A combination of multiple markers including low-serum 25(OH)D and high levels of proinflammatory cytokines characterized those subjects who responded to a vitamin D intervention with respect to improved insulin sensitivity and C-reactive protein status. This metabolic phenotyping approach, in combination with a more extensive understanding of genetic components, may help to identify specific genotype/phenotypes that are indicative of dietary intervention success for subgroups who should receive a more personalized approach within the larger population.

PERSONALIZED NUTRITION BASED ON GENE–DIET INTERACTIONS IN OBESITY, METABOLIC SYNDROME, AND TYPE 2 DIABETES MELLITUS

The ever-increasing global prevalence of obesity, MetS, and T2DM indicates that environmental factors are likely to be major contributors to the diabesity pandemic. According to the "thrifty genotype" hypothesis proposed by geneticist James Neel in 1962 [114], evolutionary selection of genes (obesity genes) that were originally beneficial for energy storage and which conferred a protective effect in times of food deprivation by promoting fat deposition, might, at least in part, explain the current escalating incidence of obesity in a modern environment of physical inactivity and easy access to and excessive consumption of calorie-dense processed foods. This makes sense and is supported by the finding that obesity and T2DM reaches epidemic proportions in certain ethnic groups such as Pima Indians, Pacific Islanders, African-Americans, and Hispanic-Americans [115]. Indeed, the much lower prevalence of obesity, insulin resistance, and T2DM observed in Pima Indians in Mexico compared to their counterparts in America illustrates that even in populations who are genetically predisposed to these conditions, their development is largely determined by environmental factors [116,117]. Such data indicate that dietary and lifestyle changes associated with Westernization are key players in the global epidemic of T2DM. Data from the Diabetes Prevention Program and the Diabetes Prevention Study indicate that lifestyle or environmental factors can modulate the genetic effects of *TCF7L2* polymorphisms [28,35]. In the Diabetes Prevention Study, overweight individuals with impaired glucose tolerance were allocated to an intensive diet and lifestyle intervention group or a control group. After a mean 4-year follow-up period, they found that *TCF7L2* polymorphisms were associated with the incidence of diabetes in the control group, but not the intervention group, suggesting that environmental factors can reduce genetic susceptibility even when risk genotypes are related to impaired insulin secretion. In addition to variation at the DNA level, epigenetic events are also considered to be important contributors to the obesity epidemic [118]. Twin studies in particular have provided evidence that environmental factors associated with modern-day living could affect methylation patterns of certain genes, which could lead to increased obesity risk [119]. Thus, heritability may not only be limited to DNA sequence variations, and it is clear that environmental factors play a key role in driving the diabesity epidemic.

Nutrigenetics: Gene–Diet Interactions

It is becoming increasingly obvious that an individual's phenotype represents a complex interaction between the genetic and environmental factors over the course of an individual's lifetime. Nutrition is a key environmental factor in the pathogenesis and progression of common polygenic, diet-related diseases. As discussed already, dietary fat is an important environmental factor and current evidence to support the nutrigenetics concept with respect to obesity, MetS, and T2DM is largely based on data relating to dietary fat [120–122]. The concept of gene–diet interaction describes dietary modulation of the effect of genotype on a particular phenotype (e.g., obesity, insulin resistance, and dyslipidemia) and/or modulation of the effect of a dietary factor on a particular phenotype by a genetic variant. It is generally accepted that the effect of dietary changes on plasma biomarker concentrations differs significantly between individuals. Such interindividual variability in response to dietary modification is, to a large extent, determined by genetic factors. A personalized nutrition approach based on identification of nutrient-sensitive or responsive genotypes, whereby nutrient intake is manipulated or optimized based on an individuals' genetic profile to reduce disease risk or improve effectiveness of dietary recommendations, offers the potential to break the traditional public health "one size fits all" approach, which clearly has not been successful to date within the context of obesity and metabolic health.

Nutrigenetic Evidence from Studies Investigating Dietary Fat–Gene Interactions

The *PPARγ* Pro12Ala polymorphism provides an excellent example of the relevance of gene–nutrient interactions in the development of obesity, MetS, and T2DM. In a prospective population-based cohort study, researchers showed an important interaction between habitual dietary fat composition and this SNP [123]. As the PUFA/SFA ratio increased, a significant inverse relationship was shown for both fasting insulin concentrations and BMI in the Ala carriers. These data suggest that the potential protective effect of the Ala allele may be lost in the presence of a high-SFA diet. More recently, an inverse relationship between Ala frequency and T2DM prevalence has been observed in populations where energy from lipids exceeded 30% of the total energy intake [124]. In recent years, a number of well-designed studies (LIPGENE dietary intervention of MetS cases, LIPGENE-SU.VI.MAX MetS case–control study, Genetics of Lipid Lowering Drugs and Diet Network [GOLDN], etc.) have examined interactions between dietary and/or plasma fatty acid composition and genotype in these diet-related conditions. Some of the key findings from these studies are presented.

Inflammatory Genotypes and Interactions with Diet in Obesity and Insulin Resistance

IL-6, TNF-α, and LTA

As already eluded to, inflammation plays a key role in insulin resistance. Our group has shown that plasma PUFA/SFA levels modified the observed additive genetic effects of *IL-6*, *TNF*-α, and *LTA* [62]. When stratified according to median plasma PUFA/SFA levels, MetS risk was fourfold higher in the three SNP risk genotype carriers with the lowest PUFA/SFA levels compared to noncarriers and was thought to be driven by the SFA content, with high SFA levels alone accounting for five-fold increased MetS risk. A low PUFA/SFA ratio also exacerbated their increased risk of several phenotypes (abdominal obesity, fasting hyperglycemia, hypertension, and proinflammatory profile). Interestingly, when risk genotype carriers with the lowest PUFA/SFA levels were compared with their risk genotype carriers with the highest PUFA/SFA levels, significant improvements to their metabolic profile were noted. Most importantly, a high PUFA/SFA ratio attenuated genetic predisposition to MetS risk. Moreover, risk genotype carriers with the highest PUFA/SFA levels had reduced proinflammatory status, lower triacylglycerol (TAG) levels, and insulin resistance determined by homeostasis model assessment (HOMA-IR) values than risk genotype carriers with the lowest PUFA/SFA levels. These findings support current guidelines to reduce dietary SFA intake and increase PUFA consumption.

STAT3

Data from the LIPGENE-SU.VI.MAX study identified a gene–nutrient interaction with SFAs. High dietary SFA intake (≥15.5% of energy) modulated the genetic association between *STAT3* polymorphisms with obesity [72]; carriers of more than two risk alleles with the highest SFA consumption further increased their risk of abdominal obesity by 32% compared to those carrying one or fewer risk alleles. These data suggest that individuals with certain STAT3 genotypes are more sensitive to SFAs and that these individuals may derive the most benefit from dietary manipulation and current guidelines to reduce dietary SFA intake. Although the mechanisms underlying these findings are unknown, it is possible that TLR4, the molecular link between fatty acids, obesity, inflammation, and insulin resistance [12], may play a role. Interestingly, hypothalamic FTO overexpression has been shown to result in a fourfold increase in STAT3 expression [125]. Given the importance of STAT3 in the LEP-signaling pathway, these data suggest a potential mechanism for mediating FTO's actions and potential modulation by SFAs.

Complement C3

The increased MetS risk associated with the rs2250656 A allele in the LIPGENE-SU.VI.MAX study may be explained by their classic MetS profile and raised inflammatory status [81]. Interestingly, plasma PUFA modified MetS risk whereby the combination of carrying two "risk" A alleles and having low *n*-6 or total PUFA (below the median) exacerbated MetS risk, suggesting that these individuals, who represent approximately half of the population and who are genetically predisposed to MetS, are also more sensitive to PUFA. Similarly reduced MetS risk associated with the rs11569562 polymorphism was subject to a significant effect modification by PUFA, with the greatest protection from MetS being achieved by GG homozygotes with the highest PUFA status [81]. Likewise, GG homozygotes with the highest LC *n*-3 PUFAs had the lowest risk of hypertriglyceridemia. In keeping with these findings, in the LIPGENE dietary intervention study, the "protective" rs11569562GG genotype was associated with enhanced insulin sensitivity and these individuals were more responsive to LC *n*-3 PUFA, compared to the A allele carriers. Following a 12-week low-fat (28% energy), high-complex carbohydrate diet intervention supplemented with 1.24 g/day LC *n*-3 PUFA, GG homozygotes displayed beneficial changes to their lipid profile (10% reduction in nonesterified fatty acid (NEFA), 8% nonsignificant reduction in TAG, 5% reduction in total cholesterol, and 17% reduction in low-density lipoprotein concentrations), compared to the A allele carriers. No changes were observed between genotypes when subjects on the same diet received a 1 g/day high oleic acid control supplement. In addition, the "at risk" rs2250656 A allele carriers had reduced insulin sensitivity and increased BMI, relative to the GG homozygotes. Again, genetic influences were modified by LC *n*-3 PUFA supplementation, whereby the A allele carriers achieved a 35% improvement in insulin sensitivity following intervention whereas no changes were noted between genotypes following oleic acid supplementation. Interestingly, PUFAs are ligands of FXR [126], a nuclear receptor that regulates *C3* expression [119]. Thus, it is possible that alteration of *C3* expression via modulation of FXR is a potential mechanism by which gene–nutrient interaction of *C3* genotype and dietary PUFAs could influence C3 levels and thus MetS risk. Although speculative, it may be worthy of further investigation to help elucidate the molecular basis of such gene–nutrient interactions and their impact on markers of inflammation and insulin resistance.

Adiponectin

A potential gene–nutrient interaction was found between the rs266729 polymorphism of *ADIPOQ* and the percentage energy derived from fat in the diet for the development of obesity [127]. Investigation of the effect of *ADIPOQ* SNPs, rs266729 and rs17300539, on metabolic-related traits, and their modulation by dietary fat in white Americans in the GOLDN study, revealed significant interaction with MUFA intake [128]. In subjects with high MUFA intake (>median), rs17300539 A allele carriers had lower BMI and decreased obesity risk [128]. Dietary intervention analysis has shown that CC homozygotes for rs266729 were less insulin resistant after consumption of MUFA and carbohydrate-rich diets compared to the SFA-rich diet [129]. Furthermore in the LIPGENE dietary intervention study, two SNPs (rs266729 in *ADIPOQ* and rs10920533 in *ADIPOR1*) interacted with plasma SFAs to alter insulin and HOMA-IR [130]. This study showed that a reduction in plasma SFAs decreased insulin resistance in carriers of the minor allele of rs266729 *ADIPOQ* and rs10920533 *ADIPOR1*. Personalized nutrition advice based on these data would recommend a decrease in SFAs consumption in the diet of MetS subjects carrying the minor allele of rs266729 *ADIPOQ* and/or rs10920533 *ADIPOR1*.

TCF7L2

In the GOLDN study, dietary PUFA modulated the genetic effects of the *TCF7L2* rs7903146 polymorphism on postprandial lipemia [37]. In the LIPGENE dietary intervention study, *TCF7L2* SNPs were associated with plasma lipid concentrations, carbohydrate metabolism, blood pressure, and inflammatory markers. Interactions with SFAs were noted. For example, among the rs11196224 major homozygotes elevated plasma SFA was associated with increased insulin resistance [131]. Along the same lines, in the LIPGENE-SU.VI.MAX study rs7903146 was associated with increased MetS risk, arising from their impaired insulin sensitivity, greater insulin resistance, and increased abdominal obesity and hypertension [41]. Interestingly, dietary fat intake, recorded 7.5 years prior to MetS case–control selection, modulated the genetic influence on MetS risk. In particular, high dietary SFA intake (≥15.5% of energy) accentuated the deleterious effects of rs7903146 on MetS risk, suggesting that the long-term effect of dietary fatty acid composition and consumption may have the potential to modify the genetic susceptibility of developing MetS.

FTO

Limited cross-sectional analysis of the influence of dietary factors on BMI according to *FTO* rs9939609 genotype indicates that high-fat diets increase obesity risk [132,133]. However, these studies did not investigate specific effects of dietary fat type or fatty acid composition. Recent data from a study of 354 children identified an interaction between dietary SFA and the PUFA/SFA ratio and obesity associated with *FTO* rs9939609 [134]. Similar data for adults are only emerging. In the LIPGENE-SU.VI.MAX study, *FTO* rs9939609 was associated with increased risk of having a BMI in the overweight or obese category and of being abdominally obese. Increased obesity risk was maintained over the 7.5-year follow-up period and while rs9939609 was not associated with MetS risk, risk of these obesity-related measures was higher in the risk allele carrying MetS cases relative to their nonrisk allele carrying counterparts. A novel finding in that study was that high habitual dietary SFA consumption (≥15.5% of energy) and low PUFA/SFA ratio accentuates obesity risk in the *A* allele carriers but not in the *TT* homozygotes in this adult European population, suggesting that genetic predisposition to obesity may be modulated by dietary SFA intake. This may be particularly relevant to individuals with diet-related metabolic disease who are at increased cardiometabolic risk. Recent data from the GOLDN study also identified an interaction between rs9939609 and SFA intake, whereby homozygous participants in this American population had a higher BMI only when they had a high SFA intake (>mean) [135]. Interestingly, hypothalamic FTO overexpression has been shown to result in a fourfold increase in STAT3 expression [125]. Given the importance of STAT3 in the LEP-signaling pathway, these data suggest a potential mechanism for mediating FTO's actions and potential modulation by SFAs.

FUTURE PERSPECTIVES: CHALLENGES AND OPPORTUNITIES

The search for genetic factors and gene–nutrient interactions associated with diabesity risk is challenging. Undoubtedly, advances in high-throughput genetic analysis have improved our understanding of the contribution of genetics to these diet-related conditions. Nutrition is probably the most important environmental factor that modulates genes and the variety of phenotypes associated with obesity, MetS, and T2DM. However, the molecular mechanisms underlying many of the genetic associations and gene–nutrient interactions remain unclear. The situation is further compounded by genetic heterogeneity, exposure to a complex range of environmental factors, and wide interindividual phenotypic variation. Nutrigenetics is a rapidly developing field that needs to move forward with nutritional genomics to translate observational findings into molecular mechanisms. Nutrigenetics has the potential to change diet-related disease prevention and therapy. To turn this potential to reality, we must consider the complexity of the "real-life" situation. Humans do not eat nutrients, they eat food. Therefore, more holistic methods that incorporate an individuals' whole diet or dietary patterns, rather than selecting individual dietary components, need to be developed to advance the state of the art. The combined application of nutritional and genetic epidemiology, proteomics, metabolomics, transcriptomics, lipidomics, epigenetics, and gut microbiota profiling will be crucial in this regard and will lead to a more highly integrated understanding of the complex interaction between genetic and environmental factors relevant to diabesity. Nevertheless, current data provide proof of concept. Whether personalized risk assessment, personalized nutritional advice, and genome-customized diets will be feasible for the population at large in the twenty-first century remains to be seen. Future research will have to provide solid evidence for associations between genotype, diet, and disease or risk factors.

REFERENCES

1. Eckel, R.H., S.M. Grundy, and P.Z. Zimmet. The metabolic syndrome. *Lancet* 2005, 365(9468): 1415–28.
2. Anderson, J.W., C.W. Kendall, and D.J. Jenkins. Importance of weight management in type 2 diabetes: review with meta-analysis of clinical studies. *J Am Coll Nutr* 2003, 22(5): 331–9.
3. Nishimura, S. et al. CD8+ effector T cells contribute to macrophage recruitment and adipose tissue inflammation in obesity. *Nat Med* 2009, 15(8): 914–20.
4. Winer, S. et al. Normalization of obesity-associated insulin resistance through immunotherapy. *Nat Med* 2009, 15(8): 921–9.
5. Lumeng, C.N., J.L. Bodzin, and A.R. Saltiel. Obesity induces a phenotypic switch in adipose tissue macrophage polarization. *J Clin Invest* 2007, 117(1): 175–84.
6. Weisberg, S.P. et al. Obesity is associated with macrophage accumulation in adipose tissue. *J Clin Invest* 2003, 112(12): 1796–808.
7. Hotamisligil, G.S. et al. Tumor necrosis factor alpha inhibits signaling from the insulin receptor. *Proc Natl Acad Sci U S A* 1994, 91(11): 4854–8.
8. Jager, J. et al. Interleukin-1beta-induced insulin resistance in adipocytes through down-regulation of insulin receptor substrate-1 expression. *Endocrinology* 2007, 148(1): 241–51.
9. Tanaka, T. et al. Down regulation of peroxisome proliferator-activated receptor-gamma expression by inflammatory cytokines and its reversal by thiazolidinediones. *Diabetologia* 1999, 42(6): 702–10.
10. Harford, K.A. et al. Fats, inflammation and insulin resistance: insights to the role of macrophage and T-cell accumulation in adipose tissue. *Proc Nutr Soc* 2011, 70(4): 408–17.
11. McGillicuddy, F.C. et al. Lack of interleukin-1 receptor I (IL-1RI) protects mice from high-fat diet-induced adipose tissue inflammation coincident with improved glucose homeostasis. *Diabetes* 2011, 60(6): 1688–98.

12. Shi, H. et al. TLR4 links innate immunity and fatty acid-induced insulin resistance. *J Clin Invest* 2006, 116(11): 3015–25.
13. Uysal, K.T. et al. Protection from obesity-induced insulin resistance in mice lacking TNF-alpha function. *Nature* 1997, 389(6651): 610–4.
14. Goossens, G.H. et al. Increased adipose tissue oxygen tension in obese compared with lean men is accompanied by insulin resistance, impaired adipose tissue capillarization, and inflammation. *Circulation* 2011, 124(1): 67–76.
15. Jocken, J.W. et al. Skeletal muscle lipase content and activity in obesity and type 2 diabetes. *J Clin Endocrinol Metab* 2010, 95(12): 5449–53.
16. Jans, A. et al. Transcriptional metabolic inflexibility in skeletal muscle among individuals with increasing insulin resistance. *Obesity (Silver Spring)* 2011, 19(11): 2158–66.
17. Barbarroja, N. et al. The obese healthy paradox: is inflammation the answer? *Biochem J* 2010, 430(1): 141–9.
18. Allison, D.B., M.S. Faith, and J.S. Nathan. Risch's lambda values for human obesity. *Int J Obes Relat Metab Disord* 1996, 20(11): 990–9.
19. Maes, H.H., M.C. Neale, and L.J. Eaves. Genetic and environmental factors in relative body weight and human adiposity. *Behav Genet* 1997, 27(4): 325–51.
20. Stunkard, A.J. et al. An adoption study of human obesity. *N Engl J Med* 1986, 314(4): 193–8.
21. Bouchard, C. et al. Inheritance of the amount and distribution of human body fat. *Int J Obes* 1988, 12(3): 205–15.
22. Vogler, G.P. et al. Influences of genes and shared family environment on adult body mass index assessed in an adoption study by a comprehensive path model. *Int J Obes Relat Metab Disord* 1995, 19(1): 40–5.
23. Bellia, A. et al. "The Linosa Study": epidemiological and heritability data of the metabolic syndrome in a Caucasian genetic isolate. *Nutr Metab Cardiovasc Dis* 2009, 19(7): 455–61.
24. Henneman, P. et al. Prevalence and heritability of the metabolic syndrome and its individual components in a Dutch isolate: the Erasmus Rucphen Family study. *J Med Genet* 2008, 45(9): 572–7.
25. Florez, J.C., J. Hirschhorn, and D. Altshuler. The inherited basis of diabetes mellitus: implications for the genetic analysis of complex traits. *Annu Rev Genomics Hum Genet* 2003, 4: 257–91.
26. Gloyn, A.L. The search for type 2 diabetes genes. *Ageing Res Rev* 2003, 2(2): 111–27.
27. Andreasen, C.H. and G. Andersen. Gene-environment interactions and obesity—further aspects of genomewide association studies. *Nutrition* 2009, 25(10): 998–1003.
28. Florez, J.C. et al. TCF7L2 polymorphisms and progression to diabetes in the Diabetes Prevention Program. *N Engl J Med* 2006, 355(3): 241–50.
29. Grant, S.F. et al. Variant of transcription factor 7-like 2 (TCF7L2) gene confers risk of type 2 diabetes. *Nat Genet* 2006, 38(3): 320–3.
30. Cauchi, S. et al. TCF7L2 is reproducibly associated with type 2 diabetes in various ethnic groups: a global meta-analysis. *J Mol Med* 2007, 85(7): 777–82.
31. Cauchi, S. et al. Transcription factor TCF7L2 genetic study in the French population: expression in human beta-cells and adipose tissue and strong association with type 2 diabetes. *Diabetes* 2006, 55(10): 2903–8.
32. Chandak, G.R. et al. Common variants in the TCF7L2 gene are strongly associated with type 2 diabetes mellitus in the Indian population. *Diabetologia* 2007, 50(1): 63–7.
33. Hayashi, T. et al. Replication study for the association of TCF7L2 with susceptibility to type 2 diabetes in a Japanese population. *Diabetologia* 2007, 50(5): 980–4.
34. Humphries, S.E. et al. Common variants in the TCF7L2 gene and predisposition to type 2 diabetes in UK European Whites, Indian Asians and Afro-Caribbean men and women. *J Mol Med* 2006, 84(12 Suppl): 1–10.

35. Wang, J. et al. Variants of transcription factor 7-like 2 (TCF7L2) gene predict conversion to type 2 diabetes in the Finnish Diabetes Prevention Study and are associated with impaired glucose regulation and impaired insulin secretion. *Diabetologia* 2007, 50(6): 1192–200.
36. Melzer, D. et al. Effects of the diabetes linked TCF7L2 polymorphism in a representative older population. *BMC Med* 2006, 4: 34.
37. Warodomwichit, D. et al. Polyunsaturated fatty acids modulate the effect of TCF7L2 gene variants on postprandial lipemia. *J Nutr* 2009, 139(3): 439–46.
38. Sjogren, M. et al. The search for putative unifying genetic factors for components of the metabolic syndrome. *Diabetologia* 2008, 51(12): 2242–51.
39. Marzi, C. et al. Variants of the transcription factor 7-like 2 gene (TCF7L2) are strongly associated with type 2 diabetes but not with the metabolic syndrome in the MONICA/KORA surveys. *Horm Metab Res* 2007, 39(1): 46–52.
40. Saadi, H. et al. Association of TCF7L2 polymorphism with diabetes mellitus, metabolic syndrome, and markers of beta cell function and insulin resistance in a population-based sample of Emirati subjects. *Diabetes Res Clin Pract* 2008, 80(3): 392–8.
41. Phillips, C.M. et al. Dietary saturated fat, gender and genetic variation at the TCF7L2 locus predict the development of metabolic syndrome. *J Nutr Biochem* 2011, 23(3): 239–44.
42. Povel, C.M. et al. Genetic variants and the metabolic syndrome: a systematic review. *Obes Rev* 2011, 12(11): 952–67.
43. Frayling, T.M. et al. A common variant in the FTO gene is associated with body mass index and predisposes to childhood and adult obesity. *Science* 2007, 316(5826): 889–94.
44. Haupt, A. et al. Variation in the FTO gene influences food intake but not energy expenditure. *Exp Clin Endocrinol Diabetes* 2009, 117(4): 194–7.
45. Speakman, J.R., K.A. Rance, and A.M. Johnstone. Polymorphisms of the FTO gene are associated with variation in energy intake, but not energy expenditure. *Obesity (Silver Spring)* 2008, 16(8): 1961–5.
46. Tanofsky-Kraff, M. et al. The FTO gene rs9939609 obesity-risk allele and loss of control over eating. *Am J Clin Nutr* 2009, 90(6): 1483–8.
47. Dina, C. et al. Variation in FTO contributes to childhood obesity and severe adult obesity. *Nat Genet* 2007, 39(6): 724–6.
48. Hinney, A. et al. Genome wide association (GWA) study for early onset extreme obesity supports the role of fat mass and obesity associated gene (FTO) variants. *PLoS One* 2007, 2(12): e1361.
49. Hunt, S.C. et al. Association of the FTO gene with BMI. *Obesity (Silver Spring)* 2008, 16(4): 902–4.
50. Horikawa, Y. et al. Genetic variation in the gene encoding calpain-10 is associated with type 2 diabetes mellitus. *Nat Genet* 2000, 26(2): 163–75.
51. Saez, M.E. et al. The CAPN10 gene is associated with insulin resistance phenotypes in the Spanish population. *PLoS One* 2008, 3(8): e2953.
52. Carlsson, E. et al. Variation in the calpain-10 gene is associated with elevated triglyceride levels and reduced adipose tissue messenger ribonucleic acid expression in obese Swedish subjects. *J Clin Endocrinol Metab* 2004, 89(7): 3601–5.
53. Garant, M.J. et al. SNP43 of CAPN10 and the risk of type 2 diabetes in African-Americans: the Atherosclerosis Risk in Communities Study. *Diabetes* 2002, 51(1): 231–7.
54. Shima, Y. et al. Association of the SNP-19 genotype 22 in the calpain-10 gene with elevated body mass index and hemoglobin A1c levels in Japanese. *Clin Chim Acta* 2003, 336(1–2): 89–96.
55. Dalziel, B. et al. Association of the TNF-alpha-308 G/A promoter polymorphism with insulin resistance in obesity. *Obes Res* 2002, 10(5): 401–7.

56. Hamid, Y.H. et al. Variations of the interleukin-6 promoter are associated with features of the metabolic syndrome in Caucasian Danes. *Diabetologia* 2005, 48(2): 251–60.
57. Huth, C. et al. IL6 gene promoter polymorphisms and type 2 diabetes: joint analysis of individual participants' data from 21 studies. *Diabetes* 2006, 55(10): 2915–21.
58. Shen, J. et al. The effect of IL6-174C/G polymorphism on postprandial triglyceride metabolism in the GOLDN studyboxs. *J Lipid Res* 2008, 49(8): 1839–45.
59. Sookoian, S. et al. The G-308A promoter variant of the tumor necrosis factor-alpha gene is associated with hypertension in adolescents harboring the metabolic syndrome. *Am J Hypertens* 2005, 18(10): 1271–5.
60. Meirhaeghe, A. et al. Lack of association between certain candidate gene polymorphisms and the metabolic syndrome. *Mol Genet Metab* 2005, 86(1–2): 293–9.
61. Qi, L. et al. Interleukin-6 genetic variability and adiposity: associations in two prospective cohorts and systematic review in 26,944 individuals. *J Clin Endocrinol Metab* 2007, 92(9): 3618–25.
62. Phillips, C.M. et al. Additive effect of polymorphisms in the IL-6, LTA, and TNF-{alpha} genes and plasma fatty acid level modulate risk for the metabolic syndrome and its components. *J Clin Endocrinol Metab* 2010, 95(3): 1386–94.
63. Aaronson, D.S. and C.M. Horvath. A road map for those who don't know JAK-STAT. *Science* 2002, 296(5573): 1653–5.
64. Cernkovich, E.R. et al. Adipose-specific disruption of signal transducer and activator of transcription 3 increases body weight and adiposity. *Endocrinology* 2008, 149(4): 1581–90.
65. Cui, Y. et al. Essential role of STAT3 in body weight and glucose homeostasis. *Mol Cell Biol* 2004, 24(1): 258–69.
66. Gao, Q. et al. Disruption of neural signal transducer and activator of transcription 3 causes obesity, diabetes, infertility, and thermal dysregulation. *Proc Natl Acad Sci U S A* 2004, 101(13): 4661–6.
67. Gorogawa, S. et al. Insulin secretory defects and impaired islet architecture in pancreatic beta-cell-specific STAT3 knockout mice. *Biochem Biophys Res Commun* 2004, 319(4): 1159–70.
68. Inoue, H. et al. Role of STAT-3 in regulation of hepatic gluconeogenic genes and carbohydrate metabolism in vivo. *Nat Med* 2004, 10(2): 168–74.
69. Vaisse, C. et al. Leptin activation of Stat3 in the hypothalamus of wild-type and ob/ob mice but not db/db mice. *Nat Genet* 1996, 14(1): 95–7.
70. Gianotti, T.F. et al. Study of genetic variation in the STAT3 on obesity and insulin resistance in male adults. *Obesity (Silver Spring)* 2008, 16(7): 1702–7.
71. Jamshidi, Y. et al. Common STAT3 variants are not associated with obesity or insulin resistance in female twins. *Obesity (Silver Spring)* 2007, 15(7): 1634–9.
72. Phillips, C.M. et al. Dietary saturated fat modulates the association between STAT3 polymorphisms and abdominal obesity in adults. *J Nutr* 2009, 139(11): 2011–7.
73. Weedon, M.N. et al. Combining information from common type 2 diabetes risk polymorphisms improves disease prediction. *PLoS Med* 2006, 3(10): e374.
74. Arita, Y. et al. Paradoxical decrease of an adipose-specific protein, adiponectin, in obesity. *Biochem Biophys Res Commun* 1999, 257(1): 79–83.
75. Menzaghi, C., V. Trischitta, and A. Doria. Genetic influences of adiponectin on insulin resistance, type 2 diabetes, and cardiovascular disease. *Diabetes* 2007, 56(5): 1198–209.
76. Sheng, T. and K. Yang. Adiponectin and its association with insulin resistance and type 2 diabetes. *J Genet Genomics* 2008, 35(6): 321–6.
77. Engstrom, G. et al. Complement C3 is a risk factor for the development of diabetes: a population-based cohort study. *Diabetes* 2005, 54(2): 570–5.

78. Halkes, C.J. et al. Postprandial increase of complement component 3 in normolipidemic patients with coronary artery disease: effects of expanded-dose simvastatin. *Arterioscler Thromb Vasc Biol* 2001, 21(9): 1526–30.
79. Muscari, A. et al. Relationship of serum C3 to fasting insulin, risk factors and previous ischaemic events in middle-aged men. *Eur Heart J* 2000, 21(13): 1081–90.
80. van Oostrom, A.J. et al. The metabolic syndrome in relation to complement component 3 and postprandial lipemia in patients from an outpatient lipid clinic and healthy volunteers. *Atherosclerosis* 2007, 190(1): 167–73.
81. Phillips, C.M. et al. Complement component 3 polymorphisms interact with polyunsaturated fatty acids to modulate risk of metabolic syndrome. *Am J Clin Nutr* 2009, 90(6): 1665–73.
82. Deeb, S.S. et al. A Pro12Ala substitution in PPARgamma2 associated with decreased receptor activity, lower body mass index and improved insulin sensitivity. *Nat Genet* 1998, 20(3): 284–7.
83. Altshuler, D. et al. The common PPARgamma Pro12Ala polymorphism is associated with decreased risk of type 2 diabetes. *Nat Genet* 2000, 26(1): 76–80.
84. Andrulionyte, L. et al. Common polymorphisms of the PPAR-gamma2 (Pro12Ala) and PGC-1alpha (Gly482Ser) genes are associated with the conversion from impaired glucose tolerance to type 2 diabetes in the STOP-NIDDM trial. *Diabetologia* 2004, 47(12): 2176–84.
85. Ghoussaini, M. et al. Implication of the Pro12Ala polymorphism of the PPAR-gamma 2 gene in type 2 diabetes and obesity in the French population. *BMC Med Genet* 2005, 6: 11.
86. Knowler, W.C. et al. Reduction in the incidence of type 2 diabetes with lifestyle intervention or metformin. *N Engl J Med* 2002, 346(6): 393–403.
87. Flegal, K.M. et al. Prevalence and trends in obesity among US adults, 1999–2008. *JAMA* 2010, 303(3): 235–41.
88. Mokdad, A.H. et al. The spread of the obesity epidemic in the United States, 1991–1998. *JAMA* 1999, 282(16): 1519–22.
89. Phillips, C.M., A.C. Tierney, and H.M. Roche. Gene-nutrient interactions in the metabolic syndrome. *J Nutrigenet Nutrigenomics* 2008, 1(3): 136–51.
90. Meyer, K.A. et al. Dietary fat and incidence of type 2 diabetes in older Iowa women. *Diabetes Care* 2001, 24(9): 1528–35.
91. van Greevenbroek, M.M. et al. The cross-sectional association between insulin resistance and circulating complement C3 is partly explained by plasma alanine aminotransferase, independent of central obesity and general inflammation (the CODAM study). *Eur J Clin Invest* 2011, 41(4): 372–9.
92. Wang, L. et al. Plasma fatty acid composition and incidence of diabetes in middle-aged adults: the Atherosclerosis Risk in Communities (ARIC) Study. *Am J Clin Nutr* 2003, 78(1): 91–8.
93. Hu, F.B., R.M. van Dam, and S. Liu. Diet and risk of Type II diabetes: the role of types of fat and carbohydrate. *Diabetologia* 2001, 44(7): 805–17.
94. Melanson, E.L., A. Astrup, and W.T. Donahoo. The relationship between dietary fat and fatty acid intake and body weight, diabetes, and the metabolic syndrome. *Ann Nutr Metab* 2009, 55(1–3): 229–43.
95. Warensjo, E., U. Riserus, and B. Vessby. Fatty acid composition of serum lipids predicts the development of the metabolic syndrome in men. *Diabetologia* 2005, 48(10): 1999–2005.
96. Perez-Jimenez, F. et al. A Mediterranean and a high-carbohydrate diet improve glucose metabolism in healthy young persons. *Diabetologia* 2001, 44(11): 2038–43.
97. Due, A. et al. Comparison of 3 ad libitum diets for weight-loss maintenance, risk of cardiovascular disease, and diabetes: a 6-mo randomized, controlled trial. *Am J Clin Nutr* 2008, 88(5): 1232–41.

98. Due, A. et al. Comparison of the effects on insulin resistance and glucose tolerance of 6-mo high-monounsaturated-fat, low-fat, and control diets. *Am J Clin Nutr* 2008, 87(4): 855–62.
99. Vessby, B. et al. Substituting dietary saturated for monounsaturated fat impairs insulin sensitivity in healthy men and women: the KANWU study. *Diabetologia* 2001, 44(3): 312–9.
100. Tierney, A.C. et al. Effects of dietary fat modification on insulin sensitivity and on other risk factors of the metabolic syndrome—LIPGENE: a European randomized dietary intervention study. *Int J Obes (Lond)* 2011, 35(6): 800–9.
101. Jenkins, D.J. et al. Glycemic index of foods: a physiological basis for carbohydrate exchange. *Am J Clin Nutr* 1981, 34(3): 362–6.
102. Oh, K. et al. Dietary fat intake and risk of coronary heart disease in women: 20 years of follow-up of the nurses' health study. *Am J Epidemiol* 2005, 161(7): 672–9.
103. Sun, Q. et al. White rice, brown rice, and risk of type 2 diabetes in US men and women. *Arch Intern Med* 2010, 170(11): 961–9.
104. Wolever, T.M. et al. Low glycaemic index diet and disposition index in type 2 diabetes (the Canadian trial of carbohydrates in diabetes): a randomised controlled trial. *Diabetologia* 2008, 51(9): 1607–15.
105. Jebb, S.A. et al. Effect of changing the amount and type of fat and carbohydrate on insulin sensitivity and cardiovascular risk: the RISCK (Reading, Imperial, Surrey, Cambridge, and Kings) trial. *Am J Clin Nutr* 2010, 92(4): 748–58.
106. Larsen, T.M. et al. Diets with high or low protein content and glycemic index for weight-loss maintenance. *N Engl J Med* 2010, 363(22): 2102–13.
107. Gogebakan, O. et al. Effects of weight loss and long-term weight maintenance with diets varying in protein and glycemic index on cardiovascular risk factors: the diet, obesity, and genes (DiOGenes) study: a randomized, controlled trial. *Circulation* 2011, 124(25): 2829–38.
108. Goldfine, A.B. et al. The effects of salsalate on glycemic control in patients with type 2 diabetes: a randomized trial. *Ann Intern Med* 2010, 152(6): 346–57.
109. Abete, I. et al. Obesity and metabolic syndrome: potential benefit from specific nutritional components. *Nutr Metab Cardiovasc Dis* 2011, 21(Suppl 2): B1–15.
110. Bakker, G.C. et al. An antiinflammatory dietary mix modulates inflammation and oxidative and metabolic stress in overweight men: a nutrigenomics approach. *Am J Clin Nutr* 2010, 91(4): 1044–59.
111. Moloney, F. et al. Antidiabetic effects of cis-9, trans-11-conjugated linoleic acid may be mediated via anti-inflammatory effects in white adipose tissue. *Diabetes* 2007, 56(3): 574–82.
112. Oliver, E. et al. Docosahexaenoic acid attenuates macrophage-induced inflammation and improves insulin sensitivity in adipocytes-specific differential effects between LC n-3 PUFA. *J Nutr Biochem* 2012, 23(9): 1192–200.
113. O'Sullivan, A. et al. Biochemical and metabolomic phenotyping in the identification of a vitamin D responsive metabotype for markers of the metabolic syndrome. *Mol Nutr Food Res* 2011, 55(5): 679–90.
114. Neel, J.V. Diabetes mellitus: a "thrifty" genotype rendered detrimental by "progress"? *Am J Hum Genet* 1962, 14: 353–62.
115. Wild, S. et al. Global prevalence of diabetes: estimates for the year 2000 and projections for 2030. *Diabetes Care* 2004, 27(5): 1047–53.
116. Esparza-Romero, J. et al. Differences in insulin resistance in Mexican and U.S. Pima Indians with normal glucose tolerance. *J Clin Endocrinol Metab* 2010, 95(11): E358–62.
117. Schulz, L.O. et al. Effects of traditional and western environments on prevalence of type 2 diabetes in Pima Indians in Mexico and the U.S. *Diabetes Care* 2006, 29(8): 1866–71.

118. Newnham, J.P. et al. Early life origins of obesity. *Obstet Gynecol Clin North Am* 2009, 36(2): 227–44, xii.
119. Fraga, M.F. et al. Epigenetic differences arise during the lifetime of monozygotic twins. *Proc Natl Acad Sci U S A* 2005, 102(30): 10604–9.
120. Phillips, C. et al. Genetic and nutrient determinants of the metabolic syndrome. *Curr Opin Cardiol* 2006, 21(3): 185–93.
121. Phillips, C.M., A.C. Tierney, and H.M. Roche. Gene-nutrient interactions in the metabolic syndrome. *J Nutrigenet Nutrigenomics* 2008, 1(3): 136–51.
122. Roche, H.M., C. Phillips, and M.J. Gibney. The metabolic syndrome: the crossroads of diet and genetics. *Proc Nutr Soc* 2005, 64(3): 371–7.
123. Luan, J. et al. Evidence for gene-nutrient interaction at the PPARgamma locus. *Diabetes* 2001, 50(3): 686–9.
124 Scacchi, R. et al. An analysis of peroxisome proliferator-activated receptor gamma (PPAR-gamma 2) Pro12Ala polymorphism distribution and prevalence of type 2 diabetes mellitus (T2DM) in world populations in relation to dietary habits. *Nutr Metab Cardiovasc Dis* 2007, 17(9): 632–41.
125. Gutierrez-Aguilar, R. et al. Expression of new loci associated with obesity in diet-induced obese rats: from genetics to physiology. *Obesity (Silver Spring)* 2012, 20(2): 306–12.
126. Zhao, A. et al. Polyunsaturated fatty acids are FXR ligands and differentially regulate expression of FXR targets. *DNA Cell Biol* 2004, 23(8): 519–26.
127. Santos, J.L. et al. Genotype-by-nutrient interactions assessed in European obese women. A case-only study. *Eur J Nutr* 2006, 45(8): 454–62.
128. Warodomwichit, D. et al. ADIPOQ polymorphisms, monounsaturated fatty acids, and obesity risk: the GOLDN study. *Obesity (Silver Spring)* 2009, 17(3): 510–7.
129. Perez-Martinez, P. et al. Adiponectin gene variants are associated with insulin sensitivity in response to dietary fat consumption in Caucasian men. *J Nutr* 2008, 138(9): 1609–14.
130. Ferguson, J.F. et al. Gene-nutrient interactions in the metabolic syndrome: single nucleotide polymorphisms in ADIPOQ and ADIPOR1 interact with plasma saturated fatty acids to modulate insulin resistance. *Am J Clin Nutr* 2010, 91(3): 794–801.
131. Delgado-Lista, J. et al. Pleiotropic effects of TCF7L2 gene variants and its modulation in the metabolic syndrome: from the LIPGENE study. *Atherosclerosis* 2011, 214(1): 110–6.
132. Lee, H.J. et al. Effects of common FTO gene variants associated with BMI on dietary intake and physical activity in Koreans. *Clin Chim Acta* 2010, 411(21–22): 1716–22.
133. Sonestedt, E. et al. Fat and carbohydrate intake modify the association between genetic variation in the FTO genotype and obesity. *Am J Clin Nutr* 2009, 90(5): 1418–25.
134. Moleres, A. et al. Dietary fatty acid distribution modifies obesity risk linked to the rs9939609 polymorphism of the fat mass and obesity-associated gene in a Spanish case-control study of children. *Br J Nutr* 2012, 107(4): 533–8.
135. Corella, D. et al. A high intake of saturated fatty acids strengthens the association between the fat mass and obesity-associated gene and BMI. *J Nutr* 2011, 141(12): 2219–25.

7 Nutrigenetics and Crohn's Disease

Lynnette R. Ferguson

CONTENTS

INTRODUCTION

Inflammatory bowel disease (IBD) is a collective term for a crippling group of disorders, characterized by bowel disfunction and food intolerances. Crohn's disease (CD) and ulcerative colitis (UC) are important forms of this disease. Both conditions are characterized by chronic inflammation of the gastrointestinal tract, involving an overreactive immune response to certain dietary items and/or commensal microorganisms, in a genetically susceptible host. We have previously summarized the factors involved in disease susceptibility, including genetics, diet, and microbiota [1–3]. It is not altogether clear whether malnutrition is a cause or effect of CD. However, malnourishment is common, and nutritional support often becomes important during the progression of the disease [4].

Risk factors triggering disease symptoms in individuals who have already developed the disease, but are in remission, may be different from those originally initiating the disease. It is also important to recognize the individual nature of patient response to diet, and that what is beneficial to one patient may be detrimental to another [5]. This almost certainly relates to the genetic nature of the condition [1]. If appropriately managed, nutrition can be an important factor in disease remission. Tighe et al. [6] ask whether nutrition should be primary or adjuvant therapy in IBD. This includes treatment of malnutrition and micronutrient deficiencies, as well as prevention of osteoporosis. In children, nutritional intervention, often with enteral nutrition, is essential for promotion of optimal growth and development. Indeed, one of the most sustainable approaches to reducing the symptoms of IBD in both children and adults involves putting them on an elemental formula, often over several weeks, until symptoms abate. Whole foods can then be gradually and cautiously introduced back into the diet. It is essential that people with the disease identify and avoid foods that worsen symptoms. For example, a number of CD patients may be dairy intolerant. Other general recommendations made are to limit excess saturated fats, reduce carbohydrates generally, and more specifically reduce high-fiber foods during disease flares. Some, but not all, subjects seem to benefit from probiotics [7].

The basis of genetic susceptibility to IBD has now been extensively studied. More than 160 genes are involved in susceptibility to the diseases, many of them overlapping between the two forms. In essence, these are genes involved in response to bacteria, in innate and adaptive immunity, and in barrier function [8,9]. Foods that have the potential to affect those functions might be considered as potentially beneficial (or detrimental) in CD.

LESSONS FROM ANIMAL STUDIES

Effect of Genotype on Intestinal Inflammation

Several different kinds of animal models have been used to study IBD and are generally classed into chemically induced, cell-transfer, congenial mutant, and genetically engineered models [10]. The most informative may be rodent models that knockout certain known IBD susceptibility genes, since these are better in line with human studies. Two of these (multidrug resistant [mdrla(–/–)] and interleukin-10 deficient [IL10(–/–)]) mice may be of particular interest, and will be considered in the subsequent discussion.

Dommels et al. [11] studied intestinal inflammation in mdrla(–/–) mice. These animals spontaneously develop intestinal inflammation, and the study was designed to measure inflammation and gene expression changes over time. Initial signs of inflammation occurred around 16 weeks of age, and most of the knockout mice developed inflammation between 16 and 27 weeks of age. The lesions identified were transmural and discontinuous, making this very similar to human IBDs. In colonic epithelial cell scrapings from the inflamed area of 25-week-old mdrla(–/–), genes involved in inflammatory response pathways were upregulated, whereas genes involved in biotransformation and transport were downregulated.

Subsequent studies on the same mouse model showed an altered caecal microbiota in these mice, which preceded the onset of intestinal inflammation [12]. Caecal microbiota of mdr1a(–/–) and their control counterparts were studied at 12 weeks (with no intestinal inflammation) and 25 weeks of age (when inflammation had developed). Denaturing gradient gel electrophoresis fingerprints of control and mdr1a(–/–) mice revealed significant differences in the presence of bacterial DNA fragments at these two time points. The authors suggested that the lack of Abcb1 transporters in intestinal cells, resulting from the disruption of the *mdr1a* gene, might be the cause of changes in the caecal microbiota. These could have an additive effect to the genetic defect, in the development of intestinal inflammation in mdr1a(–/–) mice.

IL10(–/–) mice provide another model of particular relevance to human IBD [13]. In this example, the disease does not reproducibly develop unless the mice are inoculated with pathogenic bacteria. These gene-deficient mice develop colitis, mainly in the colon, with symptoms similar to human CD. Barnett et al. [14] compared the responses of IL10(–/–) and C57BL/6J (control) mice to oral bacterial inoculation with 12 strains of *Enterococcus faecalis* and *E. faecium* isolated from calves or poultry, complex intestinal flora collected from healthy control mice, or a mixture of the two. Their endpoint showed changes in colonic gene expression levels.

A vitamin D deficiency, especially coupled with one or more single nucleotide polymorphisms (SNPs) in the vitamin D receptor (VDR) leads to serious colitis symptoms in several different animal models [15]. The small intestine contains large numbers of CD8αα(+) T cells that suppress immune response, and the VDR plays a role in the development of CD8αα(+) T cells. Decreased maturation and proliferation of CD8αα(+) cells in VDR knockout (KO) mice results in fewer functional CD8αα(+), and thereby leads to increased inflammation in the gastrointestinal tract of these mice, especially when dietary vitamin D is also low. More generally, VDR KO and vitamin D-deficient mice have a surplus of effector T cells that have been implicated in the pathology of autoimmune diseases, including multiple sclerosis and IBD. Conventional T cells develop normally in VDR KO mice, but there is overproduction of interferon gamma (IFN-γ) and IL17.

Goff et al. [16] used β-glucuronides of vitamin D to target delivery to the colon, and showed therapeutic effects against induced colitis in a dextran sodium sulfate-induced murine model of IBD. Potentially of even more interest is the way in which bacteria regulate VDR, and how this in turn affects the nuclear factor (NF)-κB pathway in intestinal epithelial cells. The effects of an inactive VDR receptor on NF-κB activation in intestinal epithelia was studied using VDR(–/–) mice [17]. This study also considered the role of enteric bacteria on VDR expression. The data showed that commensal and pathogenic bacteria regulate colonic epithelial VDR expression. Perhaps even more importantly, the VDR receptor appears to negatively regulate bacterial-induced intestinal NF-κB activation, thereby modulating host response to infections. This work emphasized the importance of VDR as a contributor to intestinal homeostasis, and in protecting the host from bacterial invasion and infection. The hypothesis generated is illustrated in Figure 7.1.

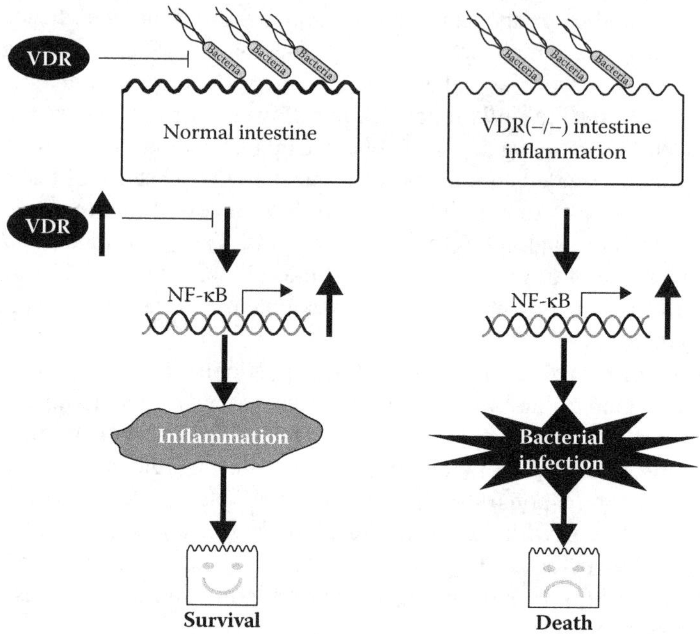

FIGURE 7.1 The VDR, gut microbiota, and intestinal inflammation in IBD. This working model of VDR in the regulation of bacterial invasion and thereby of NF-κB activity, leading to host protection, and intestinal homeostasis, was developed by Wu et al. (Data from Wu, S. et al., *American Journal of Pathology*, 177, 2, 686–97, 2010.)

Effects of Whole Foods and Dietary Components on Inflammation in Animal Models of IBD

Knoch et al. [18] hypothesized that dietary arachidonic acid (AA), an omega-6 (n-6) polyunsaturated acid (PUFA) would aggravate colon inflammation in the IL10(–/–) mouse model, in comparison to an oleic acid control diet. They studied the effects of AA on gene expression profiles during colitis, using whole genome microarray analysis. Contrary to their hypothesis, their findings suggested that dietary AA protected colonocytes from oxidative stress in IL10(–/–) mice.

When IL10(–/–) mice are raised under conventional, but not germ-free, conditions, they show an inflammatory reaction to intestinal bacteria, and develop spontaneous colitis, with characteristics similar to that of human CD. Both dietary omega-3 (n-3) and n-6 PUFA have direct anti-inflammatory effects, and affect colonic gene expression profiles in this model [18,19]. In addition to direct anti-inflammatory effects, another primary effect of these foods in the IL10(–/–) model is to modulate the diversity of caecal bacteria. Similar effects were obtained in the MDR(–/–) model through feeding broccoli or blueberry [20], or the dietary supplement, curcumin [21].

Bacteria and Intestinal Barrier Function

An intact intestinal barrier function is important for preserving health, as a compromised barrier allows antigen entry and can induce inflammatory diseases. Alteration of tight junction (TJ) signaling in healthy humans is a potential mechanism that could lead to the strengthening of the intestinal barrier, resulting in limiting the ability of antigens to enter the body and potentially triggering undesirable immune responses. Probiotic bacteria can play a role in enhancing intestinal barrier function, although the mechanisms are not fully understood. A number of animal studies have shown the ability of certain probiotics to prevent alterations to TJs in the IL10(–/–) mouse model [22,23]. Ulluwishewa et al. [24] expanded these studies to the effect of probiotic bacteria on healthy intestinal epithelial cell genes involved in the whole TJ signaling pathway, including those encoding for bridging, plaque, and dual-location TJ proteins.

LESSONS FROM HUMAN STUDIES

Role of Genotype in Crohn's Disease

The first gene associated with CD susceptibility, nucleotide oligomerization domain 2 (*NOD*2), was discovered in 2001, through candidate gene studies [25,26]. This was an important discovery, for several reasons. The gene pointed to two different events associated with CD—recognition of microbiota and human immune response. Subsequent candidate gene studies confirmed the importance of this gene in different populations, and also associated related genes with CD susceptibility [3,27–33].

One of the problems with early candidate gene studies is that individual groups had small study numbers, and data were often difficult to reproduce. Thus work prior to 2001 had linked around 8 genetic regions with disease susceptibility, but the causal genes were elusive. Since 2006, genome-wide association studies (GWAS) have dominated the literature on genetic susceptibility to disease. These use a non-hypothesis-directed approach to gene discovery in disease. A key part of the success of these studies is large population numbers, from international consortia. This leads to high statistical significance, and results that reproduce in comparable population studies. By 2010, the number of genes unequivocally associated with IBD generally had risen to 99, and five main pathways were apparent. These involved innate immunity, adaptive immunity, autophagy, intestinal barrier function, and IL10 signaling [8,34]. Many components of the IL23 pathway, including *IL*23R, *IL*12B, *STAT*3, *JAK*2, and *TYK*2, appear as true IBD susceptibility genes. This pathway is thought to play a critical role in maintaining intestinal immune homeostasis through adaptive response mechanisms [8]. *JAK2*/*STAT*3 signaling may act somewhat distinctly in its own right [2]. It also appears that IL10 signaling per se increasingly plays a central role in IBD pathogenesis, possibly acting somewhat distinctly from the IL23 pathway above [13] (Figure 7.2).

The International Immunochip Consortium developed a gene chip, highly preselected for genes and gene regions relevant to autoimmune diseases, and established collaborations among 87 different laboratories. This permitted an association analysis of 1.23 million SNPs, and imputed genotype data, from 15 IBD studies [9]. The authors then performed a meta-analysis of data from more than 75,000 cases and controls. This approach permitted identification of 71 new loci among a total of 163 loci with genome-wide significance. Most loci contributed to both forms of IBD. They observed striking overlap between susceptibility loci for IBD and mycobacterial infection. Gene expression network analysis confirmed this relationship. Collectively, these

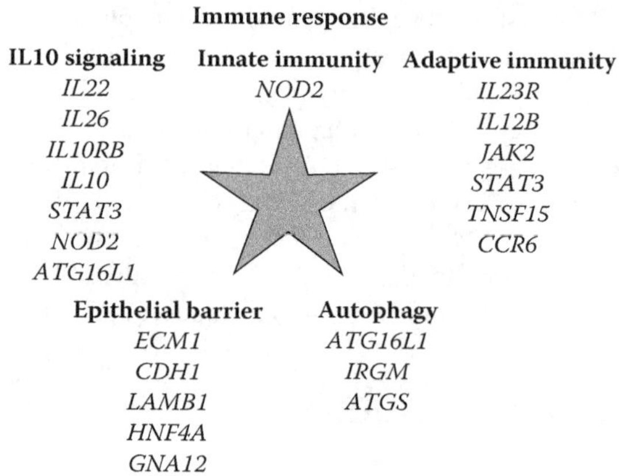

FIGURE 7.2 Key genes and gene pathways in Crohn's disease. (Modified from Lees, C.W. et al., 60, 12, 1739–53, *Gut*, 2011.)

findings shed light on the genetic and environmental interactions underlying these diseases. The work confirms the key importance of *Mycobacterium* in the diseases, and validates a role for autophagy in generally suppressing bacterial overgrowth in those who do not carry the genetic variant.

The other major pathway affected in IBD involves genes in barrier function [8]. If these are affected, they are likely to lead to a leaky gut and ineffective barrier control of permeability. A diagrammatic context is provided in Figure 7.2.

GENE–DIET INTERACTIONS IN CROHN'S DISEASE

Examples of Interactions Relevant to Innate Immune Response

Various SNPs, including a frameshift mutation in *NOD*2, are well recognized to contribute to susceptibility to CD [8,25,26]. There is evidence that vitamin D signaling can directly induce *NOD*2 expression, lending support to the hypothesis that vitamin D insufficiency/deficiency plays a causative role in CD [35].

Vitamin D is a hormone precursor present in two forms, ergocalciferol and cholecalciferol. While ergocalciferol (vitamin D2) is present in plants, yeast, and fungi, cholecalciferol (vitamin D3) is synthesized in the skin during exposure to sunlight. Thus, vitamin D requirements may be fulfilled from diet and/or from sun exposure. Some nontraditional roles have been recently ascribed to vitamin D, including anti-inflammatory and immune-modulating effects. These effects have led to possible implications in the pathophysiology of immune-mediated diseases such as both forms of IBD. Cholecalciferol is converted by hepatic vitamin D 25-hydroxylase to 25-hydroxyvitamin D (25OHD), the major circulating metabolite. Although 25OHD is largely inactive, it has a long half-life that makes it a useful indicator of overall vitamin D status. In the kidneys, 25OHD is converted by 25-hydroxyvitamin D 1α-hydroxylase to produce the active vitamin D metabolite, 1,25-dihydroxyvitamin D3 (calcitriol or $1,25(OH)_2D_3$). Serum calcium regulates the activity of la-hydroxylase, as also do fibroblast growth factor 23, phosphate, and $1,25(OH)_2D_3$ itself.

There is a close connection between vitamin D and calcium status in the body. $1,25(OH)_2D_3$ stimulates the intestinal absorption of orally ingested calcium, the tubular reabsorption of calcium filtered in the kidney, and mobilization of calcium stores from the skeleton by stimulating the maturation of osteoclasts. Chronic vitamin D deficiency results in undermineralization of bones. In association with the reduced calcium status that many of them have, through being advised against dairy products, this is highly relevant to the high risk of osteoporosis in CD patients [36–39].

The VDR has been identified in cells of the human immune system, and established as an important target of active $1,25(OH)_2D_3$. The active form of vitamin D enters the target cells from serum, autocrine, or paracrine sources, where it binds to the VDR. VDR is a member of a superfamily of nuclear hormone receptors that includes the peroxisome proliferator-activated and glucocorticoid receptors whose actions interact with both dietary and harmaceutical interventions in CD [40–42]. The conformational change thus induced promotes heterodimerization with the retinoid X receptor (RXR). This heterodimer has high affinity for the vitamin D responsive element (VDRE), and the association of the VDR/RXR complex with the VDRE leads to the attraction of a complex of co-activator proteins. On target cell entry, $1,25(OH)_2D_3$ binds with the VDR, leading to a conformational change and heterodimerization with the RXR. This increases the affinity of the VDR/RXR complex for the VDRE, a specific promoter region in vitamin D responsive genes, thereby turning on gene transcription (Figure 7.3) [43].

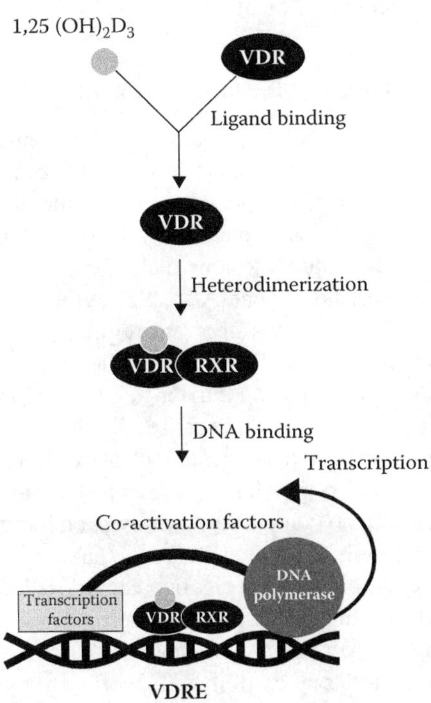

FIGURE 7.3 Proposed mechanisms of regulation of gene transcription by $1,25(OH)_2D_3$.

The active form of vitamin D suppresses the function of pathogenic T cells, while at the same time inducing several regulatory T cells that suppress IBD development and progression [15,44,45]. Vitamin D deficiency appears to play a role in the development of several immune-mediated diseases, including CD. Vitamin D deficiency has been regularly shown in CD patients [3]. Therefore, improving vitamin D status, and/or possibly using VDR agonists, has been suggested to be useful in CD treatment [7]. This would be especially relevant in those patients identified as having functional SNPs in the VDR [46].

Examples of Interactions Relevant to Adaptive Immune Function

Nutritional interventions that act through the peroxisome proliferator-activated receptors (PPARs) such as dietary conjugated linoleic acid (CLA) and long-chain n-3 PUFA have demonstrated anti-inflammatory efficacy in animal models of CD [40,41,47]. Clinical data on n-3 PUFA in IBD remains generally controversial, although results of a recent human study show that IBD remission can be maintained by maintaining the n-3:n-6 ratio more than 0.65 via n-3 PUFA intervention. We have pointed out that many of the different results may be because of the very different natures of the sources and products used [48]. In mice, CLA prevented inflammation-driven colorectal cancer by activating PPAR γ and modulating regulatory T cells and macrophages. CLA is the subject of an ongoing clinical study in patients with CD. For both compounds, there is an urgent need for placebo-controlled, large-scale, multicenter clinical trials [41,47].

Interactions Relevant to Leaky Barrier Function

Epithelial barrier function is typically impaired in CD, contributing to diarrhea and also enhancing inflammation by increased luminal antigen uptake. This intestinal epithelial barrier is composed of an apical enterocyte membrane, and the epithelial TJ. It is vulnerable to changes in TJ, through the induction of epithelial apoptosis, and/or by the appearance of inflammatory lesions such as erosions or ulcers. TJ strands are reduced in CD, and strand breaks appear. Also, Th1 cytokines such as tumor necrosis factor-alpha (TNF-α) and IFN-γ are important regulators for CD. Therapeutically, anti-inflammatory remedies such as TNF-α antibodies are most effective in improving active CD in parallel with repairing barrier function. This has been attributed to reduced cytokine release in active CD, because of immune cell apoptosis. A number of therapeutic compounds and nutrients can also directly affect barrier function. Several probiotics and also transforming growth factor-β have shown beneficial effects in animal models, but no comparable data exist on human CD. The two groups of dietary components for which human data are available are the micronutrient (zinc [49–51]) and the flavonoids (quercetin, epigallocatechin gallate, genistein, quercetin, and myricetin [51]), all of which have protective properties related to the intestinal TJ barrier. Soybean-derived genistein, enhances the TJ barrier and protects against oxidative stress and inflammatory cytokines. It works by blocking tyrosine kinase phosphorylation caused by oxidative stress, which, if allowed to proceed, would lead to the disassembly of the TJ. Quercetin, on the other hand, stabilizes the TJ barrier through an increase of TJ proteins and their assembly [52].

Zinc and Intestinal Barrier Function

Ringstad et al. [53] measured serum zinc, copper, and selenium levels in 74 children with IBD in the Gastroenterology Unit of Great Ormond Street Children's Hospital, London, UK. They showed that those children with CD had significantly lower levels of each of these trace elements as compared with those with UC, or age- and sex-matched normal controls. A small trial of 15 children, ages 8–18 years, with stable CD, and 15 healthy matched controls suggested that low plasma zinc concentrations could be caused by reduced zinc absorption [54]. The effects of oral zinc sulfate supplementation (110 mg three times a day) were considered for 8 weeks in 12 patients with quiescent CD [55]. This treatment significantly improved intestinal barrier function in 10 of those patients, and this treatment appeared to prevent relapse in those whose intestine did show a response.

GWAS studies have identified multiple CD susceptibility loci, including association with noncoding intergenic SNPs at 10q21 [56]. These authors fine-mapped the 10q21 locus, by genotyping 86 SNPs in 1632 CD cases and 961 controls and by performing single-marker and conditional analyses using logistic regression. The most significant association observed was at the nonsynonymous SNP, rs7076156 (Ala62Thr), in *ZNF*365. Conditional analysis on rs7076156 nullified all other significant associations, suggesting that this is the causative variant. Four isoforms of ZNF365 have previously been identified. The authors used reverse transcription-PCR to show differential expression of *ZNF*365D in intestinal resections from both CD subjects and controls. These data support the hypothesis that this nonsynonymous Ala62Thr SNP explains the association between 10q21 and CD risk, probably by altering expression of genes under the control of *ZNF*365 isoform D.

Modulation of the Gut Microbiota

A distinctive characteristic of both forms of IBD is their microbiota [3,28,57]. Although it is not clear whether it is cause or effect of the disease, significant differences in gut microbiota between control subjects and those with IBD have been observed in both animal models and humans [58,59]. The role of diet in the regulation of the immune response against gut microbiota is the subject of current intensive evaluation [58]. An effective short-term method to both control the disease and modulate the microbiota is via enteral or parenteral nutrition. However, since most of the currently used formulas reduce the diversity of bacteria, long-term usage is not likely to be beneficial [60].

A number of dietary components, including various antioxidants, plant flavonoids, and long-chain n-3 PUFA have been shown to reduce symptoms of CD in many individuals [61,62]. These seem to act through various mechanisms including a reduction of free radicals, decreased production of proinflammatory molecules and the promotion of anti-inflammatory responses leading to more efficient gut barrier functioning, which in turn will have positive effects on control of the gut microflora.

Probiotics, Prebiotics, and Synbiotics

One of the most obvious dietary items being promoted as modulating the gut microbiota is probiotics [63]. These are live bacteria, often used as natural therapies by patients, despite failure by any of the companies to achieve a health claim on these. Several different types of probiotics have been tested for efficacy in IBD [64,65]. While there is some suggestion of benefit when UC patients are treated with a range of different probiotics, including the mixture VSL#3 [66], sample sizes have been too small and methodological flaws in study designs mean that more data are necessary before probiotics could be routinely recommended in clinical practice of UC. The data for probiotics are less convincing for CD than for UC, since these tend to enhance diarrhea, which is already a problem for these subjects [67]. Despite this lack of convincing evidence, consumer surveys have shown that more subjects with active IBD are taking pro- or prebiotics than does the general population [68].

In healthy individuals, regular consumption of prebiotic carbohydrates such as fructooligosaccharides (FOS) can substantially influence the intestinal microbiota [69]. Benjamin et al. [69] sought to study whether FOS had beneficial activity in CD patients with active disease, using a randomized double-blind placebo-controlled trial design. A total of 103 CD subjects with active disease were randomized for 4 weeks to 15 g/day FOS or nonprebiotic placebo for 4 weeks. The primary endpoint was the clinical evidence of a significant fall in CD Activity Index. More patients on the FOS arm (14 [26%] vs. 4 [8%]; $p = .018$) withdrew before the scheduled endpoint of the trial. The trial showed an impact on dendritic cell function but no clinical benefit in patients with active CD. UC may be more responsive to prebiotics, but there have been no convincing well-designed clinical trials, with sufficient numbers of subjects to draw conclusions for probiotics, prebiotics, or their combination at this time [70].

Phenolics and Other Plant Pigments

Dietary phenolic compounds are typically metabolized before absorption. *Clostridium* and *Eubacterium* genera are involved in the metabolism of many phenolic compounds, and their growth will be promoted by this means. The health benefits from phenolic consumption will thus be attributable not only to their bioactive metabolites but also to their effects on modulation of the intestinal bacterial population [71]. There is also particular interest in cocoa flavones for their effects on the microbiota [72]. As Qin recently concluded, the effect of dietary chemicals on gut bacteria and IBD demands further study [73].

Macronutrients and Micronutrients

Wu and co-workers showed both short-term and long-term dietary responses of the human intestinal microbiota to specific classes of nutrients [24]. They tested the effects of long-term dietary habits on the intestinal microbiota in 98 healthy volunteers. Their analysis revealed that the human intestinal microbiota is characterized by bacterial groups that relate to the nature of dietary fats, proteins, and/or carbohydrates. Inverse correlations were observed for proteins versus carbohydrates, and fats versus carbohydrates. Ten subjects, in a hospital environment, were randomized to high-fat and low-fiber or low-fat and high-fiber diets. Their intestinal microbiota changed significantly within the first 24 hours of the controlled dietary regime. However, identical short-term diets did not overcome the high degree of inter-individual variations. It appears that the intestinal microbiota consists of some bacterial groups affected by short-term dietary changes, and others that can only be changed by long-term dietary habits, such as those referred to as human enterotypes. In this particular study, ten days of dietary intervention was not sufficient to switch individuals between the enterotypes [74]. At this stage, however, the necessary length of time is not clear.

Micronutrients may provide some of the most potentially useful approaches to modulating CD in patients. The one which provides some of the most elegant (and potentially applicable) examples is, again, vitamin D. Ly et al. [75] discuss the increasing body of evidence for the importance of the vitamin D pathway, not only in gut homeostasis but also in signaling between the microbiota and the host. Weiss [76] goes further to suggest that bacterial components plus vitamin D may prove the ultimate solution to autoimmune disease. Also of interest are data from Sakaki et al. [77] showing that bacterial Cytochrome P450 enzymes may be able to convert vitamin D into its "active" form. It has been proposed that that the vitamin D often observed in autoimmune disease is not a sign of deficiency because of inadequate intake. Instead, there is reason to believe that the lower levels come about through chronic infection with intracellular bacteria leading to malfunctions in vitamin D metabolism, by causing VDR dysfunction within phagocytes [78].

There is increasing evidence to suggest that the symptoms of many CD patients who were administered vitamin D may be caused by the ability of this nutrient to help regulate bacteria-induced inflammation [79]. Liu et al. [80] suggest that this occurs through Toll-like receptor triggering. Their data confirm the possibility that differences in the ability of genetically predisposed individuals to produce vitamin D, may contribute to susceptibility to microbial infection.

CONCLUSIONS

CD is a form of IBD, characterized by chronic inflammation in the colon and often other parts of the gastrointestinal tract, genetics and environmental susceptibility factors, and a number of food intolerances. These intolerances, however, differ among individuals, making CD a potential example of nutrigenetics. Although there are now more than 160 genes that have been associated with these diseases, which fall into distinct pathways, related to response to microbiota, immune response, and intestinal barrier function, there is good evidence from both animal and human studies to suggest some specific dietary interventions for each of these.

An increasing number of genes associated with the disease are found to affect the gut microbiota. The environment also has an impact. Thus, early attempts to link susceptibility genes with dietary factors may have been confused by the microbiota. Research attempts must be directed toward establishing the effects of macro- and micronutrients, and plant pigments on the gut microbiota, and hence on symptoms and long-term implications of CD. Vitamin D may be an especially important micronutrient, especially in the presence of VDR mutations.

REFERENCES

1. Ferguson, L.R., Nutrigenomics and inflammatory bowel diseases. *Expert Review of Clinical Immunology*, 2010. 6(4): 573–83.
2. Ferguson, L.R. et al., Genetic factors in chronic inflammation: single nucleotide polymorphisms in the STAT-JAK pathway, susceptibility to DNA damage and Crohn's disease in a New Zealand population. *Mutation Research*, 2010. 690(1–2): 108–15.
3. Gentschew, L. and L.R. Ferguson, Role of nutrition and microbiota in susceptibility to inflammatory bowel diseases. *Molecular Nutrition & Food Research*, 2012. 56(4): 524–35.
4. Yakut, M. et al., Serum vitamin B12 and folate status in patients with inflammatory bowel diseases. *European Journal of Internal Medicine*, 2010. 21(4): 320–3.
5. Petermann, I. et al., Mushroom intolerance: a novel diet-gene interaction in Crohn's disease. *British Journal of Nutrition*, 2009. 102(4): 506–8.
6. Tighe, M.P., J.R.F. Cummings, and N.A. Afzal, Nutrition and inflammatory bowel disease: primary or adjuvant therapy. *Current Opinion in Clinical Nutrition & Metabolic Care*, 2011. 14(5): 491–6.
7. Brown, A.C., S.D. Rampertab, and G.E. Mullin, Existing dietary guidelines for Crohn's disease and ulcerative colitis. *Expert Review of Gastroenterology & Hepatology*, 2011. 5(3): 411–25.
8. Lees, C.W. et al., New IBD genetics: common pathways with other diseases. *Gut*, 2011. 60(12): 1739–53.
9. Jostins, L. et al., Host-microbe interactions have shaped the genetic architecture of inflammatory bowel disease. *Nature*, 2012. 491: 119–24.
10. Mizoguchi, A., Animal models of inflammatory bowel disease. *Progress in Molecular Biology & Translational Science*, 2012. 105: 263–320.
11. Dommels, Y.E.M. et al., Characterization of intestinal inflammation and identification of related gene expression changes in mdr1a(–/–) mice. *Genes & Nutrition*, 2007. 2(2): 209–23.
12. Nones, K. et al., Multidrug resistance gene deficient (mdr1a–/–) mice have an altered caecal microbiota that precedes the onset of intestinal inflammation. *Journal of Applied Microbiology*, 2009. 107(2): 557–66.
13. Wang, A.H. et al., The effect of IL-10 genetic variation and interleukin 10 serum levels on Crohn's disease susceptibility in a New Zealand population. *Human Immunology*, 2011. 72(5): 431–5.
14. Barnett, M.P.G. et al., Changes in colon gene expression associated with increased colon inflammation in interleukin-10 gene-deficient mice inoculated with Enterococcus species. *BMC Immunology*, 2010. 11: 39.
15. Bruce, D. and M.T. Cantorna, Intrinsic requirement for the vitamin D receptor in the development of CD8alphaalpha-expressing T cells. *Journal of Immunology*, 2011. 186(5): 2819–25.
16. Goff, J.P. et al., Targeted delivery of vitamin D to the colon using beta-glucuronides of vitamin D: therapeutic effects in a murine model of inflammatory bowel disease. *American Journal of Physiology - Gastrointestinal & Liver Physiology*, 2012. 302(4): G460–9.
17. Wu, S. et al., Vitamin D receptor negatively regulates bacterial-stimulated NF-kappaB activity in intestine. *American Journal of Pathology*, 2010. 177(2): 686–97.
18. Knoch, B. et al., Genome-wide analysis of dietary eicosapentaenoic acid- and oleic acid-induced modulation of colon inflammation in interleukin-10 gene-deficient mice. *Journal of Nutrigenetics & Nutrigenomics*, 2009. 2(1): 9–28.
19. Knoch, B. et al., Dietary arachidonic acid-mediated effects on colon inflammation using transcriptome analysis. *Molecular Nutrition & Food Research*, 2010. 54 Suppl 1: S62–74.

20. Paturi, G. et al., Influence of dietary blueberry and broccoli on caecal microbiota activity and colon morphology in mdr1a(−/−) mice, a model of inflammatory bowel diseases. *Nutrition*, 2012. 28(3): 324–30.
21. Nones, K. et al., The effects of dietary curcumin and rutin on colonic inflammation and gene expression in multidrug resistance gene-deficient (mdr1a−/−) mice, a model of inflammatory bowel diseases. *British Journal of Nutrition*, 2009. 101(2): 169–81.
22. Anderson, R.C. et al., Lactobacillus plantarum DSM 2648 is a potential probiotic that enhances intestinal barrier function. *FEMS Microbiology Letters*, 2010. 309(2): 184–92.
23. Anderson, R.C. et al., Lactobacillus plantarum MB452 enhances the function of the intestinal barrier by increasing the expression levels of genes involved in tight junction formation. *BMC Microbiology*, 2010. 10: 316.
24. Ulluwishewa, D. et al., Regulation of tight junction permeability by intestinal bacteria and dietary components. *Journal of Nutrition*, 2011. 141(5): 769–76.
25. Hugot, J.P. et al., Association of NOD2 leucine-rich repeat variants with susceptibility to Crohn's disease. *Nature*, 2001. 411(6837): 599–603.
26. Ogura, Y. et al., A frameshift mutation in NOD2 associated with susceptibility to Crohn's disease. *Nature*, 2001. 411(6837): 603–6.
27. Van Heel, D.A., D.P. McGovern, and D.P. Jewell, Crohn's disease: genetic susceptibility, bacteria, and innate immunity. *Lancet*, 2001. 357(9272): 1902–4.
28. Baker, P.I., D.R. Love, and L.R. Ferguson, Role of gut microbiota in Crohn's disease. *Expert Review of Gastroenterology & Hepatology*, 2009. 3(5): 535–46.
29. Browning, B.L. et al., Has toll-like receptor 4 been prematurely dismissed as an inflammatory bowel disease gene? Association study combined with meta-analysis shows strong evidence for association. *American Journal of Gastroenterology*, 2007. 102(11): 2504–12.
30. Browning, B.L. et al., Association of DLG5 variants with inflammatory bowel disease in the New Zealand Caucasian population and meta-analysis of the DLG5 R30Q variant. *Inflammatory Bowel Diseases*, 2007. 13(9): 1069–76.
31. Ferguson, L.R. et al., Single nucleotide polymorphisms in human Paneth cell defensin A5 may confer susceptibility to inflammatory bowel disease in a New Zealand Caucasian population. *Digestive & Liver Disease*, 2008. 40(9): 723–30.
32. Ferguson, L.R. et al., Single nucleotide polymorphism in the tumor necrosis factor-alpha gene affects inflammatory bowel diseases risk. *World Journal of Gastroenterology*, 2008. 14(29): 4652–61.
33. Huebner, C. et al., Nucleotide-binding oligomerization domain containing 1 (NOD1) haplotypes and single nucleotide polymorphisms modify susceptibility to inflammatory bowel diseases in a New Zealand caucasian population: a case-control study. *BMC Research Notes*, 2009. 2: 52.
34. Franke, A. et al., Genome-wide meta-analysis increases to 71 the number of confirmed Crohn's disease susceptibility loci. *Nature Genetics*, 2010. 42(12): 1118–25.
35. Wang, T.-T. et al., Direct and indirect induction by 1,25-dihydroxyvitamin D3 of the NOD2/CARD15-defensin beta2 innate immune pathway defective in Crohn disease. *Journal of Biological Chemistry*, 2010. 285(4): 2227–31.
36. Bours, P.H.A. et al., Seasonal variation of serum 25-hydroxyvitamin D levels in adult patients with inflammatory bowel disease. *Osteoporosis International*, 2011. 22(11): 2857–67.
37. Cravo, M. et al., Risk factors for metabolic bone disease in Crohn's disease patients. *Inflammatory Bowel Diseases*, 2010. 16(12): 2117–24.
38. Kumari, M. et al., Vitamin D-mediated calcium absorption in patients with clinically stable Crohn's disease: a pilot study. *Molecular Nutrition & Food Research*, 2010. 54(8): 1085–91.
39. Orlic, Z.C. et al., How activity of inflammatory bowel disease influences bone loss. *Journal of Clinical Densitometry*, 2010. 13(1): 36–42.

40. Evans, N.P. et al., Conjugated linoleic acid ameliorates inflammation-induced colorectal cancer in mice through activation of PPARgamma. *Journal of Nutrition*, 2010. 140(3): 515–21.
41. Bassaganya-Riera, J. and R. Hontecillas, CLA and n-3 PUFA differentially modulate clinical activity and colonic PPAR-responsive gene expression in a pig model of experimental IBD. *Clinical Nutrition*, 2006. 25(3): 454–65.
42. Mencarelli, A. et al., Probiotics modulate intestinal expression of nuclear receptor and provide counter-regulatory signals to inflammation-driven adipose tissue activation. *PLoS ONE* [Electronic Resource], 2011. 6(7): e22978.
43. Carlberg, C. and P. Polly, Gene regulation by vitamin D3. *Critical Reviews in Eukaryotic Gene Expression*, 1998. 8(1): 19–42.
44. Cantorna, M.T., Vitamin D and its role in immunology: multiple sclerosis, and inflammatory bowel disease. *Progress in Biophysics & Molecular Biology*, 2006. 92(1): 60–4.
45. Cantorna, M.T., Mechanisms underlying the effect of vitamin D on the immune system. *Proceedings of the Nutrition Society*, 2010. 69(3): 286–9.
46. Eloranta, J.J. et al., Association of a common vitamin D-binding protein polymorphism with inflammatory bowel disease. *Pharmacogenetics and Genomics*, 2011. 21(9): 559–64.
47. Bassaganya-Riera, J. and R. Hontecillas, Dietary conjugated linoleic acid and n-3 polyunsaturated fatty acids in inflammatory bowel disease. *Current Opinion in Clinical Nutrition & Metabolic Care*, 2010. 13(5): 569–73.
48. Ferguson, L.R., B.G. Smith, and B.J. James, Combining nutrition, food science and engineering in developing solutions to inflammatory bowel diseases— omega-3 polyunsaturated fatty acids as an example. *Food & Function*, 2010. 1(1): 60–72.
49. El-Tawil, A.M., Zinc supplementation tightens leaky gut in Crohn's disease. *Inflammatory Bowel Diseases*, 2012. 18(2): E399.
50. Ainley, C. et al., The influence of zinc status and malnutrition on immunological function in Crohn's disease. *Gastroenterology*, 1991. 100(6): 1616–25.
51. Hering, N.A. and J.-D. Schulzke, Therapeutic options to modulate barrier defects in inflammatory bowel disease. *Digestive Diseases*, 2009. 27(4): 450–4.
52. Suzuki, T. and H. Hara, Role of flavonoids in intestinal tight junction regulation. *Journal of Nutritional Biochemistry*, 2011. 22(5): 401–8.
53. Ringstad, J., S. Kildebo, and Y. Thomassen, Serum selenium, copper, and zinc concentrations in Crohn's disease and ulcerative colitis. *Scandinavian Journal of Gastroenterology*, 1993. 28(7): 605–8.
54. Griffin, I.J. et al., Zinc metabolism in adolescents with Crohn's disease. *Pediatric Research*, 2004. 56(2): 235–9.
55. Sturniolo, G.C. et al., Zinc supplementation tightens "leaky gut" in Crohn's disease. *Inflammatory Bowel Diseases*, 2001. 7(2): 94–8.
56. Haritunians, T. et al., Variants in ZNF365 isoform D are associated with Crohn's disease. *Gut*, 2011. 60(8): 1060–7.
57. Sartor, R.B., Key questions to guide a better understanding of host-commensal microbiota interactions in intestinal inflammation. *Mucosal immunology*, 2011. 4(2): 127–32.
58. Haller, D., Nutrigenomics and IBD: the intestinal microbiota at the cross-road between inflammation and metabolism. *Journal of Clinical Gastroenterology*, 2010. 44 Suppl 1: S6–9.
59. Hammer, H.F., Gut microbiota and inflammatory bowel disease. *Digestive Diseases*, 2011. 29(6): 550–3.
60. Albenberg, L.G., J.D. Lewis, and G.D. Wu, Food and the gut microbiota in inflammatory bowel diseases: a critical connection. *Current Opinion in Gastroenterology*, 2012. 28(4): 314–20.

61. Calder, P.C., Fatty acids and inflammation: the cutting edge between food and pharma. *European Journal of Pharmacology*, 2011. 668 Suppl 1: S50–8.
62. Calder, P.C., The role of marine omega-3 (n-3) fatty acids in inflammatory processes, atherosclerosis and plaque stability. *Molecular Nutrition & Food Research*, 2012. 56(7): 1073–80.
63. Cain, A.M. and K.D. Karpa, Clinical utility of probiotics in inflammatory bowel disease. *Alternative Therapies in Health & Medicine*, 2011. 17(1): 72–9.
64. D'Inca, R. et al., Rectal administration of Lactobacillus casei DG modifies flora composition and Toll-like receptor expression in colonic mucosa of patients with mild ulcerative colitis. *Digestive Diseases & Sciences*, 2011. 56(4): 1178–87.
65. Do, V.T., B.G. Baird, and D.R. Kockler, Probiotics for maintaining remission of ulcerative colitis in adults. *Annals of Pharmacotherapy*, 2010. 44(3): 565–71.
66. Jackson, E.L., P.J. Hamlin, and A.C. Ford, VSL#3 and remission in active ulcerative colitis: larger studies required. *American Journal of Gastroenterology*, 2011. 106(3): 547; author reply 547–8.
67. Doherty, G.A. et al., Meta-analysis: targeting the intestinal microbiota in prophylaxis for post-operative Crohn's disease. *Alimentary Pharmacology & Therapeutics*, 2010. 31(8): 802–9.
68. Hedin, C.R.H. et al., Probiotic and prebiotic use in patients with inflammatory bowel disease: a case-control study. *Inflammatory Bowel Diseases*, 2010. 16(12): 2099–108.
69. Benjamin, J.L. et al., Randomized, double-blind, placebo-controlled trial of fructo-oligosaccharides in active Crohn's disease. *Gut*, 2011. 60(7): 923–9.
70. Quigley, E.M.M., Prebiotics and probiotics: their role in the management of gastrointestinal disorders in adults. *Nutrition in Clinical Practice*, 2012. 27(2): 195–200.
71. Selma, M.V., J.C. Espin, and F.A. Tomas-Barberan, Interaction between phenolics and gut microbiota: role in human health. *Journal of Agricultural & Food Chemistry*, 2009. 57(15): 6485–501.
72. Tzounis, X. et al., Prebiotic evaluation of cocoa-derived flavanols in healthy humans by using a randomized, controlled, double-blind, crossover intervention study. *American Journal of Clinical Nutrition*, 2011. 93(1): 62–72.
73. Qin, X., The effect of dietary chemicals on gut bacteria and IBD demands further study. *Journal of Crohn's and Colitis*, 2011. 5(2): 175.
74 Wu, H.-J. and E. Wu, The role of gut microbiota in immune homeostasis and autoimmunity. *Gut Microbes*, 2012. 3: 4–14.
75. Ly, N.P. et al., Gut microbiota, probiotics, and vitamin D: interrelated exposures influencing allergy, asthma, and obesity? *Journal of Allergy and Clinical Immunology*, 2011. 127(5): 1087–94; quiz 1095–6.
76. Weiss, S.T., Bacterial components plus vitamin D: the ultimate solution to the asthma (autoimmune disease) epidemic? *Journal of Allergy and Clinical Immunology*, 2011. 127(5): 1128–30.
77. Sakaki, T. et al., Bioconversion of vitamin D to its active form by bacterial or mammalian cytochrome P450. *Biochimica et Biophysica Acta*, 2011. 1814(1): 249–56.
78. Waterhouse, J.C., T.H. Perez, and P.J. Albert, Reversing bacteria-induced vitamin D receptor dysfunction is key to autoimmune disease. *Annals of the New York Academy of Sciences*, 2009. 1173: 757–65.
79. Albert, P.J., A.D. Proal, and T.G. Marshall, Vitamin D: the alternative hypothesis. *Autoimmunity Reviews*, 2009. 8(8): 639–44.
80. Liu, P.T. et al., Toll-like receptor triggering of a vitamin D-mediated human antimicrobial response. *Science*, 2006. 311(5768): 1770–3.

8 Microbiome and Host Interactions in Inflammatory Bowel Diseases
Relevance for Personalized Nutrition

Wayne Young, Bianca Knoch, and Nicole C. Roy

CONTENTS

INTRODUCTION

The human gastrointestinal tract is home to an estimated 100 trillion microorganisms. Collectively referred to as the intestinal microbiota, they are thought to outnumber the cells of their host 10 fold and represent by far the largest microbial community associated with the human body [1]. The intestinal bacteria in humans comprise 500–1000 bacterial species and complex metabolic relationships exist between bacterial communities and their host [2]. Figure 8.1 illustrates the different compartments of the human gastrointestinal tract, physiological processes and conditions, and the major bacteria genera found therein [3]. Very little is known about these interbacterial relationships and how they relate to host health, but it is known that increasing diversity of the large bowel bacteria promotes metabolic homeostasis and the ability to resist invading pathogens [4].

This complex ecosystem represents a huge reservoir of metabolic capability and plays a crucial role in a number of developmental and nutritional processes in the

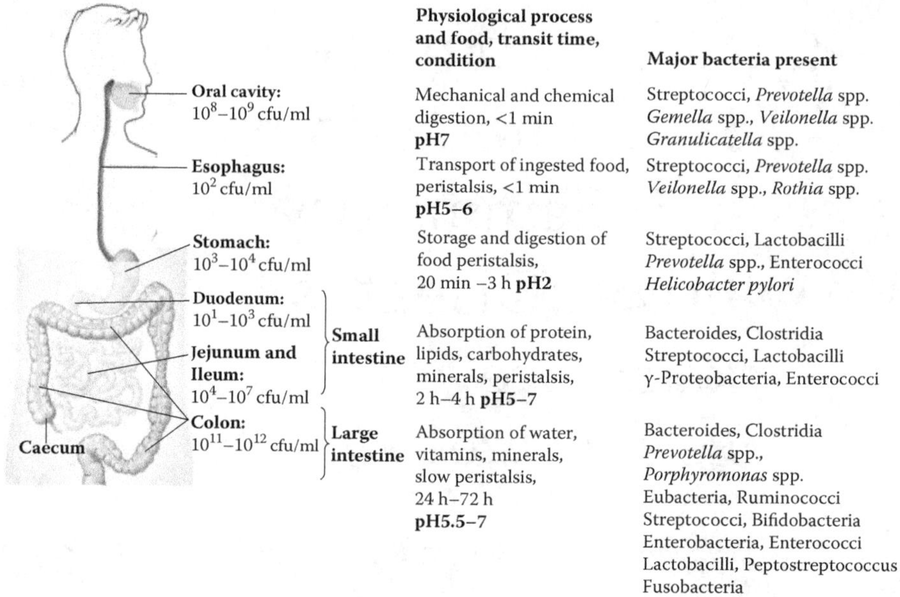

FIGURE 8.1 Compartments of the human gastrointestinal tract, physiological processes and conditions, and the major bacteria genera found herein. (From Manson et al., The commensal microbiology of the gastrointestinal tract, in: G.B. Huffnagle and M.C. Noverr (Eds.), *Advances in Experimental Medicine and Biology, GI Microbiota and Regulation of the Immune System*, Landes Bioscience and Springer Science + Business Media, pp. 15–28, 2008.)

intestine. The adaptive coevolution of the microbial community and its host has enabled humans to harvest nutrients from sources that they would otherwise lack the ability to utilize [5]. The intestinal microbiota also stimulates development of the immune system and assists the host by excluding pathogens. Studies have revealed how members of the intestinal microbiota are able to manipulate host physiology to the benefit of both microbe and host [6]. Community composition and metabolic activity of the microbiota are influenced by a variety of factors including the diet and health status of the host [7,8]. Likewise, the resident microbiota may also be an important factor in a number of diseases or conditions, including colon cancer, inflammatory bowel diseases (IBD), and obesity [9–11].

Intestinal bacteria live in an endosymbiotic relationship with a healthy host and regulate vital processes in the host related to metabolism (e.g., fermentation of digestion resistant carbohydrates leading to production of short-chain fatty acids [SCFAs]), mucosal barrier function (e.g., inhibition of pathogen invasion and enhancement of epithelial barrier integrity), and immunity (e.g., priming mucosal immune system to maintain intestinal epithelium homeostasis) [12]. In a healthy intestine, the fine balance between these processes determines the immune tolerance of the host toward its commensal bacteria. In IBD patients, it is hypothesized that there is an abnormal microbial composition with an increased prevalence of detrimental microbes and a concomitant decrease in beneficial microbial populations. There is evidence that an aberrant mucosal immune response to normal intestinal bacteria underlies mucosal inflammation in human disease [13]. Animal models of IBD show that induction of inflammation involves activation of innate immune factors such as pattern-recognition receptors, example, toll-like receptors (TLR), which recognize molecular bacterial motifs at intestinal mucosal surfaces to mount antigen-specific adaptive immune responses [13,14]. However, it is still unclear whether this dysbiosis is cause or consequence of the disease [12,15].

Prebiotic (i.e., nondigestible nutrients), probiotic (i.e., beneficial microbes), and synbiotic (i.e., synergistic combination of pro- and prebiotics) approaches present promising nutritional strategies in IBD to target changes in intestinal microbial composition [8,12,16,17]. Nutrients interact directly with the host genome and indirectly through the collective genomes of the entire intestinal microbial community, commonly referred to as the metagenome, which therefore acts as an interface between food and host genome. Nutrients can be metabolized by intestinal microbes to produce metabolites that regulate target genes in the host metabolism [17]. The use of high-throughput next generation sequencing (NGS) technologies enables comprehensive analyses of the effects of nutrients on mucosal immune responses (host genome) and microbial communities (microbiome) of the intestinal tract.

This chapter summarizes approaches to the qualitative and quantitative analyses of the microbial communities of the large bowel, mainly focusing on interactions between microbial communities and mucosal metabolism and how these differ between healthy individuals and individuals with IBD, and discusses the relevance of these interactions to nutrigenomic studies.

QUALITATIVE AND QUANTITATIVE ANALYSES OF THE LARGE BOWEL MICROBIOTA

An understanding of the large bowel microbial composition and activity can be accomplished through a variety of methods ranging from culture-based methods to molecular fingerprinting methods such as temperature or denaturing gradient gel electrophoresis (TGGE or DGGE) [18–20]. Advances in NGS technologies have enabled a highly detailed examination of the microbiota to a level not previously possible. The application of NGS allows not only the identification of bacterial taxa that make up the microbiota, but also the genetic composition of metagenome [21–24].

Most of the bacteria in the human gastrointestinal tract are anaerobes, and only an estimated 20%–40% are cultivable in the laboratory using classical plating and speciation techniques [25]. Traditional culture methods based on phenotypic characterization are insufficient to detect the whole bacterial community in the intestine, due to low coverage, low reproducibility, low sensitivity, and being time consuming and laborious [26,27]. Nevertheless, traditional cultivation techniques provided early insights into the physiology of cultivable bacteria in the intestine and are still applied in clinical microbiology.

Culture-independent and higher resolution molecular methods have become an important tool in studying the diversity, abundance, and population dynamics of complex bacterial communities [28]. These molecular methods are based mainly on the detection of 16S ribosomal RNA (rRNA) or the DNA that makes up the genes encoding the rRNA [29]. The use of RNA isolated from bacterial cells indicates the metabolic activity, because the number of ribosomes per cell is approximately proportional to bacterial growth rate [30]. In contrast, analysis of DNA provides a phylogenetic overview of the community that encompasses living, dormant, lysed, or dead cells [18]. The 16S rRNA gene has become a key bacterial marker due to its unique composition of highly conserved as well as variable genomic regions, its evolutionary stability and its high copy number within bacterial cells [31]. Differences in base pair sequence within the variable regions are used to distinguish between bacterial genera and species. Highly conserved regions of the ribosomal RNA or DNA can be used to design universal probes targeting all bacteria (Eubacteria), whereas variable regions are used for targeting specific groups of bacteria. Numerous 16S rRNA gene sequences including uncultured bacterial clones are available in the database of the National Centre for Biotechnology Information, which allows for sequence comparisons across the world.

The bacterial community in a sample can be analyzed using untargeted community profiling methods such as polymerase chain reaction (PCR) combined with TGGE or DGGE, or DNA-arrays (DNA chips) (Figure 8.2). Targeted analysis methods include fluorescent in situ hybridization (FISH) with specific synthetic oligonucleotide probes combined with flow cytometry or microscopic analysis [25,31–34] and quantitative PCR quantification of DNA fragments [35]. Multiplex PCR even allows the amplification of several target regions of the 16S rRNA gene in a single reaction with multiple primer pairs [36].

More recently, analysis of the microbiota in colonic digesta has been carried out using NGS of barcode-tagged 16S rRNA gene amplicons, providing detailed taxonomic and abundance information [10,24,37]. Using NGS, it is also possible to characterize the metagenome and metatranscriptome of the microbiota to gain insight into the genetic activity of the community [38,39]. Studying the metagenome and metatranscriptome in parallel with taxonomic profiling can provide important information on the activity of the microbiota as the most abundant molecular functions may be provided by several different taxa or by those that are not necessarily the most abundant (Figure 8.3) [40,41]. The major advantage offered by NGS technologies over traditional capillary sequencing platforms is the generation of much greater numbers of sequences without cloning bias by parallelizing the sequencing process, enabling the production of thousands or millions of sequences at once. The use of NGS platforms has transformed the study of microbial communities in the large bowel by providing detailed insights into the community structure and activity beyond what was possible with traditional Sanger sequencing. For example, the Roche 454 Titanium platform is capable of generating up to one million sequences in one run, with a read length of 500 bases. However, the use of NGS platforms presents unique challenges.

Analysis of the large datasets generated is computationally intensive and the error rate is higher than with traditional Sanger sequencing, which have been reported between 0.001% and 1%, while 454 sequencing has had reported error rates between 0.49% and 2.8% [42]. Due to the large number of sequences generated, an increase in error rate can result in a major overestimation of community diversity [43]. Therefore, stringent filtering of sequences based on quality score or complex algorithms for minimizing the effects of sequencing errors is often required [44]. Despite

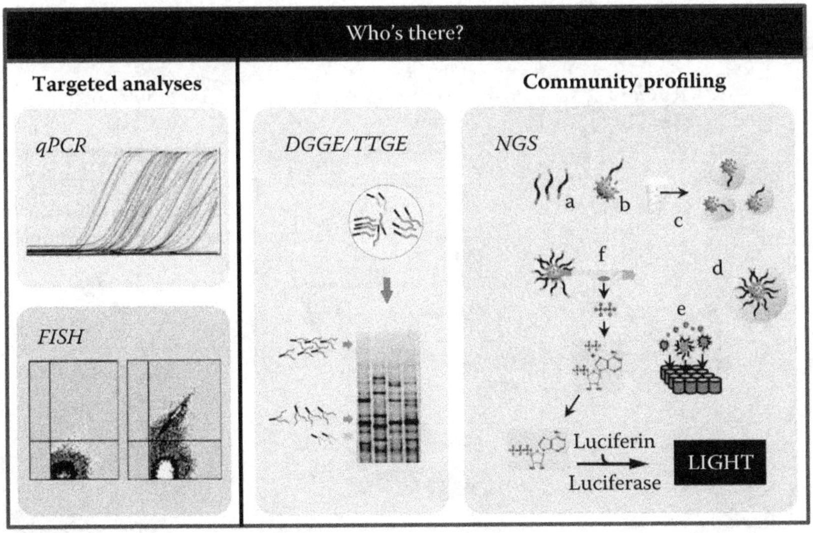

FIGURE 8.2 Methods for identifying microbiota composition. Targeted analyses include qPCR and FISH, using primers or fluorescent probes directed at functional or 16S rRNA genes. Community profiling methods include DGGE/TTGE, which provide a molecular fingerprint of community composition, or NGS methods, which can provide highly detailed taxonomic information. Both community profiling methods typically target the 16S rRNA gene, but other polymorphic genes may also be analyzed. DGGE/TTGE distinguishes community profiles based on differential migration of partially denatured PCR products. NGS methods using technologies such as the Roche GS FLX Titanium sequencer identify PCR products present in a mixed population; (a) Sample DNA is amplified using fusion PCR primers ligated with A and B adapters specific to the 5' and 3' ends. (b) PCR amplicons are captured on microbeads. Concentrations of microbeads and DNA are optimized such that one microbead will have one captured DNA fragment. (c) Microbeads are suspended in a water-in-oil emulsion with amplification reagents, such that each microbead is contained within its own mini breactor. (d) Each captured DNA fragment is amplified by emulsion PCR. (e) Microbeads with clonally amplified DNA are loaded onto a sequencing plate with a well diameter that allows only one microbead to fit in each well. Individual nucleotides are flowed across the plate in a fixed order to facilitate sequencing-by-synthesis. (f) Within each well, the introduction of a nucleotide complementary to the microbead bound DNA template results on the extension of a DNA strand by DNA polymerase. This results in the release of pyrophosphate, which is detected as a light signal following a chain of chemical reactions involving sulfurylase and luciferase.

these limitations, NGS platforms have proven to be invaluable for the compositional and metagenomic analysis of the large bowel microbiota [21,45,46].

Valuable insight into the interactions between microbiota, host genetic factors, and food components can also be gained by analysis of metabolite profiles (metabolome) in a variety of biological compartments such as urine, plasma, and liver [47]. Although an understanding of the microbiota taxonomic and genetic composition can be thought of as knowledge of the metabolic and functional potential of the microbial community, the metabolome provides a snapshot of biological processes that have actually occurred. Because some metabolites are produced by interactions

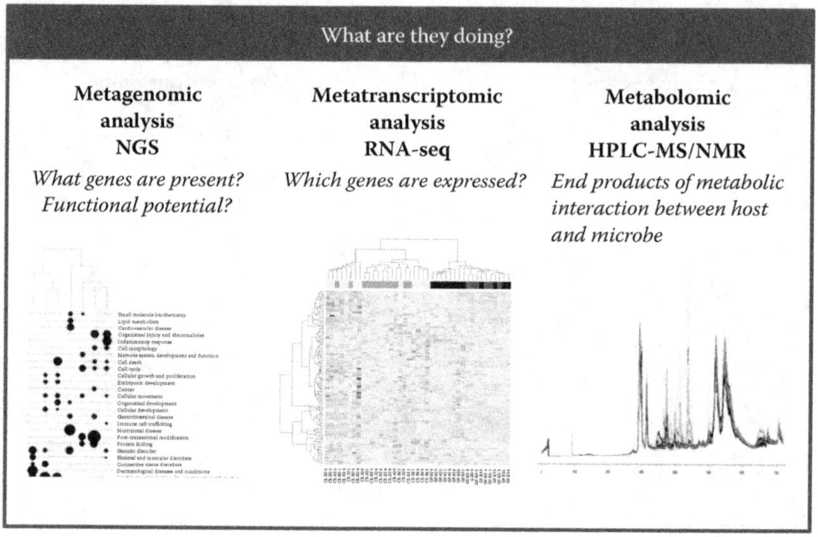

FIGURE 8.3 Methods for analysis of microbiota biological function and capability. Metagenomic analysis of all bacterial genes present in microbiota indicates the most abundant molecular functions. Metatranscriptomic analysis using NGS of mRNA (RNA-seq) identifies genes that are most highly expressed in the community. Metabolomic analyses provide a snapshot of metabolites resulting from host and microbiota interactions.

between gene products from the host and microbiota, analysis of the metabolome provides knowledge that could not be gained by studying the host and bacterial genetic components in isolation [48,49]. Commonly used techniques for metabolomic analyses include liquid chromatography–mass spectrometry and nuclear magnetic resonance [50–52].

LARGE BOWEL MICROBIAL ECOSYSTEM OF HEALTHY INDIVIDUALS

The steady supply of nutrients and physical protection offered by the host makes the large bowel an ideal habitat for microbes to flourish. However, despite the suitability of this environment for microbial life, selection pressures within the adult human intestine result in a microbiota predominantly comprised of members from just two bacterial phyla—the Gram-negative Bacteroidetes and low G+C content, Gram-positive Firmicutes [5,21]. Of the 55 known bacterial phyla, only a further 6 have been identified in the adult human gastrointestinal tract [5,37]. In contrast, ecosystems such as soil are known to harbor 20 or more bacterial phyla [5]. Although microbial diversity at the phyla level is limited in the large bowel, there is broad phylogenetic diversity within the phyla present. The human intestine is thought to be inhabited by over 800 bacterial species, most of which belong to the clostridial cluster XIVa group, clostridial cluster IV group, and Bacteroides-Prevotella group [45]. Also resident, but in smaller numbers, are members of the Actinobacteria and Proteobacteria phyla. Fungi and Archaea can also be found, but collectively they account for only 1% of the microbiota in the large bowel [53,54]. Furthermore, diversity of the Archaea in the human large bowel is limited to only two described species, *Methanobrevibacter smithii* and *Methanosphaera stadtmanae* [53,54].

The large bowel is the primary site of microbial colonization with bacterial concentrations reaching 10^{11}–10^{12} per gram of content [56]. In contrast, due to low pH and rapid flow rate, the stomach and proximal ileum contain far fewer bacteria; concentrations in this region are typically 10^3–10^5 per gram of content and are mainly composed of acid-tolerant lactobacilli and streptococci [56,57]. Bacterial diversity and densities increase dramatically further down the intestinal tract. The distal ileum contains up to 10^8 microbes per gram of content and is considered a transitional zone between the small intestine and large bowel. Within the large bowel itself, three distinctive habitats have been described. Firstly, there is the firmly attached layer of mucus that covers the epithelium forming a protective barrier that is sparsely populated with bacteria [58]. Above the firmly attached mucus is a loosely adherent layer of mucus that is densely populated with mucus-associated bacteria [58]. Finally, the large bowel lumen and digestive residues contain vast numbers of microbes that collectively function as an anaerobic bioreactor capable of harvesting carbon and energy from indigestible plant-derived polysaccharides [59].

Most studies indicate that the majority of bacterial species identified in the large bowel are yet to be cultured [45,60,61]. There is considerable variation in the relative abundance of species present between individuals. Even within the large bowel, variation in species diversity and abundance has been identified in different compartments, such as the ascending colon, descending colon, rectum, and feces [53]. Although fecal samples are often collected when studying the intestinal microbiota, fecal bacteria merely represent the community in the distal colon, not that of the proximal colon or terminal ileum. Such samples most likely do not accurately represent the upper intestinal bacteria or their collective metabolic activity.

The source of bacterial variation within the large bowel is not yet fully understood and is the subject of extensive study. However, a number of factors have been shown to influence the microbial community structure including diet, host phenotype, and kinship [7,24,62,63]. Community composition of the cecum in mice has been shown to be more similar between mothers and their offspring compared to unrelated mice [24]. Furthermore, this similarity is shared between offspring of the same mother from different litters [24]. Similarly, fecal community profiles in humans have a more similar structure between related individuals, regardless of whether they live together or in separate residences [10]. However, it is apparent that factors other than host genotype play a major role in shaping the microbial community. Surprisingly, studies examining fecal microbial communities show profiles between monozygotic twins are no more similar to each other than those from dizygotic twins [10], suggesting environmental factors may play a larger role than genotype in dictating microbiota composition under some circumstances.

Current diversity estimates of the microbiota vary between surveys, but a recent study of the microbial community in twins using deep pyrosequencing of the V2 region of the 16S rRNA gene indicates approximately 800 phylotypes are present in the large bowel [45]. A remarkable aspect of the human bacterial community is the distinctiveness of profiles between individuals. Analysis of over 10^6 sequences from a pair of identical twins indicated that only 39% and 53% of species detected in the feces were shared between the two communities [45]. A wider survey examining 31 monozygotic and 23 dizygotic twin pairs and their mothers was unable to characterize a core set of bacterial species shared between all individuals [45]. Of the most abundant species-level phylotypes across all community sets, only 37 were present in >50% of the samples, and only one species, a member of the Lachnospiraceae family, was found in 99% of individuals [45]. In a recent study of 124 European individuals, metagenomic sequencing of large bowel communities produced a catalogue of 3.3 million microbial genes assembled from 576.7 gigabases of sequence [21]. Despite such broad sequence coverage, phylogenetic analysis showed only 18 species that were present in all individuals [21]. However, this study was able to identify 75 bacterial species that were common to >50% of the sample group and 57 species that were shared by >90% [21]. Although the large bowel microbial community structure is highly variable between individuals, it is remarkably stable over time in adults [37,62]. The stability of the microbial community suggests its structure is shaped by strong selective and homeostatic mechanisms present in the large bowel.

In order to understand the relationship between the substantial diversity present in the large bowel community and its function, a number of metagenomic studies have been carried out relating community phylotype composition to the collective genomes of the microbiota [10,21]. These studies have shown that despite the absence of an obvious core microbial community, individuals shared an extensive collection of microbial genes that form a core microbiome at the gene level [10]. Analysis of the microbiome revealed a common pool of housekeeping genes required for bacterial function and a set of genes that appear to facilitate bacterial adaptation to the large bowel environment [10,21]. This second category included genes that encode for an extensive collection of carbohydrate-active enzymes, factors for binding to host proteins, synthesis of SCFA, and the production of essential amino acids and vitamins [10,21,64]. From these studies, it appears that the diversity in the microbiota is underpinned by a set of core functional processes that is shared across communities of varying composition. These results also suggest a functional plasticity among members of the microbiota; different members of the community are able to undertake similar roles under different conditions.

MUCOSAL AND BACTERIAL INTERACTIONS IN INDIVIDUALS WITH IBD

The health status of the host has been shown to influence the large bowel microbiota profile in a number of studies. Both human clinical and animal studies have provided evidence that differences exist in bacterial communities of individuals with IBD compared to control subjects, which suggests luminal bacteria and bacterial products may be involved in initiation and progression of intestinal inflammation [65,66]. For example, antibiotic treatment decreased intestinal bacteria concentrations and attenuated colitis in CD patients [67,68]. Mouse models showed that the interaction between genetic susceptibility and bacteria is important in the etiology of IBD (Table 8.1). Some mice do not develop IBD when maintained in germ-free conditions and in others the disease development was reduced in specific pathogen-free

TABLE 8.1
Interaction of the Host Genotype with Bacterial and Environmental Factors

Model	Reference
No colitis in germ-free condition	
IL2-deficient mouse	[78]
IL10-deficient mouse	[74]
TCRα-deficient mouse	[79]
Reduced colitis in specific pathogen-free condition or after antibiotic treatment	
IL2-deficient mouse	[78]
IL10-deficient mouse	[72,80]
Mdr1α-deficient mouse	[81]
TGFβ dnRII transgenic mouse	[82]
Bacteria with anti-inflammatory effects	
Lactobacillus sp. in IL10-deficient mouse	[83,84]
Bacteria with proinflammatory effects	
Bacteroides vulgatus in HLA-B27/β2m transgenic rats	[69]
Enterococcus faecalis in IL10-deficient mouse	[71,75]
Escherichia coli in IL10-deficient mouse	[71]
Helicobacter hepaticus in IL10-deficient and TGFαβ dnRII transgenic mouse	[85,86]

conditions or by antibiotic administration. On the other hand, it has been shown that colonization of the gastrointestinal tract with specific bacteria can have anti-inflammatory effects, whereas others can induce colitis. Colonization studies with germ-free rodent models indicate that enteric bacteria vary in their ability to induce colitis and specifically interact with the genetically susceptible host [69–71]. Probiotic bacteria, such as *Lactobacillus* spp., were able to prevent colitis in an interleukin-10 gene-deficient (*Il10*$^{-/-}$) mouse model of IBD [72]. *Enterococcus* spp. are common intestinal bacteria of healthy humans and animals [73,74], but *E. faecalis* has been shown to induce IBD in germ-free *Il10*$^{-/-}$ mice [75] and *E. faecalis* and *E. faecium* isolates combined with a mixed "complex intestinal flora" derived from healthy C57BL/6J mice raised under conventional conditions can induce a more consistent intestinal inflammation [76,77].

Intestinal inflammation influences the gastrointestinal environment, where some bacterial species flourish and others decrease in numbers [87]. In contrast to healthy individuals, colon biopsy samples from CD patients are characterized by a higher load of mucosa-associated bacteria. However, the overall bacterial diversity appears to be reduced in individuals with CD whose communities shows higher prevalence of Proteobacteria and Bacteroidetes phyla when compared with UC patients and healthy subjects. It remains to be elucidated which bacterial populations are most important in the etiology of CD or UC and whether a certain degree of variation in the community profile reflects interindividual differences among intestinal bacteria. In order to address these important questions in more detail, NGS and robust statistical methods for analysis of large data sets will be required. Furthermore, a consistent use of the phylotype definition would facilitate more productive comparisons of results from different studies.

A variety of bacteria, including *Escherichia coli, Pseudomonas aeruginosa, Helicobacter pylori, Bacteroides vulgatus,* and *Clostridium difficile,* have been linked to the pathogenesis of IBD [88–91]. *Bacteroides* spp., *Bifidobacterium animalis, C. cocleatum,* and *Enterococcus* spp. are also more prevalent in the large bowel of colitic *Il10*$^{-/-}$ mice [65]. A decrease in the abundance and diversity of the Firmicutes has been demonstrated in fecal samples from patients with CD [63]. Furthermore, postoperative recurrence of ileal CD is higher in patients with lower proportions of mucosa-associated *Faecalibacterium prausnitzii* [9]. Cluster analysis of the community profiles obtained by NGS of normal individuals or patients with CD or UC also shows a clear delineation based on disease status [21].

Colonic bacteria metabolize mainly carbohydrates and proteins and host-produced substances (e.g., mucin) to salvage energy by anaerobic fermentation. Protein fermentation metabolites such as phenolic and indolic compounds, branched-chain fatty acids, sulfur-containing compounds, and ammonia seem to affect IBD by damaging epithelial cells in genetically susceptible hosts, thereby resulting in inflammation [92,93]. Butyrate, a SCFA produced by bacteria and a major fermentation product in the large bowel, is an important energy source for colonocytes. Inhibition of butyrate metabolism by reduced sulfide-containing compounds from luminal bacteria can lead to loss of epithelial barrier integrity and induce inflammatory lesions similar to those seen in UC [4,94–96]. Products of bacterial metabolism have also been shown to affect processes implicated in the development of cancer [11].

Certain butyrate-producing bacteria may have a role in modulating IBD. Metagenomic studies have shown that the diversity and prevalence of the Firmicutes, and the clostridial cluster IV group in particular, are reduced in patients with CD [63]. *Faecalibacterium prausnitzii* has also been shown to reduce the production of inflammatory cytokines in peripheral blood mononuclear cells [9]. Furthermore, a reduction in severity of 2,4,6-trinitrobenzenesulfonic acid-induced colitis has been observed in mice receiving an intragastric dose of *F. prausnitzii* [9]. The possible reduction in butyrate available for intestinal epithelial cells may be a factor that influences IBD, as butyrate exhibits anti-inflammatory properties and is an important energy source for colonocytes [97,98]. However, the explanation for the reduced diversity and numbers of Firmicutes in IBD remains unknown. It seems likely that mucosal immune regulation and changes in the intestinal environment play a role in determining the microbial community composition.

Nucleotide-binding and oligomerization domain 1 (NOD1) and 2 (NOD2) are intracellular receptors for bacterial components that have an important role in innate immunity through the detection of bacterial components derived from peptidoglycans [99]. NOD2 responds to muramyl dipeptide, a specific motif of peptidoglycan, whereas NOD1 reacts to a Gram-negative peptidoglycan derivative, γ-D-glutamyl-meso-diamino-pimelic acid [100,101]. Mutations in NOD2 have been associated with

CD, which suggest NOD2 may have an important role in regulating inflammatory diseases [102]. However, the microbiota and host interactions underlying the mechanisms by which this may occur are not yet fully understood. Studies using NOD2-deficient mice have shown that stimulation of NOD2 inhibits proinflammatory responses mediated by TLR2 due to defective activation of the nuclear factor kappa in B-cells (NF-κB) signaling pathway [101]. Wild-type antigen present cells (APCs) stimulated by peptidoglycans show increased production of proinflammatory IL-12 compared to APCs from NOD2-deficient mice. Furthermore, cells from NOD2-deficient mice were shown to have elevated levels of NF-κB. Another study using NOD2-deficient mice showed an increased susceptibility to Listeria monocytogenes infection given orally, but not by intravenous or intraperitoneal delivery [103]. Although it is apparent that TLR and NOD-mediated sensing of bacterial molecular motifs is crucial for modulating inflammatory and homeostatic responses to the intestinal microbiota, their exact role and mechanisms of action are not yet fully understood.

The epithelium of the large bowel forms a protective barrier that may be as little as a single cell thick, which has a critical role for excluding exogenous pathogens and antigens, yet at the same time allowing the passage of water and nutrients. It is a site characterized by a high rate of cell turnover where the entire epithelium is replaced every five to seven days [104]. A characteristic feature of germ-free rats is a reduction in epithelial cell proliferation compared to conventionally raised rats [105]. Therefore, bacterial-induced increases in cell proliferation in the large bowel may be mediated by TLR signaling. However, in the absence of intestinal injury, epithelial cell proliferation in MyD88- or TLR4-deficient mice is similar to that in wild-type mice, which suggests some other bacterial factor(s) are involved in their proliferation [106]. In contrast, intestinal epithelial cell proliferation is reduced in MyD88-, TLR4-, or TLR2-deficient mice when intestinal injury is induced using dextran sulfate sodium (DSS) [107,108]. Injury to colonic epithelial cells allows the resident microbiota access to the lamina propria that results in an acute inflammatory response. Moreover, MyD88$^{-/-}$ mice show increased mortality and morbidity after DSS administration compared to wild-type mice [107]. This increase in mortality was not due to an overgrowth in commensal bacteria and was found to be independent of T, B, and NK cell activity [107]. Wild-type mice given broad-spectrum antibiotics or antibodies targeting TLR2 or TLR4 resulted in similar DSS-induced injury severity in the colon [107,108]. Administration of DSS to wild-type germ-free mice also produces greater colonic injury compared to mice that have a conventional microbiota [109].

At first, these findings seem counter-intuitive as it would be expected that mice that are unable to mount a TLR-dependent immune response to the resident bacterial community would exhibit reduced intestinal pathology following administration of DSS. These studies show that under normal conditions, a lack of TLR signaling is tolerated for normal intestinal epithelial cell proliferation. However, in the presence of injury, both the intestinal bacterial community and their detection by TLR-mediated signaling are required for optimal cell proliferation.

Epithelial barrier function may also be influenced by products of bacterial metabolism. Butyrate has been shown to increase cell layer integrity in cultured epithelial colorectal adenocarcinoma (Caco-2) cells, as measured by transepithelial electrical resistance (TEER) [110]. This increase in barrier function was attributed to an increase in AMP-activated protein kinase K (AMPK) levels, which resulted in an accelerated assembly of tight junction proteins [110]. Furthermore, the butyrate-induced activation of AMPK and increased TEER was eliminated by the addition of a specific inhibitor of AMPK. Acetate has also been shown to play an important role in the amelioration of intestinal injury following DSS administration in mice. Treatment with acetate following DSS administration was shown to reduce colonic inflammation [109]. However, mice deficient in G Protein-Coupled Receptor (GPR43), a receptor that binds SCFA, displayed increased injury following DSS administration, which could not be abrogated by acetate treatment [109]. DSS-induced intestinal injury in germ-free mice was reduced by treatment with acetate, indicating the presence of a TLR-independent mechanism for protection against epithelial damage [109].

Studies using germ-free mice have also shown that colonization with *B. thetaiotaomicron* increases expression levels of genes involved in enhancing barrier integrity in the intestinal epithelium [111]. In further studies, confocal microscopy of cultured Caco-2 cells stimulated with a TLR2 ligand revealed an apical tightening and sealing of ZO-1, a tight junction molecule [112]. Furthermore, stimulation of TLR2 resulted in enhanced TEER, indicating an increase in barrier function [112]. These studies suggest that barrier integrity and repair in intestinal epithelial cells is mediated by receptors that sense bacterial components and metabolic products. Upon signaling, they activate downstream events that limit the extent of damage by increasing proliferation, reducing apoptosis, and regulating inflammatory pathways.

ROLE OF MICROBIOTA IN ASSESSING NUTRIENT AND GENE INTERACTIONS IN IBD

The interaction of dietary components with the host's mucosa and alteration of resident intestinal microbiota provides new insights into its mechanism of action in IBD pathogenesis. Changes in dietary intake of food components (e.g., fatty acids, carbohydrates, proteins and peptides, prebiotics, and probiotics) modulate gene expression in host intestine, as well as in liver, adipose tissue, and muscle and change the intestinal microbiota composition [17]. The binding of dietary polyunsaturated fatty acids (PUFAs), particularly n-3 PUFA, to the nuclear transcription factor peroxisome proliferator-activated receptor alpha (PPARA) to regulate the expression of genes mostly involved in lipid metabolism represents a direct nutrient-gene interaction [113]. The study by [114] have shown that in response to dietary n-3 PUFA eicosapentaenoic acid, the expression levels of the *Ppara* gene and some of its target genes were increased in the colon of *Il10*$^{-/-}$ mice. This anti-inflammatory effect of n–3 PUFAs in the intestine had previously been linked to a PPARα-mediated inhibition of NF-κB and associated proinflammatory events [115]. The same investigators have also shown that these n-3 and n-6 PUFAs differentially alter the cecal microbial community composition associated with the host genotype of wild-type and *Il10*$^{-/-}$ mice [116].

The study by Bassaganya-Riera and Hontecillas [117] suggested that dietary n-3 PUFAs and conjugated linoleic acid might be able to reduce endotoxin levels by changing the intestinal microbial composition and thus its metabolic activity to decrease inflammatory disease risk. However, evidence demonstrating the extent to which intestinal microbes may modulate the interaction between nutrients and host in IBD remains scarce. The study by Hildebrandt et al. [46] showed a high-fat diet affected the composition of the murine intestinal microbiome (i.e., decrease in *Bacteroidetes* and increase in *Firmicutes* and *Proteobacteria*) independently of obesity.

Dietary carbohydrates may also have major effects on the microbiome in the large bowel. In particular, nondigestible dietary carbohydrates (which escape degradation in the upper intestinal tract) are able to alter the composition of the microbiota and its fermentation products in the large bowel and feces [118,119]. For example, feeding inulin and fructo-oligosaccharides, commonly used as prebiotics, increases large bowel abundance of bifidobacteria and lactobacilli [118,120,121]. The specific changes observed are dependent on the type and quantity of nondigestible carbohydrates. Although feeding maize resistant starch or inulin to newly weaned rats results in similar alterations in colonic SCFA concentrations, the microbiota underwent different compositional changes [122]. Newly weaned rats fed with resistant starch showed an expansion of bifidobacteria, whereas inulin-fed rats exhibited an increased abundance of bacteria belonging to clostrial cluster XIVa [122]. Changes in host tissue expression in response to dietary nondigestible carbohydrates are also specific to the type of carbohydrate, with inulin, resistant starch, and konjac flour all resulting in distinct transcriptional profiles [122]. These examples represent indirect nutrient-host gene interactions mediated by intestinal microbes and could be used to favor the enrichment of the intestinal community with beneficial bacteria that in turn might positively regulate the IBD host metabolism.

Previous studies have shown that a high carbohydrate intake might be associated with increased risk for CD as well as UC [123–125]. These studies suggest that microbial sensing and processing of carbohydrates might be involved in IBD, and further investigations are warranted to define sugar-sensitive and sugar-insensitive microbiomes and their relationship to IBD. An understanding of these factors could lead to the development of specific personalized diets for individual IBD patients.

Much attention has been given to prebiotics, probiotics, or synbiotics, but variable results have been described, particularly for applications of probiotics in the treatment of IBD [8,126–128], likely due to genetic heterogeneity of the study subjects. Despite the tremendous market value of the functional foods industry [129], claims of efficacy are often not supported by scientific evidence. In particular, it is now recognized that additional studies are required to support many of the health claims attributed to prebiotics and probiotics [130]. Indeed, the European Food Safety Authority (EFSA) issued negative opinions on the health claims of 416 products in 2010, including claims for the use of several probiotic products for maintaining digestive health and β-glucans for maintaining healthy blood glucose levels [131–133]. Therefore, studies that investigate the biological mechanisms of action have a crucial role in providing information to enable informed decisions to be made on supplement use.

SUMMARY AND CONCLUDING REMARKS

It is clear that the progression and incidence of IBD is influenced by interactions that occur between host genetic factors, the resident microbiota, and diet. However, elucidating the precise mechanisms governing these highly complex interactions is a challenging task.

Alterations in the host or microbiota transcriptome may not always result in changes in the proteome or metabolome in response to diet. Analysis of the metabolite profile in urine or blood may further elucidate the interactions between microbiota and host and how microbial activities are related to host phenotype and metabolism [52,134]. Characterizing host or microbiota proteomes may also reveal changes in gene products that cannot be explained by alterations in transcription, such as those resulting from posttranslational modifications or alternate splicing of transcripts. Metagenomic analysis of the bacterial genes present in the large bowel may provide useful information regarding the selection pressures exerted in this ecosystem by determining which genes are enriched under certain situations [40].

Characterization of responses in other tissue compartments such as the mesenteric lymph nodes or the metabolite profile of the portal and hepatic system may also help to provide a better understanding of how the interplay between nutrients and intestinal microbes influences host health, particularly in the context of IBD. The decreasing costs associated with high throughput technologies and the advent of new single molecule sequencing platforms provide great potential for extending existing knowledge.

Despite the complex nature of food, host, and microbe interactions, an integrated nutrigenomic-based approach for studying these systems offers the potential for effective and personalized strategies for alleviating IBD.

REFERENCES

1. Savage, D. C. (1977). Microbial ecology of the gastrointestinal tract. *Annu Rev Microbiol 31*: 107–133.
2. Macdonald, T. T. and Monteleone, G. (2005). Immunity, inflammation, and allergy in the gut. *Science 307*: 1920–1925.
3. Manson, J. M., Rauch, M., and Gilmore, M. S. (2008). The commensal microbiology of the gastrointestinal tract, in: G.B. Huffnagle and M.C. Noverr (Eds.), *Advances in Experimental Medicine and Biology, GI Microbiota and Regulation of the Immune System*, Austin, TX: Landes Bioscience and Springer Science + Business Media, pp. 15–28.
4. Macfarlane, S., Steed, H., and Macfarlane, G. T. (2009). Intestinal bacteria and inflammatory bowel disease. *Crit Rev Clin Lab Sci 46*: 25–54.
5. Backhed, F., Ley, R. E., Sonnenburg, J. L., Peterson, D. A. and Gordon, J. I. (2005). Host-bacterial mutualism in the human intestine. *Science 307*: 1915–1920.
6. Kelly, D., Campbell, J. I., King, T. P., Grant, G., Jansson, E. A. et al. (2004). Commensal anaerobic gut bacteria attenuate inflammation by regulating nuclear-cytoplasmic shuttling of PPAR-gamma and RelA. *Nat Immunol 5*: 104–112.
7. De Filippo, C., Cavalieri, D., Di Paola, M., Ramazzotti, M., Poullet, J. B. et al. (2010). Impact of diet in shaping gut microbiota revealed by a comparative study in children from Europe and rural Africa. *Proc Natl Acad Sci U S A 107*: 14691–14696.
8. Lindsay, J. O., Whelan, K., Stagg, A. J., Gobin, P., Al-Hassi, H. O. et al. (2006). Clinical, microbiological, and immunological effects of fructo-oligosaccharide in patients with Crohn's disease. *Gut 55*: 348–355.
9. Sokol, H., Pigneur, B., Watterlot, L., Lakhdari, O., Bermudez-Humaran, L. G. et al. (2008). Faecalibacterium prausnitzii is an anti-inflammatory commensal bacterium identified by gut microbiota analysis of Crohn disease patients. *Proc Natl Acad Sci U S A 105*: 16731–16736.

10. Turnbaugh, P. J., Hamady, M., Yatsunenko, T., Cantarel, B. L., Duncan, A. et al. (2009). A core gut microbiome in obese and lean twins. *Nature 457*: 480–484.
11. O'Keefe, S. J., Ou, J., Aufreiter, S., O'Connor, D., Sharma, S. et al. (2009). Products of the colonic microbiota mediate the effects of diet on colon cancer risk. *J Nutr 139*(11): 2044–2048.
12. Fava, F. and Danese, S. (2011). Intestinal microbiota in inflammatory bowel disease: friend or foe? *World J Gastroenterol 17*: 557–566.
13. Strober, W., Fuss, I., and Mannon, P. (2007). The fundamental basis of inflammatory bowel disease. *J Clin Investig 117*:514–521.
14. Honda, K. and Takeda, K. (2009). Regulatory mechanisms of immune responses to intestinal bacteria. *Mucosal Immunol 2*: 187–196.
15. Sun, L., Nava, G. M., and Stappenbeck, T. S. (2011). Host genetic susceptibility, dysbiosis, and viral triggers in inflammatory bowel disease. *Curr Opin Gastroenterol 27*: 321–327.
16. Furrie, E., Macfarlane, S., Thomson, G., and Macfarlane, G. T. (2005). Toll-like receptors-2, -3 and -4 expression patterns on human colon and their regulation by mucosal-associated bacteria. *Immunology 115*: 565–574.
17. Delzenne, N. M., Neyrinck, A. M., and Cani, P. D. (2011). Modulation of the gut microbiota by nutrients with prebiotic properties: consequences for host health in the context of obesity and metabolic syndrome. *Microb Cell Fact 10 Suppl 1*: S10.
18. Tannock, G. W., Munro, K., Bibiloni, R., Simon, M. A., Hargreaves, P. et al. (2004). Impact of consumption of oligosaccharide-containing biscuits on the fecal microbiota of humans. *Appl Environ Microbiol 70*: 2129–2136.
19. Walter, J., Tannock, G. W., Tilsala-Timisjarvi, A., Rodtong, S., Loach, D. M. et al. (2000). Detection and identification of gastrointestinal Lactobacillus species by using denaturing gradient gel electrophoresis and species-specific PCR primers. *Appl Environ Microbiol 66*: 297–303.
20. Simpson, J. M., McCracken, V. J., White, B. A., Gaskins, H. R., and Mackie, R. I. (1999). Application of denaturant gradient gel electrophoresis for the analysis of the porcine gastrointestinal microbiota. *J Microbiol Methods 36*: 167–179.
21. Qin, J., Li, R., Raes, J., Arumugam, M., Burgdorf, K. S. et al. (2010). A human gut microbial gene catalogue established by metagenomic sequencing. *Nature 464*: 59–65.
22. Muegge, B. D., Kuczynski, J., Knights, D., Clemente, J. C., Gonzalez, A. et al. (2011). Diet drives convergence in gut microbiome functions across mammalian phylogeny and within humans. *Science 332*: 970–974.
23. Claesson, M. J., Cusack, S., O'Sullivan, O., Greene-Diniz, R., de Weerd, H. et al. (2011). Composition, variability, and temporal stability of the intestinal microbiota of the elderly. *Proc Natl Acad Sci U S A 108 Suppl 1*: 4586–4591.
24. Ley, R. E., Backhed, F., Turnbaugh, P., Lozupone, C. A., Knight, R. D. et al. (2005). Obesity alters gut microbial ecology. *Proc Natl Acad Sci U S A 102*: 11070–11075.
25. Tannock, G. (2005). Microbiota of mucosal surfaces in the gut of monogastric animals, in: J. Nataro, P. Cohen, H. Mobley, and J. Weiser (Eds.), *In Colonization of Mucosal Surfaces*, 1st Edition, ASM Press, Washington, DC, pp. 163–178.
26. Furham, J. A., MacCallum, K., and Davis, A. A. (1992). Novel major archebacterial group from marine plankton. *Nature 356*: 148–149.
27. Dutta, S., Chatterjee, A., Dutta, P., Rajendran, K., Roy, S. et al. (2001). Sensitivity and performance characteristics of a direct PCR with stool samples in comparison to conventional techniques for diagnosis of Shigella and enteroinvasive Escherichia coli infection in children with acute diarrhoea in Calcutta, India. *J Med Microbiol 50*: 667–674.
28. Amor, K. B. and Vaughan, E. E. (2006). Molecular ecology of the human intestinal microbiota, in: A.C. Ouwehand and E. Vaughan (Eds.), *Gastrointestinal Microbiology*, 1st Edition, Taylor & Francis Group, LLC, New York, USA, pp. 1–23.

29. Franks, A. H., Harmsen, H. J. M., Raangs, G. C., Jansen, G. J. et al. (1998). Variations in bacterial populations in human feces measured by fluorescent in situ hybridization with group-specific 16S rRNA-targeted oligonucleotide probes. *Appl Environ Microbiol 64*: 3336–3345.
30. Felske, A., Rheims, H., Wolterink, A., Stackebrandt, E., and Akkermans, A. D. (1997). Ribosome analysis reveals prominent activity of an uncultured member of the class Actinobacteria in grassland soils. *Microbiology 143 (Pt 9)*: 2983–2989.
31. Amann, R. I., Ludwig, W., and Schleifer, K. H. (1995). Phylogenetic identification and in-situ detection of individual microbial-cells without cultivation. *Microbiol Rev 59*: 143–169.
32. Wang, R. F., Cao, W. W., and Cerniglia, C. E. (1996). PCR detection and quantitation of predominant anaerobic bacteria in human and animal fecal samples. *Appl Environ Microbiol 62*: 1242–1247.
33. Wilson, K. H. and Blitchington, R. B. (1996). Human colonic biota studied by ribosomal DNA sequence analysis. *Appl Environ Microbiol 62*: 2273–2278.
34. Yu, Z. T. and Morrison, M. (2004). Comparisons of different hypervariable regions of rrs genes for use in fingerprinting of microbial communities by PCR-denaturing gradient gel electrophoresis. *Appl Environ Microbiol 70*: 4800–4806.
35. Rinttila, T., Kassinen, A., Malinen, E., Krogius, L., and Palva, A. (2004). Development of an extensive set of 16S rDNA-targeted primers for quantification of pathogenic and indigenous bacteria in faecal samples by real-time PCR. *J Appl Microbiol 97*: 1166–1177.
36. Garcia, L., Tercero, J. C., Legido, B., Ramos, J. A., Alemany, J. et al. (1998). Rapid detection of Actinobacillus actinomycetemcomitans, Prevotella intermedia and Porphyromona gingivalis by multiplex PCR. *J Periodontal Res 33*: 59–64.
37. Costello, E. K., Lauber, C. L., Hamady, M., Fierer, N., Gordon, J. I. et al. (2009). Bacterial community variation in human body habitats across space and time. *Science 326*: 1694–1697.
38. McNulty, N. P., Yatsunenko, T., Hsiao, A., Faith, J. J., Muegge, B. D. et al. (2011). The impact of a consortium of fermented milk strains on the Gut Microbiome of Gnotobiotic Mice and Monozygotic Twins. *Sci Transl Med 3*: 106ra106.
39. Booijink, C. C., Boekhorst, J., Zoetendal, E. G., Smidt, H., Kleerebezem, M. et al. (2010). Metatranscriptome analysis of the human fecal microbiota reveals subject-specific expression profiles with genes encoding proteins involved in carbohydrate metabolism being dominantly expressed. *Appl Environ Microbiol 76*: 5533–5540.
40. Turnbaugh, P. J., Backhed, F., Fulton, L., and Gordon, J. I. (2008). Diet-induced obesity is linked to marked but reversible alterations in the mouse distal gut microbiome. *Cell Host Microbe 3*: 213–223.
41. Arumugam, M., Raes, J., Pelletier, E., Le Paslier, D., Yamada, T. et al. (2011). Enterotypes of the human gut microbiome. *Nature 473*: 174–180.
42. Hoff, K. J. (2009). The effect of sequencing errors on metagenomic gene prediction. *BMC Genomics 10*: 520.
43. Quince, C., Lanzen, A., Curtis, T. P., Davenport, R. J., Hall, N. et al. (2009). Accurate determination of microbial diversity from 454 pyrosequencing data. *Nat Methods 6*: 639–641.
44. Johnson, P. L. and Slatkin, M. (2008). Accounting for bias from sequencing error in population genetic estimates. *Mol Biol Evol 25*: 199–206.
45. Turnbaugh, P. J., Quince, C., Faith, J. J., McHardy, A. C., Yatsunenko, T. et al. (2010). Organismal, genetic, and transcriptional variation in the deeply sequenced gut microbiomes of identical twins. *Proc Natl Acad Sci U S A 107*: 7503–7508.
46. Hildebrandt, M. A., Hoffmann, C., Sherrill-Mix, S. A., Keilbaugh, S. A., Hamady, M. et al. (2009). High-fat diet determines the composition of the murine gut microbiome independently of obesity. *Gastroenterology 137*: 1716–1724, e1711–e1712.

47. Martin, F. P., Wang, Y., Sprenger, N., Yap, I. K., Lundstedt, T. et al. (2008). Probiotic modulation of symbiotic gut microbial-host metabolic interactions in a humanized microbiome mouse model. *Mol Syst Biol 4*: 157.
48. Clayton, T. A., Baker, D., Lindon, J. C., Everett, J. R., and Nicholson, J. K. (2009). Pharmacometabonomic identification of a significant host-microbiome metabolic interaction affecting human drug metabolism. *Proc Natl Acad Sci 106*: 14728–14733.
49. Claus, S. P., Ellero, S. L., Berger, B., Krause, L., Bruttin, A. et al. (2011). Colonization-induced host-gut microbial metabolic interaction. *MBio 2*: e00271–e00210.
50. Llorach, R., Urpi-Sarda, M., Jauregui, O., Monagas, M., and Andres-Lacueva, C. (2009). An LC-MS-based metabolomics approach for exploring urinary metabolome modifications after cocoa consumption. *J Proteome Res 8*: 5060–5068.
51. Wikoff, W. R., Anfora, A. T., Liu, J., Schultz, P. G., Lesley, S. A. et al. (2009). Metabolomics analysis reveals large effects of gut microflora on mammalian blood metabolites. *Proc Natl Acad Sci U S A 106*: 3698–3703.
52. Martin, F. P., Dumas, M. E., Wang, Y., Legido-Quigley, C., Yap, I. K. et al. (2007). A top-down systems biology view of microbiome-mammalian metabolic interactions in a mouse model. *Mol Syst Biol 3*: 112.
53. Eckburg, P. B., Bik, E. M., Bernstein, C. N., Purdom, E., Dethlefsen, L. et al. (2005). Diversity of the human intestinal microbial flora. *Science 308*: 1635–1638.
54. Palmer, C., Bik, E. M., Digiulio, D. B., Relman, D. A., and Brown, P. O. (2007). Development of the human infant intestinal microbiota. *PLoS Biol 5*: e177.
55. Duncan, S. H., Louis, P. and Flint, H. J. (2007). Cultivable bacterial diversity from the human colon. *Lett Appl Microbiol 44*: 343–350.
56. Leser, T. D. and Molbak, L. (2009). Better living through microbial action: the benefits of the mammalian gastrointestinal microbiota on the host. *Environ Microbiol 11*: 2194–2206.
57. Hayashi, H., Takahashi, R., Nishi, T., Sakamoto, M., and Benno, Y. (2005). Molecular analysis of jejunal, ileal, caecal and recto-sigmoidal human colonic microbiota using 16S rRNA gene libraries and terminal restriction fragment length polymorphism. *J Med Microbiol 54*: 1093–1101.
58. Johansson, M. E., Phillipson, M., Petersson, J., Velcich, A., Holm, L. et al. (2008). The inner of the two Muc2 mucin-dependent mucus layers in colon is devoid of bacteria. *Proc Natl Acad Sci U S A 105*: 15064–15069.
59. Louis, P., Scott, K. P., Duncan, S. H., and Flint, H. J. (2007). Understanding the effects of diet on bacterial metabolism in the large intestine. *J Appl Microbiol 102*: 1197–1208.
60. Rajilic-Stojanovic, M., Smidt, H., and de Vos, W. M. (2007). Diversity of the human gastrointestinal tract microbiota revisited. *Environ Microbiol 9*: 2125–2136.
61. Hayashi, H., Sakamoto, M., Kitahara, M., and Benno, Y. (2006). Diversity of the Clostridium coccoides group in human fecal microbiota as determined by 16S rRNA gene library. *FEMS Microbiol Lett 257*: 202–207.
62. Ley, R. E., Turnbaugh, P. J., Klein, S., and Gordon, J. I. (2006). Microbial ecology: human gut microbes associated with obesity. *Nature 444*: 1022–1023.
63. Manichanh, C., Rigottier-Gois, L., Bonnaud, E., Gloux, K., Pelletier, E. et al. (2006). Reduced diversity of faecal microbiota in Crohn's disease revealed by a metagenomic approach. *Gut 55*: 205–211.
64. Turnbaugh, P. J., Ley, R. E., Mahowald, M. A., Magrini, V., Mardis, E. R. et al. (2006). An obesity-associated gut microbiome with increased capacity for energy harvest. *Nature 444*: 1027–1031.
65. Bibiloni, R. Simon, M. A., Albright, C., Sartor, B., and Tannock, G. W. (2005). Analysis of the large bowel microbiota of colitic mice using PCR/DGGE. *Lett Appl Microbiol 41*: 45–51.

66. Mangin, I., Bonnet, R., Seksik, P., Rigottier-Gois, L., Sutren, M. et al. (2004). Molecular inventory of faecal microflora in patients with Crohn's disease. *FEMS Microbiol Ecol 50*: 25–36.
67. Colombel, J. F., Lemann, M., Cassagnou, M., Bouhnik, Y., Duclos, B. et al. (1997). A controlled trial comparing ciprofloxacin with trial mesalazine for the treatment of active Crohn's disease. *Gastroenterology 112*: A951–A951.
68. Gui, G. P. H., Thomas, P. R. S., Tizard, M. L. V., Lake, J., Sanderson, J. D. et al. (1997). Two-year-outcomes analysis of Crohn's disease treated with rifabutin and macrolide antibiotics. *J Antimicrob Chemother 39*: 393–400.
69. Rath, H. C., Wilson, K. H. and Sartor, R. B. (1999). Differential induction of colitis and gastritis in HLA-B27 transgenic rats selectively colonized with Bacteroides vulgatus or Escherichia coli. *Infect Immun 67*: 2969–2974.
70. Waidmann, M., Bechtold, O., Frick, J. S., Lehr, H. A., Schubert, S. et al. (2003). Bacteroides vulgatus protects against Escherichia coli-induced colitis in gnotobiotic interleukin-2-deficient mice. *Gastroenterology 125*: 162–177.
71. Kim, S. C., Tonkonogy, S. L., Albright, C. A., Tsang, J., Balish, E. J. et al. (2005). Variable phenotypes of enterocolitis in interleukin 10-deficient mice monoassociated with two different commensal bacteria. *Gastroenterology 128*: 891–906.
72. Madsen, K. L., Doyle, J. S., Tavernini, M. M., Jewell, L. D., Rennie, R. P. et al. (2000). Antibiotic therapy attenuates colitis in interleukin 10 gene-deficient mice. *Gastroenterology 118*: 1094–1105.
73. Jett, B. D., Huycke, M. M., and Gilmore, M. S. (1994). Virulence of enterococci. *Clin Microbiol Rev 7*: 462–478.
74. Sellon, R. K., Tonkonogy, S., Schultz, M., Dieleman, L. A., Grenther, W. et al. (1998). Resident enteric bacteria are necessary for development of spontaneous colitis and immune system activation in interleukin-10-deficient mice. *Infect Immun 66*: 5224–5231.
75. Balish, E. and Warner, T. (2002). Enterococcus faecalis induces inflammatory bowel disease in interleukin-10 knockout mice. *Am J Pathol 160*: 2253–2257.
76. Roy, N., Barnett, M., Knoch, B., Dommels, Y., and McNabb, W. (2007). Nutrigenomics applied to an animal model of Inflammatory Bowel Diseases: transcriptomic analysis of the effects of eicosapentaenoic acid- and arachidonic acid-enriched diets. *Mutat Res 622*: 103–116.
77. Barnett, M. P., McNabb, W. C., Cookson, A. L., Zhu, S., Davy, M. et al. (2010). Changes in colon gene expression associated with increased colon inflammation in interleukin-10 gene-deficient mice inoculated with Enterococcus species. *BMC Immunol 11*: 39.
78. Sadlack, B., Merz, H., Schorle, H., Schimpl, A., Feller, A. C. et al. (1993). Ulcerative colitis-like disease in mice with a disrupted interleukin-2 gene. *Cell 75*: 253–261.
79. Dianda, L., Hanby, A. M., Wright, N. A., Sebesteny, A., Hayday, A. C. et al. (1997). T cell receptor-alpha beta-deficient mice fail to develop colitis in the absence of a microbial environment. *Am J Pathol 150*: 91–97.
80. Kuhn, R., Lohler, J., Rennick, D., Rajewsky, K. and Muller, W. (1993). Interleukin-10-deficient mice develop chronic enterocolitis. *Cell 75*: 263–274.
81. Panwala, C. M., Jones, J. C. and Viney, J. L. (1998). A novel model of inflammatory bowel disease: mice deficient for the multiple drug resistance gene, mdr1a, spontaneously develop colitis. *J Immunol 161*: 5733–5744.
82. Hahm, K. B., Im, Y. H., Parks, T. W., Park, S. H., Markowitz, S. et al. (2001). Loss of transforming growth factor beta signalling in the intestine contributes to tissue injury in inflammatory bowel disease. *Gut 49*: 190–198.
83. Madsen, K. L., Malfair, D., Gray, D., Doyle, J. S., Jewell, L. D. et al. (1999). Interleukin-10 gene-deficient mice develop a primary intestinal permeability defect in response to enteric microflora. *Inflamm Bowel Dis 5*: 262–270.

84. Schultz, M. and Sartor, R. B. (2000). Probiotics and inflammatory bowel diseases. *Am J Gastroenterol 95*: S19–S21.
85. Kullberg, M. C., Ward, J. M., Gorelick, P. L., Caspar, P., Hieny, S. et al. (1998). Helicobacter hepaticus triggers colitis in specific-pathogen-free interleukin-10 (IL-10)-deficient mice through an IL-12- and gamma interferon-dependent mechanism. *Infect Immun 66*: 5157–5166.
86. Chin, E. Y., Dangler, C. A., Fox, J. G., and Schauer, D. B. (2000). Helicobacter hepaticus infection triggers inflammatory bowel disease in T cell receptor alphabeta mutant mice. *Comp Med 50*: 586–594.
87. McBurney, W., Mangold, M., Munro, K., Schultz, M., Rath, H. C. et al. (2006). PCR/DGGE and 16S rRNA gene library analysis of the colonic microbiota of HLA-B27/beta2-microglobulin transgenic rats. *Lett Appl Microbiol 42*: 165–171.
88. Chadwick, V. S. and Anderson, R. P. (1992). Microorganisms and their products in inflammatory bowel disease, in: R. MacDermott (Ed.), *Inflammatory Bowel Disease*, Elsevier, New York, USA, pp. 241–258.
89. Darfeuille-Michaud, A., Neut, C., Barnich, N., Lederman, E., Di Martino, P. et al. (1998). Presence of adherent Escherichia coli strains in ileal mucosa of patients with Crohn's disease. *Gastroenterology 115*: 1405–1413.
90. Linskens, R. K., Huijsdens, X. W., Savelkoul, P. H., Vandenbroucke-Grauls, C. M., and Meuwissen, S. G. (2001). The bacterial flora in inflammatory bowel disease: current insights in pathogenesis and the influence of antibiotics and probiotics. *Scand J Gastroenterol Suppl 234*: 29–40.
91. Eckburg, P. B. and Relman, D. A. (2007). The role of microbes in Crohn's disease. *Clin Infect Dis 44*: 256–262.
92. Gottschalk, G. (1986). Bacterial fermentation, in: *Bacterial Metabolism*, 1st Edition, Springer-Verlag, New York, USA, pp. 210–282.
93. Macfarlane, G. T., Gibson, G. R., and Cummings, J. H. (1992). Comparison of fermentation reactions in different regions of the human colon. *J Appl Bacteriol 72*: 57–64.
94. Roediger, W. E., Duncan, A., Kapaniris, O., and Millard, S. (1993). Reducing sulfur compounds of the colon impair colonocyte nutrition: implications for ulcerative colitis. *Gastroenterology 104*: 802–809.
95. Mariadason, J. M., Barkla, D. H., and Gibson, P. R. (1997). Effect of short-chain fatty acids on paracellular permeability in Caco-2 intestinal epithelium model. *Am J Physiol 272*: G705–G712.
96. Wachtershauser, A. and Stein, J. (2000). Rationale for the luminal provision of butyrate in intestinal diseases. *Eur J Nutr 39*: 164–171.
97. Saemann, M. D., Bohmig, G. A., Osterreicher, C. H., Burtscher, H., Parolini, O. et al. (2000). Anti-inflammatory effects of sodium butyrate on human monocytes: potent inhibition of IL-12 and up-regulation of IL-10 production. *FASEB J 14*: 2380–2382.
98. Roediger, W. E. (1982). Utilization of nutrients by isolated epithelial cells of the rat colon. *Gastroenterology 83*: 424–429.
99. Cario, E. (2005). Bacterial interactions with cells of the intestinal mucosa: toll-like receptors and NOD2. *Gut 54*: 1182–1193.
100. Kim, J. G., Lee, S. J., and Kagnoff, M. F. (2004). Nod1 is an essential signal transducer in intestinal epithelial cells infected with bacteria that avoid recognition by toll-like receptors. *Infect Immun 72*: 1487–1495.
101. Watanabe, T., Kitani, A., Murray, P. J., and Strober, W. (2004). NOD2 is a negative regulator of Toll-like receptor 2-mediated T helper type 1 responses. *Nat Immunol 5*: 800–808.
102. Strober, W., Murray, P. J., Kitani, A., and Watanabe, T. (2006). Signalling pathways and molecular interactions of NOD1 and NOD2. *Nat Rev Immunol 6*: 9–20.

103. Kobayashi, K. S., Chamaillard, M., Ogura, Y., Henegariu, O., Inohara, N. et al. (2005). Nod2-dependent regulation of innate and adaptive immunity in the intestinal tract. *Science 307*: 731–734.
104. Cliffe, L. J., Humphreys, N. E., Lane, T. E., Potten, C. S., Booth, C. et al. (2005). Accelerated intestinal epithelial cell turnover: a new mechanism of parasite expulsion. *Science 308*: 1463–1465.
105. Goodlad, R. A., Ratcliffe, B., Fordham, J. P., and Wright, N. A. (1989). Does dietary fibre stimulate intestinal epithelial cell proliferation in germ free rats? *Gut 30*: 820–825.
106. Fukata, M., Michelsen, K. S., Eri, R., Thomas, L. S., Hu, B. et al. (2005). Toll-like receptor-4 is required for intestinal response to epithelial injury and limiting bacterial translocation in a murine model of acute colitis. *Am J Physiol Gastrointest Liver Physiol 288*: G1055–G1065.
107. Rakoff-Nahoum, S., Paglino, J., Eslami-Varzaneh, F., Edberg, S., and Medzhitov, R. (2004). Recognition of commensal microflora by toll-like receptors is required for intestinal homeostasis. *Cell 118*: 229–241.
108. Silva, M. A., Jury, J., Porras, M., Vergara, P., and Perdue, M. H. (2008). Intestinal epithelial barrier dysfunction and dendritic cell redistribution during early stages of inflammation in the rat: role for TLR-2 and -4 blockage. *Inflamm Bowel Dis 14*: 632–644.
109. Maslowski, K. M., Vieira, A. T., Ng, A., Kranich, J., Sierro, F. et al. (2009). Regulation of inflammatory responses by gut microbiota and chemoattractant receptor GPR43. *Nature 461*: 1282–1286.
110. Peng, L., Li, Z. R., Green, R. S., Holzman, I. R., and Lin, J. (2009). Butyrate enhances the intestinal barrier by facilitating tight junction assembly via activation of AMP-activated protein kinase in Caco-2 cell monolayers. *J Nutr 139*: 1619–1625.
111. Hooper, L. V. and Gordon, J. I. (2001). Commensal host-bacterial relationships in the gut. *Science 292*: 1115–1118.
112. Cario, E., Gerken, G., and Podolsky, D. K. (2004). Toll-like receptor 2 enhances ZO-1-associated intestinal epithelial barrier integrity via protein kinase C. *Gastroenterology 127*: 224–238.
113. Price, P. T., Nelson, C. M., and Clarke, S. D. (2000). Omega-3 polyunsaturated fatty acid regulation of gene expression. *Curr Opin Lipidol 11*: 3–7.
114. Knoch, B., Barnett, M. P., Zhu, S., Park, Z. A., Nones, K. et al. (2009). Genome-wide analysis of dietary eicosapentaenoic acid- and oleic acid-induced modulation of colon inflammation in interleukin-10 gene-deficient mice. *J Nutrigenet Nutrigenomics 2*: 9–28.
115. Wild, G. E., Drozdowski, L., Tartaglia, C., Clandinin, M. T., and Thomson, A. B. (2007). Nutritional modulation of the inflammatory response in inflammatory bowel disease—from the molecular to the integrative to the clinical. *World J Gastroenterol 13*: 1–7.
116. Knoch, B., Barnett, M. P., McNabb, W. C., Zhu, S., Park, Z. A. et al. (2010). Dietary arachidonic acid-mediated effects on colon inflammation using transcriptome analysis. *Mol Nutr Food Res 54 Suppl 1*: S62–S74.
117. Bassaganya-Riera, J. and Hontecillas, R. (2010). Dietary conjugated linoleic acid and n-3 polyunsaturated fatty acids in inflammatory bowel disease. *Curr Opin Clin Nutr Metab Care 13*: 569–573.
118. Kruse, H. P., Kleessen, B., and Blaut, M. (1999). Effects of inulin on faecal bifidobacteria in human subjects. *Br J Nutr 82*: 375–382.
119. Macfarlane, S. and Macfarlane, G. T. (2006). Composition and metabolic activities of bacterial biofilms colonizing food residues in the human gut. *Appl Environ Microbiol 72*: 6204–6211.
120. Kleessen, B., Hartmann, L., and Blaut, M. (2003). Fructans in the diet cause alterations of intestinal mucosal architecture, released mucins and mucosa-associated bifidobacteria in gnotobiotic rats. *Br J Nutr 89*: 597–606.

121. Kleessen, B., Hartmann, L., and Blaut, M. (2001). Oligofructose and long-chain inulin: influence on the gut microbial ecology of rats associated with a human faecal flora. *Br J Nutr 86*: 291–300.
122. Young, W. (2010). *The Effects of Digestion Resistant Carbohydrates on the Colon Microbiota and Colon Tissue Transcriptome of Weanling Rats, Department of Microbiology and Immunology*, University of Otago, Dunedin.
123. Reif, S., Klein, I., Lubin, F., Farbstein, M., Hallak, A. et al. (1997). Pre-illness dietary factors in inflammatory bowel disease. *Gut 40*: 754–760.
124. Sakamoto, N., Kono, S., Wakai, K., Fukuda, Y., Satomi, M. et al. (2005). Dietary risk factors for inflammatory bowel disease: a multicenter case-control study in Japan. *Inflamm Bowel Dis 11*: 154–163.
125. VerBerkmoes, N. C., Denef, V. J., Hettich, R. L., and Banfield, J. F. (2009). Systems biology: functional analysis of natural microbial consortia using community proteomics. *Nat Rev Microbiol 7*: 196–205.
126. Butterworth, A. D., Thomas, A. G., and Akobeng, A. K. (2008). Probiotics for induction of remission in Crohn's disease. *Cochrane Database Syst Rev 16*: CD006634.
127. Schultz, M. and Lindstrom, A. L. (2008). Rationale for probiotic treatment strategies in inflammatory bowel disease. *Expert Rev Gastroenterol Hepatol 2*: 337–355.
128. Kaur, I. P., Kuhad, A., Garg, A., and Chopra, K. (2009). Probiotics: delineation of prophylactic and therapeutic benefits. *J Med Food 12*: 219–235.
129. PriceWaterhouseCoopers (2009). Leveraging growth in the emerging functional foods industry: trends and market opportunities. *Functional Foods Report*. pp. 1–22.
130. Sanders, M. E., Tompkins, T., Heimbach, J. T., and Kolida, S. (2005). Weight of evidence needed to substantiate a health effect for probiotics and prebiotics: regulatory considerations in Canada, E.U., and U.S. *Eur J Nutr 44*: 303–310.
131. EFSA Panel on Dietetic Products, N. a. A. N. (2010). Scientific Opinion on the substantiation of health claims related to Lactobacillus rhamnosus LB21 NCIMB 40564 and decreasing potentially pathogenic intestinal microorganisms (ID 1064), digestive health (ID 1064), and reduction of mutans streptococci in the oral cavity (ID 1064) pursuant to Article 13(1) of Regulation (EC) No 1924/2006. *EFSA Journal 8*: 1487.
132. EFSA Panel on Dietetic Products, N. a. A. N. (2010). Scientific Opinion on the substantiation of health claims related to beta-glucans and maintenance or achievement of normal blood glucose concentrations (ID 756, 802, 2935) pursuant to Article 13(1) of Regulation (EC) No 1924/2006. *EFSA Journal 8*: 1482.
133. EFSA Panel on Dietetic Products, N. a. A. N. (2010). Scientific Opinion on the substantiation of health claims related to Lactobacillus plantarum 299v (DSM 9843) and "immune system" (ID 1081), pursuant to Article 13(1) of Regulation (EC) No 1924/2006. *EFSA Journal 8*: 1488.
134. Velagapudi, V. R., Hezaveh, R., Reigstad, C. S., Gopalacharyulu, P., Yetukuri, L. et al. (2010). The gut microbiota modulates host energy and lipid metabolism in mice. *J Lipid Res 51*: 1101–1112.

9 Importance of Cell-Specific Gene Expression Patterns for Understanding Nutrient and Gene Interactions in Inflammatory Bowel Diseases

Anna E. Russ, Jason S. Peters, Warren C. McNabb, and Nicole C. Roy

CONTENTS

INTRODUCTION

The majority of the digestion and absorption of food is carried out by the small intestine. However, some intact or partially digested food components reach the large intestine, notably the colon, where the majority of the enteric microbiota is found. The colon has a major role in absorption of electrolytes and fluid, but other components such as oligosaccharides are absorbed in small quantities [1]. Other food components (e.g., fiber) reaching the colon are metabolized by the intestinal microbiota into different components that may be absorbed across the epithelium [2]. The colon is therefore the site of a complex interplay between food components, the intestinal microbiota, and the intestinal mucosal (epithelial and immune) system. Despite the challenges in understanding how these three components interact, the colon is an important tissue in which to study the role of nutrition in health and disease, particularly intestinal inflammatory conditions.

The colon is a complex tissue composed of multiple layers: the mucosa, submucosa, muscularis externa, and serosa (Figure 9.1). Each layer may be involved in inflammation, but interactions between cells in the mucosa are particularly important. The mucosa consists of the epithelial cell layer, the lamina propria, and a thin layer of muscle—the muscularis mucosae. The submucosa is a layer of connective tissue beneath the mucosa that, like the lamina propria of the mucosa, may contain recruited immune cells when inflammation is present [3]. Colonic epithelial cells are the first line of defense against enteric antigens and bacteria with lymphoepithelial interactions in the intestine helping to promote mucosal homeostasis [4]. Epithelial cells in the adult mammalian small intestine include absorptive enterocytes (>80%), secretory goblet cells (16%), enteroendocrine cells (1%) and Paneth cells (at the bottom of the crypts) derived from stem cells located at the crypt base [5], and cells that have migrated to the epithelium (e.g., intraepithelial lymphocytes). The colon differs from the small intestine (duodenum, jejunum, and ileum) in that it has no Paneth cells and when mature, no villi [6].

Biopsy specimens obtained from inflammatory bowel disease (IBD) patients or tissue samples from mouse models of IBD have been studied to better understand changes in intestinal tissues and the pathogenesis of IBD, and ultimately to contribute to the development of treatments for this group of diseases. The role of various immune cell types already present in the tissue before inflammation or recruited from the blood has been studied, as have the profiles of secreted cytokines in inflamed intestinal tissue and their role in inflammation development and maintenance [7–10]. Studying changes in global gene expression in the inflamed intestine

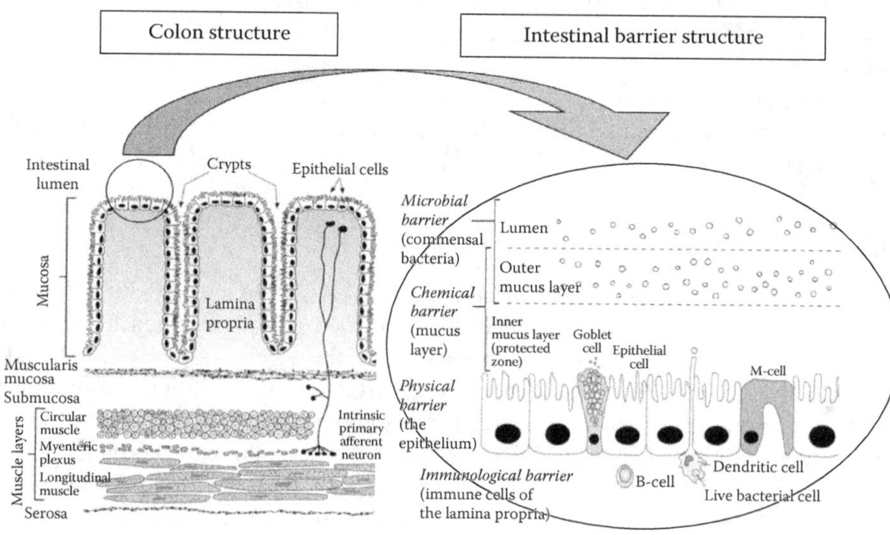

FIGURE 9.1 Diagram showing the structure of the colon and intestinal barrier. (Adapted from Anderson, R.C. et al., *Colitis*, Intech, 2012.)

of IBD models has also been useful in identifying the likely mechanisms underlying the initiation and maintenance of inflammation in the intestinal mucosa [11,12]. However, in whole colon gene expression profiles, it is difficult (if not impossible) to determine which regions of tissue or cell type(s) are contributing to the observed changes in gene expression in response to inflammatory stimuli, as the presence of healthy tissue or cell type(s) in the sample may confound the data.

Identifying and isolating the regions of tissue or specific cell types that are involved in inflammation, as opposed to the whole tissue or cell type(s), and measuring their gene expression profiles may be important for more accurately defining the complex interplay between nutrients and gene expression changes in the intestine. Understanding these may enable the discovery of mechanisms by which food components are able to interact with specific intestinal cells and impact the inflammatory process, whether negatively or positively [13]. This inflamed tissue or cell type–specific approach can allow us to study the interactions between particular patient genotypes, resulting alterations in intestinal gene expression, and how these impact the action of food components on molecular pathways leading to changes in susceptibility to inflammation [14]. This could lead to new nutrition-based treatments for IBD, or enable the development of recommendations for optimal nutrition for people at risk of intestinal or other regions of inflammation [15].

Laser microdissection (LMD) is a technique that allows specific regions of tissues and/or phenotypically similar populations of cells to be removed from frozen tissue, enabling subsequent molecular profiling of these cells, which is reflective of their in vivo state [16–18]. Examining cells dissected from frozen tissue preserves the influence of surrounding cells and the luminal environment on gene expression [6]. Studying gene expression changes in specific cell types or regions of the colon may contribute to a better understanding of the role of particular cells in the complex processes involved in colon inflammation and may identify new roles for some cell types. LMD combined with gene expression profiling has not yet been applied to the study of cell function in the healthy and diseased intestinal tract. Furthermore, the potential role of food components in modifying gene expression patterns observed in IBD has yet to be explored.

The scope of this review is to (1) outline the methods by which RNA is harvested from selected tissue areas and cell types in the colon for effective LMD, based on our experiences in optimizing this process in our laboratory for intestinal tissues; and (2) describe how transcriptomic data obtained through LMD can contribute to our understanding of the roles of specific cell types in the pathogenesis of IBD. These approaches are reviewed with a focus on how they are used to improve our understanding of how nutrients interact with genes associated with the IBD phenotype.

INSIGHTS INTO LASER MICRODISSECTION OF SPECIFIC TISSUE AREAS OR CELL TYPES

With the completion of the human genome initiative, the ability to link phenotype and genotype through molecular analysis now means that obtaining anatomically specific signals from molecules isolated from tissues of interest is becoming more important [19]. Capturing such molecules from heterogeneous tissue can be somewhat challenging when the focal point is mRNA. In the first years of the developing LMD technology, the number of cells required for a methodology such as DNA methylation was approximately 200 cells while approximately 2,000–20,000 cells were required to extract an adequate quantity of RNA for downstream analysis [16]. Current RNA extraction kits describe small quantities of cells giving a sufficient quantity of RNA for downstream analyses, but this must be under the most ideal circumstances, which are rarely the case in the laboratory. Although LMD is a powerful technique that has enhanced many molecular biological techniques, it is heavily dependent on procuring excellent cellular material.

The LMD technique requires several steps to be performed efficiently to generate RNA of sufficient quality for transcriptomic analysis such as microarrays (Figure 9.2). Briefly, tissue dissection, freezing, cryosectioning, and section staining are far more important in terms of procuring good-quality RNA than how the LMD itself is performed [20]. All of the steps performed before LMD are time-consuming, and thus any steps that can be removed from the method will reduce the amount of nuclease activity and ultimately increase the likelihood of isolating RNA of the highest possible quality. The isolation of pure populations of cell types will often mean that the material available for RNA extractions is very small. However, many proprietary extraction kits are designed to work with limited starting material, and are therefore suitable for LMD samples. The goal of staining slides for LMD is to allow for identification of the target tissue areas or cell types from the surrounding tissue. Avoiding excessive water washes and hydration/dehydration steps (which are important for histological diagnoses) is essential in the preparation of samples for LMD to minimize RNA degradation. Ironically, the actual time spent on the laser dissector appears insignificant after the lengthy sample preparation. While literature reports rarely present discussions of detailing the important aspects of tissue sample preparation, understanding these basic requirements is crucial for any new researchers in this field.

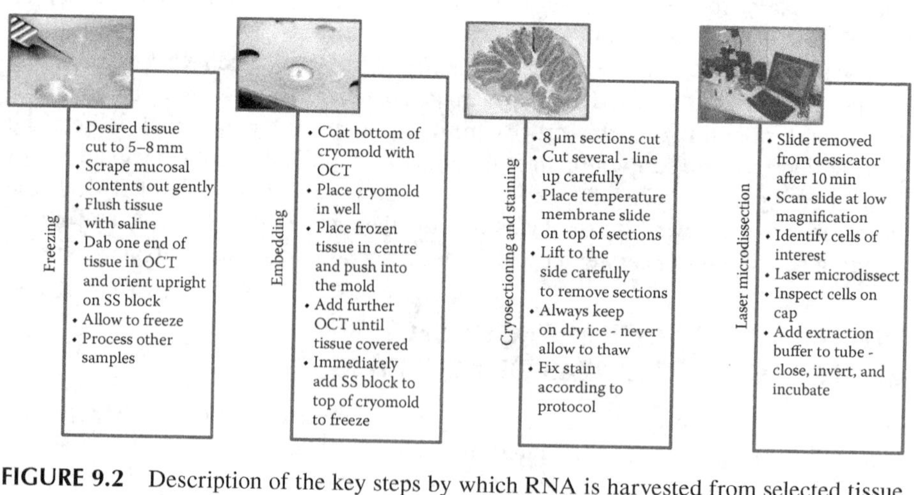

FIGURE 9.2 Description of the key steps by which RNA is harvested from selected tissue areas and cell types for effective LMD.

Adequate tissue sampling requires a variety of equipment and reagents. Those used in our laboratory are summarized in Table 9.1. Briefly, surgical instruments and bench surfaces used for sampling were cleaned with 100% ethanol at the beginning of the process and again in between each animal sampled. Cleaned instruments were dried with lint-free Kimwipes™ to avoid residual tissue. Similarly, the embedding block was sprayed with 100% ethanol and wiped clean with Kimwipes just before freezing the samples to clear ice from the block. The embedding block was also placed on dry ice, low in the container, to allow the gas phase to keep the samples frozen and protect them from the ambient air temperature.

Tissue samples for LMD and transcriptomic analysis were removed rapidly from animals and processed immediately to minimize time as a contributing factor for loss of tissue RNA integrity. Freezing soft tissue samples, such as the intestine, in liquid nitrogen may distort their physical appearance and hinder effective cross-sectioning using a cryostat. To avoid this, 5–8 mm tissue samples were dipped in Tissue-Tek® OCT (optimal cutting temperature) Compound (Sakura Finetek USA Inc.) and then oriented on a stainless steel block maintained in dry ice. Our embedding block was designed and modified from the cryoembedding system designed by pathologist Stephen Peters [21]. These modifications include 18-mm round cryomolds (Sakura Finetek USA Inc.) and a stainless steel block with machined round inserts that allow the cryomolds to sit neatly while allowing for heat extraction from the bottom and sides of the mold to freeze the OCT more effectively. With intestinal tissues, the digesta was gently removed with a spatula and the remaining tissue flushed with chilled 0.9% sterile saline before freezing. Using this technique, we froze intestinal tissues for sufficient time to maintain their shape and RNA integrity. Longer lengths of intestine such as jejunum samples were held in place with tweezers or a probe to

TABLE 9.1
Materials Required for Tissue Sampling for LMD of Tissue Areas or Specific Cells

Equipment or Solutions	Use
Angled forceps, probe, iris scissors	Tissue dissection for embedding
Stainless steel embedding block and weight	Freezing tissue and embedding
Dry ice	Freezing and storage of samples
Sterile 70% ethanol or AR 100% ethanol	Cleaning instruments/cry molds/bench
Small plastic spatula	Scrapping mucosa clean
Small polystyrene box	Embedding block
Larger polystyrene box	Sample storage
Tissue freezing media (e.g., OCT)	Embedding
Tissue-Tekcryomolds—15 × 15 mm or round	Embedding
MMI Membrane Slides	Mounting of sections
MMI Isolation Caps	LMD
Histogene LCM Frozen Section Stain	Staining
RNaseZap (or RNase Away)	General cleaning
PicoPure RNA Extraction Kit	RNA extraction

ensure that the tissue did not fold down on itself before freezing is complete. Once frozen, tissues were mounted into a cryomold (precleaned with RNaseZAP or RNase Away followed by sterile 70% ethanol) with a small amount of OCT. Once secured, additional OCT was added until the cryomold was full. A small stainless steel block was then added to the top of the cryomold to enable further heat extraction of OCT into the tissue and rapidly decrease the temperature, avoiding possible tissue thawing. Samples were kept on dry ice until transferred into the −80°C freezer for longer-term storage.

The next step is the cryosectioning of the embedded tissue. Cryosectioning uses a cryostat or freezing microtome, in which the temperature is regulated appropriately for the tissue being sectioned; for intestinal tissue this is −20°C. The embedded samples (−80°C) were kept on dry ice throughout this procedure. To remove the embedded sample from the cryomold, we placed a small amount of OCT on the cryostat chuck, then placed the cryomold containing the embedded sample onto this. To expose the inside edge of the block containing the sample, we pulled the tab on the cryomold away from the block. The temperature of the embedded block was allowed to equilibrate to that of the cryostat chamber temperature for approximately 15 minutes before 8-μm-thick sections were cut. Two-to-four sections were then mounted onto a membrane slide (Molecular Machines and Industries, Zurich Switzerland) and the slides were placed into an RNase-free container kept on dry ice and later stored at −80°C until staining was performed. During the cryosectioning step, slides must remain frozen at all times. Although one section was often sufficient, variations with sectioning and possible damage of the section during the staining procedure may occur and it is therefore advisable to prepare additional sections on one slide. Mounting the section onto the membrane slide as described in the preceding discussion is always more difficult when compared with mounting onto glass slides for histology. This is because the membrane slides are kept in the cryostat before the mount to avoid thawing of the section.

Staining is a time-sensitive process therefore speed is paramount, but care must also be taken when staining to avoid the section sliding off the slide into the staining solutions. Slides were gently immersed into stain solutions rather than vigorously rinsed as would be standard for glass slides. Some minor alterations to the Arcturus® HistoGene® LCM Frozen Section Staining Kit protocol were necessary for preparing colonic tissues for LMD in our laboratory; the main modification was to the dehydration of sections using xylene washes. Xylene often dried out the membrane increasing the risk of tearing during LMD. In our laboratory, effective dehydration was achieved using 100% ethanol without damaging the membrane supporting the section. Water rinses were also omitted. Stained and dehydrated sections were kept in a desiccator until LMD was performed. Many LMD users (including those from our laboratory) recommend dissecting cells within 20 minutes of removal from the desiccator [20].

Several brands of the LMD system are commercially available. In our laboratory, the microdissection steps were performed using the MMI® CellCut Plus® laser microdissection system (Molecular Machines and Industries), with a motorized Olympus IX81 microscope. The MMI CellCut Plus laser microdissection system uses membrane slides where the cryosection is placed on the underside, and the membrane slide sits against a glass slide for support. The advantage of this configuration is contamination-free isolation of cell types or tissue areas, as the isolation cap never comes into contact with the section.

As mentioned earlier, the actual time spent on the laser microdissector is minimal relative to the time and effort required to obtain a quality section. Nevertheless, this final step must also be undertaken rapidly. Camera configurations, preferences, and laser dissection parameters were optimized with practice samples before any experimental samples were used. Sample slides were quickly moved from the desiccator to the microscope stage. Cells of interest were identified and dissection was performed rapidly, that is, within 20–30 minutes of removal from the desiccator. Excessive time spent on the microscope can lead to the uptake of atmospheric moisture, which will increase nuclease activity, while also preventing the adhesion of dissected cells to the isolation cap. Once cells or tissue regions were isolated using LMD and harvested in the isolation cap, extraction buffer was added to the cells until RNA extraction was performed. After dissection, cells on the isolation cap were examined in the same spatial orientation as the original slide, and any cells identified as mistakenly cut or undesirable for RNA extraction were ablated with further laser shots; these cells were removed by centrifugation in the subsequent extraction protocol. Sample tubes were incubated at 42°C for 30 minutes (according to the PicoPure™ kit protocol) with the extraction buffer completely covering the tube cap containing the sample. This step reflects that of other extraction methods reported in the literature, which include an incubation step to improve cell lysis. The cell lysate was then collected at the bottom of the tube through centrifugation as per the manufacturer's protocol and the RNA sample was extracted immediately or stored at −80°C.

A limited number of RNA isolation kits can provide reliable RNA preparations compatible with the downstream steps for transcriptomic analysis using microarray, such as the PicoPure® RNA Isolation Kit (MDS Analytical Technologies Inc., Sunnyvale, CA), the Absolutely RNA™ Microprep Kit (Agilent Technologies, Santa Clara, CA), and the RNeasy Plus Micro Kit (Qiagen, Hilden, Germany). In our laboratory, several of these kits have been tested using mouse colon tissues. The Arcturus® PicoPure® RNA Isolation Kit (Arcturus Engineering Inc., catalog no. KIT0202, 0204; MDS Analytical Technologies Inc.) has been validated for small cell samples such as those obtained by LMD [22,23]. Most importantly, it allows for elution in a small volume (11–30 μL), which is essential for the small sample sizes typically collected from the mouse intestine and associated LMD samples. This kit provided the best results when RNA was extracted from colon sections using the manufacturer's instructions (User Guide Version D) and included the recommended DNase treatment (RNase-free DNase Set, catalog no. 79254; Qiagen). These findings were in agreement with literature reports [6,24]. DNase treatment was a prerequisite if the Agilent Bioanalyzer Total RNA Pico Kit was used to verify RNA integrity, as without DNase treatment of the samples, this kit cannot perform satisfactorily.

The integrity of the extracted total RNA (RNA integrity number; RIN) was verified using the RNA 6000 Pico Chip Kit for the 2100 Bioanalyzer (Agilent Technologies). Many researchers report the Bioanalyzer electropherograms or gel-like images but do not report an RIN for each sample, making it difficult to compare protocols. However, RINs obtained using the Pico Chip Kit for the Agilent

Bioanalyzer have not yet been validated for gene expression analysis to the same extent as those obtained using the higher-input Nano Kit. This made it difficult to judge how appropriate the RNA quality of our samples was for downstream transcriptomic analysis based on RIN value alone. As a general rule, the key criteria included the presence of two very strong ribosomal RNA peaks, or RINs, within the range of 4.0–7.0 (higher values are much more difficult to obtain and ideally the samples used for one experiment should have similar RINs). Samples with RINs in this range performed well in microarray experiments.

Yields from microdissected cells are often insufficient to measure total RNA concentration and purity by spectrophotometric methods such as the NanoDrop 1000 (Thermo Scientific, Wilmington, DE). However, even though RNA purity was not measured in these small samples, the PicoPure™ RNA Isolation Kit was designed to yield high-purity RNA, which was ready for amplification. The DNase and subsequent wash steps were used to ensure the RNA was free from contaminants such as genomic DNA. High-quality gene expression data were obtained from these samples, which is supportive of the RNA sample purity being adequate.

The Qubit® 2.0 Fluorometer was used in addition to the Bioanalyzer concentration estimate to quantify the levels of total RNA present in the LMD samples. The Qubit™ RNA Assay Kit is able to measure smaller amounts of RNA (initial sample concentration range of 250 pg/μL to 100 ng/μL) than the spectrophotometric NanoDrop method. It is also more accurate than the spectrophotometric and Bioanalyzer methods as it directly measures RNA even in the presence of other molecules (DNA, salts, solvents, proteins, and free nucleotides), which is impossible with spectrophotometric methods. However, RNA quantity in some samples was still too low to enable accurate measurement with the Qubit 2.0 Fluorometer. The fluorometer measurements were used to calculate RNA input for the amplification except when the sample was too low in concentration to be measured (<4 ng/μL); in these cases, the maximum volume (10 μL) of sample was used.

Following the guidelines outlined here, our laboratory has yielded high-quality RNA from colon epithelial cells isolated from a mouse model of IBD. The RNA was of sufficient quantity for downstream global gene expression (microarray) and performed well in this analysis. These techniques provided high-quality microarray data that will help us to understand the function of the colon epithelium in intestinal inflammation in mouse models of IBD.

TRANSCRIPTOMIC ANALYSIS OF MICRODISSECTED CELLS OF THE COLON: INFLAMMATION AND NUTRITION

Studying gene expression provides a unique insight into the function of a tissue or cell that can be obtained with very small amounts of sample, more so than studies of DNA or protein. The development of these techniques for microdissecting cells and measuring global gene expression is likely to provide new insights into the role different types of intestinal cells have in the function of the intestine in health and disease. It may also make a valuable contribution to the study of how they respond to nutritional factors and how they are involved in processes such as inflammation, which can cause disease when dysregulated. Throughout this section, the term "inflammation" will be used in the context of intestinal inflammatory disease such as IBD.

Besides the maintenance of barrier function, intestinal epithelial cells play a role in the tissue's response to bacteria and the initiation of inflammation [25,26]. Changes in the colonic epithelium, such as increased paracellular permeability and mucosal immune defense malfunction, are thought to be important in the initiation of inflammation [27,28].

The different cell types in the epithelium all have actions that may impact on intestinal inflammation and the digestion and absorption of food components. Changes in secretion of mucus by goblet cells [29] and changes in enteroendocrine cell function [30] are often involved in IBD. Paneth cells of the terminal ileum, which is often affected in IBD, have an important role in innate immunity and defense from the intestinal microbiota [31]. Absorptive enterocytes, which make up the majority of the epithelium, are involved in the recognition, processing, and presentation of luminal antigens [32]. Enterocytes also secrete immunoglobulins and antimicrobial proteins that are transported into the intestinal lumen [32] as well as a range of chemokines in response to inflammatory stimuli [11]. LMD could be useful in understanding the different roles that these cells have in IBD and also in response to nutritional stimuli.

Intestinal immune responses take place in the epithelium, lamina propria, and gut-associated lymphoid tissue. Intraepithelial lymphocytes are much more common in the colon than the small intestine, at least in mouse models [32]. These lymphocytes are interspersed between the epithelial cells and monitor for damaged or stressed epithelial cells [32]. During inflammation, the lamina propria may contain a large number of immune cells recruited from the blood, such as T and B lymphocytes, neutrophils, and macrophages [7,11,33]. There are many T-cell subsets and many complex interactions between immune cells occur in healthy tissue and in intestinal inflammation [33]. Further research is required to understand these interactions and the role of specific T-cell subsets in inflammation and LMD could be a useful technique to achieve that in combination with transcriptomics.

In intestinal inflammation, the function of smooth muscle contraction and intestinal motility is negatively affected [34]. Intestinal motility may also be affected by the enteric nervous system in inflammation [34]. Human colonic smooth muscle cells were found to be able to synthesize pro-inflammatory mediators [35], suggesting these muscles in the colon may actually have an active role in colitis besides their role in intestinal motility.

Clearly, many intestinal cells are involved in inflammation, creating a very complex tissue environment in which to study the development and maintenance of IBD. In addition, some cell types in the colon may have as-yet undefined actions in IBD. Understanding the actions of specific cells and tissue regions and determining how they are altered by particular food components is an important step toward elucidating the ways in which the inflammatory process is affected by dietary factors. These processes must be understood before the ultimate goal of being able to make dietary recommendations for people with genetic susceptibility to IBD can be achieved.

Analysis of microdissected cells can provide a more detailed, tissue region–specific understanding of how a disease develops and progresses. The development of *Helicobacter*-induced gastric lymphomas has been studied using LMD of mucosal cells and immune infiltrates from stomach sections followed by microarray analysis [24]. Gene expression pattern differences between specific stomach cell types and whole stomach characterized different stages of *Helicobacter* infection in vivo [24]. Molecular signatures in endogenous mucosal cells and immune cell infiltrates were identified: in the mucosal fraction, the expression levels of mucosal defense genes was increased, while in the lymphocytic fraction the expression levels of many B-cell and some T-cell genes were increased [24]. This study demonstrated that gene expression patterns in lymphocytic and mucosal fractions differed from each other, and from expression patterns in whole stomach. These findings confirm that the likely cellular origin of particular transcripts could be identified by transcriptomic analysis in specific cell fractions.

LMD is also an important tool for studying the role of cell types in IBD that are difficult to study in vitro. Paneth cells secrete α-defensins and other antimicrobial proteins including lysozyme and secretory phospholipase A2 [31]. They, therefore, have an important role in innate immune responses to luminal microbiota. Paneth cells and the defensins they secrete have been shown to play a role in ileal Crohn's disease (CD), one of the IBDs [31]. There are no cultured cell lines available to model Paneth cells, so they cannot be studied in vitro, but LMD allows the study of Paneth cell function in vivo [36]. Lala et al. [36] harvested relatively pure populations of Paneth cells and villus epithelial cells from the terminal ileum from CD-affected tissues of patients undergoing surgical resection. In situ hybridization and immunohistochemical localization of the nucleotide-binding oligomerization domain-containing protein 2 (NOD2; a known IBD susceptibility gene) expression in Paneth cells confirmed that NOD2 mRNA was most abundant in the Paneth cell fraction, which was consistent with the LMD gene expression analysis and confirmed that the cell fraction harvested was likely to be the desired Paneth cells [36]. Such studies provide valuable insights into the role of gene expression differences between individuals and the mechanisms by which they affect a person's susceptibility to IBD [37,38].

Analysis of microdissected cells also enables the gene expression profile of a specific cell type to be studied in detail. Many studies into the function of the epithelium in colitis have used techniques such as *in vitro* cell lines, the isolation of live epithelial cells from fresh tissue, or *in situ* hybridization in tissue sections [39–41]. Studies that include analysis of gene expression typically use whole intestinal tissue and/or intestinal mucosa as a proxy for the epithelial cell fraction [42]. These techniques all have limitations that can be overcome by analysis of the gene expression of epithelial cells isolated by LMD. Findings in epithelial cell lines can be specific to the cell line and affected by the culture conditions, and therefore may not be representative of epithelial cells *in vivo*. *In situ* hybridization is limited to a few specific molecules of interest. LMD allows the study of cells in their in vivo state in stored tissue, and allows for analysis of global gene expression.

Flanagan et al. [11] used LMD and microarray techniques to discover novel molecules expressed by intestinal epithelial cells that are dysregulated in colitis in a mouse model of IBD and associated with the expression of other inflammatory molecules. LY6 molecules are used as markers of immune cell differentiation [43] but their functions are difficult to elucidate. The presence of LY6 molecules on epithelial cell surfaces is regulated by inflammatory cytokines [43]. Microarray analysis of microdissected colon epithelial cells in inflamed colons of adult *Il10*$^{-/-}$ mice showed that the expression of the LY6 family of molecules was specific to the diseased state of colitis and not expressed on healthy intestinal epithelial cells [11]. Formation of cross-links between LY6 molecules on the surface of epithelial cells resulted in increased production of many chemokines, which suggests that LY6 molecules may be an upstream switch in the expression of chemokine genes in colitis [11]. The epithelial cell microarray analysis showed that expression of the LY6 family and chemokine genes was increased in these cells confirming the coexistence of these two findings in the same analysis [11]. This suggests that enterocytes have a direct role in affecting chemokine synthesis, which in turns affects immune cell recruitment into the area. This suggests that enterocytes have an active role in inflammation besides barrier function, antigen processing, and secretion of immunoglobulins and antimicrobial proteins.

LMD followed by transcriptome profiling has yet to be fully utilized in the study of nutrient and gene interactions in the intestine. Few studies have investigated the role of intestinal cells in inflammation using LMD [11,44] although the role of epithelial cells in intestinal inflammation has been studied using various other techniques [42,45]. Differences between cells in specific crypt regions of the intestine have been studied in healthy adult human colon tissue [46], in developing gastrointestinal tissues [47], and interactions between the intestinal microbiota and intestinal cells have also been studied [48]. One example of the use of LMD to study interactions between nutritional factors and gene expression is a study by Jovanovic et al. [49]. Mice were fed *ad libitum* or fasted, dosed with leptin or saline by intraperitoneal administration, and their arcuate nucleus was microdissected for gene expression analysis: this study identified leptin-regulated genes within the arcuate nucleus of the hypothalamus [49]. Overall, there seems to be a lack of research into nutrient–gene interactions using LMD in the intestine, in either health or inflammation.

SUMMARY AND CONCLUSIONS

Understanding the function of intestinal cells and their gene expression changes in response to dietary factors and the inflammatory processes may be important for understanding the interplay between intestinal tissue and dietary factors in inflammatory disease of the intestine. LMD is a useful technique that allows the capture and downstream gene expression analysis of specific cell fractions or tissue regions. Advantages of this technique are (1) the use of stored frozen tissue rather than fresh, and (2) the ability to study cells captured at a single time point in their in vivo state. Cells studied through LMD have been subjected to their in vivo environment throughout their life span and are not influenced by in vitro culture methods. Findings regarding cell function obtained through the use of this technology are therefore likely to be more reflective of the in vivo function of the cell of interest than similar types of analysis performed on in vitro cell lines or on cells cultured from a mixed population in live tissue. However, gene expression profiling of microdissected cells poses a number of challenges, including maintenance of RNA integrity during tissue staining, which is necessary to visualize the cell types of interest, and during the time taken to identify and dissect the cells. Working with small amounts of RNA poses additional challenges to those expected with RNA work. This review summarizes the methods that provide good results in our laboratory, in terms of obtaining adequate cell visualization, good RNA quality and yield, and describes how these techniques may contribute to the study of intestinal cell function in inflammation, and nutrient and gene interactions that may play a part in intestinal homeostasis.

ACKNOWLEDGMENTS

The authors thank Drs Matthew Barnett, Shalome Bassett, Mark McCann, and Emma Bermingham for the constructive review of this manuscript.

REFERENCES

1. Bode, L., Kunz, C., Muhly-Reinholz, M., Mayer, K., Seeger, W. et al. (2004). Inhibition of monocyte, lymphocyte, and neutrophil adhesion to endothelial cells by human milk oligosaccharides. *Thromb. Haemost. 92*: 1402–1410.
2. Hamer, H. M., Jonkers, D., Venema, K., Vanhoutvin, S., Troost, F. J. et al. (2008). Review article: the role of butyrate on colonic function. *Aliment. Pharmacol. Ther. 27*: 104–119.
3. Anderson, R. C., Dalziel, J. E., Gopal, P. K., Bassett, S., Ellis, A. et al. The role of intestinal barrier function in early life in the development of colitis, in: M. Fukata (Ed.), *Colitis*, Intech, 2011, pp. 3–30. ISBN 978-953-307-799-4, InTech, January 1, 2012. Book published online: http://www.intechopen.com/books/colitis.
4. Dahan, S., Roth-Walter, F., Arnaboldi, P., Agarwal, S. and Mayer, L. (2007). Epithelia: lymphocyte interactions in the gut. *Immunol. Rev. 215*: 243–253.
5. van der Flier, L. G. and Clevers, H. (2009). Stem cells, self-renewal, and differentiation in the intestinal epithelium. *Annu. Rev. Physiol. 71*: 241–260.
6. Stappenbeck, T. S., Hooper, L. V., Manchester, J. K., Wong, M. H. and Gordon, J. I. Laser capture microdissection of mouse intestine: characterizing mRNA and protein expression, and profiling intermediary metabolism in specified cell populations, in: *Laser Capture Microscopy and Microdissection*, 2002, pp. 167–196.
7. Baumgart, D. C., McVay, L. D. and Carding, S. R. (1998). Mechanisms of immune cell-mediated tissue injury in inflammatory bowel disease (Review). *Int. J. Mol. Med. 1*: 315–332.
8. Berg, D. J., Davidson, N., Kuhn, R., Muller, W., Menon, S. et al. (1996). Enterocolitis and colon cancer in interleukin-10-deficient mice are associated with aberrant cytokine production and CD4+ TH1-like responses. *J. Clin. Invest. 98*: 1010–1020.
9. DiFedele, L. M., He, J., Bonkowski, E. L., Han, X., Held, M. A. et al. (2005). Tumor necrosis factor alpha blockade restores growth hormone signaling in murine colitis. *Gastroenterology 128*: 1278–1291.
10. Leon, A. J., Garrote, J. A. and Arranz, E. (2006). Cytokines in the pathogenesis of inflammatory bowel diseases. *Med. Clin. (Barc) 127*: 145–152.
11. Flanagan, K., Modrusan, Z., Cornelius, J., Chavali, A., Kasman, I. et al. (2008). Intestinal epithelial cell up-regulation of LY6 molecules during colitis results in enhanced chemokine secretion. *J. Immunol. 180*: 3874–3881.
12. Te Velde, A. A., De Kort, F., Sterrenburg, E., Pronk, I., Ten Kate, F. J. W. et al. (2007). Comparative analysis of colonic gene expression of three experimental colitis models mimicking inflammatory bowel disease. *Inflamm. Bowel Dis. 13*: 325–330.
13. Lucendo, A. J. and De Rezende, L. C. (2009). Importance of nutrition in inflammatory bowel disease. *World J. Gastroenterol. 15*: 2081–2088.

14. Chapman-Kiddell, C. A., Davies, P. S., Gillen, L. and Radford-Smith, G. L. (2010). Role of diet in the development of inflammatory bowel disease. *Inflamm. Bowel Dis. 16*: 137–151.
15. Ferguson, L. R. (2006). Nutrigenomics: integrating genomic approaches into nutrition research. *Mol. Diagn. Ther. 10*: 101–108.
16. Espina, V., Wulfkuhle, J. D., Calvert, V. S., VanMeter, A., Zhou, W. et al. (2006). Laser-capture microdissection. *Nat. Protoc. 1*: 586–603.
17. Hooper, L. V. (2004). Laser microdissection: exploring host–bacterial encounters at the front lines. *Curr. Opin. Microbiol. 7*: 290–295.
18. Walch, A., Specht, K., Smida, J., Aubele, M., Zitzelsberger, H. et al. (2001). Tissue microdissection techniques in quantitative genome and gene expression analyses. *Histochem. Cell Biol. 115*: 269–276.
19. Bova, G. S., Eltoum, I. A., Kiernan, J. A., Siegal, G. P., Frost, A. R. et al. (2005). Optimal molecular profiling of tissue and tissue components: defining the best processing and microdissection methods for biomedical applications. *Mol. Biotechnol. 29*: 119–152.
20. Clement-Ziza, M., Munnich, A., Lyonnet, S., Jaubert, F. and Besmond, C. (2008). Stabilization of RNA during laser capture microdissection by performing experiments under argon atmosphere or using ethanol as a solvent in staining solutions. *RNA 14*: 2698–2704.
21. Peters, S. R. (2003). The art of embedding tissue for frozen section. Part I: a system for precision face down cryoembedding of tissues using freezing temperature-embedding wells. *J. Histotechnol. 26*: 11–19.
22. Caretti, E., Devarajan, K., Coudry, R., Ross, E., Clapper, M. L. et al. (2008). Comparison of RNA amplification methods and chip platforms for microarray analysis of samples processed by laser capture microdissection. *J. Cell Biochem. 103*: 556–563.
23. Lang, J., Magbanua, M., Scott, J., Makrigiorgos, G. M., Wang, G. et al. (2009). A comparison of RNA amplification techniques at sub-nanogram input concentration. *BMC Genomics 10*: 326.
24. Mueller, A., O'Rourke, J., Grimm, J., Guillemin, K., Dixon, M. F. et al. (2003). Distinct gene expression profiles characterize the histopathological stages of disease in helicobacter-induced mucosa-associated lymphoid tissue lymphoma. *Proc. Natl. Acad. Sci. U. S. A. 100*: 1292–1297.
25. Cario, E. and Podolsky, D. K. (2000). Differential alteration in intestinal epithelial cell expression of toll-like receptor 3 (TLR3) and TLR4 in inflammatory bowel disease. *Infect. Immun. 68*: 7010–7017.
26. Laukoetter, M. G., Nava, P., Lee, W. Y., Severson, E. A., Capaldo, C. T. et al. (2007). JAM-A regulates permeability and inflammation in the intestine in vivo. *J. Exp. Med. 204*: 3067–3076.
27. McGuckin, M. A., Eri, R., Simms, L. A., Florin, T. H. J. and Radford-Smith, G. (2009). Intestinal barrier dysfunction in inflammatory bowel diseases. *Inflamm. Bowel Dis. 15*: 100–113.
28. Nenci, A., Becker, C., Wullaert, A., Gareus, R., Van Loo, G. et al. (2007). Epithelial NEMO links innate immunity to chronic intestinal inflammation. *Nature 446*: 557–561.
29. Moehle, C., Ackermann, N., Langmann, T., Aslanidis, C., Kel, A. et al. (2006). Aberrant intestinal expression and allelic variants of mucin genes associated with inflammatory bowel disease. *J. Mol. Med. 84*: 1055–1066.
30. O'Hara, J. R., Lomax, A. E., Mawe, G. M. and Sharkey, K. A. (2007). Ileitis alters neuronal and enteroendocrine signalling in guinea pig distal colon. *Gut 56*: 186–194.
31. Bevins, C. L. (2006). Paneth cell defensins: key effector molecules of innate immunity. *Biochem. Soc. Trans. 34*: 263–266.
32. Henderson, P., van Limbergen, J. E., Schwarze, J. and Wilson, D. C. (2011). Function of the intestinal epithelium and its dysregulation in inflammatory bowel disease. *Inflamm. Bowel Dis. 17*: 382–395.

33. Izcue, A., Coombes, J. L. and Powrie, F. (2009). Regulatory lymphocytes and intestinal inflammation. *Annu. Rev. Immunol. 27*: 313–338.
34. Ohama, T., Hori, M. and Ozaki, H. (2007). Mechanism of abnormal intestinal motility in inflammatory bowel disease: how smooth muscle contraction is reduced? *J. Smooth Muscle Res. 43*: 43–54.
35. Salinthone, S., Singer, C. A. and Gerthoffer, W. T. (2004). Inflammatory gene expression by human colonic smooth muscle cells. *Am. J. Physiol. Gastrointest. Liver Physiol. 287*: G627–G637.
36. Lala, S., Ogura, Y., Osborne, C., Hor, S. Y., Bromfield, A. et al. (2003). Crohn's disease and the *NOD2* gene: a role for paneth cells. *Gastroenterology 125*: 47–57.
37. Rogler, G. (2007). The effects of *NOD2/CARD15* mutations on the function of the intestinal barrier. *J. Crohns Colitis. 1*: 53–60.
38. Wehkamp, J., Harder, J., Weichenthal, M., Schwab, M., Schäffeler, E. et al. (2004). *NOD2* (CARD15) mutations in Crohn's disease are associated with diminished mucosal α-defensin expression. *Gut 53*: 1658–1664.
39. Brand, S., Beigel, F., Olszak, T., Zitzmann, K., Eichhorst, S. T. et al. (2006). IL-22 is increased in active Crohn's disease and promotes proinflammatory gene expression and intestinal epithelial cell migration. *Am. J. Physiol. Gastrointest. Liver Physiol. 290*: G827–G838.
40. Fahlgren, A., Hammarstrom, S., Danielsson, A. and Hammarstrom, M.-L. (2004). β-Defensin-3 and -4 in intestinal epithelial cells display increased mRNA expression in ulcerative colitis. *Clin. Exp. Immunol. 137*: 379–385.
41. Ruiz, P. A., Shkoda, A., Kim, S. C., Sartor, R. B. and Haller, D. IL-10 gene-deficient mice lack TGF-beta/Smad-mediated TLR2 degradation and fail to inhibit proinflammatory gene expression in intestinal epithelial cells under conditions of chronic inflammation, in: W. W. Domschke, M. F. Kagnoff, T. F. Kucharzik, L. Mayer and S. R. Targan (Eds.), *Inflammatory Bowel Disease: Genetics, Barrier Function, Immunologic Mechanisms, and Microbial Pathways*, New York Academy of Sciences, New York, NY, 2006, vol. 1072, pp. 389–394..
42. Kwon, J. H., Keates, S., Bassani, L., Mayer, L. F. and Keates, A. C. (2002). Colonic epithelial cells are a major site of macrophage inflammatory protein 3α (MIP-3α) production in normal colon and inflammatory bowel disease. *Gut 51*: 818–826.
43. Bamezai, A. (2004). Mouse Ly-6 proteins and their extended family: markers of cell differentiation and regulators of cell signaling. *Arch. Immunol. Ther. Exp. 52*: 255–266.
44. Funke, B., Lasitschka, F., Roth, W., Penzel, R., Meuer, S. et al. (2011). Selective down-regulation of retinoic acid-inducible gene I within the intestinal epithelial compartment in Crohn's disease. *Inflamm. Bowel Dis. 17*: 1943–1954.
45. Ruiz, P. A., Anna, S., Kim, S. C., Sartor, R. B. and Haller, D. (2005). IL-10 gene-deficient mice lack TGF-beta/smad signaling and fail to inhibit proinflammatory gene expression in intestinal epithelial cells after the colonization with colitogenic enterococcus faecalis. *J. Immunol. 174*: 2990–2999.
46. George, M., Wehkamp, J., Kays, R., Leutenegger, C., Sabir, S. et al. (2008). In vivo gene expression profiling of human intestinal epithelial cells: analysis by laser microdissection of formalin fixed tissues. *BMC Genomics 9*: 209.
47. Giannakis, M., Stappenbeck, T. S., Mills, J. C., Leip, D. G., Lovett, M. et al. (2006). Molecular properties of adult mouse gastric and intestinal epithelial progenitors in their niches. *J. Biol. Chem. 281*: 11292–11300.
48. Hooper, L. V., Wong, M. H., Thelin, A., Hansson, L., Falk, P. C. et al. (2001). Molecular analysis of commensal host–microbial relationships in the intestine. *Science 291*: 881–884.
49. Jovanovic, Z., Tung, Y. C. L., Lam, B. Y. H., O'Rahilly, S. and Yeo, G. S. H. (2010). Identification of the global transcriptomic response of the hypothalamic arcuate nucleus to fasting and leptin. *J. Neuroendocrinol. 22*: 915–925.

Section III

Technologies in Nutrigenetics/ Nutrigenomics

10 Data Mining and Network Analysis

Potential Importance in Nutrigenomics Research

Vijayalakshmi Varma and Jim Kaput

CONTENTS

INTRODUCTION

Nutrients and Biological Processes

Nutrients and bioactive components of food constitute the most important environmental factor that influences the health or disease status of an individual. Nutrients alter biological processes by influencing the expression of genetic information either in a direct or indirect manner. Individual genetic variability produce differences in physiological responses to the same nutrients resulting in differences in the ability to maintain health or in the initiation, progression, and severity of a disease (Kaput 2008).

Biological processes are integrated and regulated at the cellular, tissue, and systems level. The mechanisms by which cellular regulation and modulation of function take place by integration of signals that include RNA, protein, and metabolites still remain to be fully identified (Parker et al. 2009). Such knowledge is critical to provide an improved understanding of the physiological processes as it relates to maintenance of health or disease pathogenesis. Much of the research in the area of nutrition has historically focused on the role of deficiencies of single micronutrients, overnutrition of macronutrients, or the toxicities from food components. Virtually all of these studies use intervention—control groups that produce the population-attributable risk rather than individual risk (or benefit) factors (Kaput 2008). Further understanding of the molecular functions of the food components, their mechanism of action, and their physiological effects in individuals requires not only technological advances but also new scientific approaches.

New Technologies and Impact on Nutrigenomics

The emergence of high-throughput technologies enabled the sequencing of entire genomes and led to the development of genomics (study of genomes). A major emphasis in nutrigenomics has been to examine interactions between genes and the environment using transcriptomics (Afman and Muller 2006). High-throughput methodologies for simultaneous evaluation of other downstream biomolecular components and effectors, such as regulatory microRNA (miRNA) (microNomics), DNA and chromatin modifications (epigenomics), proteins (proteomics), metabolites (metabolomics), and the interaction within each biomolecular level and between these levels (interactomes), has deepened understanding of how the expression of genetic information is controlled (Altshuler et al. 2008; Garcia-Canas et al. 2010; Hocquette et al. 2009; Kandpal et al. 2009; Vidal et al. 2011). With these advancements, biological research in general and nutrigenomics in particular are providing an enhanced ability to decipher genes, proteins, or metabolites that play a role in modulating function at the cellular or systems level and providing a molecular link between nutrition and physiology.

OMIC TECHNOLOGIES

While many of the OMIC techniques will be discussed in further detail in Chapters 11 through 14, a brief outline of what these technologies entail is presented here to put into perspective the sequential steps from individual biomolecules to biological pathways, networks, and eventually interactomes. This progressive buildup of information and its integration is represented in Figure 10.1.

TRANSCRIPTOMICS

This technique uses array or sequencing-based high-throughput methodology to examine the expression of genes at the mRNA level (Garcia-Canas et al. 2010). An alteration of mRNA expression is one of the first steps affected by nutrients in the flow of molecular information from the genome to the proteome and sequentially

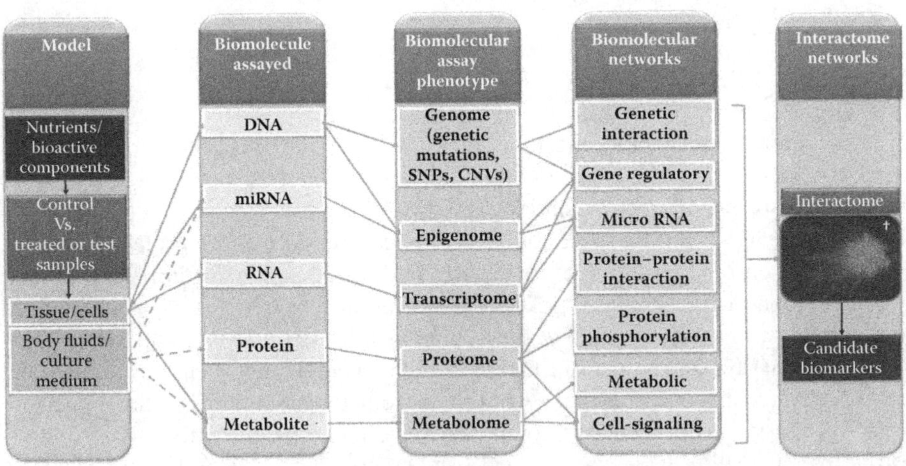

FIGURE 10.1 Example of a network-based modeling approach to examine the effects of nutrients or bioactive components. Cells/media or tissues/body fluids obtained following in vitro or in vivo treatments respectively with nutrients and bioactive components can be profiled using high-throughput techniques to assay biomolecules that reveal the biomolecular phenotype. Information acquired can further be used to examine biomolecular networks at each biomolecular level and integrated cellular networks such as the interactome encompassing different biomolecular levels so as to reveal potential biomarkers in response to the nutrients or bioactive components of interest. The symbol "†" indicates the representative interactome image obtained from http://en.wikipedia.org/wiki/File:Human_interactome.jpg#filelinks (Human Interactome network visualized by Cytoscape 2.5).

down to the metabolome (Garcia-Canas et al. 2010). Microarray technologies replaced the single gene/candidate gene approach of examining the effects of nutrients or bioactives and enabled a systems approach that interrogates the effects of thousands of genes in a larger context of other genes simultaneously. This resulted in the identification of co-regulated sets of genes and generation of new biological hypothesis (Gohil and Chakraborty 2004; Hu and Kong 2004). A number of studies have applied microarrays technology to nutrigenomics studies (Kato and Kimura 2003; Sparks et al. 2006; Tsuda et al. 2006) to examine the effects of nutrients and bioactive compounds.

Mirnomics

It is now recognized that more than half of the cellular transcripts expressed are regulated by miRNAs (Friedman et al. 2009). miRNAs are posttranscriptional regulators that bind to complementary sequences on target messenger RNA transcripts (mRNAs) resulting either in translational repression or degradation of the target with consequent gene silencing (Bartel 2009). High-throughput methodologies for detecting global miRNA alterations are now available although it is more complex to elucidate the function of miRNA compared to mRNA, since a single miRNA may be responsible for regulating several target sequences and thus many gene transcripts. Studies examining the role of nutrients and bioactive components in modulating miRNAs are now being actively explored (Mathers et al. 2010; Romao et al. 2012; Witzany 2012).

Epigenomics

It is the study of reversible and inheritable modifications that occur on the cellular DNA or proteins involved in chromatin structure. DNA methylation (methylation of cytosines) and posttranslational modifications of chromosomal proteins that include acetylation and methylation of lysine residues in histone proteins combine to influence chromatin architecture. These modifications play an important role in the regulation of the expression of genes and cellular processes and are influenced by nutrients and several bioactive food components (Ong and Perusse 2011). High-throughput assays for the determination of the epigenetic modifications on a global level have recently been developed improving our understanding of the epigenetic effect of nutrients and bioactive components and their specific effects (Laird 2010; Milagro et al. 2012; Stefanska et al. 2012).

Proteomics

It encompasses the study of the entire proteome that includes the measurable set of expressed proteins at a given time. Compared to the genes in the genome (~25,000), the human proteome is estimated to be fourfold greater because of alternative splicing of mRNA and posttranslational modifications. The proteome exhibits differences depending on the cell type as well as the status or activity of the cell (Garcia-Canas et al. 2010). Proteomic profiling in response to nutrition has been done on many tissues (Bondia-Pons et al. 2011; Cooney et al. 2012; Cruz-Topete et al. 2011) and cells (Magdalon et al. 2011) and is continuing to be explored.

METABOLOMICS

It is a rapidly emerging field that identifies and quantifies the metabolome that includes the complete set of endogenous or exogenous metabolites (≤1000 Da) present in biological systems such as a cell, tissue organ, or organism under a given set of conditions (Garcia-Canas et al. 2010). As metabolites are considered the true endpoints of the expression and regulation of genes, some consider it the most relevant for understanding physiological processes (Rimbach et al. 2008). Metabolomic approaches are increasingly being explored to investigate the impact of nutrient fluxes on different metabolic pathways whose availability in turn regulate the storage or expenditure of energy (Moazzami et al. 2011). Metabolomic analyses have enabled the identification of several plasma components related to the dietary intervention (Ovesna et al. 2008), and metabolites such as glucose, cholesterol, and triglycerides are routinely used as biomarkers of health and disease state (Kussmann et al. 2008).

BIOLOGICAL NETWORKS AND PATHWAYS

The biomolecular players identified, using high-throughput analytical technologies of genes, transcripts through metabolites reveal their fragmented physiological profiles under a given set of experimental conditions unless the components are analyzed in one biological source. However, to fully understand the spatial and functional aspects associated with the expression profiles of the different biomolecules, knowledge of the molecular interactions that occur between them is essential. Molecular interactions within a cell occur at different levels (1) between the same biomolecules at each level (e.g., protein–protein interaction) or (2) interactions between different biomolecules (e.g., gene–protein, protein–metabolite, and other combinations). Interactions between these different biomolecules of genes, proteins, metabolites, and their modifications have been analyzed using bioinformatics and computational approaches to reveal complex molecular interactions of networks. Such networks are usually built using data derived from experiments that analyze small sets of proteins and their interactions. The resulting networks are representations of the interactome, the complex molecular interactions that regulate cellular functions (Vidal et al. 2011). Interactomes are static representations of dynamic processes since metabolic processes continuously alter the concentrations of interacting components.

Biological networks are generated and analyzed on the basis of modern graph theory (Pavlopoulos et al. 2011) where the vertices of the graphs represent nodes and the edges represent the connections between nodes. The resulting networks thus have topological structures where the nodes represent genes, proteins, or metabolites, which show significant biological properties (Zhu et al. 2007) and the edges represent the connections between nodes. Depending on the type of the network and the interaction of biomolecules, the graphs in the network may be undirected, directed, weighted, or bipartite. The mathematical description and characteristics of these graphs are well described elsewhere (Grigorov 2005; Ma'ayan 2008;

Pavlopoulos et al. 2011). Biological networks, unlike biological pathways that are static and predefined, can be dynamic when they are built de novo out of building blocks from binary interactions that are specific for each dataset (Ekins et al. 2007). Examples of static biological databases include enzymes and metabolic pathways (EMP)/metabolic pathway database (MPW), BRaunschweig ENzyme DAtabase (BRENDA), ERGO, a genome analysis and discovery suit (http://ergo.integratedgenomics.com/ERGO/), and Kyoto Encyclopedia of Genes and Genomes (KEGG), based primarily on metabolic pathways. GeneGo and Biocarta pathways are an example of a collation of signaling and metabolic pathways. Gene Microarray pathway Profiler is a database of gene ontology (GO) terms that is designed for viewing and analyzing gene lists from experimental data (Ekins et al. 2007). Protein lounge consists of metabolic and signaling pathway maps that can be browsed but cannot be used for mapping experimental data (Ekins et al. 2007).

Types of Biological Networks

Typical biological networks at each biomolecular and interbiomolecular level are described in excellent reviews (Vidal et al. 2011; Zhu et al. 2007) and are briefly reviewed here. In general, the networks maps are built based on function—regulatory (gene expression), protein–protein interactions, metabolic networks, transcription factor binding, protein phosphorylation, genetic interactions, signaling networks, miRNA networks, and disease–drug networks. Noticeably missing is a focused network of nutrient interactions and their effects on each of these independent networks. The different biological networks are of course not independent of each other but form a network of networks that determine the overall physiology and function of the cell. Such overarching networks constitute the interactomes. These networks are briefly described below.

Gene Regulatory Networks

In gene regulatory networks, the nodes constitute either a transcription factor or a putative DNA regulatory element, and the directed edges represent the physical binding of transcription factors to such regulatory elements indicating transcriptional regulation (Ma'ayan 2008; Vidal et al. 2011). Approaches that have enabled large-scale mapping of gene regulatory networks include yeast one-hybrid approach and chromatin immunoprecipitation (ChIP) approach. The yeast one-hybrid approach can discover novel transcription factors but rely on having known or suspected regulatory regions in the target genes. On the other hand, the ChIP approach can discover novel regulatory motifs but rely on the availability of reagents specific to transcription factors of interest (Reece-Hoyes et al. 2005; Vaquerizas et al. 2009; Vidal et al. 2011).

Protein–Protein Interaction Networks

These are the most mapped and studied networks as they are considered the main building blocks for biological function (Ekins et al. 2007). In protein–protein network maps, nodes represent proteins and a set of edges represent a physical interaction between proteins. Such multi-edge connections indicate that proteins can be linked by more than one connection. It signifies that the proteins may be evolutionarily related or be coexpressed under different conditions and reflects different types of interactions between the proteins. As the edges are nondirected, the specifics of which protein binds the other cannot be described (Ma'ayan 2008). Methodologies used to map protein–protein interactions also include the yeast two-hybrid system that maps binary interactions (Dreze et al. 2010). Mapping protein complexes that inform indirect associations between proteins is obtained by affinity or immunopurification of isolated protein complexes followed by mass spectrometric identification of proteins in these complexes (Charbonnier et al. 2008).

Metabolic Networks

Metabolic networks have been the most studied since the tools for biochemical pathway analyses emerged in the early 1900s. Metabolic pathways describe all the possible biochemical reactions for a particular cell or organism. Networks generated from the pathways have metabolites at the nodes, whereas edges represent the reactions that convert one metabolite into another or may represent an enzyme. Edges are directed or nondirected depending on whether a reaction is reversible or not (Vidal et al. 2011). While metabolic pathway charts are not new and have existed for sometime, formation of comprehensive metabolic network maps has emerged following the completion of full genome sequencing together with accurate genome annotation tools. Such maps are now being compiled for numerous species, predominantly prokaryotes and unicellular eukaryotes (Oberhardt et al. 2009) and also in humans (Ma et al. 2007).

Protein Phosphorylation Networks

About 2% of the protein coding genes are translated to protein kinases and about 30% of the cellular proteins are thought to be phosphorylated in vivo (Manning et al. 2002a,b). Enrichment of phosphor-proteins on matrices that bind phospho-modified proteins followed by mass spectroscopy analyses have been used to allow the identification of large number of phosphorylated residues. Other studies have used immunoprecipitation to enrich for tyrosine phosphoproteins followed by tyrosine mass spectrophotometry to identify serine, threonine, or tyrosine phosphorylation sites (Ballif et al. 2004; Brill et al. 2004; Tao et al. 2005).

Genetic Interaction Networks

In some cases, functionally related genes exhibit interactions at the genetic level that can be defined by comparing the phenotype produced by mutations in a pair of interacting genes (Vidal et al. 2011). The foundations for this concept were built on now classical genetic studies (reviewed in Novick et al. [1989]). Genetic interaction studies have advanced because of high-throughput mapping of genetic interactions. The technologies used to map interactions include synthetic genetic and high-density arrays of mating pairs produced from sets of single mutants (Boone et al. 2007). More recently, barcodes embedded in a set of yeast deletion mutants have been used to measure the relative growth rate in a population using hybridization to antibarcode microarrays (Costanzo et al. 2010).

Cell Signaling Networks

These networks are represented as directed graphs that indicate three types of links including activation, inhibition, or neutral state, and thus capture functional relationships (Ma'ayan 2008). Signaling networks include small molecules such as cyclic adenosine monophosphate as well as proteins. They provide information on the pathway of cell signaling where signals from the extracellular environment received at receptors transduce the information through cascades of coupled biochemical reactions (Ma'ayan 2008).

MicroRNA Networks

miRNAs play a role in cellular regulation processes, and networks of the interactions of the miRNA with the expressed genome are now a major focus of study. Knowledge of the sequence of the miRNA makes it computationally possible to identify the network of interactions between miRNA and the expressed genome. Some studies have used text mining or have developed and analyzed a network of transcription factors and miRNAs to better understand how endogenous miRNA plays a role in intracellular regulation (Ma'ayan 2008).

Disease–Drug Networks

Data generated from high-throughput technologies including genomics, proteomics, metabolomics, and so on have enabled monitoring the alterations in the molecular components associated with different disease states and drug treatments and the generation of disease–disease, disease–drug, and drug–drug networks (Hu and Agarwal 2009; Suthram et al. 2010). Such integrated drug–drug, disease–drug, or drug–disease interactions are represented as complex maps of nodes interconnected via edges, where the nodes represent the drugs or gene or protein products and the edges specify the physical interactions or the other biologically relevant associations (Azuaje 2012). Networks such as these provide insights to improve identification of new drug targets in the drug discovery process, provide a way for systematic drug repositioning, unveil disease mechanisms and disease pathways, and better understand any potential side effects of drugs (Hu and Agarwal 2009).

Interactome Networks

In addition to networks that link the biomolecules within each biomolecular/macromolecular level, cellular systems can also be visualized as a complex web of interactions between different macromolecules such as RNA, proteins, and genes each of which constitute the nodes while the edges represent physical, biochemical, or functional interactions between these cellular components. Such interactions constitute the interactome, which is an integration of all the interactions. An interactome is a dynamic network and reveals how complex biological processes may be controlled providing information at the systems level as opposed to the analysis at each biomolecular level of genes or proteins or metabolites or linear pathways. Vidal et al. (2011) have enumerated distinct approaches that have been pursued to capture interactome networks that include (1) compilation or curation of existing data in literature, obtained from one or a few types of physical or biochemical interactions, (2) computational predictions based on available "orthogonal" information apart from physical or biochemical interactions or similarities, gene order conservation, copresence and coabsence of genes in completely sequenced genomes or proteomes, and protein structural information, and (3) systematic unbiased high-throughput experimental mapping strategies applied at the scale of whole genomes or proteomes (Marcotte and Date 2001; Roberts 2006; Walhout and Vidal 2001; Vidal et al. 2011). In addition, the mapping and analysis of interactome networks in different organisms further enables transfer of biological information from one well-characterized species to another not well characterized one (Vidal et al. 2011).

Network Analysis

Networks exist ubiquitously throughout biology and can be visualized to represent the relationships between genes and gene products (Berger and Iyengar 2009). To analyze and unravel the complex organization of the cellular networks, a number of statistical and computational tools are necessary to effectively extract the networks and the information it embeds from experimentally determined molecular data. Computational biology attempts to offer much of the needed methodology to better understand the resulting biomolecular interactions and networks. Such a process is called network analysis and it involves approaches that take different kinds of entities (nodes), modeling the relationships (edges) between the entities, and generating hypotheses from the resulting network (Ekins et al. 2007). The need to access biological data of different types is further stimulating the development of a number of data sources that can be interrogated to identify new and unknown links. A list of some of the databases and tools for pathways and network analyses are listed in Table 10.1. Some of the popular well-described tools for visualization of generated data that provide data integration capabilities include Cytoscape, VisANT, Pathway Studio, and PATIKA. These tools provide a more dynamic model of cellular processes through incorporation of gene expression data, subcellular localization information, and time-dependent behavior (Suderman and Hallett 2007).

TABLE 10.1
Examples of Database Tools for Pathway and Network Analysis[a]

Transcription Factors/Gene Regulatory Networks	
DPInteract—DNA–Protein Interactions Database	http://arep.med.harvard.edu/dpinteract/
miRBase—MicroRNA Database	http://www.mirbase.org/
pSTIING—Protein, Signaling, Transcriptional Interactions and Inflammation Network Gateway	http://pstiing.licr.org/
TRANSFAC—Transcription Factor Database	http://www.biobase-international.com/gene-regulation
Pathways Knowledge Base—Ingenuity Pathways Knowledge Base	http://www.ingenuity.com/
Protein–Protein Interactions	
BIND—Biomolecular Interaction Network Database	http://bond.unleashedinformatics.com/
BioGrid—Biological General Repository of interaction Datasets	http://thebiogrid.org/

(Continued)

TABLE 10.1 (*Continued*)
Examples of Database Tools for Pathway and Network Analysis[a]

DIP—Database of Interacting Proteins	http://dip.doe-mbi.ucla.edu/dip/Main.cgi
Interactome—Krogan Lab Interactome Database	http://interactome-cmp.ucsf.edu/
Pathways Knowledge Base—Ingenuity Pathways Knowledge Base	http://www.ingenuity.com/
STRING—Search Tool for the Retrieval of Interacting Genes/Proteins	http://string.embl.de/
MINT—Molecular Interaction Database	http://mint.bio.uniroma2.it/mint/Welcome.do
Metabolic Pathways	
BioPath—Biochemical Pathways Database	http://www.molecular-networks.com/databases/biopath
ExPASy—Biochemical Pathway Maps	http://web.expasy.org/pathways/
GeneNet—Genetic Networks	http://wwwmgs.bionet.nsc.ru/mgs/gnw/genenet/
GenMAPP—Gene Map Anotator and Pathway Profiler	http://www.genmapp.org/showcase.html
KEGG—Kyoto Encyclopedia of Genes and Genomes	http://www.genome.jp/kegg/
MetaCore—MetaCore Pathway Database	http://www.genego.com/metacore.php
HMDB—Human Metabolome Database	http://www.hmdb.ca/
PATIKA—Pathway Analysis Tools for Integration and Knowledge Acquisition	http://www.patika.org/
Protein Lounge	http://www.proteinlounge.com/
Reactome—Reactome Knowledge Base	http://www.reactome.org/ReactomeGWT/entrypoint.html
Genetic Interactions Network	
BIND—Biomolecular Interaction Network Database	http://bond.unleashedinformatics.com/
BioGrid—Biological General Repository of Interaction Datasets	http://thebiogrid.org/
Interactome—Krogan Lab Interactome Database	http://interactome-cmp.ucsf.edu/
GeneMANIA–GeneMANIA	http://www.genemania.org/
GeneNet—Genetic Networks	http://wwwmgs.bionet.nsc.ru/mgs/gnw/genenet/
GenePath–GenePath	http://www.genepath.org/
Cytoscape	http://www.cytoscape.org/
Signaling Pathways	
BioModels—BioModels Database	http://www.ebi.ac.uk/biomodels-main/
MetaCore—MetaCore Pathway Database	http://www.genego.com/metacore.php
PATIKA—Pathway Analysis Toos for Integration and Knowledge Acquisition	http://www.patika.org/
SPIKE—Signaling Pathway Integrated Knowledge Engine	http://www.ariadnegenomics.com/products/databases/resnet/
Wiki Pathways—WikiPathways	http://wikipathways.org/index.php/WikiPathways

[a] A more comprehensive list of resources for pathway and network analysis can be found at http://www.pathguide.org/.

DATA MINING

With the advancement of these multiomic high-throughput technologies, unprecedented amounts of biological data are constantly generated that populate many different types of databases that store genomic, chemical, proteomic, and metabolomic data (Yang et al. 2012). These data include comprehensive information obtained about genome sequences, gene expression, polymorphisms, epigenetic modifications, proteins and metabolites, and the interactions between them constituting the interactomes. Such data collection has initiated new methodologies and approaches in data mining (DM), a science that seeks to find new interesting patterns and relationships in huge amounts of data. DM involves the bioinformatics approaches that combine biological data using computational tools and statistical methods to analyze data and summarize it into useful information. Such systematic approach facilitates the extraction and correlation of patterns of knowledge that is implicit in the stored databases (Cheung 2012), and enables discovery and prioritization of downstream targets of interest and a better understanding of the molecular mechanisms relating to nutrient, drug, or toxicant. DM is also rightly referred to as knowledge discovery from data. Efficient DM methods of the large amounts of data are key to fueling discovery in the post-genomic era.

Types of Data Mining

Popular DM approaches include text mining of literature databases and microarray DM (Sakharkar and Sakharkar 2007; Yang et al. 2012).

Text Mining

It is defined as the computational discovery of previously unknown information using bioinformatic and computational approaches to extract information from written resources (Jensen et al. 2006). Text mining involves two major steps consisting of information retrieval followed by information extraction (Ananiadou et al. 2006; Hirschman et al. 2002; Rebholz-Schuhmann et al. 2005). Information retrieval examines literature or abstracts related to a particular topic using gene search engines or information retrieval searching tools. Information extraction uses two approaches: (1) co-occurrence to extract relationships of a particular type as in the case of interactions of two proteins and (2) co-occurrence to extract relationships such as gene–gene or protein–protein interactions and biological pathways beyond recognition of terms, and includes technologies that combine syntax and semantics to reveal interactions (Yang et al. 2012). Based on the type of data generated by the high-throughout techniques, the DM approaches developed include microarray DM, proteomic DM, chemogenomic DM, and integrated DM (Yang et al. 2012).

Microarray Data Mining

It refers to bioinformatics approaches in microarray data analysis to discover entities and biological pathways that define phenotype (Butte 2002; Desany and Zhang 2004; Ricke et al. 2006; Yang et al. 2012) and is achieved either by unsupervised clustering or by supervised classification (Mount and Pandey 2005). Unsupervised clustering determines if a group of genes share coherent expression across a subset of conditions such as hierarchical clustering, principle component analysis, and self-organizing maps. Supervised analysis approach searches genes that can distinguish between samples, for example, between normal controls and disease conditions in question (Yang et al. 2012). Two important limitations involving DM of microarray samples are (1) that gene expression does not always correlate with protein levels and (2) that gene expression analyses are a snapshot of a point in time and in a specific physiological and nutritional state. Ideally, multiple samples in time and under different conditions with analyses of protein levels would provide the types of datasets to analyze biological processes at the systems level (Desany and Zhang 2004; Ricke et al. 2006).

Proteomic Data Mining

Several technologies are being explored to produce high-throughput proteomic data. Advances in mass spectrometry that allow for untargeted analyses of samples provide qualitative datasets for analyses. More recently, barcoded DNA aptamers that recognize individual proteins to allow for the simultaneous identification and quantification of over 1000 proteins (Gold et al. 2010) are extending high-throughput proteomic analyses. Proteomic DM methods are necessary to analyze and extract useful information (Gerling et al. 2006; Hanash et al. 2008; Siepen et al. 2008). The open proteomic database (www.proteomecommons.org) and EMBL databases have become available to protein mine data. However, better computational methods are still needed for the integration, for mining results of comparative analysis, and for functional interpretation of high-throughput proteomic data (Yang et al. 2012).

Chemogenomic Data Mining

Chemical genomics is a technology that enables analyses of phenotypes by integrating small molecules from chemical libraries to the analyses of cells (Bredel and Jacoby 2004; Wuster and Madan Babu 2008). For example, data mined from a 2D matrix resulting from chemogenomics screening, where one dimension is the chemical library and the second is the library of different cell types, can enable the identification of cellular drug targets with impact on understanding a chemical's influence on pathways. In addition, the individual results from cell-based assays with discrete endpoints or from specific enzymatic reactions may be analyzed with system level network analyses to create interactomes of chemical targets within biological processes (Yang et al. 2012). Challenges associated with this chemogenomic DM include better methods to mine, profile, and analyze data (Yang et al. 2012).

Integrated Data Mining

To effectively understand the cellular mechanisms, DM using an integrated approach encompassing different levels of molecular information is needed. Approaches that can integrate different sources of data including genome, proteome, and metabolome will enhance the discovery of valuable targets (Kim et al. 2007).

EXAMPLES OF STUDIES USING DATA MINING AND NETWORK ANALYSIS IN NUTRIGENOMICS STUDIES

A number of nutrigenomics studies are beginning to successfully use DM or the network analysis tools or a combination of the two to advance our knowledge of the role and mechanism of action of nutrients in cellular dysfunction or disease development. Some examples of such studies will be discussed in this section. The popular approaches used in these studies include

1. In silico methods that use DM to examine a number of existing studies to arrive at potential candidate biomarkers for a cell, tissue, or an organism, for a disease, or for development or enrichment of an existing pathway
2. Analyses of the many pathways known to be associated with a disease process. In this approach the gene dataset of interest obtained from the control and test samples are used to align with the multiple pathways to identify potential downstream markers
3. Use of multi-omics approach to obtain data on genomics, transcriptomics, proteomics, and metabolomics with integration of the dataset using appropriate bioinformatics and statistical tools

Examples of studies using such approaches will be described.

Text Mining Study for Pathway Enrichment and Validation

Updated representations of pathways and biological networks are essential to integrate different types of genomic results in a systems biology approach that enable the understanding of the effect of a nutrients and bioactive components in health (van Ommen et al. 2008). Waagmeester et al. conducted a text mining study to examine and enrich existing pathways in carotenoid metabolism, as although the key players in the carotenoid metabolic pathway are known, a clear understanding of the pathway is far from complete (Waagmeester et al. 2009). Hence, to enrich and update carotenoid and vitamin A metabolic pathway, a text mining approach was used for finding potential pathway entities in the literature for carotenoid as well as vitamin A. The authors first generated a seed corpus (SC) from the comprehensive review publication by Balmer and Bloomhoff (2002), which provided 1191 references. They then generated a second corpus (QSC) by querying for "carotenoids" using PubMed that resulted in a set of 51,628 references of which 34,682 contained an abstract. The abstracts from the QSC were assessed for relevance to the topic of interest by measuring the similarity to SC and then given a similarity score to generate a similarity extended corpus (SEC) when the score was greater than the selected threshold. This process resulted in the selection of 13,579 abstracts as the SEC that was considered to be relevant to the construction of the vitamin A metabolism pathway. As a next step, a set of 89,086 unique terms were extracted from the 13,579 abstracts of SEC, of which 6,515 potential entities for vitamin A pathway were identified for contextual evaluation. These entities were integrated in the carotenoid pathways on wikipathways and validated by two curators who were involved with the creation of the initial pathways. Of 226 potential pathway entities that were identified, a semi-automatic extraction method was used to generate a smaller number of 37 pathway entities. Of these, 13 were included in the pathway for vitamin A metabolism. Of the remaining 24 pathway entities, 14 were attributed to processes related to metabolic pathways and 10 of the remaining terms were categorized as nutrients and biomarkers. Thus, in this study using a text mining approach, Waagmeester et al. were able to identify and include 13 new entities to the vitamin A metabolic pathway and thus enrich the pathway for carotenoid and vitamin A metabolism.

Combinatorial Approach of Text/Data Mining and Pathway or Network Analysis of the Mined Data to Identify Candidate Genes Related to Disease States

Kim et al. (2010) performed in silico studies using combined text/DM to discover obesity-specific candidate genes expressed in the liver of C57BL/6J mouse in response to a high-fat diet. Most of the efforts in different published studies in identifying genes responsible for obesity development have been from microarray data. The authors (Kim et al. 2010) chose to interpret the functional relationship among genes that they data mined from literature and public databases using the STRING database (http://string-db.org/), a database of known and predicted protein–protein interactions to examine if obesity-related genes are functionally related. Using this approach, they shortlisted 31 genes that were based on the regulation of gene expression in the liver and their specific cellular function. The selected genes were classified using the KEGG pathway and GO. This in silico DM study revealed that 50% of the identified potential candidate genes for obesity were involved in the pathway of lipid metabolism suggesting that a diet high in fat mostly affects lipid metabolism. Their search also determined that 20 out of the 31 input obesity genes were very closely connected with each other.

Another study used a similar text/DM approach followed by pathway analyses of extracted data to identify carbohydrate metabolic genes that map to quantitative trait loci (QTLs) that are associated with obesity and type 2 diabetes mellitus (T2DM) (Varma et al. 2010). Both obesity and T2DM are complex polygenic diseases with a phenotype that depends on the interactions of multiple genes and is influenced by varied environmental factors. Although genome-wide association studies (GWAS) have identified approximately 20 loci of T2DM and about 13 for obesity (at the time of analyses), these studies are limited in identifying the key genes that may be responsible for the disease condition since environmental variables were not measured but known to contribute to these phenotypes. In addition, differences in allele frequencies among ancestral populations would change the impact of individual alleles (Myles et al. 2008). Most of the early GWAS also neglected to analyze copy number variations (CNVs) that account for 13% of the genetic variation between individuals (Freeman et al. 2006). To provide an example of the connections between publically available datasets, our group manually retrieved data on CNVs and single nucleotide polymorphisms (SNPs) among carbohydrate metabolic genes initially obtained using pathway maps such as wikipathways, GeneGo Pathway maps, and text mining methods. SNPs and CNVs to these genes were mined from public domain databases using gene ID and NCBI entrez gene database for information on the chromosome. Coding SNPs and CNVs for a particular gene were obtained from the NCBI SNP page accessed from the SNP:GENEVIEW link option and from the database for genomic variants (DGV-TORR, http://projects.tcgag.ca/variation/) and CNV project (CNV-CHOP, http:cnv.chop.edu/) sites, respectively. Potential candidate genes were then electronically mapped to QTLs related to obesity and T2DM and their intermediate phenotypes using the Arraytrack QTL library that yields associations of genes to QTLs (Xu et al. 2010). This study identified candidate genes that link genetic data to nutrients metabolized by carbohydrate metabolic pathways. The approach is hypothesis driven and examines and analyzes sets of genes and seeks to link genetic data to nutrition through identification of cofactors and substrates derived from diet.

A similar approach was used in another DM exercise (Wise and Kaput 2009) that sought to map genes involved in micronutrient metabolism to genetic regions involved in chronic disease. This study provided a priority list of 54 candidate micronutrient genes that mapped to QTLs. However, experimental confirmation of these candidate gene lists has not been done.

Network-Based Approaches to Analyze Experimental Data

Morine et al. (2011) used new analysis incorporating a joint multivariate and network-based approach to analyze experimental data that included dietary records, adipose tissue transcriptomics data, and a comprehensive plasma marker profile obtained in a study examining human volunteers with metabolic syndrome. This study aimed to better understand the link between diet and health using a nutritional systems biology approach at the tissue level. While transcriptomics has become a key technology to better understand molecular nutrition, the appropriate techniques to extract data from high-throughput datasets are still limiting. The authors suggested that although pathway analysis using gene set enrichment analysis is a popular approach to analyzing transcriptomic data, there exists technical issues including inherent redundancy among pathways and interconnectedness between pathways when not accounted for, which can limit biological interpretations of high-throughput datasets. The data were further analyzed in the context of a global interaction network that is partitioned into functionally related clusters/modules of genes. However, the authors suggest that when modeling transcriptomic activity in metabolic networks, path constructs instead of clusters should be used as paths match the native pattern of energy flux through a metabolic network. They defined a method to identify altered transcriptomic activity in the context of network paths rather than clusters to identify local coexpressed paths in the metabolic network that show covariance with recorded dietary intake of omega-3 polyunsaturated fatty acids (*n*-3 PUFA) and correlation with a urinary marker of oxidative stress. They also simultaneously analyzed promoter regions of *n*-3 PUFA-correlated genes and detected significantly overrepresented binding sites for transcription factors related to adipogenesis. This study included a final set of microarray data containing 10,618 genes. For metabolic network analysis, the Edinburgh human metabolic network reconstruction (www.ehmm.bioinformatics.ed.ac.uk/), which contains information for 1627 unique metabolites and 1371 unique metabolic enzymes was used. For the study analysis, the network was first transformed to an enzyme-centric construction where two genes/protein are linked if gene A produces a metabolite that is used as a metabolic substrate by gene B. Coexpression of each gene–gene pair in the metabolic network construction was assessed using Akaike's information criterion. Significantly overrepresented transcription factor binding sites among genes with the expression showing positive correlation with *n*-3-PUFA were identified. They performed promoter analysis using the transcription factor matrix (TFM)-explorer tool (Tonon et al. 2010). Using this new approach, Morine et al. highlighted coexpressed regions of the metabolic network with opposing direction of correlation with habitual *n*-3 PUFA intake and urinary isoprotane levels. This was a novel result that was not previously identified when traditional enrichment pathways were examined.

USEFULNESS OF DATA MINING AND NETWORK ANALYSIS IN NUTRIGENOMICS STUDIES

The post-genomic era has presented biological research with immense opportunities for exploratory research. Advanced methods of data extraction and interpretation using network and interactome analysis are beginning to allow for the examination of mechanisms of action of different nutrients, bioactives, toxicants, or drugs, or the specific compound of interest and to explore their physiological effects in health and disease states. Koyuturk (2012) has described many of the efforts that have led to novel insights into the complexity of living systems and understanding cellular regulation and function at a systems level by the use of sophisticated abstraction algorithms and analytical techniques that address a broad range of problems including (1) inference and reconstruction of complex cellular networks, (2) identification of common and coherent patterns in cellular networks to better understand the organizing principles and building blocks of cellular signaling, regulation, and metabolism, and (3) characterization of cellular mechanisms that underlie the differences between living systems of evolutionary diversity development and differentiation and complex phenotypes in terms of disease (Koyuturk 2010).

Progress in the field of nutritional research has accelerated with the advent of new and improved high-throughput technologies leading to the development of nutritional genomics or nutrigenomics. Applications of network analysis may aid in determining a protein's or gene's function and response to nutrients or bioactive components and for designing effective strategies for treating diseases or prognosis or early diagnosis of a disease (Pavlopoulos et al. 2011). Network analysis promises to greatly increase our knowledge of mechanisms underlying the multiple actions of nutrients and bioactives.

CONCLUSION

Bioinformatic tools have enabled DM and network-based approaches to analyze the large amounts of existing data in curated databases to provide valuable information to better understand biological processes. These can be utilized to provide additional support for experimental results and develop new hypotheses. Important targets that may determine the downstream molecular mechanisms and be modulated by nutrients or dietary components may include moieties from different biomolecular levels such as genes, proteins, metabolites, or disease markers in biological pathways or in crucial nodes of a regulatory network (Chen and Chen 2008). While data mining methodologies are very promising and may enable the identification of important potential targets, wet lab validations of these targets are still necessary as data mining methods may sometimes incorrectly associate molecules.

Similarly, although network analyses may provide a more complete view of biological process, these visualizations are just that static representations of dynamic systems with metabolite fluxes and changing interactions. Pathway maps and network maps provide what is called the illusion of explanatory depth (Rozenblit and Keil 2002)—the concept that once we visualize knowledge, humans tend to believe they understand the process or system. Network analyses is a more in-depth view of biological systems compared to two-dimensional pathway maps of linear interactions, the networks are nonetheless imperfect representations of dynamic, living organisms. Computational systems may someday be able to model the dynamics of those systems.

REFERENCES

Afman, L., and M. Muller. 2006. Nutrigenomics: from molecular nutrition to prevention of disease. *J Am Diet Assoc* 106: 569–76.

Altshuler, D., M.J. Daly, and E.S. Lander. 2008. Genetic mapping in human disease. *Science* 322: 881–8.

Ananiadou, S., D.B. Kell, and J. Tsujii. 2006. Text mining and its potential applications in systems biology. *Trends Biotechnol* 24: 571–9.

Azuaje, F. 2012. Drug interaction networks: an introduction to translational and clinical applications. *Cardiovasc Res* 97: 631–41.

Ballif, B.A., J. Villen, S.A. Beausoleil, D. Schwartz, and S.P. Gygi. 2004. Phosphoproteomic analysis of the developing mouse brain. *Mol Cell Proteomics* 3: 1093–101.

Balmer, J.E., and R. Blomhoff. 2002. Gene expression regulation by retinoic acid. *J Lipid Res* 43: 1773–808.

Bartel, D.P. 2009. MicroRNAs: target recognition and regulatory functions. *Cell* 136: 215–33.

Berger, S.I., and R. Iyengar. 2009. Network analyses in systems pharmacology. *Bioinformatics* 25: 2466–72.

Bondia-Pons, I., N. Boque, L. Paternain, E. Santamaria, J. Fernandez, J. Campion, F. Milagro, F. Corrales, and J.A. Martinez. 2011. Liver proteome changes induced by a short-term high-fat sucrose diet in wistar rats. *J Nutrigenet Nutrigenomics* 4: 344–53.

Boone, C., H. Bussey, and B.J. Andrews. 2007. Exploring genetic interactions and networks with yeast. *Nat Rev Genet* 8: 437–49.

Bredel, M., and E. Jacoby. 2004. Chemogenomics: an emerging strategy for rapid target and drug discovery. *Nat Rev Genet* 5: 262–75.

Brill, L.M., A.R. Salomon, S.B. Ficarro, M. Mukherji, M. Stettler-Gill, and E.C. Peters. 2004. Robust phosphoproteomic profiling of tyrosine phosphorylation sites from human T cells using immobilized metal affinity chromatography and tandem mass spectrometry. *Anal Chem* 76: 2763–72.

Butte, A. 2002. The use and analysis of microarray data. *Nat Rev Drug Discov* 1: 951–60.

Charbonnier, S., O. Gallego, and A.C. Gavin. 2008. The social network of a cell: recent advances in interactome mapping. *Biotechnol Annu Rev* 14: 1–28.
Chen, Y.P., and F. Chen. 2008. Identifying targets for drug discovery using bioinformatics. *Expert Opin Ther Targets* 12: 383–9.
Cheung, J.Y. 2012. Data mining: concepts and techniques. *Choice: Curr Rev Acad Libr* 49: 1100.
Cooney, J.M., M.P. Barnett, D. Brewster, B. Knoch, W.C. McNabb, W.A. Laing, and N.C. Roy. 2012. Proteomic analysis of colon tissue from interleukin-10 gene-deficient mice fed polyunsaturated fatty acids with comparison to transcriptomic analysis. *J Proteome Res* 11: 1065–77.
Costanzo, M., A. Baryshnikova, J. Bellay, Y. Kim, E.D. Spear, C.S. Sevier, H. Ding et al. 2010. The genetic landscape of a cell. *Science* 327: 425–31.
Cruz-Topete, D., E.O. List, S. Okada, B. Kelder, and J.J. Kopchick. 2011. Proteomic changes in the heart of diet-induced pre-diabetic mice. *J Proteomics* 74: 716–27.
Desany, B., and Z. Zhang. 2004. Bioinformatics and cancer target discovery. *Drug Discov Today* 9: 795–802.
Dreze, M., D. Monachello, C. Lurin, M.E. Cusick, D.E. Hill, M. Vidal, and P. Braun. 2010. High-quality binary interactome mapping. *Methods Enzymol* 470: 281–315.
Ekins, S., Y. Nikolsky, A. Bugrim, E. Kirillov, and T. Nikolskaya. 2007. Pathway mapping tools for analysis of high content data. *Methods Mol Biol* 356: 319–50.
Freeman, J.L., G.H. Perry, L. Feuk, R. Redon, S.A. McCarroll, D.M. Altshuler, H. Aburatani et al. 2006. Copy number variation: new insights in genome diversity. *Genome Res* 16: 949–61.
Friedman, R.C., K.K. Farh, C.B. Burge, and D.P. Bartel. 2009. Most mammalian mRNAs are conserved targets of microRNAs. *Genome Res* 19: 92–105.
Garcia-Canas, V., C. Simo, C. Leon, and A. Cifuentes. 2010. Advances in Nutrigenomics research: novel and future analytical approaches to investigate the biological activity of natural compounds and food functions. *J Pharm Biomed Anal* 51: 290–304.
Gerling, I.C., S. Singh, N.I. Lenchik, D.R. Marshall, and J. Wu. 2006. New data analysis and mining approaches identify unique proteome and transcriptome markers of susceptibility to autoimmune diabetes. *Mol Cell Proteomics* 5: 293–305.
Gohil, K., and A.A. Chakraborty. 2004. Applications of microarray and bioinformatics tools to dissect molecular responses of the central nervous system to antioxidant micronutrients. *Nutrition* 20: 50–5.
Gold, L., D. Ayers, J. Bertino, C. Bock, A. Bock, E.N. Brody, J. Carter et al. 2010. Aptamer-based multiplexed proteomic technology for biomarker discovery. *PLoS One* 5: e15004.
Grigorov, M.G. 2005. Global properties of biological networks. *Drug Discov Today* 10: 365–72.
Hanash, S.M., S.J. Pitteri, and V.M. Faca. 2008. Mining the plasma proteome for cancer biomarkers. *Nature* 452: 571–9.
Hirschman, L., J.C. Park, J. Tsujii, L. Wong, and C.H. Wu. 2002. Accomplishments and challenges in literature data mining for biology. *Bioinformatics* 18: 1553–61.
Hocquette, J.F., I. Cassar-Malek, A. Scalbert, and F. Guillou. 2009. Contribution of genomics to the understanding of physiological functions. *J Physiol Pharmacol* 60 Suppl 3: 5–16.
Hu, G., and P. Agarwal. 2009. Human disease-drug network based on genomic expression profiles. *PLoS One* 4: e6536.
Hu, R., and A.N. Kong. 2004. Activation of MAP kinases, apoptosis and nutrigenomics of gene expression elicited by dietary cancer-prevention compounds. *Nutrition* 20: 83–8.
Jensen, L.J., J. Saric, and P. Bork. 2006. Literature mining for the biologist: from information retrieval to biological discovery. *Nat Rev Genet* 7: 119–29.
Kandpal, R., B. Saviola, and J. Felton. 2009. The era of 'omics unlimited. *Biotechniques* 46: 351–2, 354–5.

Kaput, J. 2008. Nutrigenomics research for personalized nutrition and medicine. *Curr Opin Biotechnol* 19: 110–20.
Kato, H., and T. Kimura. 2003. Evaluation of the effects of the dietary intake of proteins and amino acids by DNA microarray technology. *J Nutr* 133: 2073S–7S.
Kim, B., H.J. Lee, H.Y. Choi, Y. Shin, S. Nam, G. Seo, D.S. Son et al. 2007. Clinical validity of the lung cancer biomarkers identified by bioinformatics analysis of public expression data. *Cancer Res* 67: 7431–8.
Kim, E.J., E. Kim, E.Y. Kwon, H.S. Jang, C.G. Hur, and M.S. Choi. 2010. Network analysis of hepatic genes responded to high-fat diet in C57BL/6J mice: nutrigenomics data mining from recent research findings. *J Med Food* 13: 743–56.
Koyuturk, M. 2010. Algorithmic and analytical methods in network biology. *Wiley Interdiscip Rev Syst Biol Med* 2: 277–92.
Kussmann, M., S. Rezzi, and H. Daniel. 2008. Profiling techniques in nutrition and health research. *Curr Opin Biotechnol* 19: 83–99.
Laird, P.W. 2010. Principles and challenges of genomewide DNA methylation analysis. *Nat Rev Genet* 11: 191–203.
Ma'ayan, A. 2008. Network integration and graph analysis in mammalian molecular systems biology. *IET Syst Biol* 2: 206–21.
Ma, H., A. Sorokin, A. Mazein, A. Selkov, E. Selkov, O. Demin, and I. Goryanin. 2007. The Edinburgh human metabolic network reconstruction and its functional analysis. *Mol Syst Biol* 3: 135.
Magdalon, J., E. Hatanaka, T. Romanatto, H.G. Rodrigues, W.M. Kuwabara, C. Scaife, P. Newsholme, and R. Curi. 2011. A proteomic analysis of the functional effects of fatty acids in NIH 3T3 fibroblasts. *Lipids Health Dis* 10: 218.
Manning, G., G.D. Plowman, T. Hunter, and S. Sudarsanam. 2002a. Evolution of protein kinase signaling from yeast to man. *Trends Biochem Sci* 27: 514–20.
Manning, G., D.B. Whyte, R. Martinez, T. Hunter, and S. Sudarsanam. 2002b. The protein kinase complement of the human genome. *Science* 298: 1912–34.
Marcotte, E., and S. Date. 2001. Exploiting big biology: integrating large-scale biological data for function inference. *Brief Bioinform* 2: 363–74.
Mathers, J.C., G. Strathdee, and C.L. Relton. 2010. Induction of epigenetic alterations by dietary and other environmental factors. *Adv Genet* 71: 3–39.
Milagro, F.I., M.L. Mansego, C. De Miguel, and J.A. Martinez. 2012. Dietary factors, epigenetic modifications and obesity outcomes: progresses and perspectives. *Mol Aspects Med* (In press).
Moazzami, A.A., R. Andersson, and A. Kamal-Eldin. 2011. Changes in the metabolic profile of rat liver after alpha-tocopherol deficiency as revealed by metabolomics analysis. *NMR Biomed* 24: 499–505.
Morine, M.J., A.C. Tierney, B. van Ommen, H. Daniel, S. Toomey, I.M. Gjelstad, I.C. Gormley et al. 2011. Transcriptomic coordination in the human metabolic network reveals links between n-3 fat intake, adipose tissue gene expression and metabolic health. *PLoS Comput Biol* 7: e1002223.
Mount, D.W., and R. Pandey. 2005. Using bioinformatics and genome analysis for new therapeutic interventions. *Mol Cancer Ther* 4: 1636–43.
Myles, S., D. Davison, J. Barrett, M. Stoneking, and N. Timpson. 2008. Worldwide population differentiation at disease-associated SNPs. *BMC Med Genomics* 1: 22.
Novick, P., B.C. Osmond, and D. Botstein. 1989. Suppressors of yeast actin mutations. *Genetics* 121: 659–74.
Oberhardt, M.A., B.O. Palsson, and J.A. Papin. 2009. Applications of genome-scale metabolic reconstructions. *Mol Syst Biol* 5: 320.
Ong, T.P., and L. Perusse. 2011. Impact of nutritional epigenomics on disease risk and prevention: introduction. *J Nutrigenet Nutrigenomics* 4: 245–7.

Ovesna, J., O. Slaby, O. Toussaint, M. Kodicek, P. Marsik, V. Pouchova, and T. Vanek. 2008. High throughput 'omics' approaches to assess the effects of phytochemicals in human health studies. *Br J Nutr* 99 E Suppl 1: ES127–34.

Parker, A., I. McCaffery, and S. Patterson. 2009. Examining molecular biology in humans. *Biotechniques* 46: 358–60.

Pavlopoulos, G.A., M. Secrier, C.N. Moschopoulos, T.G. Soldatos, S. Kossida, J. Aerts, R. Schneider, and P.G. Bagos. 2011. Using graph theory to analyze biological networks. *BioData Min* 4: 10.

Rebholz-Schuhmann, D., H. Kirsch, and F. Couto. 2005. Facts from text—is text mining ready to deliver? *PLoS Biol* 3: e65.

Reece-Hoyes, J.S., B. Deplancke, J. Shingles, C.A. Grove, I.A. Hope, and A.J. Walhout. 2005. A compendium of Caenorhabditis elegans regulatory transcription factors: a resource for mapping transcription regulatory networks. *Genome Biol* 6: R110.

Ricke, D.O., S. Wang, R. Cai, and D. Cohen. 2006. Genomic approaches to drug discovery. *Curr Opin Chem Biol* 10: 303–8.

Rimbach, G., C. Boesch-Saadatmandi, J. Frank, D. Fuchs, U. Wenzel, H. Daniel, W.L. Hall, and P.D. Weinberg. 2008. Dietary isoflavones in the prevention of cardiovascular disease—a molecular perspective. *Food Chem Toxicol* 46: 1308–19.

Roberts, P.M. 2006. Mining literature for systems biology. *Brief Bioinform* 7: 399–406.

Romao, J.M., W. Jin, M. He, T. McAllister, and L. Guan le. 2012. Altered microRNA expression in bovine subcutaneous and visceral adipose tissues from cattle under different diet. *PLoS One* 7: e40605.

Rozenblit, L., and F. Keil. 2002. The misunderstood limits of folk science: an illusion of explanatory depth. *Cogn Sci* 26: 521–62.

Sakharkar, M.K., and K.R. Sakharkar. 2007. Targetability of human disease genes. *Curr Drug Discov Technol* 4: 48–58.

Siepen, J.A., J.N. Selley, and S.J. Hubbard. 2008. PepSeeker: mining information from proteomic data. *Methods Mol Biol* 484: 319–32.

Sparks, L.M., H. Xie, R.A. Koza, R. Mynatt, G.A. Bray, and S.R. Smith. 2006. High-fat/low-carbohydrate diets regulate glucose metabolism via a long-term transcriptional loop. *Metabolism* 55: 1457–63.

Stefanska, B., H. Karlic, F. Varga, K. Fabianowska-Majewska, and A. Haslberger. 2012. Epigenetic mechanisms in anti-cancer actions of bioactive food components - the implications in cancer prevention. *Br J Pharmacol* 167: 279–97.

Suderman, M., and M. Hallett. 2007. Tools for visually exploring biological networks. *Bioinformatics* 23: 2651–9.

Suthram, S., J.T. Dudley, A.P. Chiang, R. Chen, T.J. Hastie, and A.J. Butte. 2010. Network-based elucidation of human disease similarities reveals common functional modules enriched for pluripotent drug targets. *PLoS Comput Biol* 6: e1000662.

Tao, W.A., B. Wollscheid, R. O'Brien, J.K. Eng, X.J. Li, B. Bodenmiller, J.D. Watts, L. Hood, and R. Aebersold. 2005. Quantitative phosphoproteome analysis using a dendrimer conjugation chemistry and tandem mass spectrometry. *Nat Methods* 2: 591–8.

Tonon, L., H. Touzet, and J.S. Varre. 2010. TFM-Explorer: mining cis-regulatory regions in genomes. *Nucleic Acids Res* 38: W286–92.

Tsuda, T., Y. Ueno, T. Yoshikawa, H. Kojo, and T. Osawa. 2006. Microarray profiling of gene expression in human adipocytes in response to anthocyanins. *Biochem Pharmacol* 71: 1184–97.

van Ommen, B., S. Fairweather-Tait, A. Freidig, A. Kardinaal, A. Scalbert, and S. Wopereis. 2008. A network biology model of micronutrient related health. *Br J Nutr* 99 Suppl 3: S72–80.

Vaquerizas, J.M., S.K. Kummerfeld, S.A. Teichmann, and N.M. Luscombe. 2009. A census of human transcription factors: function, expression and evolution. *Nat Rev Genet* 10: 252–63.

Varma, V., C. Wise, and J. Kaput. 2010. Carbohydrate metabolic pathway genes associated with quantitative trait loci (QTL) for obesity and type 2 diabetes: identification by data mining. *Biotechnol J* 5: 942–9.

Vidal, M., M.E. Cusick, and A.L. Barabasi. 2011. Interactome networks and human disease. *Cell* 144: 986–98.

Waagmeester, A., P. Pezik, S. Coort, F. Tourniaire, C. Evelo, and D. Rebholz-Schuhmann. 2009. Pathway enrichment based on text mining and its validation on carotenoid and vitamin A metabolism. *OMICS* 13: 367–79.

Walhout, A.J., and M. Vidal. 2001. Protein interaction maps for model organisms. *Nat Rev Mol Cell Biol* 2: 55–62.

Wise, C., and J. Kaput. 2009. A strategy for analyzing gene-nutrient interactions in type 2 diabetes. *J Diabetes Sci Technol* 3: 710–21.

Witzany, G. 2012. Do we eat gene regulators? *Commun Integr Biol* 5: 230–2.

Wuster, A., and M. Madan Babu. 2008. Chemogenomics and biotechnology. *Trends Biotechnol* 26: 252–8.

Xu, J., C. Wise, V. Varma, H. Fang, B. Ning, H. Hong, W. Tong, and J. Kaput. 2010. Two new ArrayTrack libraries for personalized biomedical research. *BMC Bioinformatics* 11 Suppl 6: S6.

Yang, Y., S.J. Adelstein, and A.I. Kassis. 2012. Target discovery from data mining approaches. *Drug Discov Today* 17 Suppl: S16–23.

Zhu, X., M. Gerstein, and M. Snyder. 2007. Getting connected: analysis and principles of biological networks. *Genes Dev* 21: 1010–24.

11 Metabolomics

An Important Tool for Assessing State of Health and Risk of Disease in Nutrigenomics Research

Hui-Ming Lin and Daryl Rowan

CONTENTS

INTRODUCTION

Metabolomic analysis has been defined as "a comprehensive and quantitative analysis of the metabolome" [1], where the metabolome is the full suite of metabolites contained within a biological system. Because of the diversity of the chemical properties of metabolites and the limitations of analytical techniques, it is presently impossible to measure the complete metabolome. Therefore, the definition for a similar term, metabonomic analysis, appears more appropriate—"the quantitative measurement of the time-related multi-parametric metabolic response of living systems to pathophysiological stimuli or genetic modification" [2]. Currently, the terms "metabolomic" and "metabonomic" are considered to be synonymous. In short, metabolomic analysis refers to the comprehensive study of the responses of small molecules (metabolites) to experimental or environmental challenge. High-throughput analytical techniques (e.g., gas chromatography–mass spectrometry [GC-MS], capillary electrophoresis–mass spectrometry [CE-MS], liquid chromatography–mass spectrometry [LC-MS], and nuclear magnetic resonance [NMR]) are used to measure multiple metabolites simultaneously in biological samples.

In nutrigenetic and nutrigenomic research, metabolomic analysis can be used to determine how food-derived metabolites are modified by the consumer, including by the intestinal microbiota, and how they may influence gene expression to produce a certain phenotype. Metabolomic analysis can also be used to identify metabolite biomarkers that indicate consumption of particular foods or the consumer's state of health and risk of disease. This chapter provides a brief introduction to metabolomic methodologies and explains how metabolomic analysis can be applied in nutrigenomic and nutrigenetic research. Some examples of applications of metabolomics analysis to nutrigenetic and nutrigenomic research are provided.

METABOLOMIC METHODOLOGIES

Analytical Platforms

Metabolomic analysis requires analytical technologies that are capable of the precise quantification of numerous and diverse metabolites in biological samples. No single analytical technique can measure the complete metabolome because of the diverse chemical properties of metabolites and the limitations of the analytical technologies presently available. The use of different biological samples, sample processing methods, and analytical technologies (platforms and instruments) results in the measurement of a broad range of metabolites and is required for comprehensive analysis of the metabolome.

The choice of analytical platforms and instruments depends on the classes of metabolites that may, a priori, be of interest, and whether a targeted or nontargeted approach to their measurement is to be taken. In a nontargeted approach, no prior selection of metabolites for precise quantification is made and the methodology focuses on the measurement of the maximum number of metabolites rather than on the type or chemical identity of these metabolites. This approach may measure metabolites of unknown chemical structure and allows for the discovery of experimental effects on novel metabolites of as yet unknown function. Thus, sample preparation is usually minimal to enable the retention in the sample extract of as many metabolites as possible. This nontargeted approach is more suitable for metabolite profiling studies that do not require metabolite identification and where the pattern of metabolites' level, rather than biochemical processes, is of interest or will be used to discriminate between classes of samples. In contrast, a targeted approach involves the precise measurement of specific metabolites or classes of metabolites (e.g., B-group vitamins and tryptophan metabolites [3]). Sample preparation is usually more extensive to preserve and enrich for these metabolites, and instrument settings are optimized for enhanced and selective detection to aid accurate quantification of the metabolites.

The major analytical platforms used to measure metabolites in metabolomic analysis are MS (usually coupled with chromatographic instruments, e.g., the hyphenated techniques of GC-MS, LC-MS, CE-MS) and NMR spectroscopy, described in the following subsections.

Mass Spectrometry

MS refers to the measurement of the apparent masses (technically the mass/charge ratios) of metabolites or the products of their fragmentation. Metabolites are introduced into the high vacuum of the mass spectrometer where they are ionized (converted into charged ions) or are broken into smaller ionized fragments that can be manipulated and measured by the instrument. The fragmentation of a metabolite is generally dependent on its chemical structure, thus unique mass spectra (graphs of mass fragment ions and their abundance) can be generated for most metabolites and used for compound identification.

For metabolomic analysis, mass spectrometers are usually coupled to chromatographic instruments to give a separation of the metabolites in a sample before mass spectrometric detection. This increases the number of individual metabolites that can be detected and measured. The type of chromatographic instrument interfaced to the mass spectrometer depends on the metabolites of interest, but is typically a gas or liquid chromatograph or uses CE.

In GC-MS analysis, liquid samples are vaporized in the injector and carried in a flow of helium gas through a capillary column that is coated internally with an adsorbent film. The temperature of the column is varied during the chromatographic run. Thus, the separation of chemical compounds is mainly influenced by their boiling points, as well as their chemical affinity with the internal coating in the capillary. This technique is ideal for analyzing volatile compounds such as flavor volatiles and fatty acids that are sufficiently thermally stable to be easily vaporized for entry into the GC column. For nonvolatile polar metabolites such as simple sugars and amino acids, a chemical derivatization (e.g., conversion to their trimethylsilyl ethers) is required to increase their thermal stability and volatility before they can be analyzed in this way [4].

In LC-MS, a liquid mobile phase (solvent) is used to carry compounds through a column packed with fine particles coated with an adsorbent surface. Separation of metabolites is achieved through the different affinities of metabolites for the chemical surface of the particles in the column and by progressively changing the composition of the liquid solvent phase. A wide range of both polar and nonpolar metabolites, including structural and stereoisomers, can be separated by using different combinations of chromatographic LC columns and mobile phases.

The third MS-coupled chromatographic technique with increasing use and significance in metabolomic analysis is CE-MS. CE-MS is generally used for the measurement of charged compounds [5] where the metabolites are separated according to the charge and size in the electroosmotic flow generated by the application of a high voltage to a buffered solution in a silica capillary.

Further information about mass spectrometric metabolomic analysis and the types of mass spectrometers can be found in other more extensive reviews [6–8].

Nuclear Magnetic Resonance Spectroscopy

Atoms whose nuclei possess appropriate magnetic properties, such as the stable isotopes ^{1}H and ^{13}C, absorb radiofrequency energy when subjected to a magnetic field. This energy absorption, which occurs at particular radiofrequencies, is referred to as NMR and is reported as the chemical shift. Energy absorption by the various nuclei in a metabolite depends on the type of nuclei and the structural arrangement of the atoms (the chemical environment). Metabolites can therefore be identified according to the pattern of their chemical shifts. Where these patterns of chemical shifts do not totally overlap, prior separation of the metabolites in the sample is not required for quantification. This enables multiple metabolites to be measured with minimal sample processing in complex samples such as urine or serum. NMR procedures for metabolomic analysis of biological samples are described in detail by Beckonert et al. [9].

Mass Spectrometry Compared to Nuclear Magnetic Resonance

The relative advantages and limitations of the various hyphenated MS and NMR spectroscopy techniques provide different opportunities for surveying the complexity of the metabolome (Table 11.1). All these techniques are widely used in metabolomic analysis. In terms of reproducibility and ease of quantification, NMR performs better than MS. However, NMR is a relatively insensitive technique that generally provides information about only the more highly abundant metabolites. The measurement and identification of low-concentration metabolites are hindered by the presence of metabolites of higher concentrations in the sample, as the NMR resonances of the less abundant metabolites are frequently overshadowed by those of the more abundant metabolites. Since NMR is nondestructive to samples, these less abundant metabolites can however be recovered for analysis by more sensitive and selective mass spectrometric methods.

The coupling of mass spectrometers to chromatographic instruments for prior separation of metabolites in a complex sample increases the number of detectable metabolites. In addition, MS is better suited to detecting low abundant metabolites, provided that suitable operating parameters (e.g., chromatographic separation from interfering metabolites and appropriate ionization conditions) are found. This is especially in the case of LC-MS where efficient ionization of metabolites is required for high sensitivity. When mixtures of metabolites are analyzed by LC-MS, selective ionization of the more easily ionized metabolites commonly occurs (ion suppression) resulting in poor quantitation or even failure to detect particular metabolites. This problem is usually overcome by chromatographic separation of metabolites.

Chemical derivatization (e.g., formation of trimethylsilyl ether derivatives) is required before nonvolatile metabolites such as sugars and organic and amino acids can be analyzed by GC-MS. Such derivatizations are not generally used in LC-MS analysis, although they can be used to enhance the detection of specific classes of metabolites. Chemical derivatization can complicate the analysis through formation of multiple chemical derivatives and the production of chemical artifacts. Thus, LC-MS analysis offers faster sample throughput and greater flexibility compared to GC-MS analysis that involves chemical derivatization.

TABLE 11.1
Comparison of Different Technologies for Performing Metabolomic Analysis

	Mass Spectrometry			NMR
	Measures mass of ionized molecules or molecular fragments resulting from fragmentation of metabolites in a vacuum			Measures energy absorption of atomic nuclei in metabolites at a certain radiofrequency in a magnetic field
	Gas Chromatography	**Liquid Chromatography**	**Capillary Electrophoresis**	
	Separation of metabolites using a gas mobile phase and a stationary phase in a capillary column	Separation of metabolites using a liquid mobile phase and a stationary phase in a packed column	Separation of metabolites in an electrically charged liquid phase in a silica capillary	
Type of metabolites detected	Volatile compounds	Various	Charged compounds	Various
Quantification	Optimization of chromatographic separation and ionization conditions required for precise quantification of a wide range of metabolites			Easy and accurate for abundant metabolites
Reproducibility	Highly reproducible mass spectra that can be used to identify compounds by matching to mass spectral libraries	Mass spectra influenced by ionization technique and sample matrix		High reproducibility for abundant metabolites
Sensitivity	High sensitivity for metabolites that can be ionized			Low sensitivity
Sample treatment	Chemical derivatization required for nonvolatile compounds. Small amounts required	Minimal preparation. Small amounts required	Minimal preparation. Small amounts required	Minimal preparation. Nondestructive, sample can be reused

However, metabolite identification for GC-MS is greatly aided using computer-based matching to published mass spectral libraries and databases, as the use of electron ionization at a standard 70 eV ionization energy results in highly reproducible mass spectra. In comparison, the reproducibility of LC-MS mass spectra is poor because of the use of different ionization techniques, energies, and effects of the sample matrix [4].

Overall, the respective chromatographic-coupled MS techniques each have their own advantages and limitations. Ultimately, the choice of analytical platforms and instruments depends on their availability and the particular classes of metabolites that may be of interest. Ideally, more than one platform or instrument should be used for a more comprehensive coverage of the metabolome.

Data Analysis

The data generated from metabolomic analysis of biological samples consist of measurements of the absolute and relative concentrations of many metabolites. These measurements collectively represent the metabolite profile of the sample. Depending on the type of instrument, data processing is required to convert the information about metabolites from the raw data files into a form suitable for statistical analysis. For example, relevant quantitative measures such as the areas of mass spectral peaks must be extracted from GC-MS or LC-MS data. The peak areas from the spectrum of several samples have to be aligned (corrected for differences in chromatographic retention times between samples) and collated into a single data file for statistical analysis. Data processing software is usually provided with the instrument but may be instrument dependent or limited in function. Open source software that is instrument independent is also available, such as XCMS and MZmine [10,11].

Normalization is an essential data processing step that is required to correct for factors that could bias the interpretation of the data, such as variation arising from analytical processing (e.g., batch differences) or the biological condition of the samples (e.g., urine concentration). Various data normalization techniques are available [12,13]. The inclusion of quality control samples throughout the process of sample analysis assists in monitoring and correcting for any changes in analytical performance. Recommended quality control samples are pooled aliquots of all the samples in an experiment, as every metabolite present in any sample will have its corresponding reference in the pooled quality control samples [14].

Metabolomic data consist of measurements of multiple metabolites together with values for relatively few other experimental parameters (treatments, time points). Such data can be analyzed using multivariate statistical techniques, which consist of unsupervised and supervised classification methods [15]. Unsupervised classification methods, such as principal component analysis and hierarchical clustering, analyze the variation in the data without prior designation of samples into their classes [16,17]. Such methods are useful for identifying unexpected variations and trends in the data. Supervised classification methods, such as multiple *t*-tests and partial least squares discriminant analysis (PLS-DA), compare the variation of samples according to their designated classes. Such methods are used for identifying the variables (metabolites) that contribute to the differences between the sample classes. Free Web-based metabolomic data analysis software incorporating these statistical analyses, such as MetaboAnalyst, are now available [18].

Public mass spectral databases of metabolites, such as Golm, Metlin, and MassBank, are available to assist in structure identification [19–21]. Public websites with information on metabolites and metabolic pathways are also available to assist in the interpretation of the function of metabolites of interest [10]. Examples include the Human Metabolome Database [22] and the KEGG Pathway Database (www.genome.jp/kegg).

METABOLOMIC APPLICATIONS IN NUTRIGENOMICS/NUTRIGENETICS

Nutrigenetic and nutrigenomic research seeks to increase our understanding of the interaction between foods, genes, and nutrition by studying the effects of diet on gene expression and by studying genetic differences in dietary response. Knowledge gained from nutrigenetic and nutrigenomic research can be used to develop personalized nutrition strategies for optimum health. To achieve all these aims, an understanding of the metabolism of the food of interest and the identification of the bioactive food compound is necessary. Quantification of exposure to the bioactive compound is required to study its molecular and physiological effects. Biomarkers to assess health response to bioactive food components are also required to evaluate beneficial effects. These requirements can be achieved using metabolomic analysis, as the technology enables multiple metabolites to be screened in parallel in biofluids, tissues, or food (Figure 11.1).

IDENTIFICATION OF BIOACTIVE FOOD COMPONENTS

The use of metabolomic techniques to profile food metabolites is not a novel concept as chromatography-coupled MS techniques and high-performance liquid chromatography (HPLC) have been used to characterize the composition of plant-based foods long before the term "metabolomic" was coined. Over the years, instrument technologies are becoming more powerful with increasing sensitivity to identify bioactive compounds in foods. The process of identifying bioactive compounds in a food may involve separating the components of the food into fractions according to solvent solubility or chromatography, followed by testing of the fractions for bioactivity in in vitro cell-based assays or in vivo animal feeding studies (bioassay-guided fractionation). Metabolomic analysis can then be performed on the bioactive fractions to identify the metabolites that are present. For example, fractionation of extracts from raspberry fruit by preparative HPLC by

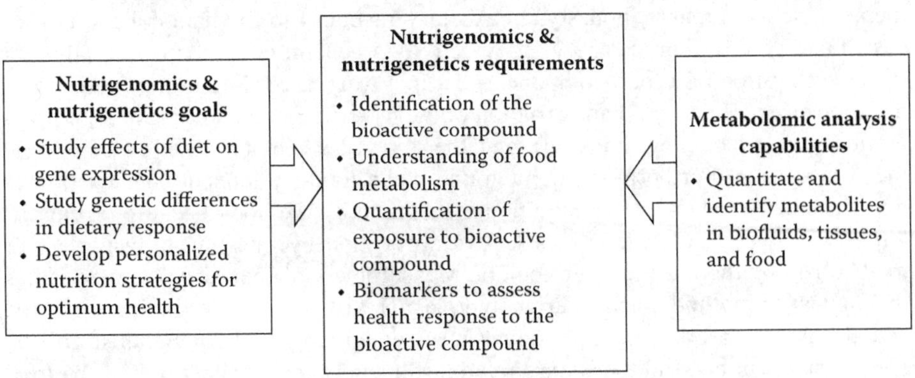

FIGURE 11.1 Contributions of metabolomic analysis to nutrigenomic and nutrigenetic research.

Mullen et al. [23], and gel filtration by Ross et al. [24], led to a partial discrimination of metabolites responsible for the antioxidant and cellular antiproliferative properties of these extracts.

Isolation or synthesis of the tentatively identified bioactive compounds may need to be carried out to confirm chemical identity. These samples can then be tested using the in vitro or in vivo models to confirm their bioactivity. Where the bioactivity of a food is ill-defined or is not related in a simple way to one or a few food constituents, the bioassay-guided approach fails. In this case, bioactivity may have to be represented by the metabolite profile of the food, which may be all the metabolites measured, or a subset of metabolites that best discriminates the food according to its bioactivity.

Metabolomic analysis may also be used to probe the relationship between food composition or bioactivity and the genetic variation of the plants or animals that the food was derived from [25,26]. For example, LC-MS metabolite profiles of cooked rice from diverse rice varieties, performed by Heuberger et al. [25], could differentiate the rice varieties according to their subspecies classification. The total phenolics and vitamin E levels were linked to single nucleotide polymorphisms of genes in the biosynthesis pathways of these compounds. In another example, LC-MS profiling of polyphenolic levels of raspberry fruits, performed by Stewart et al. [26], showed that the metabolites levels were influenced by either environmental conditions or genetic variety, indicating that the levels of some polyphenols were regulated by rigorous genetic control. Overall, these studies show that metabolomic analysis in conjunction with genomic analysis can uncover genetic influences on the regulation of the levels of bioactive or nutritional metabolites in the food. This knowledge can be used to optimize food composition through environmental or genetic manipulation of the plant or animal.

Quantification of Dietary Exposure

Accurate quantification of both food composition and of bioactive food components is required to study the molecular or physiological effects of foods. Conventional methods of measuring dietary exposure such as self-reporting of dietary intakes by study participants and the use of food composition databases are inadequate and widely acknowledged to be flawed [27]. Self-reporting depends on the individual's memory, self-awareness, honesty, and dietary response to the data collection process. Food composition databases provide only a general or standardized value for the concentration of a food component that may vary according to the food source (e.g., the effect of natural plant variation or the use of different cultivars), food preparation (e.g., processing, cooking), and the analytical methods used to determine the composition. Furthermore, the amount of the food component consumed does not necessarily reflect the actual amount absorbed by the body because of the differences between individuals in selective absorption by intestinal transporters or metabolism by the intestinal microbiota. Measurement of food-derived metabolites that appear in biofluids such as urine and plasma will give a better indication of the actual amount absorbed by the body. An understanding of the metabolism of the food component and time–response relationships between consumption of the food component and the appearance of metabolites in biofluids is thus required to select a suitable metabolite biomarker of exposure to the food component.

The ability of metabolomic analysis to screen multiple metabolites in parallel makes the technique suitable for analyzing biofluids and tissues for metabolites produced by the metabolism of food components [28–33] or by the action of the intestinal microbiota on nondigestible food components [34]. Fardet et al. [28] used LC-MS to analyze urine collected from rats fed with diets supplemented with lignins or phenolic acids. Data analysis using PLS-DA showed that the metabolic fingerprints of the urine samples were similar between lignin-supplemented diets and control diets, confirming that lignins are largely inert to digestion and are not absorbed into the body. In contrast, various metabolites arising from the metabolism of the phenolic acids were identified.

In a further example, Stalmach et al. [29] studied the metabolism of coffee polyphenols in humans by using LC-MS to analyze urine and plasma collected at several time points within 24 hours after drinking coffee. Coffee components that were absorbed by the small intestine or large intestine could be differentiated according to their presence in urine and plasma samples at different time points. Metabolites that were quickly excreted were also identified according to their absence in plasma and presence in urine. Urinary dihydrocaffeic acid-3-*O*-sulfate and feruloylglycine were proposed as potential and sensitive biomarkers for coffee consumption.

Overall, these studies show that metabolomic analysis of biofluids can be used to understand the metabolism of food components and to identify biomarkers of food intake.

Assessment of Dietary Intervention

The goal of nutrigenetics and nutrigenomic research is to develop personalized dietary strategies for the optimal health of human individuals. Biomarkers of health status and of responsiveness to dietary components are therefore required to evaluate the efficacy of nutrigenomic and nutrigenetic dietary regimes. The metabolite profile of an organism is closely associated with its genotype [35,36], as genes code for proteins that participate in metabolic pathways. The influence of external factors on gene expression and biochemical pathways, such as diet and pathogens, will lead to changes in the metabolite profile. Therefore, the levels of metabolites in biofluids can provide information about the health status of an organism and their response to diet. Metabolite biomarkers of diseases are already successfully used in clinical practice—elevated glucose levels in blood after fasting as an indicator of diabetes and creatinine levels in blood as an indicator of renal function. Nevertheless, new and more accurate biomarkers of diseases and therapeutic response are always sought after.

Metabolomic analysis of biofluids and tissues has the potential for biomarker discovery. Ideally, large well-characterized cohorts with longitudinal samples should be used for biomarker discovery. The accuracy of potential biomarkers must be validated in independent cohorts. A few noteworthy examples of biomarker discovery by metabolomic analysis are described as follows.

Wang et al. [37] identified a metabolite profile that predicted future diabetes by performing LC-MS metabolomic analysis on plasma samples of 189 nondiabetic individuals who later developed diabetes within 12 years and 189 matched controls.

Approximately 60 metabolites were measured using a targeted approach. Elevated levels of five amino acids, isoleucine, leucine, valine, tyrosine, and phenylalanine, predicted future diabetes. This result was validated in a further study comprising 163 cases and 163 controls. The authors cited other studies that supported the role of amino acids in pathogenesis of diabetes, such as the development of insulin resistance in animals and humans supplemented with branched-chain amino acids, and correlation of fasting concentrations of amino acid with obesity and insulin levels.

Holmes et al. [38] identified potential urinary biomarkers of cardiovascular disease risk by performing NMR metabolomic analysis of urine samples from 4630 individuals from East Asian and Western populations. The urinary metabolite profiles discriminated populations according to geographical regions, diets, and blood pressure. Formate, alanine, and hippuric acid were associated with blood pressure and were identified as potential biomarkers of cardiovascular disease risk.

The identification of accurate biomarkers for disease is challenging due, in part, to the genetic variation that occurs within human populations. Distinct metabolite profiles, associated with specific genetic variants, can be determined by combined genome-wide association studies and metabolomic analysis as shown by Gieger et al., Illig et al., and Suhre et al. [39–41]. The cumulative work of these three studies revealed associations between blood metabolite levels and genetic loci related to disease and of pharmaceutical relevance. Overall, the levels of over 250 metabolites from 60 biochemical pathways were measured in serum samples from 2820 individuals in two large population-based European cohorts (German KORA and British TwinsUK studies), using LC–tandem mass spectrometry (LC-MS-MS). Geiger et al. [39] established that the ratios of metabolites as a surrogate for enzymatic activity explained a higher proportion of genetic variance than the use of single metabolite concentrations alone. Illig et al. [40] showed that for 8 of 9 genetic loci, the genetic variant is located in or near genes encoding enzymes or solute carriers with biochemical relevance to the metabolites. Finally, Suhre et al. [41] identified 37 genetic loci that were associated with metabolite concentrations, of which 25 of the loci account for 10%–60% of the differences in metabolite levels per allele copy. Cross-reference of these genetic loci to databases of disease-related and pharmaceutically relevant genetic associations provided new insights into the functions of these loci and confirmed previous associations. For example, SLC2A9 gene variants were associated with uric acid concentrations and self-reported gout [42].

Even when genetic variants are not known, metabolite profiles can identify subgroups that are likely to respond differently to a diet. Clayton et al. [43] showed that the urinary metabolite profiles of rats prior to drug treatment could predict their response toward paracetamol. The urinary profiles were generated by NMR analysis. In another example, Rezzi et al. [44] showed that metabolite profiles could be linked to dietary preference, where chocolate-loving and chocolate-indifferent individuals have metabolite differences that are present even in the absent of chocolate stimulation. The metabolite profiles of the individuals were measured by NMR analysis. Some of the differential metabolites were derived from intestinal microbiota metabolism, suggesting that dietary habits may influence intestinal microbiota profile. Dietary preference can affect health and is influenced by taste response that is genetically mediated [44].

Overall, these studies show the potential of metabolomic analysis in identifying biomarkers of disease that may be used to assess the efficacy of dietary interventions. The advantage of using metabolites as biomarkers in biofluids to assess health status is that these fluids can be sampled repetitively without dire consequences to the animal or human subject. This is useful in both animal and human studies, as the effect of dietary intervention can be monitored over time and the outcome of the experiment may be quickly determined through early changes in metabolite biomarkers. Repetitive sampling of biofluids is also required for monitoring human patients and provides a form of biological replication to confirm findings.

Discovery of Food and Gene Interactions

The identification of metabolite biomarkers of dietary exposure or disease risk can provide insights into the pathways of the disease process and their modulation by food components. Specific genotypes associated with these pathways that may benefit from dietary modulation can be determined. These points are shown by a noteworthy study by Wang et al. [45] who performed nontargeted metabolomic analysis of plasma samples to identify metabolite profiles that could predict the risk of cardiovascular disease. The plasma of 50 stable patients who later suffered a heart attack, stroke, or death within 3 years and of 50 matched controls was analyzed by LC-MS. A further cohort of 25 cases and 25 controls was used to validate the results and to narrow down the number of metabolites to 18 metabolites associated with cardiovascular risk. Of these 18 metabolites, 3 were strongly correlated to each other. Further structural elucidation analysis using NMR, MS, LC-MS-MS, and GC-MS-MS identified these three metabolites as trimethylamine *N*-oxide (TMAO), choline, and betaine. Further validation using an independent cohort of 1876 subjects confirmed that fasting plasma levels of these three metabolites were associated with risk of cardiovascular disease. Animal feeding studies with isotope-labeled compounds or antibiotics showed that TMAO is derived from trimethylamine, which is produced by intestinal microbial metabolism of betaine and choline, where the latter is derived from dietary phosphatidylcholine (lecithin). TMAO is produced from trimethylamine through the action of hepatic flavin monooxygenases. The authors found that TMAO plasma levels correlated with the size of artherosclerotic plaques in artherosclerotic-prone mice supplemented with choline. Furthermore, TMAO plasma levels, aortic lesion formation, and HDL cholesterol concentrations are correlated with the expression of hepatic flavin monooxygenases in mice. A genetic locus containing the flavin monooxygenase gene cluster had a strong effect on atherosclerosis in the mice. Examination of plasma TMAO levels in humans showed correlations to hepatic expression levels of flavin monooxygenase. Overall, these findings by Wang et al. [45] indicate that the cardiovascular risk of individuals with certain flavin monooxygenase genetic variants may be modulated by their dietary choline and that plasma level of TMAO may be a potential biomarker of cardiovascular health status.

Metabolomic analysis can also be used to understand the differential effects of specific genotypes on the absorption and metabolism of foods. For example, Lin et al. [46] performed nontargeted GC-MS analysis of urine samples from interleukin-10-deficient ($IL10^{-/-}$) mice fed with extracts of the fruits of yellow- and green-fleshed kiwifruits. The $IL10^{-/-}$ mouse is a model of inflammatory bowel disease and develops intestinal inflammation in the presence of intestinal microbiota. The authors found that $IL10^{-/-}$ mice had a higher excretion of metabolites associated with the kiwifruit diet compared with the wild-type mice. These differences in the excretion of diet-associated metabolites possibly arise through differences in intestinal microbial metabolism or through an increase in intestinal permeability, which are both known consequences of *IL10* gene deficiency and of inflammatory bowel disease [47,48]. In this example, the effect of the gene variant on food metabolites was not through the direct interaction of the gene with the food metabolites, showing the usefulness of metabolomic analysis in identifying unexpected effects of gene variants on food metabolism.

SUMMARY

Metabolomic analysis is the comprehensive study of small molecule metabolites using technologies such as MS and NMR, which enable high-throughput parallel measurements of the many metabolites in a complex biological sample. Applications of metabolomic analysis in nutrigenetic and nutrigenomic research include the identification of bioactive food components and food-derived metabolites, the quantification of dietary exposure to metabolites, the identification of biomarkers to assess the efficacy of dietary interventions, and the discovery of novel food–gene interactions.

REFERENCES

1. Fiehn, O., Combining genomics, metabolome analysis, and biochemical modelling to understand metabolic networks. *Comp Funct Genomics* 2001, 2(3): 155–68.
2. Nicholson, J.K., J.C. Lindon, and E. Holmes, 'Metabonomics': understanding the metabolic responses of living systems to pathophysiological stimuli via multivariate statistical analysis of biological NMR spectroscopic data. *Xenobiotica* 1999, 29(11): 1181–9.
3. Midttun, O., S. Hustad, and P.M. Ueland, Quantitative profiling of biomarkers related to B-vitamin status, tryptophan metabolism and inflammation in human plasma by liquid chromatography/tandem mass spectrometry. *Rapid Commun Mass Spectrom* 2009, 23(9): 1371–9.
4. Halket, J.M. et al., Chemical derivatization and mass spectral libraries in metabolic profiling by GC/MS and LC/MS/MS. *J Exp Bot* 2005, 56(410): 219–43.
5. Monton, M.R. and T. Soga, Metabolome analysis by capillary electrophoresis-mass spectrometry. *J Chromatogr A* 2007, 1168(1–2): 237–46.
6. Dettmer, K., P.A. Aronov, and B.D. Hammock, Mass spectrometry-based metabolomics. *Mass Spectrom Rev* 2007, 26(1): 51–78.
7. Kind, T. and O. Fiehn, Advances in structure elucidation of small molecules using mass spectrometry. *Bioanal Rev* 2010, 2(1–4): 23–60.
8. Want, E.J. et al., Global metabolic profiling procedures for urine using UPLC-MS. *Nat Protoc* 2010, 5(6): 1005–18.
9. Beckonert, O. et al., Metabolic profiling, metabolomic and metabonomic procedures for NMR spectroscopy of urine, plasma, serum and tissue extracts. *Nat Protoc* 2007, 2(11): 2692–703.

10. Tohge, T. and A.R. Fernie, Web-based resources for mass-spectrometry-based metabolomics: a user's guide. *Phytochemistry* 2009, 70(4): 450–6.
11. Smith, C.A. et al., XCMS: processing mass spectrometry data for metabolite profiling using nonlinear peak alignment, matching, and identification. *Anal Chem* 2006, 78(3): 779–87.
12. Craig, A. et al., Scaling and normalization effects in NMR spectroscopic metabonomic data sets. *Anal Chem* 2006, 78(7): 2262–7.
13. Dieterle, F. et al., Probabilistic quotient normalization as robust method to account for dilution of complex biological mixtures. Application in 1H NMR metabonomics. *Anal Chem* 2006, 78(13): 4281–90.
14. Sangster, T. et al., A pragmatic and readily implemented quality control strategy for HPLC-MS and GC-MS-based metabonomic analysis. *Analyst* 2006, 131(10): 1075–8.
15. Trygg, J., E. Holmes, and T. Lundstedt, Chemometrics in metabonomics. *J Proteome Res* 2007, 6(2): 469–79.
16. Manly, B.F.J., *Multivariate Statistical Methods: A Primer*. 3rd ed., 2005, Boca Raton, FL: Chapman & Hall/CRC Press.
17. Ringner, M., What is principal component analysis? *Nat Biotechnol* 2008, 26(3): 303–4.
18. Xia, J. et al., MetaboAnalyst: a web server for metabolomic data analysis and interpretation. *Nucleic Acids Res* 2009, 37(Web Server issue): W652–60.
19. Kopka, J. et al., GMD@CSB.DB: the Golm Metabolome Database. *Bioinformatics* 2005, 21(8): 1635–8.
20. Smith, C.A. et al., METLIN: a metabolite mass spectral database. *Ther Drug Monit* 2005, 27(6): 747–51.
21. Horai, H. et al., MassBank: a public repository for sharing mass spectral data for life sciences. *J Mass Spectrom* 2010, 45(7): 703–14.
22. Wishart, D.S. et al., HMDB: a knowledgebase for the human metabolome. *Nucleic Acids Res* 2009, 37(Database issue): D603–10.
23. Mullen, W. et al., Ellagitannins, flavonoids, and other phenolics in red raspberries and their contribution to antioxidant capacity and vasorelaxation properties. *J Agric Food Chem* 2002, 50(18): 5191–6.
24. Ross, H.A., G.J. McDougall, and D. Stewart, Antiproliferative activity is predominantly associated with ellagitannins in raspberry extracts. *Phytochemistry* 2007, 68(2): 218–28.
25. Heuberger, A.L. et al., Metabolomic and functional genomic analyses reveal varietal differences in bioactive compounds of cooked rice. *PLoS One* 2010, 5(9): e12915.
26. Stewart, D. et al., Metabolomic approach to identifying bioactive compounds in berries: advances toward fruit nutritional enhancement. *Mol Nutr Food Res* 2007, 51(6): 645–51.
27. Macdiarmid, J. and J. Blundell, Assessing dietary intake: who, what and why of under-reporting. *Nutr Res Rev* 1998, 11(2): 231–53.
28. Fardet, A. et al., Metabolomics provide new insight on the metabolism of dietary phytochemicals in rats. *J Nutr* 2008, 138(7): 1282–7.
29. Stalmach, A. et al., Metabolite profiling of hydroxycinnamate derivatives in plasma and urine after the ingestion of coffee by humans: identification of biomarkers of coffee consumption. *Drug Metab Dispos* 2009, 37(8): 1749–58.
30. Urpi-Sarda, M. et al., Targeted metabolic profiling of phenolics in urine and plasma after regular consumption of cocoa by liquid chromatography-tandem mass spectrometry. *J Chromatogr A* 2009, 1216(43): 7258–67.
31. Winning, H. et al., An exploratory NMR nutri-metabonomic investigation reveals dimethyl sulfone as a dietary biomarker for onion intake. *Analyst* 2009, 134(11): 2344–51.
32. Llorach, R. et al., Metabolomics study of human urinary metabolome modifications after intake of almond (Prunus dulcis (Mill.) D.A. Webb) skin polyphenols. *J Proteome Res* 2010, 9(11): 5859–67.

33. O'Sullivan, A., M.J. Gibney, and L. Brennan, Dietary intake patterns are reflected in metabolomic profiles: potential role in dietary assessment studies. *Am J Clin Nutr* 2011, 93(2): 314–21.
34. Jacobs, D.M. et al., Non-digestible food ingredients, colonic microbiota and the impact on gut health and immunity: a role for metabolomics. *Curr Drug Metab* 2009, 10(1): 41–54.
35. Fiehn, O. et al., Metabolite profiling for plant functional genomics. *Nat Biotechnol* 2000, 18(11): 1157–61.
36. Assfalg, M. et al., Evidence of different metabolic phenotypes in humans. *Proc Natl Acad Sci U S A* 2008, 105(5): 1420–4.
37. Wang, T.J. et al., Metabolite profiles and the risk of developing diabetes. *Nat Med* 2011, 17(4): 448–53.
38. Holmes, E. et al., Human metabolic phenotype diversity and its association with diet and blood pressure. *Nature* 2008, 453(7193): 396–400.
39. Gieger, C. et al., Genetics meets metabolomics: a genome-wide association study of metabolite profiles in human serum. *PLoS Genet* 2008, 4(11): e1000282.
40. Illig, T. et al., A genome-wide perspective of genetic variation in human metabolism. *Nat Genet* 2010, 42(2): 137–41.
41. Suhre, K. et al., Human metabolic individuality in biomedical and pharmaceutical research. *Nature* 2011, 477(7362): 54–60.
42. Doring, A. et al., SLC2A9 influences uric acid concentrations with pronounced sex-specific effects. *Nat Genet* 2008, 40(4): 430–6.
43. Clayton, T.A. et al., Pharmaco-metabonomic phenotyping and personalized drug treatment. *Nature* 2006, 440(7087): 1073–7.
44. Rezzi, S. et al., Human metabolic phenotypes link directly to specific dietary preferences in healthy individuals. *J Proteome Res* 2007, 6(11): 4469–77.
45. Wang, Z. et al., Gut flora metabolism of phosphatidylcholine promotes cardiovascular disease. *Nature* 2011, 472(7341): 57–63.
46. Lin, H.M. et al., Metabolomic analysis reveals differences in urinary excretion of kiwifruit-derived metabolites in a mouse model of inflammatory bowel disease. *Mol Nutr Food Res* 2011, 55(12): 1900–4.
47. Bibiloni, R. et al., Analysis of the large bowel microbiota of colitic mice using PCR/DGGE. *Lett Appl Microbiol* 2005, 41(1): 45–51.
48. Kennedy, R.J. et al., Interleukin 10-deficient colitis: new similarities to human inflammatory bowel disease. *Br J Surg* 2000, 87(10): 1346–51.

12 Epigenetics—What Role Could This Play in Functional Foods and Personalized Nutrition?

Matthew P.G. Barnett, Shalome A. Bassett, and Emma N. Bermingham

CONTENTS

INTRODUCTION

Hippocrates, the ancient Greek physician considered by some to be the father of modern medicine, has often been quoted as saying: "Let food be thy medicine, and medicine be thy food" [1]. Furthermore, in a wide variety of human cultures, there is a tradition of using foods for their healing properties; an obvious case is the long history of Chinese herbal medicine [2]. These two examples demonstrate that for a significant proportion of recorded human history, it has been acknowledged that food, in addition to its obvious role as a source of macronutrients, may have properties that make it beneficial to human health in ways that go "beyond nutrition." The term "functional foods" has relatively recently been applied to this very old concept in the context of physiologically active foods as a means of improving health [3]. It is now generally recognized that functional foods refer to foods with specific health benefits.

Food can have a wide range of functions in addition to supplying macronutrients. Examples include those that supply essential micronutrients, such as selenium in Brazil nuts [4] or omega-3 polyunsaturated fatty acids (n-3 PUFAs) in fish and other marine organisms [5], and those containing compounds such as glucosamine, which may improve joint health [6] (see Table 12.2 later in the chapter for a more comprehensive list of functional foods). Food components have also been identified which can interact with individual genes and thus have very specific functional outcomes, a phenomenon studied in the field of nutrigenomics and nutrigenetics [7]. Recent advances in the so-called "omics" technologies have enabled the interactions between food and genes to be studied at a genome-wide level, looking not only at relationships between food components and specific gene variants, but also measuring how foods can influence the expression of genes and proteins. The technology therefore exists to investigate the functional effects of food at an unprecedented level, with the potential for this to be applied on an individual basis. This requires comprehensive analysis and considerable computing power, and is further complicated by the role that epigenetics may play in the interactions between food and genes.

Epigenetics is a term encompassing mechanisms that enable an organism to alter its gene expression in response to environmental stimuli. Diet is one such stimulus, to which an organism is exposed on a daily basis. It therefore seems logical that epigenetic mechanisms would be relevant to changes in gene expression and phenotype in response to food consumption, and indeed there is a growing body of evidence to support this. In the field of personalized nutrition, epigenetics represents another layer of complexity in addition to that associated with food and gene variants; it may also provide an opportunity to expand the current understanding and appreciation of functional foods. A better understanding of epigenetic mechanisms and how they respond to the consumption of foods increases the possibility of identifying or developing functional foods that can target improved health through these mechanisms.

In this chapter, various epigenetic mechanisms will be described, how organisms might respond to food via epigenetic mechanisms will be explored, and the potentially important role of epigenetics in the growth of food products *per se* will be considered. Food allergies will be used as an example of food influencing epigenetic mechanisms for a specific health outcome. The concept of functional foods, and how such foods may improve human health through epigenetics, will be discussed, as will the issue of food pollutants which may lead to epigenetic changes. This chapter will conclude by looking at these issues within the global context of an increasing population and increasing competition for food.

EPIGENETICS

Since first used by Waddington in 1942 [8], the term "epigenetics" has been defined in a variety of different ways, and these definitions continue to evolve. This is in part due to the term having at least two semi-independent origins during the twentieth century [9]. Waddington's definition related the term to developmental biology, referring to the study of processes "which constitute the epigenesis which is also involved in development" [10]. This reflected Waddington's view that rather than a simple relationship between gene and phenotype, there are complex gene–gene and gene–environment interactions that play a key role in the developmental process.

Nanney had a somewhat different concept of epigenetic systems, characterizing them as "signal interpreting devices, yielding predictable results in response to specific stimuli from inside and outside the cell" [11]. A key difference of this concept was that these mechanisms were thought to be cytoplasmic rather than nuclear, although Nanney later conceded that epigenetic systems were "presumably limited by the information contained in the genetic library." One key observation made by Nanney was that "an epigenetic change should not result in a permanent loss of information and a return to a previous condition of expression is always theoretically possible." This potential reversibility of epigenetic changes is one feature that makes them relevant in human health and well-being. If epigenetic modifications, unlike genetic variants such as single nucleotide polymorphisms (SNPs), are potentially reversible despite being heritable, this plasticity then allows an organism to adapt to environmental cues and adjust its phenotypic development and evolve accordingly [12]. If poor dietary choices have led to poor health mediated by epigenetic events, the possibility remains that appropriate food choices may reverse these changes and enable an individual to come closer to achieving maximum health based on their genetic potential. For example, reduced *in utero* nutrition may result in the offspring adapting to a nutrient-poor environment, mediated by alterations in epigenetic mechanisms. If the postnatal environment which the offspring encounters has sufficient or excess nutrition, this may result in major metabolic disturbances because the offspring is not "programmed" for this level of nutrition. This phenomenon of programming may underlie many complex diseases now common in the Western world, including cardiovascular disease, type 2 diabetes, cancer, and obesity [12,13]. However, the plasticity of epigenetic mechanisms suggests that appropriate nutritional interventions may be able to act on these mechanisms to modify the long-term risk of such metabolic disturbances [14].

Having considered the definition of epigenetics, it is important to also consider its place in biology. It has been described as having two key components: as a "response" system, whereby environmental influences can be "sensed" and thereby influence the regulation and expression of the genetic code, and as a "memory" system, which through heritability of certain epigenetic "marks" can potentially pass on acquired characteristics through generations. The latter is somewhat controversial, as it hints at the views of Lamarck which suggested traits acquired by an organism could be passed on to its offspring [15], a view largely dismissed with the arrival of the concept of natural selection. Even so, the fact that epigenetic inheritance has been conclusively demonstrated suggests it may be important in the field of evolutionary biology [16].

Regardless of which of the above components is considered, it is clear that epigenetics is an important factor in all biological systems, in the same way as genetics, due to the universal nature of epigenetic mechanisms in both plants and animals.

For the purposes of this chapter, the role of epigenetics as a response mechanism, in which gene expression can be influenced in response to environmental cues, will be the primary focus. The definition of Riggs et al. will therefore be used, being "the study of mitotically and/or meiotically heritable changes in gene function that cannot be explained by changes in DNA sequence" [17]. This includes modifications of DNA, DNA-binding proteins, and histones that alter the structure of chromatin without altering the DNA nucleotide sequence, as well as non-coding RNA (ncRNA) molecules such as micro-RNAs (miRNAs), which can alter regulation of gene expression.

DNA Methylation

DNA methylation is the attachment of a methyl (CH_3) group to a cytosine at the CpG dinucleotide, forming 5-methyl-2-deoxycytidine (5-mdC), a modification so frequent that 5-mdC has been referred to as the fifth nucleotide [18]. An abundance of methyl groups (hypermethylation) in the promoter region of a gene is associated with so-called "silencing" or inactivation of that gene. Conversely, genes that are transcriptionally active have a deficit of methyl groups (hypomethylation) in their promoter regions. However, DNA hypermethylation not only occurs in single CpG islands or single genes—often multiple adjacent CpG-rich regions are affected, resulting in gene silencing across large chromosomal domains [19].

This long-range epigenetic silencing is well documented, for example, in colon [20] and breast [21] cancers, and in differentiation of T-helper cells [22]. It demonstrates that the regulation of gene expression by DNA methylation is not simple; both global hypomethylation of genomic DNA and hypermethylation of specific gene promoters have been implicated in carcinogenesis [23,24].

While DNA methylation is the most common epigenetic modification, it has recently become clear that there is at least one other alteration occurring at the cytosine residue as part of the epigenetic machinery of the cell. The oxidation of 5-mdC results in the formation of 5-hydroxymethylcytosine (5-hmC), which appears to play a role in demethylation (the process by which methyl groups are removed from cytosine) [25] and to be important in DNA methylation-related plasticity [26]. Levels of 5hmC may be highly variable according to the tissue type and transcriptional activity [27], and while there is still much uncertainty as to the precise role(s) of 5hmC, it has already been referred to as the "sixth base" [28].

Histone Modifications

Modification of histone proteins (including methylation and acetylation as well as the less-common phosphorylation, ubiquination, and sumoylation) represents another key epigenetic mechanism. As with changes to DNA methylation, many histone modifications are potentially reversible and are regulated by enzymes that either add or remove these covalent modifications. However, while DNA methylation is generally associated with repression of gene expression, histone modifications can lead to either gene activation or repression depending on the type of modification and the amino acid residue involved. For example, lysine acetylation is associated with transcriptional activation, while lysine methylation results in either activation or repression [29]. Acetyl and methyl groups are added to the N-terminal "histone tails" by histone acetyltransferases (HATs) and histone methyltransferases

(HMTs), respectively, while histone deacetylases (HDACs) and histone demethylases (HDMs) remove these groups. Acetylation of histones is important in the regulation of gene expression and is normally associated with transcriptionally active gene-dense regions, referred to as euchromatin. Addition of acetyl ($COCH_3$) groups to the histone tail causes the chromatin to relax and allow transcription to occur. Conversely, removal of the acetyl group by HDACs causes the chromatin to compress and prevent transcription from occurring and is commonly associated with gene silencing. Histone acetylation can be transient and must be maintained by enzymatic activity. Similarly, arginine methylation can also be temporary and may play a role in inflammation, whereas lysine methylation is relatively stable.

Non-Coding RNA

Another epigenomic modification is ncRNA, which includes miRNA and short interfering RNA (siRNA) molecules. miRNAs are highly stable small ncRNA molecules that regulate gene expression and protein production in cells. Due to their unique interaction with mRNA, miRNAs may regulate as much as 30% of all human genes [30]. While this interaction typically involves miRNAs binding to the 3′ untranslated region (UTR) of target mRNA and thus directing their post-transcriptional repression [31], there is evidence that they can also bind to the 5′ UTR and act as either activators or repressors of gene expression [32,33]. Hence, miRNAs play a key role in regulation of gene expression and are also being recognized for their potential importance in extracellular signaling [34] and development of disease [35]. In transient biological responses, such as the immune response, where temporary miRNA modulation occurs, influencing this modulation may have profound biological effects. As described in more detail later in this chapter, there is growing evidence that compounds found within foods can influence miRNA expression, thereby influencing gene expression with consequent physiological outcomes.

EPIGENETIC MECHANISMS IN PLANTS AND ANIMALS

Before discussing functional foods and their potential role in modulating epigenetic mechanisms, it is important to first consider the relationship between food and epigenetics on a more general level. As Figure 12.1 suggests, the potential relationship between the foods we eat and epigenetic mechanisms represents a highly complex network of interactions. Consideration must be given not only to the interactions between environment, genotype, and epigenetic mechanisms within an individual, but also to the possibility that epigenetic changes occurring within a food (be it plant or animal) may interact with and influence gene expression of the consumer of that food.

Because of this complexity, when considering the possible role epigenetics may have in functional foods, it is necessary to consider the role that epigenetic mechanisms may play at each point within the food chain, taking into account epigenetic changes within the plant or animal food source, as well as those that occur in the animal or human which consumes that food.

The epigenetic mechanisms which allow organisms to respond to their environment (including diet) are also active within the plants, fungi, and animals which

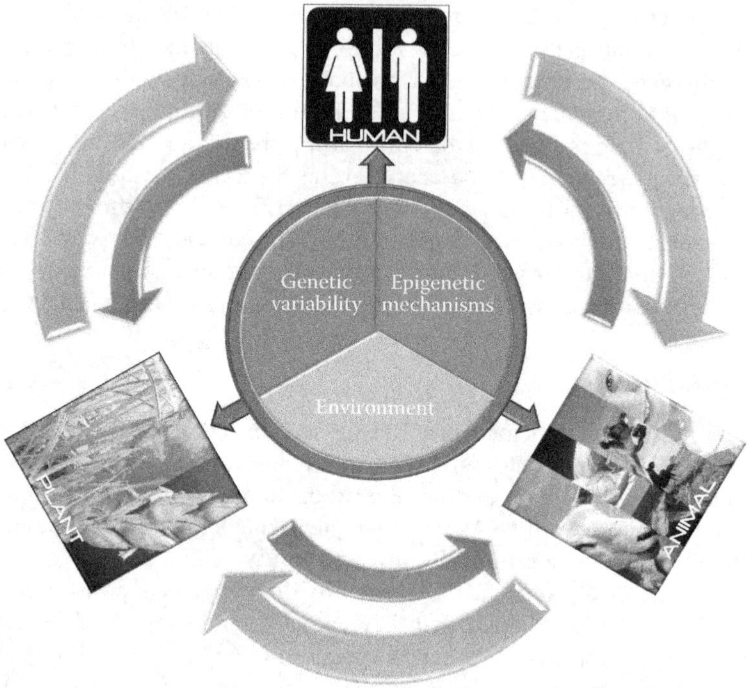

FIGURE 12.1 Complex interactions between plants, animals, and humans which can influence epigenetic mechanisms in each. This figure demonstrates the fundamental role of epigenetic mechanisms in the interactions between plants, animals, and humans. For example, in humans, the impact of environmental factors (including the foods ingested as part of the diet) interacts with the genetic variability of the human, and with the various epigenetic mechanisms, to produce a phenotypic outcome. In addition, because the plant or animal source of the food also responds to its environment via epigenetic mechanisms, the epigenetics of the plant and/or animal may play an important role in the human phenotypic outcome. Furthermore, the environmental interactions between plant, animal, and human (e.g., grazing of a plant by an herbivore; selective breeding strategies of plants and animals; use of pesticides) may also modulate the phenotype via epigenetic mechanisms, with potential outcomes of relevance to human health.

are consumed as part of the diet. The phenotypic outcomes of these environmental responses may have profound effects on their properties as food. This is the case for both plants and animals, as the following examples demonstrate.

Research in the field of plant epigenetics is relatively scarce (as an example, a PubMed search for "plant epigenetics" returned 338 references, compared to 4.384 references on "human epigenetics"; April 2013), with the focus being on either model organisms such as *Arabidopsis*, or staple food plants such as rice and wheat. Nonetheless, research has clearly shown the importance of epigenetic mechanisms in plants. Examples include studies in rice demonstrating heritable changes in nitrogen deficiency tolerance accompanied by modified DNA methylation [36] and promoter DNA methylation conferring pathogen resistance [37]; evidence implicating a developmental role of DNA methylation in regulating tissue-specific gene expression in sorghum [38]; and changes in the genomic distribution of methylation in tomato in response to water stress [39]. These data suggest that understanding epigenetic regulation within plants may enable improvements in their yield and/or nutrient content, and thus make an important contribution to making the best use of these as food sources.

There is a larger body of research on epigenetic mechanisms in animals than in plants (2,318 references from a PubMed search for "animal epigenetics"; April 2013); as in the case of plants, much of this involves model organisms, in particular mice and rats, while research into animals such as cattle and sheep, which are regularly consumed by humans, is not comprehensive. Particular examples include effects on embryogenesis and assisted reproduction using a variety of models, including bovine [40–42] and the role of epigenetic factors in pre-natal programming in the pig [43].

These examples demonstrate that epigenetics can have a major role in phenotypic outcomes of plants and animals; when these are used as food sources, these altered phenotypes may in turn lead to epigenetic changes within the human consumer, with consequent outcomes of relevance to the health of that consumer.

INFLUENCE OF NUTRITION ON EPIGENETICS

The food in our diets is one of the key environmental influences to which we, as consumers of that food, may respond through epigenetic mechanisms. While research into the role of diet in miRNA regulation in particular is relatively novel, there is clear evidence to demonstrate dietary effects on a variety of epigenetic mechanisms, with relevant outcomes in terms of health and well-being in the consumer. Some examples of this research are summarized in Table 12.1.

Evidence of the ability of nutrition to interact with dietary HDAC inhibitors and miRNAs will be described as two examples of nutrient–epigenetic interactions, and the case of food allergy will be used as an example where nutrition may have an important health outcome via epigenetic mechanisms.

Dietary HDAC Inhibitors

Over recent years, a number of different compounds have been identified that possess the ability to either inhibit or activate groups of histone-modifying enzymes, primarily HDACs and HATs. HDAC inhibitors represent a promising therapeutic approach for diseases including cancer [75], and dietary compounds that can alter histone acetylation offer novel strategies for preventing, delaying, or reversing these diseases through simple dietary choices. Dietary manipulation of histone structure and function through specific nutrients and other compounds has been gaining increasing interest particularly due to their accessibility to the general population as well as their ability to act as primary protective agents [76,77]. For instance, in the case of inflammatory bowel diseases, particular food constituents may be important for modulating specific epigenetic changes to reduce inflammation and ultimately lower the risk of colon cancer; all by making subtle modifications to the histone code.

Some food components have the ability to influence histone acetylation either via inhibition of HATs or type I, II, and III HDAC enzymes; several of which are outlined in Table 12.1. Curcumin and copper have been shown to induce histone

TABLE 12.1
Food Components for Which There Is Evidence of an Influence on Epigenetic Mechanisms

	Dietary Component	Food Source	Epigenetic Mechanism	References
DNA Methylation	Apigenin	Celery, parsley	Inhibits DNMT-mediated DNA methylation	[44]
	Betanin	Red beetroot	Inhibits DNMT-mediated DNA methylation	[45]
	Bioflavonoids (fisetin, myricetin, quercitin)	Poison ivy, berries and citrus (respectively)	Inhibits DNMT-1-mediated DNA methylation	[46]
	Caffeic acid	Coffee	Inhibits DNMT-mediated DNA methylation	[47]
	Coumaric/ hydroxycinnamic acid	Cinnamon	Inhibits DNMT-mediated DNA methylation	[44]
	Curcumin	Tumeric	Inhibits DNMT-mediated DNA methylation	[44,48]
	Ellagic acids	Berries	Inhibits DNMT-mediated DNA methylation	[45]
	Genistein	Soy	Inhibits DNMT-mediated DNA methylation	[44,49]
	Isothiocyanates (e.g., sulforaphane)	Broccoli, cruciferous vegetables	Unknown but results in reduced methylation of *GSTP1* Sulforaphane - decreased expression of DNMTs	[50]
	Lycopene	Tomatoes	Unknown but results in reduced methylation of *GSTP1, RARβ and HIN-1*	[49]
	Protocatechuric acid	Olives	Inhibits DNMT-mediated DNA methylation	[45]
	Resveratrol	Grapes, wine, eucalyptus	Inhibits DNMT-mediated DNA methylation	[45]
	Sinapic acid	Mustard	Inhibits DNMT-mediated DNA methylation	[45]
	Tea polyphenols (catechin, epicatechin, etc.)	Green tea	Inhibits DNMT-mediated DNA methylation	[51]
Histone Modifications	Allicin	Garlic	H4 acetylation	[52]
	Anacardic acid	Cashew nuts	HAT inhibitor; results in H3K9 and H3K14 deacetylation	[53,54]
	Coumaric/ hydroxycinnamic acid	Cinnamon	HDAC inhibitor; results in histone acetylation	[55]
	Curcumin	Turmeric	HAT inhibitor; results in H3/H4 deacetylation	[53]
	Diallyl disulfide	Garlic	HDAC inhibitor; results in increased H3/H4 acetylation	[56,57]

	Equol	Soy	HDAC inhibitor; results in H2A/H2B/H3/H4 acetylation	[58]
	Flavone	Feijoa	HDAC inhibitor; results in histone acetylation	[59]
	Genistein	Soy	HAT activator/HDAC inhibitor; results in H2A/H2B/H3/H4 acetylation	[58,60]
	Isothiocyanates (e.g., sulforaphane)	Broccoli, cruciferous vegetables	HDAC inhibitor; results in H3/H4 acetylation	[61,62]
	Quercitin	Citrus, apple, berries	HAT inhibitor, SIRT1 activator; influences expression of *IP-10, MIP-2*	[63]
	Resveratrol	Grapes, wine, eucalyptus	SIRT1 activator; influences expression of *TNFα*, *IL-8*, *RBP*	[63,64]
	Sanguinarine	Opium poppy	HAT inhibitor; results in H3/H4 deacetylation; histone methylation inhibitor; results in H3K9/H3K4 demethylation	[65]
	Tea polyphenols (catechin, epicatechin, etc.)	Green tea	HAT inhibitor; results in reduced histone acetylation	[66]
	Ursolic acid	Basil	HDAC inhibitor; results in histone acetylation	[67]
	Curcumin	Turmeric	Up-regulation of miRNA-22; leads to suppression of *SP1* and *ESR1*	[68]
	Epigalocatechin-3-gallate	Green tea	Up-regulation of miR-16 and modified expression of at least 60 other miRNAs	[69]
	Ethanol	Alcohol	Up-regulation of miR-212 in human colon; up-regulation of several miRNA and reduction of others in mouse fetal brain	[70,71]
Micro RNAs	Fat		High fat diet up-regulates expression of miR-143 in mesenteric fat	[72]
	Genistein	Soy	Modulates expression of miR-27a; up-regulates expression of miR-146a	[73]
	Vitamin E deficiency	Sunflower seeds, almonds	Reduced expression of miR-122a and miR-122b	[74]

hypoacetylation by inhibiting HAT activity *in vitro* thereby triggering oxidative stress resulting in the arrest of cell proliferation [78,79]. Studies in animal models have also shown that curcumin acts as a protective agent against cardiac hypertrophy, inflammation, and fibrosis through both suppression of HAT activity and down-regulation of several key signaling pathways [80,81]. Of the green tea polyphenols, epigalocatechin-3-gallate is the most potent HAT inhibitor displaying great potential as a chemopreventative agent for chronic inflammation [66]. Likewise, quercitin, found in a variety of different fruits, also displays HAT inhibition [82] as well as the dual role of activating sirtuin 1 (SIRT1), a class III HDAC [83]. Caloric restriction has also been shown to decrease cancer susceptibility by increasing the activity of type III HDACs. For example, resveratrol, a polyphenolic compound found in grapes, wine, and peanuts, has been shown to increase expression of the NAD-dependent HDAC SIRT1 and mimic the caloric restriction pathways for longevity in *Caenorhabditis elegans* and *Drosophila melanogaster* [63]. However, this compound is more likely to play a role in aging and neurodegenerative diseases.

Butyrate, the smallest known HDAC inhibitor formed from the fermentation of dietary fiber by colonic microbiota, has been shown to exert anti-inflammatory and anti-proliferative effects, particularly in ulcerative colitis [84]. Although micromolar to low millimolar concentrations are required for HDAC inhibition *in vitro*, these levels are considered to be achievable in the gastrointestinal tract, where butyrate serves as the principal oxidative fuel for colonocytes. Diallyl disulfide—among the first compounds to be described as having an impact on histone acetylation [56]—and sulforaphane (found in cruciferous vegetables) also act as HDAC inhibitors and have been shown to inhibit cell proliferation and stimulate apoptosis in a manner analogous to other clinical HDAC inhibitors [85]. Healthy human volunteers fed broccoli sprouts (1 cup/day), which naturally contain high-level sulforaphane, showed hyperacetylation of histones H3 and H4 in normal circulating blood cells. The level of HDAC inhibition was greater than, or equal to, that achieved with the clinically used HDAC inhibitor vorinostat. Sulforaphane has also been shown to inhibit HDAC activity in human colon cancer cells accompanied by both global and localized histone hyperacetylation, G2/M cell cycle arrest, and increased apoptosis [86]. Studies have also demonstrated that sulforaphane inhibits HDAC activity *in vivo* and suppresses tumor development with significant inhibition of spontaneous intestinal polyps in Apc^{min} mice, which have been used extensively in studies with chemopreventive agents [61].

Molecular modeling studies also suggest that dietary compounds such as vitamin H (biotin), lipoic acid, and metabolites of vitamin E and conjugated linoleic acids may be HDAC inhibitors [87]. For example, biotinylation of histone 4 (at lysine 8 and 12) has been associated with heterochromatin structures, gene silencing, mitotic condensation of chromatin, and DNA repair [88,89]. Histone biotinylation appears to be a reversible process and depends on an exogenous biotin supply which suggests that foods rich in biotin may play an important role in maintaining "normal" chromatin structure.

While *in vitro* evidence has made significant contributions to the understanding of the epigenetic mechanisms associated with dietary agents, additional clinical studies are still required to examine the safety profiles of various doses of these compounds together with the possible interactions between different food components. An important consideration is whether or not the concentrations of these dietary compounds required for inhibition of HDAC activity are achievable under normal physiological conditions or whether it is more feasible to extract these compounds from natural sources and use them to fortify existing foods or beverages.

Non-Coding RNA

ncRNAs such as miRNAs may be the epigenetic mechanism with the greatest potential by which nutrition can act to influence health. They are able to respond very rapidly to external stimuli and influence gene expression. Some examples of nutritional influences on miRNAs include the polyphenolic compound curcumin (found in the spice turmeric) and genistein from soy. Curcumin has been shown to alter miRNA expression in human pancreatic cells, increasing the abundance of miRNA-22 and decreasing miRNA-199a*. The up-regulation of miRNA-22 in turn suppresses the expression of its target genes SP1 transcription factor (SP1) and estrogen receptor 1 (ESR1) [68]. In the case of genistein, in human uveal melanoma cells, it has been shown to reduce levels of microRNA-27a (miR-27a) with a consequent increase in expression of one of its target genes, zinc finger and BTB domain containing 10 (ZBTB10), which may be a mechanism by which cell growth is inhibited [73]. More examples of food compounds for which evidence of an effect on miRNA function exists are shown in Table 12.1.

An important point to consider is the highly stable nature of miRNAs. Recent research has clearly shown that miRNAs found in foods are sufficiently stable to survive cooking and digestion, and they have been identified intact in human plasma following ingestion [90]. Not only that, but these intact plant miRNAs are able to directly act to influence the expression of genes within the human host [90]. Thus, when endeavoring to establish the potential effects of miRNAs on human health, it is not only necessary to consider the influence that miRNAs may be having on the phenotype of the food and the role that food components may have on miRNA expression in the consumer, but the possibility that miRNAs from the food (be it plant or animal) may be making their way intact through the digestion process and subsequently directly influencing gene expression in the consumer.

Food Allergies

There has been a dramatic increase in the prevalence of food allergies over recent years, particularly in westernized countries with high rates of respiratory and skin allergies. For instance, in Australia, food allergy now affects up to 10% of infants [91]. Food allergy susceptibility and early immune function have been linked to a combination of maternal phenotype, infant genotype, and environmental exposures during critical periods of development (e.g., *in utero* or early postnatal life) that affect early gene expression [92]. For example, environmental exposure during pregnancy to dietary changes, microbial burden, medications, smoking, and other pollutants have all been shown to have effects on the fetal immune function in pregnancy [93]. As is the case for cardiovascular disease, type II diabetes, obesity, and hypertension [14], the rise in allergic disease has occurred faster than that can be explained by genetic factors alone. Epigenetic mechanisms are a likely means by which these environmental exposures can alter gene expression and disease risk [91] and because these changes can be inherited across subsequent generations, there is the potential for an allergy risk to be amplified [92].

Although there are very limited studies that have investigated the role of epigenetics in food allergy, inferences can be made from studies of other allergic reactions, such as asthma and eczema, which are strongly associated with food allergies [94]. Several asthma studies suggest a link between epigenetic gene regulation, immunity, and physiological development. For instance, pregnant mice fed a methyl donor-enriched diet had offspring with enhanced allergic airway disease [95]. This demonstrates that dietary factors can modify the heritable risk of allergies during fetal development, in this case by enhancing DNA methylation at specific CpG motifs to alter gene expression. There is also considerable evidence that epigenetic regulation mechanisms, such as histone modifications and DNA methylation patterns, play a central role in T-cell development where an altered Th1 (proinflammatory)/Th2 (anti-inflammatory) balance results in allergic disease [96]. Because recent studies indicate that epigenetic changes are responsible for differentiation of key regulatory (Treg) and inflammatory (Th17) immune T-cells [97] and other cell types and cellular processes may also be regulated by genes under epigenetic control, this process may play a key role in a broad range of immune-related processes [96].

A variety of maternal nutritional changes during pregnancy have been implicated in immune development and allergic risk, including a reduction in the intake of n-3 PUFAs [98], antioxidants [99], and a range of specific vitamins and micronutrients [93]. These changes associated with the "modern," more processed diet, appear to affect the composition of intestinal microbiota as well as tolerance development [100]. Whereas avoidance of specific "allergenic" foods is no longer recommended for allergy prevention, preliminary investigations of maternal supplementation with fish oil [101], pre- and probiotics [102], and vitamins such as vitamin D [103] suggest that these may have some beneficial effect on immune function by inducing tolerance and reducing the risk of allergic disease [100]. Thus, through epigenetic mechanisms, nutrition offers promising opportunities for re-programming gene expression to both prevent and at least partially ameliorate food allergy and this may represent a key target for epigenetic functional foods.

EPIGENETICS AND FUNCTIONAL FOODS

As noted earlier, the concept of functional foods has been around since at least the time of the ancient Greeks [1]. The term "functional food" was much more recently coined by the Japanese [104] and has since been the focus of many reviews [104,105]. While it has been suggested that functional foods can only be classed as such if they provide nutrients which are non-essential and provide health benefits [106], functional foods are typically described as foods that provide benefits (health and physiological) above and beyond simply providing nutrients and energy [107].

Many functional foods target digestive health (Table 12.2); however, interest in other market sectors (including obesity, aging, stress, and energy levels) is growing [108]. While the early development of an organism has been indicated as a key time during which epigenetic changes occur, aging has also been postulated as a potential key period for epigenetic change [109]. Therefore, opportunities exist to develop

TABLE 12.2
Some Examples of Currently Available Functional Foods and Their Potential Influence on Epigenetic Mechanisms

Trend	Brand	Product	Target Nutrient	Does Target Nutrient Have a Potential Epigenetic Effect?	Ref
Digestive health	Yoplait	Yoplus	Probiotic	No[a]	[128]
	Danone	Activia	Probiotic	No[a]	[128]
	General Mills	Fiber One	Fiber	Potential via breakdown products	[129]
	Yakult	Yakult	Probiotic	No[a]	[128]
		ProViva	Probiotic	No[a]	[128]
	Kellogg's	FiberPlus	Fiber	Potential via breakdown products	[129]
	Bimbo	Doble Fibra	Fiber	Potential via breakdown products	[129]
Energy	Austrian Red Bull GmbH	Red Bull	Taurine	Unknown for specific amino acids however protein can exert epigenetic effects	
			Glucuronolactone	Unknown	
			Caffeine	Yes	[130]
			B vitamins	Yes	
	5-Hour Energy		B-vitamins	Yes	
			Amino acids	Unknown for specific amino acids however protein can exert epigenetic effects	
			Caffeine	Yes	[130]
	Ocean Spray	Cranergy	Not stated		
Fruit	Ocean Spray	Craisins	Not stated		
		ProViva	Probiotic	No[a]	[128]
	Compal	Essential	Fruit	Unknown however diets high in fruit and vegetables are associated with lower levels of hypermethylation in humans	[131]

(*Continued*)

TABLE 12.2 (*Continued*)
Some Examples of Currently Available Functional Foods and Their Potential Influence on Epigenetic Mechanisms

Trend	Brand	Product	Target Nutrient	Does Target Nutrient Have a Potential Epigenetic Effect?	Ref
			Cranberry	Unknown	
			Blueberry	Unknown	
			Pomegranate	Unknown	
			Fig	Unknown	
			Prune	Unknown	
			Rhubarb	Unknown	
			Pear	Unknown	
Weight management	Kellogg's	Special K	Protein	Yes low protein diets during gestation affect epigenetic markers in offspring.	[132,133]
		NeuroTrim	Konjac	Unknown	
	Unilever	Slimfast			
Naturally healthy and ultra-convenient		Broccosprouts	Sulforaphane (broccoli)	Yes	[134]
	James White Drinks	Beet It	Nitrates (beetroot juice)	Unknown	
	Vita	Vita Coco	Electrolytes (coconut water)	Unknown	
			Almonds	Unknown	
			Pistachios	Unknown	
Antioxidants		Pom Wonderful	Antioxidants (pomegranate)	Unknown	
	Nestle	Nescafe Green Blend	Antioxidants (coffee)	Yes (coffee phenols)	[47]
Immunity	Valio	Gelfis	Probiotic (LLG)		
	Lonsdale	Oasis Health break	Juice (Blackcurrant, elderberry)	Unknown	
			Vitamin D	Yes	[135]
Bones & movement		Joint Juice	Glucosamine	Yes	[6]
		Elations			
	Danone	Densia			
	Fonterra	Anlene	Calcium	Unknown	
			Chondroitin	Unknown	

[a] This may depend on the specific strain/s included in the probiotic.

functional foods for the developing (via maternal transfer either *in utero* or via breast milk) and aging human.

With few exceptions, functional foods do not typically focus on specific nutrients, and the beneficial effects of consuming functional foods should be a part of a "normal" diet [104]. However, specific nutrients can have functional benefits (e.g., antioxidants, dietary fiber) and the inclusion of these nutrients within a food can result in them being considered "functional." These nutrients include n-3 fatty acids, vitamins A, C, D and E, and micronutrients [104,108].

The mode of action of functional nutrients may differ. For example, nutrients that are known to exert epigenetic effects include those involved in one carbon metabolism because they influence the supply of methyl groups and the biochemical pathways of methylation [107]. These include folate, vitamin B_2, vitamin B_6, vitamin B_{12}, methionine, choline, betaine, and zinc [107]. Selenium has also been of interest in terms of epigenetic regulation of disease due to the link between selenomethionine supplementation and reduction in cancer-associated morbidity [110,111] coupled with the link between DNA methylation and cancer [112]. Additionally, selenium is thought to prevent cancer and cardiovascular disease through its role in the immune response and "antioxidant" effects [113].

It is possible to manipulate the concentration of nutrients implicated in the epigenetic regulation of the host in whole foods. For example, selenium-enriched broccoli [114–116], milk [117–119], and meat [120] have been produced and tested in experimental models. Additionally, it is possible to enrich quail eggs with lycopene [121] and n-3 PUFAs [105]. It is clear that consumers prefer food that has been enriched naturally [122,123], and it is therefore important to consider the method by which a functional ingredient is incorporated into a food.

It is also clear that the bioavailability and form of nutrients can affect their functionality. For example, it is known that the form of selenium may impact its effect on selenoprotein activity or gene activity [124,125]. A study that compared the ability of different forms of selenium to reduce colon cancer showed that selenium-enriched milk was more bioavailable compared to selenium yeast and more protective against colorectal cancer [118]. However, the effects of different forms of nutrients and their bioavailability on their ability to influence epigenetic mechanisms are less well understood. For instance, in mice fed selenium in the forms of sodium selenite, selenomethionine, and yeast-derived selenium, a reduction in DNA oxidation was only observed in mice fed yeast-derived selenium [125]. This suggests that the form of selenium may impact on its ability to alter epigenetic mechanisms in the host. Similarly, the bioavailability of folate (the form that occurs naturally in foods) is 50% compared with between 70 and 85% for folic acid (the form found in supplements) [126,127], which may have implications on the ability of this supplement to influence DNA methylation via one carbon metabolism.

A range of functional foods available globally which has been recently described [108] is listed in Table 12.2. While some of these foods contain nutrients that have functional properties, it is largely unknown whether they exert their health benefits via epigenetic mechanisms. Those functional foods for which a substantiated claim of acting via an epigenetic effect can be made may increase their "point of difference" from competitors (and thereby their value), a potentially important factor given the increasingly difficult regulations surrounding health claims.

Food Pollutants

Having discussed the possible role of epigenetics in the development of functional foods, it is worth briefly mentioning the potential unintended functional role of components that may occur within foods, such as pollutants or contaminants. There is research suggesting that compounds such as genistein in soy [73,136] or bisphenol-A in plastics [137] may have epigenetic effects, at least in animal models. This is highly relevant because of the widespread use of soy as a food source and of plastics containing bisphenol-A as a packaging material for food and beverage products [138]. The health implications of these compounds, particularly over the longer term, are less clear. However, because maternal exposure to either genistein or bisphenol-A during gestation can alter DNA methylation in the offspring with associated potential health impacts [136,137] the long-term consequences may be profound. While genistein could be relevant for a specific, targeted health outcome, because it is an "invisible" ingredient of soy-containing foods [138], its presence must be taken into account for any soy-containing foods designed to modulate epigenetic targets. In the case of compounds such as bisphenol-A, there may be important implications for processing and/or packaging of foods to ensure that contamination is not occurring.

Contamination of foods by agricultural chemicals such as insecticides is also of some concern. Pesticide residues including organochlorine, organophosphorus, and pyrethroids may be found in various food commodities such as wheat [139]. While the evidence of epigenetic effects associated with exposure to such residues is scarce, it has been observed that early exposure to the pyrethroid insecticide permethrin results in heart damage in adult rats [140]. While not conclusively demonstrated, the authors of this study suggest that long-term consequences of a short period of neonatal exposure to permethrin are the result of epigenetic changes occurring during this key period of development. While these effects may not be of concern to the majority of consumers, they may be of particular relevance for foods targeted at, for example, pregnant women or newborn babies.

Finally, while many studies have assumed that environmental contaminants that enter the food chain and end up in the maternal diet are directly influencing the offspring, there is also evidence that these contaminants may influence maternal behavior toward the offspring, for which there is also evidence of potential long-term effects modulated by epigenetic mechanisms [141].

EPIGENETICS AND PERSONALIZED NUTRITION

Nutrigenomics is a field of science with the goal of understanding how foods and food components interact with different individuals, with consequent divergent effects on health due to the genetic variability of those individuals. In the longer term, the aim is to develop a personalized approach to nutrition, whereby a person's genotype could be matched to their diet for optimal health, or novel foods could be developed to target a specific health outcome. While initially focused on genetic variations such as SNPs and how these might impact on food–gene interactions, it is clear that the plasticity of epigenetic mechanisms makes these an important component of any comprehensive approach to personalized nutrition.

As is the case for nutrigenomics, any approach aimed at personalized nutrition based on influencing epigenetic mechanisms will be faced by a number of questions or issues. For example, how likely is it that "tailored nutrition" based on individual genotype and/or epigenetic characteristics will be achieved, given the enormous complexity of understanding the interactions involved? While the idea of a $1,000 genome has been a goal for some time, and according to recent reports has now been achieved [142], this does not include the cost of information technology to process the data, or of medical expertise to interpret the data [143]. Thus, the concept of having an individual genome analysis available would be well beyond the financial scope of the majority of people.

Another question is: what are the likely benefits of the personalized approach compared with more general approaches? For example, as mentioned earlier, chronic inflammation may be an underlying factor for a variety of diseases. Thus, a functional food that acts to reduce inflammation *per se*, potentially via epigenetic mechanisms, may be of greater benefit than one which targets a specific inflammatory disorder in a single person, although the benefit to that individual may be greater.

There is also a range of ethical issues associated with information on either genotype or an individual's epigenetic makeup. Who would have access to such information, and what are the potential issues relating to, for example, health insurance? Would a certain genotype or epigenetic "pattern" be cause for exclusion on the basis of disease pre-disposition?

While these issues are important, they may be considered peripheral to the central scientific question: is personalized nutrition incorporating comprehensive measurement and/or manipulation of epigenetic mechanisms possible and/or feasible? Currently, the answer to this is "no." While the pace of advances in the ability to measure genetic variation on a genome-wide scale is nothing short of remarkable, this is trailed by the computational ability to interpret this information, although development of this also proceeds at a rapid rate. Furthermore, as discussed previously with reference to the $1,000 genome, there is still a need for further reduction in cost before a truly personalized approach could be available to all but the wealthiest. Even if these issues are overcome, there remains the question of at what point a personalized food becomes economically viable. A recent report indicated that functional foods (those containing phytosterols and -staonols) were less cost effective in reducing cardiovascular disease compared to medical treatment [144]. While foods targeted based on genetic or epigenetic information would command a price premium, the idea of foods being made on an individual level seems impossible from the perspective of food production. Thus, it seems more likely that dietary advice and food choices could be targeted at an individual level, whereas foods that can influence the epigenetic machinery of the cell would be targeted at significant subgroups of the population where there is the possibility of sufficient economic return on the investment required to develop such foods.

SUMMARY AND CONCLUSIONS

It seems clear that epigenetic mechanisms are a potentially important target for functional foods, with their plasticity making them amenable to dietary modulation. However, understanding the highly complex nature of an individual's epigenome, the interactions with the large variety of compounds found within foods, and the added complexity of the underlying variation in genotype represent a difficult challenge. There is a need for further development of current high-throughput genetic tools to enable such analysis to be within the reach of individuals or sub-groups of the population. The costs currently associated with these analyses lead to the issue of whether they may only be available to the "worried well," people with sufficient income to afford them who may not have the greatest need. Associated with this is the question of whether this approach could be considered elitist. There are also ethical issues associated with the appropriateness of applying such technologies to diseases of Western society, many of which may be at least in part the result of poor lifestyle choices and thus largely self-inflicted.

It is also pertinent to consider the relevance of tailored or personalized nutrition in the context of the global increase in demand for food amid the ever-increasing human population. One could ask whether understanding epigenetic regulation within food sources which may enable development of better foods, or improved food production practices, which capitalize on epigenetic manipulation, is more important than the development of functional foods targeting a relatively small sector of the population in a global context of maintaining "food security" (i.e., ensuring that there is sufficient food available).

As is the case with so many issues, this may represent finding a balance between the needs of the many versus the needs of a few. While the study of epigenetics is clearly of potential relevance to both food production and the development of functional foods targeting personalized nutrition, a better understanding of the former would appear to be of more urgent need at the current time, and is arguably a better use of scientific resource. This would not, however, preclude the application of fundamental information concerning epigenetics and food to the issue of personalized nutrition and functional foods, and there is no reason why research into both should not proceed in parallel.

REFERENCES

1. Shivashankara, A.R. et al., Dietary agents in the prevention of alcohol-induced hepatotoxicty: preclinical observations. *Food Funct*, 2011. 3(2): p. 101–9.
2. Jiang, M. et al., The role of Chinese medicine in the treatment of chronic diseases in China. *Planta Med*, 2011. 77(9): p. 873–81.
3. Farr, D.R., Functional foods. *Cancer Lett*, 1997. 114(1–2): p. 59–63.
4. Thomson, C.D. et al., Brazil nuts: an effective way to improve selenium status. *Am J Clin Nutr*, 2008. 87(2): p. 379–84.
5. Opperman, M., W. Marais de, and A.J. Spinnler Benade, Analysis of omega-3 fatty acid content of South African fish oil supplements. *Cardiovasc J Afr*, 2011. 22(6): p. 324–9.
6. Imagawa, K. et al., The epigenetic effect of glucosamine and a nuclear factor-kappa B (NF-kB) inhibitor on primary human chondrocytes—implications for osteoarthritis. *Biochem Biophys Res Commun*, 2011. 405(3): p. 362–67.

7. Ordovas, J.M. and V. Mooser, Nutrigenomics and nutrigenetics. *Curr Opin Lipidol*, 2004. 15(2): p. 101–8.
8. Waddington, C.H., The epigenotype. *Endeavour*, 1942. 1: p. 18.
9. Haig, D., The (dual) origin of epigenetics. *Cold Spring Harb Symp Quant Biol*, 2004. 69: p. 67–70.
10. Waddington, C.H., Embryology, epigenetics and biogenetics. *Nature*, 1956. 177: p. 1241.
11. Nanney, D.L., Epigenetic factors affecting mating type expression in certain ciliates. *Cold Spring Harb Symp Quant Biol*, 1959. 23: p. 327.
12. Gluckman, P.D. et al., Epigenetic mechanisms that underpin metabolic and cardiovascular diseases. *Nat Rev Endocrinol*, 2009. 5(7): p. 401–8.
13. Waterland, R.A., Is epigenetics an important link between early life events and adult disease? *Horm Res*, 2009. 71 Suppl 1: p. 13–6.
14. Lillycrop, K.A., Effect of maternal diet on the epigenome: implications for human metabolic disease. *Proc Nutr Soc*, 2011. 70(1): p. 64–72.
15. Handel, A.E. and S.V. Ramagopalan, Is Lamarckian evolution relevant to medicine? *BMC Med Genet*, 2010. 11: p. 73.
16. Jablonka, E. and G. Raz, Transgenerational epigenetic inheritance: prevalence, mechanisms, and implications for the study of heredity and evolution. *Q Rev Biol*, 2009. 84(2): p. 131–76.
17. Riggs, A.D., R.A. Martienssen, and V.E.A. Russo, Introduction, in *Epigenetic Mechanisms of Gene Regulation*, ed. V.E.A. Russo et al., 1996, Cold Spring Harbor Laboratory Press: Cold Spring Harbor, New York. p. 1.
18. Doerfler, W., The almost-forgotten fifth nucleotide in DNA: an introduction. *Curr Top Microbiol Immunol*, 2006. 301: p. 3–18.
19. Clark, S.J., Action at a distance: epigenetic silencing of large chromosomal regions in carcinogenesis. *Hum Mol Genet*, 2007. 16 Spec No 1: p. R88–95.
20. Karpinski, P. et al., The CpG island methylator phenotype correlates with long-range epigenetic silencing in colorectal cancer. *Mol Cancer Res*, 2008. 6(4): p. 585–91.
21. Novak, P. et al., Agglomerative epigenetic aberrations are a common event in human breast cancer. *Cancer Res*, 2008. 68(20): p. 8616–25.
22. Lee, G.R. et al., T helper cell differentiation: regulation by cis elements and epigenetics. *Immunity*, 2006. 24(4): p. 369–79.
23. Mathers, J.C., Pulses and carcinogenesis: potential for the prevention of colon, breast and other cancers. *Br J Nutr*, 2002. 88 Suppl 3: p. S273–9.
24. Wilson, A.S., B.E. Power, and P.L. Molloy, DNA hypomethylation and human diseases. *Biochim Biophys Acta*, 2007. 1775(1): p. 138–62.
25. Guo, J.U. et al., Hydroxylation of 5-methylcytosine by TET1 promotes active DNA demethylation in the adult brain. *Cell*, 2011. 145(3): p. 423–34.
26. Szulwach, K.E. et al., 5-hmC-mediated epigenetic dynamics during postnatal neurodevelopment and aging. *Nat Neurosci*, 2011. 14(12): p. 1607–16.
27. Nestor, C.E. et al., Tissue-type is a major modifier of the 5-hydroxymethylcytosine content of human genes. *Genome Res*, 2012. 22(3): p. 467–77.
28. Song, C.X. and C. He, The hunt for 5-hydroxymethylcytosine: the sixth base. *Epigenomics*, 2011. 3(5): p. 521–3.
29. Martin, C. and Y. Zhang, The diverse functions of histone lysine methylation. *Nat Rev Mol Cell Biol*, 2005. 6(11): p. 838–49.
30. Filipowicz, W., S.N. Bhattacharyya, and N. Sonenberg, Mechanisms of post-transcriptional regulation by microRNAs: are the answers in sight? *Nat Rev Genet*, 2008. 9(2): p. 102–14.
31. Quinn, S.R. and L.A. O'Neill, A trio of microRNAs that control Toll-like receptor signalling. *Int Immunol*, 2011. 23(7): p. 421–5.

32. Orom, U.A., F.C. Nielsen, and A.H. Lund, MicroRNA-10a binds the 5′UTR of ribosomal protein mRNAs and enhances their translation. *Mol Cell*, 2008. 30(4): p. 460–71.
33. Roberts, A.P., A.P. Lewis, and C.L. Jopling, miR-122 activates hepatitis C virus translation by a specialized mechanism requiring particular RNA components. *Nucleic Acids Res*, 2011. 39(17): p. 7716–29.
34. Dinger, M.E., T.R. Mercer, and J.S. Mattick, RNAs as extracellular signaling molecules. *J Mol Endocrinol*, 2008. 40(4): p. 151–9.
35. Kato, M. and F.J. Slack, microRNAs: small molecules with big roles—*C. elegans* to human cancer. *Biol Cell*, 2008. 100(2): p. 71–81.
36. Kou, H.P. et al., Heritable alteration in DNA methylation induced by nitrogen-deficiency stress accompanies enhanced tolerance by progenies to the stress in rice (Oryza sativa L.). *J Plant Physiol*, 2011. 168(14): p. 1685–93.
37. Li, Y. et al., Induced pib expression and resistance to magnaporthe grisea are compromised by cytosine demethylation at critical promoter regions in rice. *J Integr Plant Biol*, 2011. 53(10): p. 814–23.
38. Zhang, M. et al., Tissue-specific differences in cytosine methylation and their association with differential gene expression in sorghum. *Plant Physiol*, 2011. 156(4): p. 1955–66.
39. Gonzalez, R.M., M.M. Ricardi, and N.D. Iusem, Atypical epigenetic mark in an atypical location: cytosine methylation at asymmetric (CNN) sites within the body of a non-repetitive tomato gene. *BMC Plant Biol*, 2011. 11(1): p. 94.
40. El Hajj, N. et al., Limiting dilution bisulfite (pyro)sequencing reveals parent-specific methylation patterns in single early mouse embryos and bovine oocytes. *Epigenetics*, 2011. 6(10): p. 1176–88.
41. Hecht, N. et al., Protamine-1 represents a sperm specific gene transcript: a study in Callithrix jacchus and Bos taurus. *Andrologia*, 2011. 43(3): p. 167–73.
42. Smith, C.S. et al., Nuclear transfer-specific defects are not apparent during the second week of embryogenesis in cattle. *Cell Reprogram*, 2010. 12(6): p. 699–707.
43. Foxcroft, G.R. et al., Prenatal programming of postnatal development in the pig. *Soc Reprod Fertil Suppl*, 2009. 66: p. 213–31.
44. Fang, M., D. Chen, and C.S. Yang, Dietary polyphenols may affect DNA methylation. *J Nutr*, 2007. 137(1 Suppl): p. 223S–8S.
45. Paluszczak, J., V. Krajka-Kuzniak, and W. Baer-Dubowska, The effect of dietary polyphenols on the epigenetic regulation of gene expression in MCF7 breast cancer cells. *Toxicol Lett*, 2010. 192(2): p. 119–25.
46. Lee, W.J., J.Y. Shim, and B.T. Zhu, Mechanisms for the inhibition of DNA methyltransferases by tea catechins and bioflavonoids. *Mol Pharmacol*, 2005. 68(4): p. 1018–30.
47. Lee, W.J. and B.T. Zhu, Inhibition of DNA methylation by caffeic acid and chlorogenic acid, two common catechol-containing coffee polyphenols. *Carcinogenesis*, 2006. 27(2): p. 269–77.
48. Liu, Z. et al., Curcumin is a potent DNA hypomethylation agent. *Bioorg Med Chem Lett*, 2009. 19(3): p. 706–9.
49. King-Batoon, A., J.M. Leszczynska, and C.B. Klein, Modulation of gene methylation by genistein or lycopene in breast cancer cells. *Environ Mol Mutagen*, 2008. 49(1): p. 36–45.
50. Traka, M. et al., Transcriptome analysis of human colon Caco-2 cells exposed to sulforaphane. *J Nutr*, 2005. 135(8): p. 1865–72.
51. Fang, M.Z. et al., Tea polyphenol (−)-epigallocatechin-3-gallate inhibits DNA methyltransferase and reactivates methylation-silenced genes in cancer cell lines. *Cancer Res*, 2003. 63(22): p. 7563–70.
52. Lea, M.A. et al., Induction of histone acetylation and inhibition of growth of mouse erythroleukemia cells by S-allylmercaptocysteine. *Nutr Cancer*, 2002. 43(1): p. 90–102.

53. Sbardella, G. et al., Identification of long chain alkylidenemalonates as novel small molecule modulators of histone acetyltransferases. *Bioorg Med Chem Lett*, 2008. 18(9): p. 2788–92.
54. Sun, Y. et al., Inhibition of histone acetyltransferase activity by anacardic acid sensitizes tumor cells to ionizing radiation. *FEBS Lett*, 2006. 580(18): p. 4353–6.
55. Waldecker, M. et al., Inhibition of histone-deacetylase activity by short-chain fatty acids and some polyphenol metabolites formed in the colon. *J Nutr Biochem*, 2008. 19(9): p. 587–93.
56. Lea, M.A., V.M. Randolph, and M. Patel, Increased acetylation of histones induced by diallyl disulfide and structurally related molecules. *Int J Oncol*, 1999. 15(2): p. 347–52.
57. Druesne, N. et al., Repetitive treatments of colon HT-29 cells with diallyl disulfide induce a prolonged hyperacetylation of histone H3 K14. *Ann N Y Acad Sci*, 2004. 1030: p. 612–21.
58. Hong, T. et al., Isoflavones stimulate estrogen receptor-mediated core histone acetylation. *Biochem Biophys Res Commun*, 2004. 317(1): p. 259–64.
59. Bontempo, P. et al., Feijoa sellowiana derived natural Flavone exerts anti-cancer action displaying HDAC inhibitory activities. *Int J Biochem Cell Biol*, 2007. 39(10): p. 1902–14.
60. Majid, S. et al., BTG3 tumor suppressor gene promoter demethylation, histone modification and cell cycle arrest by genistein in renal cancer. *Carcinogenesis*, 2009. 30(4): p. 662–70.
61. Myzak, M.C. et al., Sulforaphane inhibits histone deacetylase in vivo and suppresses tumorigenesis in Apc-minus mice. *FASEB J*, 2006. 20(3): p. 506–8.
62. Lea, M.A. et al., Induction of histone acetylation in mouse erythroleukemia cells by some organosulfur compounds including allyl isothiocyanate. *Int J Cancer*, 2001. 92(6): p. 784–9.
63. Wood, J.G. et al., Sirtuin activators mimic caloric restriction and delay ageing in metazoans. *Nature*, 2004. 430(7000): p. 686–9.
64. Yang, S.R. et al., Sirtuin regulates cigarette smoke-induced proinflammatory mediator release via RelA/p65 NF-kappaB in macrophages in vitro and in rat lungs in vivo: implications for chronic inflammation and aging. *Am J Physiol Lung Cell Mol Physiol*, 2007. 292(2): p. L567–76.
65. Selvi, B.R. et al., Sanguinarine interacts with chromatin, modulates epigenetic modifications, and transcription in the context of chromatin. *Chem Biol*, 2009. 16(2): p. 203–16.
66. Choi, K.C. et al., Epigallocatechin-3-gallate, a histone acetyltransferase inhibitor, inhibits EBV-induced B lymphocyte transformation via suppression of RelA acetylation. *Cancer Res*, 2009. 69(2): p. 583–92.
67. Chen, I.H. et al., Cytotoxic triterpenoids from the stems of Microtropis japonica. *J Nat Prod*, 2009. 72(7): p. 1231–6.
68. Sun, M. et al., Curcumin (diferuloylmethane) alters the expression profiles of microRNAs in human pancreatic cancer cells. *Mol Cancer Ther*, 2008. 7(3): p. 464–73.
69. Tsang, W.P. and T.T. Kwok, Epigallocatechin gallate up-regulation of miR-16 and induction of apoptosis in human cancer cells. *J Nutr Biochem*, 2010. 21(2): p. 140–6.
70. Tang, Y. et al., Effect of alcohol on miR-212 expression in intestinal epithelial cells and its potential role in alcoholic liver disease. *Alcohol Clin Exp Res*, 2008. 32(2): p. 355–64.
71. Wang, L.L. et al., Ethanol exposure induces differential microRNA and target gene expression and teratogenic effects which can be suppressed by folic acid supplementation. *Hum Reprod*, 2009. 24(3): p. 562–79.
72. Takanabe, R. et al., Up-regulated expression of microRNA-143 in association with obesity in adipose tissue of mice fed high-fat diet. *Biochem Biophys Res Commun*, 2008. 376(4): p. 728–32.

73. Sun, Q. et al., Genistein inhibits growth of human uveal melanoma cells and affects microRNA-27a and target gene expression. *Oncol Rep*, 2009. 22(3): p. 563–7.
74. Gaedicke, S. et al., Vitamin E dependent microRNA regulation in rat liver. *FEBS Lett*, 2008. 582(23–24): p. 3542–6.
75. Minucci, S. and P.G. Pelicci, Histone deacetylase inhibitors and the promise of epigenetic (and more) treatments for cancer. *Nat Rev Cancer*, 2006. 6(1): p. 38–51.
76. Dashwood, R.H. and E. Ho, Dietary histone deacetylase inhibitors: from cells to mice to man. *Semin Cancer Biol*, 2007. 17(5): p. 363–9.
77. Ho, E. and R.H. Dashwood, Dietary manipulation of histone structure and function. *World Rev Nutr Diet*, 2010. 101: p. 95–102.
78. Kang, J. et al., Curcumin-induced histone hypoacetylation: the role of reactive oxygen species. *Biochem Pharmacol*, 2005. 69(8): p. 1205–13.
79. Lin, C., J. Kang, and R. Zheng, Oxidative stress is involved in inhibition of copper on histone acetylation in cells. *Chem Biol Interact*, 2005. 151(3): p. 167–76.
80. Li, H.L. et al., Curcumin prevents and reverses murine cardiac hypertrophy. *J Clin Invest*, 2008. 118(3): p. 879–93.
81. Morimoto, T. et al., The dietary compound curcumin inhibits p300 histone acetyltransferase activity and prevents heart failure in rats. *J Clin Invest*, 2008. 118(3): p. 868–78.
82. Xiao, X. et al., Quercetin suppresses cyclooxygenase-2 expression and angiogenesis through inactivation of P300 signaling. *PLoS One*, 2011. 6(8): p. e22934.
83. Chung, S. et al., Regulation of SIRT1 in cellular functions: role of polyphenols. *Arch Biochem Biophys*, 2010. 501(1): p. 79–90.
84. Gibson, P.R., The intracellular target of butyrate's actions: HDAC or HDON'T? *Gut*, 2000. 46(4): p. 447–8.
85. Garfinkel, M.D. and D.M. Ruden, Chromatin effects in nutrition, cancer, and obesity. *Nutrition*, 2004. 20(1): p. 56–62.
86. Myzak, M.C. and R.H. Dashwood, Histone deacetylases as targets for dietary cancer preventive agents: lessons learned with butyrate, diallyl disulfide, and sulforaphane. *Curr Drug Targets*, 2006. 7(4): p. 443–52.
87. Vannini, A. et al., Crystal structure of a eukaryotic zinc-dependent histone deacetylase, human HDAC8, complexed with a hydroxamic acid inhibitor. *Proc Natl Acad Sci U S A*, 2004. 101(42): p. 15064–9.
88. Davis, C.D. and S.A. Ross, Dietary components impact histone modifications and cancer risk. *Nutr Rev*, 2007. 65(2): p. 88–94.
89. Hassan, Y.I. and J. Zempleni, Epigenetic regulation of chromatin structure and gene function by biotin. *J Nutr*, 2006. 136(7): p. 1763–5.
90. Zhang, L. et al., Exogenous plant MIR168a specifically targets mammalian LDLRAP1: evidence of cross-kingdom regulation by microRNA. *Cell Res*, 2011. 22(1): p. 107–26.
91. Prescott, S. and K.J. Allen, Food allergy: riding the second wave of the allergy epidemic. *Pediatr Allergy Immunol*, 2011. 22(2): p. 155–60.
92. Prescott, S.L., The influence of early environmental exposures on immune development and subsequent risk of allergic disease. *Allergy*, 2011. 66 Suppl 95: p. 4–6.
93. Prescott, S. and R. Saffery, The role of epigenetic dysregulation in the epidemic of allergic disease. *Clin Epigenetics*, 2011. 2(2): p. 223–32.
94. Tan, T.H. et al., The role of genetics and environment in the rise of childhood food allergy. *Clin Exp Allergy*, 2011. 42(1): p. 20–9.
95. Hollingsworth, J.W. et al., In utero supplementation with methyl donors enhances allergic airway disease in mice. *J Clin Invest*, 2008. 118(10): p. 3462–9.
96. Martino, D.J. and S.L. Prescott, Silent mysteries: epigenetic paradigms could hold the key to conquering the epidemic of allergy and immune disease. *Allergy*, 2010. 65(1): p. 7–15.

97. Akimzhanov, A.M., X.O. Yang, and C. Dong, Chromatin remodeling of interleukin-17 (IL-17)-IL-17F cytokine gene locus during inflammatory helper T cell differentiation. *J Biol Chem*, 2007. 282(9): p. 5969–72.
98. Dunstan, J.A. et al., Fish oil supplementation in pregnancy modifies neonatal allergen-specific immune responses and clinical outcomes in infants at high risk of atopy: a randomized, controlled trial. *J Allergy Clin Immunol*, 2003. 112(6): p. 1178–84.
99. Allan, K., F.J. Kelly, and G. Devereux, Antioxidants and allergic disease: a case of too little or too much? *Clin Exp Allergy*, 2010. 40(3): p. 370–80.
100. West, C.E., N. D'Vaz, and S.L. Prescott, Dietary immunomodulatory factors in the development of immune tolerance. *Curr Allergy Asthma Rep*, 2011. 11(4): p. 325–33.
101. Prescott, S.L. et al., Maternal fish oil supplementation in pregnancy modifies neonatal leukotriene production by cord-blood-derived neutrophils. *Clin Sci (Lond)*, 2007. 113(10): p. 409–16.
102. West, C.I. and S.L. Prescott, Prebiotics and probiotics for prevention of allergic disease, in *UpToDate*, ed. S.H. Sicherer, 2013, Wolters Kluwer Health: Waltham, MA.
103. Rochat, M.K. et al., Maternal vitamin D intake during pregnancy increases gene expression of ILT3 and ILT4 in cord blood. *Clin Exp Allergy*, 2010. 40(5): p. 786–94.
104. Lopez-Varela, S., M. Gonzalez-Gross, and A. Marcos, Functional foods and the immune system: a review. *Eur J Clin Nutr*, 2002. 56 Suppl 3: p. S29–33.
105. Surai, P.F. and N.H.C. Sparks, Designer eggs: from improvement of egg composition to functional food. *Trends Food Sci Tech*, 2001. 12(1): p. 7–16.
106. Mulry, M., Functional foods and neutraceuticals. *Nutr Sci News*, 2000. July. Available from: http://www.chiro.org/nutrition/FULL/Functional_Foods.shtml.
107. Bermingham, E.N. et al., Smart foods from the pastoral sector: implications for meat and milk producers. *Aust J Exp Agr*, 2008. 48: p. 726–34.
108. Mellentin, J., 10 key trends in food, nutrition & health 2011. *New Nutr Bus*, 2011. 16: p. 37–61.
109. Jirtle, R.L. and M.K. Skinner, Environmental epigenomics and disease susceptibility. *Nat Rev Genet*, 2007. 8(4): p. 253–62.
110. Clark, L.C. et al., Effects of selenium supplementation for cancer prevention in patients with carcinoma of the skin. A randomized controlled trial. Nutritional Prevention of Cancer Study Group. *JAMA*, 1996. 276(24): p. 1957–63.
111. Combs Jr, G.F. and W.P. Gray, Chemopreventive agents: selenium. *Pharmacol Ther*, 1998. 79(3): p. 179–192.
112. Zeng, H. et al., Dietary selenomethionine increases exon-specific DNA methylation of the p53 gene in rat liver and colon mucosa. *J Nutr*, 2011. 141(8): p. 1464–8.
113. Reilly, C., Selenium: a new entrant into the functional food arena. *Trends Food Sci Tech*, 1998. 9(3): p. 114–18.
114. Finley, J.W., Reduction of cancer risk by consumption of selenium-enriched plants: enrichment of broccoli with selenium increases the anticarcinogenic properties of broccoli. *J Med Food*, 2003. 6(1): p. 19–26.
115. Finley, J.W. and C.D. Davis, Selenium (Se) from high-selenium broccoli is utilized differently than selenite, selenate and selenomethione, but is more effective in inhibiting colon carcinogenesis. *BioFactors*, 2001. 14: p. 191–6.
116. Finley, J.W., C.D. Davis, and Y. Feng, Selenium from high selenium broccoli protects rats from colon cancer. *J Nutr*, 2000. 130: p. 2384–89.
117. Hu, Y. et al., The influence of selenium-enriched milk proteins and selenium yeast on plasma selenium levels and rectal selenoprotein gene expression in human subjects. *Br J Nutr*, 2011. 106(4): p. 572-82.
118. Hu, Y. et al., Suppression of colorectal oncogenesis by selenium-enriched milk proteins: apoptosis and K-ras mutations. *Cancer Res*, 2008. 68(12): p. 4936–44.

119. Hu, Y. et al., Selenium-enriched milk proteins and selenium yeast affect selenoprotein activity and expression differently in mouse colon. *Br J Nutr*, 2010. 104(1): p. 17–23.
120. Finley, J.W. et al., Bioavailability of selenium from meat and broccoli as determined by retention and distribution of ^{75}Se. *Biol Trace Elem Res*, 2004. 99: p. 191–209.
121. Sahin, N. et al., Lycopene-enriched quail egg as functional food for humans. *Food Res Int*, 2008. 41(3): p. 295–300.
122. Cox, D. and K. Bastiaans, Understanding Australian consumers' perceptions of selenium and motivations to consume selenium enriched foods. *Food Qual Prefer*, 2007. 18: p. 66–76.
123. Cox, D.N., Understanding consumers' perceptions of functional ingredients: Studies of selenium and protein. *Nutr & Dietetics*, 2008. 65: p. S86–8.
124. Kipp, A. et al., Four selenoproteins, protein biosynthesis, and Wnt signalling are particularly sensitive to limited selenium intake in mouse colon. *Mol Nutr Food Res*, 2009. 53(12): p. 1561–72.
125. Barger, J.L. et al., Gene expression profiling reveals differential effects of sodium selenite, selenomethionine, and yeast-derived selenium in the mouse. *Genes Nutr*, 2011. 7(2): p. 155–65.
126. Brouwer, I.A. et al., Bioavailability and bioefficacy of folate and folic acid in man. *Nutr Res Rev*, 2001. 14(2): p. 267–94.
127. Hoyo, C. et al., Folic acid supplementation before and during pregnancy in the Newborn Epigenetics STudy (NEST). *BMC Public Health*, 2011. 11: p. 46–54.
128. Worthley, D.L. et al., A human, double-blind, placebo-controlled, crossover trial of prebiotic, probiotic, and synbiotic supplementation: effects on luminal, inflammatory, epigenetic, and epithelial biomarkers of colorectal cancer. *Am J Clin Nutr*, 2009. 90(3): p. 578–86.
129. Fardet, A., New hypotheses for the health-protective mechanisms of whole-grain cereals: what is beyond fibre. *Nutr Res Rev*, 2010. 23: p. 65–134.
130. Ping, J. et al., Inheritable stimulatory effects of caffeine on steroidogenic acute regulatory protein expression and cortisol production in human adrenocortical cells. *Chem Biol Interact*, 2012. 195(1): p. 68–75.
131. Zhang, F.F. et al., Dietary patterns are associated with levels of global genomic DNA methylation in a cancer-free population. *J Nutr*, 2011. 141(6): p. 1165–71.
132. Hoile, S.P. et al., Dietary protein restriction during F_0 pregnancy in rats induces transgenerational changes in the hepatic transcriptome in female offspring. *PLoS One*, 2011. 6(7): p. e21668.
133. Zheng, S. and Y.-X. Pan, Histone modifications, not DNA methylation, cause transcriptional repression of p16 (CDKN2A) in the mammary glands of offspring of protein-restricted rats. *J Nutr Biochem*, 2011. 22(6): p. 567–73.
134. Meeran, S.M., S.N. Patel, and T.O. Tollefsbol, Sulforaphane causes epigenetic repression of *hTERT* expression in human breast cancer cell lines. *PLoS One*, 2010. 5(7): p. e11457.
135. Stefanska, B. et al., Comparative effects of retinoic acid, vitamin D and resveratrol alone and in combination with adenosine analogues on methylation and expression of phosphatase and tensin homologue tumour suppressor gene in breast cancer cells. *Br J Nutr*, 2011: p. 1–10.
136. Dolinoy, D.C. et al., Maternal genistein alters coat color and protects Avy mouse offspring from obesity by modifying the fetal epigenome. *Environ Health Perspect*, 2006. 114(4): p. 567–72.
137. Dolinoy, D.C., D. Huang, and R.L. Jirtle, Maternal nutrient supplementation counteracts bisphenol A-induced DNA hypomethylation in early development. *Proc Natl Acad Sci U S A*, 2007. 104(32): p. 13056–61.

138. Landecker, H. Food as exposure: nutritional epigenetics and the molecular politics of eating. *CSW Update Newsletter*, 2010. May 2010.
139. Riazuddin et al., Determination of multi-residue insecticides of organochlorine, organophosphorus, and pyrethroids in wheat. *Bull Environ Contam Toxicol*, 2011. 87(3): p. 303–6.
140. Vadhana, M.S. et al., Early life permethrin insecticide treatment leads to heart damage in adult rats. *Exp Gerontol*, 2011. 46(9): p. 731–8.
141. Cummings, J.A., L.G. Clemens, and A.A. Nunez, Mother counts: how effects of environmental contaminants on maternal care could affect the offspring and future generations. *Front Neuroendocrinol*, 2010. 31(4): p. 440–51.
142. Oh, G. Beyond the thousand-dollar human genome. Medill Reports, 2012 [cited 2012 12 Jan 2012]; Available from: http://news.medill.northwestern.edu/chicago/news.aspx?id=198497.
143. Harper, M. Why you can't have your $1,000 genome. *Forbes*, 2011 [cited 2012 13 Jan 2012]; Available from: http://www.forbes.com/sites/matthewherper/2011/01/06/why-you-cant-have-your-1000-genome/.
144. Eussen, S.R.B.M. et al., Costs and health effects of adding functional foods containing phytosterols/-stanols to statin therapy in the prevention of cardiovascular disease. *Eur J Pharmacol*, 2011. 668 Suppl 1(0): p. S91–100.

13 Foodomics to Study Efficacy of Human Dietary Interventions

Proof of Principle Study

Stephanie Ellett, Isobel R. Ferguson, Shuotun Zhu, Nishi Karunasinghe, Gareth Marlow, Daniel Hurley, Wen J. Lam, Dug Yeo Han, and Lynnette R. Ferguson

CONTENTS

INTRODUCTION

One of the limitations for small- to medium-sized food companies to prove efficacy of functional foods, or novel diets, is the cost of human clinical trials. Most new functional foods are developed based on a prior hypothesis. However, the food or dietary context may negate such hypotheses being correct. Thus, a costly human trial, of the standard necessary for a health claim, may fail to prove the desired effect of the new food. A variant of nutrigenomics, which is food or diet-focused, is sometimes being described as foodomics [1]. It enables non-hypothesis-based establishment of appropriate biomarkers to help reduce the test time and increase the efficacy of establishing the quickest and most effective test methods to move directly to a health claim. We have tested the ability of this approach to prove the human efficacy and to derive insights into the mechanism of action of a modified diet, in a proof of principle study in Auckland, New Zealand.

Our starting hypothesis in developing dietary intervention protocol was that the diet would be efficacious in reducing inflammation. Inflammation can be the catalyst for chronic human diseases including Alzheimer's, cardiovascular diseases, some cancers, and various autoimmune diseases, including rheumatoid arthritis, Crohn's disease (CD), type II diabetes mellitus, and so on [2–4]. Thus, reducing inflammation can be significantly beneficial to health [2,5,6]. Many studies showing the efficacy of pharmaceutical or dietary interventions in reducing inflammation have used a validated biomarker such as C-reactive protein (CRP) [7,8] or the micronucleus (MN) assay [9]. However, we sought to test the hypothesis that nutrigenomics/foodomics technologies may be more sensitive, needing fewer subject numbers, over a shorter timescale [6,10,11].

Many studies have proven that a diet high in long-chain omega-3 fatty acids, fruits, vegetables, nuts, and whole grains, and low in refined grains, saturated fats, and sugars can help in reducing inflammation [12]. Many of these dietary components are distinctive of the Mediterranean diet, whose value in protecting against chronic disease is well established [13–15]. In our ongoing studies on inflammatory bowel disease (IBD), we have also identified further beneficial and potentially detrimental dietary components in reducing inflammation [16]. Between January and March of 2012, we carried out a proof of principle pilot study to see three things:

1. Is there evidence of inflammation in apparently healthy New Zealanders?
2. Does changing their diet for 6 weeks reduce evidence of inflammation in apparently healthy New Zealanders?
3. How much intervention do New Zealanders need to successfully change their diet?

Our primary aim was to compare the efficacy of two classic biomarkers, CRP and MN, with gene expression profiles (transcriptomics) in peripheral blood mononuclear cells (PBMCs), in demonstrating the extent of the effect achieved. For this dietary intervention, we added (or subtracted) the foods we previously identified [16] to those considered typical of a Mediterranean-style diet. Full details of the diet will be published elsewhere.

PBMCs are primarily composed of lymphocytes and monocytes and are a critical component of the immune system, which can be easily obtained from a venipuncture, and as such have been used as a model to study expression of inflammatory genes [17,18]. Studies in 2009 [19] highlighted the potential of gene expression levels of PBMCs as a novel biomarker of nutritional interventions, and Theuwissen et al. [20] used PBMCs to predict inflammatory responses to functional foods. These studies provide evidence that PBMC profiling may reflect gene expression levels due to both short- and long-term nutritional changes.

METHODS

Selection of Subjects

Forty volunteers were selected from around the Auckland region. These volunteers were of any gender, ethnicity, and age. They needed to be nonsmokers, and not suffering from IBD or other chronic disorders. They all filled out a 7 day food diary to provide information about their diet prior to the study. Those diets were scored for "Mediterranean-adequacy" [21]. This scoring system involved allocating a score between 1 and 5 for: fish/seafood, fruit, vegetables, nonrefined cereals, legumes, nuts/seeds, healthy fats (olive oil and avocado), and unhealthy food (this includes anything deep fried, chocolate, lollies, muffins, cakes, biscuits). We also entered their diets into the FoodWorks database. This program offers us information on caloric intake; the average amount of fat, protein, and carbohydrates consumed daily; and a breakdown of saturated, polyunsaturated, and monounsaturated fats. From this, we were able to preselect the 30 individuals with the poorest diets, and therefore the highest levels of the two inflammatory biomarkers, who were more likely to benefit from changing their dietary habits.

Dietary Intervention Study

The preselected 30 volunteers were given (some) food weekly and asked to adhere to our dietary guidelines, as outlined in a personalized booklet given to them. This provided them with background information about what foods they were being encouraged to eat, a brief summary of their previous diet that had been entered into FoodWorks, details about what aspects of this diet should be adjusted, and an abundance of recipes that included the foods we were promoting. In this booklet, we also offered a summary of foods they were either encouraged or discouraged to eat (Table 13.1).

Summary of instructions given to trial participants:

- To change your dietary habits for a minimum of 6 weeks to include anti-inflammatory foods and cut out processed, refined white flour–based, high-sugar and high-fat foods
- To provide blood and urine samples at the beginning and end of the study
- To complete a 4 day food diary in the last week of the study
- To complete two online questionnaires about your diet and lifestyle
- To participate in one or more workshops with expert nutritionists or dieticians who can answer all diet questions and who will explain what foods we are targeting and why
- To fill in an evaluation on this study and offer feedback on what you felt did/did not work

TABLE 13.1
Foods Encouraged or Discouraged During the 6 Week Dietary Intervention

Good Foods That Relieved or Improved Inflammation from Previous Studies [15]	Foods to Avoid as They Have Shown a Negative Effect on Inflammation [15]
Blackberries	Corn
Raspberries	Red meats high in fat
Blueberries	Ground meats
Strawberries	Full fat dairy products
Red grapes	Refined and processed grains
Apples	Cakes/muffins/donuts
Apricots	Energy drinks
Cherries	Processed meats
Plums	Sweets/chocolate
Nectarines	Butter
Peaches	
Pears	
Mango	
Melon	
Bananas	
Dark green leafy vegetables	
Fish (mainly salmon)	
Grilled/roast chicken	
Honey	
Marmite/vegemite	
Boiled potatoes	
Parsnip	
Yams	
Carrots	
Kumara	
Pumpkin	
Legumes	
Hummus	
Nuts/seeds	
Avocados	
Rice crackers	
Olive oil	
Turmeric (curcumin)	
Water	
Green tea	

From the booklet given to participants of our study.

Volunteers were randomly allocated into two groups of 15: a high-intervention group and a low-intervention group. This was done to better understand how much extra input our volunteers would need to maintain the new diet. The high-intervention group received additional food each week, as well as more contact with the study coordinators to check that they are on track. All volunteers received 200 g salmon and two avocados weekly, as well as 100 green tea bags and three boxes of whole-grain cereal. In addition to this, the high-intervention group received a variety of vegetables and gluten-free bread weekly, 125 fish oil capsules, a pot of manuka honey, and two bottles of extra-virgin olive oil.

The high-intervention participants were communicated with weekly when collecting their products and were also asked to fill in a feedback form midway through the study to see how they felt they were doing, and find out what more we could do to encourage them to stay on the diet.

Sampling Procedure

Blood samples were collected before and after the 6 week intervention. The 6 mL blood samples collected in serum-separating tubes were sent away for CRP levels. Two 1 mL aliquots of blood collected in heparinized tubes were reserved for the MN assay and a 2.5 mL aliquot of whole blood was collected in a PAXgene blood RNA tube (PBRT) for gene expression arrays.

C-Reactive Protein Measurement

CRP was determined by latex-enhanced immunoturbidimetric method using the wide range CRP (wrCRP) latex reagent. The wrCRP latex reagent is a suspension of uniform polystyrene latex particles coated with anti-CRP antibody. When serum containing CRP is mixed with the latex reagent, agglutination takes place resulting in an increase in the turbidity. The turbidity is measured at 571 nm on a Siemens Advia 2400 chemistry analyzer. The CRP concentration in serum is determined from a calibration curve that is generated with the calibrators (reference range <5 mg/L).

Cytokinesis-Blocked Micronucleus Assay

Blood samples were collected into heparinized tubes and were stored at room temperature and cultured within 24 hours of initial collection. The sample was treated and harvested to permit estimation of micronuclei in cytokinesis-blocked cells, essentially as described by Thomas and Fenech [9]. Duplicate cultures were set up containing 0.6 mL whole blood and 9.25 mL alpha minimum essential medium with 15% of fetal calf serum (Gibco Ltd., New Zealand). Lymphocytes were stimulated to divide with phytohemagglutinin (PHA 15 μL/mL, Gibco) and maintained in a humidified incubator containing 5% carbon dioxide. Forty-four hours after PHA stimulation, cytochalasin B (Sigma Chemical Co., USA) was added to the cultures to give a final concentration of 4.5 μg/mL. Cultures were harvested using standard procedures involving centrifugation, swelling in hypotonic KCl, and fixation in methanol/acetic acid prior to dropping on a slide. After the slides were air dried, cells were stained with Diff–Quik stain set from Dade Behring Inc., USA. Binucleate cells were scored for MN and identified using the criteria of Thomas and Fenech [9]. At least two sets of 1000 cells have been scored, one from each harvest. Under a microscope, the amount of micronuclei, nucleoplasmic bridges, and nuclear buds were counted for every 1000 binucleated cells counted. This would give us a fair indication of chromosome breakage and DNA misrepair, providing us with an overall indication of DNA damage before and after the diet.

RNA Isolation and Storage

Following the manufacturer's recommended protocol, 2.5 mL whole blood was collected in a PBRT (PreAnalytiX). The blood was incubated at room temperature for 2 hours, after collection to improve RNA yield, before being stored at –70°C.

The PBRT was centrifuged for 10 minutes at 3000 × g, the supernatant was discarded, and the pellet was resuspended in 4 mL RNase-free water. This was centrifuged for a further 10 minutes at 3000 × g and the supernatant discarded. The pellet was resuspended in 350 μL resuspension buffer and transferred to a 2 mL processing tube. The processing tube was loaded into the QIAcube and the PAXgene Blood RNA Part A protocol was started. Once Part A was complete, the microcentrifuge tubes containing the purified RNA were transferred to the QIAcube shaker adapter and the PAXgene Blood RNA Part B protocol was started. Once complete, the RNA was placed immediately onto ice. Two aliquots of 2 μL were taken for each sample and the remainder was stored at –70°C.

The quantity of RNA was determined using the NanoDrop ND-1000 Spectrophotometer (NanoDrop Technologies) and the quality of RNA by the Experion RNA StdSens analysis kit (Bio-Rad). To proceed to gene expression microarray hybridization, a concentration of >100 ng/μL of RNA and a RNA quality indicator of >8 are required.

Gene Expression Arrays

Microarray hybridization was performed on GeneChip® PrimeView™ Human Gene Expression arrays (Affymetrix) following the manufacturer's protocol by the Centre for Genomics and Proteomics, the University of Auckland, using the Affymetrix GeneChip® Instrument System.

Gene Expression Data Analysis

Affymetrix Primeview array data in .CEL file format was read using the "affy" package in the statistical language R (*R: A Language and Environment for Statistical Computing.* R Foundation for Statistical Computing, Vienna, Austria. ISBN 3-900051-07-0, http://www.R-project.org) and normalized using the robust multiarray averaging (RMA) method. Quality assurance (QA) of the data showed that it was of good quality and free of obvious artifacts or outliers. The "limma" package in R was used to compare expression at 1 week with expression at 6 weeks for the high-intervention samples, paired by participant code. Benjamini–Hochberg false-discovery rate was used to adjust for multiple testing correction.

RESULTS

Adherence to the Diet

Out of the initial 30 volunteers for this study, 28 completed the diet for 6 weeks. We asked these 28 participants to once again fill in a food diary for the last week of their study, so that we could enter it into the FoodWorks database and compare it to their initial food record. The results we obtained from this database were very positive. In the initial food diaries, overall average daily fat intake was 68.6 g, of which 41.92% was saturated fat, 41.26% was monounsaturated fat, and 16.82% was polyunsaturated fat. In analyzing the food diaries that were filled out at the end of the study, overall average daily fat intake significantly dropped down to 43.9 g, of which only 34.4% was saturated fat, 44.7% was monounsaturated fat, and 20.9% was polyunsaturated fat. A complete record of dietary changes will be published elsewhere.

C-Reactive Protein Levels

The CRP levels, before and after intervention, are shown in Figure 13.1. There was a decreased trend in the CRP level for both high and low diets after 6 weeks intervention. CRP in high diet intervention was significantly ($p = 0.019$) lower post-intervention than those in preintervention (mean ± SE and mean ± SE, respectively) (Figure 13.1).

Cytokinesis-Blocked Micronucleus Assays

Cytokinesis-blocked MN levels, before and after the intervention, are shown in Figure 13.2. Although the levels of MN did decrease somewhat over the 6 week study, the extent of the differences before and after did not reach statistical significance.

Gene Expression Arrays

A heat map illustrating the most significant differences in gene expression is shown in Figure 13.3.

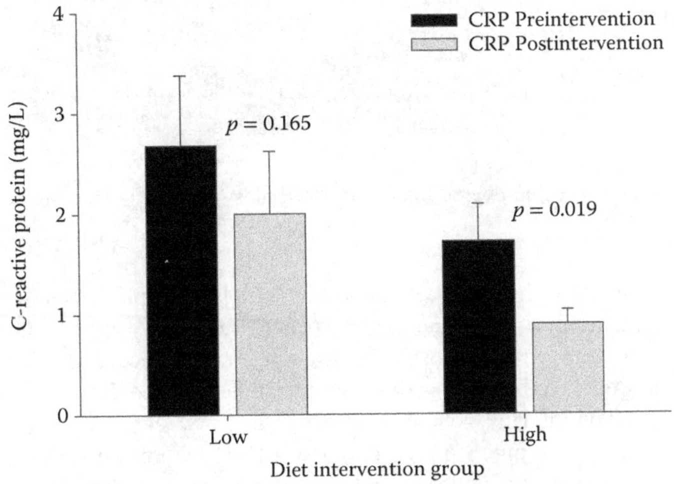

FIGURE 13.1 Average (mean ± SE) levels of C-reactive protein, measured from serum samples of all subjects, before and after the dietary intervention.

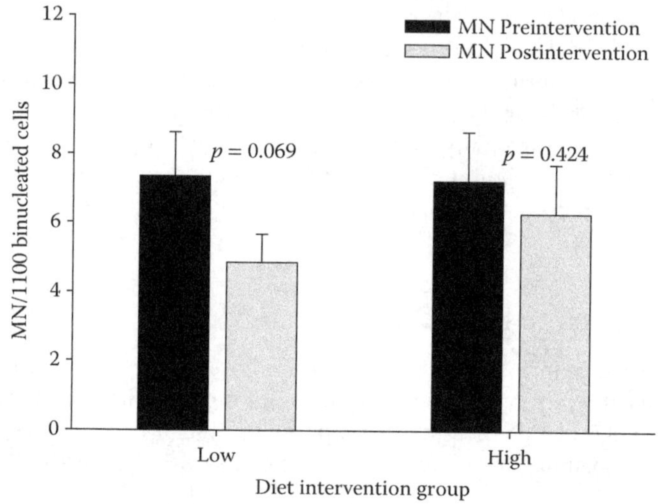

FIGURE 13.2 Micronuclei scored in 1100 cytokinesis-blocked cells for each participant. Illustrated are the averages (mean ± SE) for the two groups of participants.

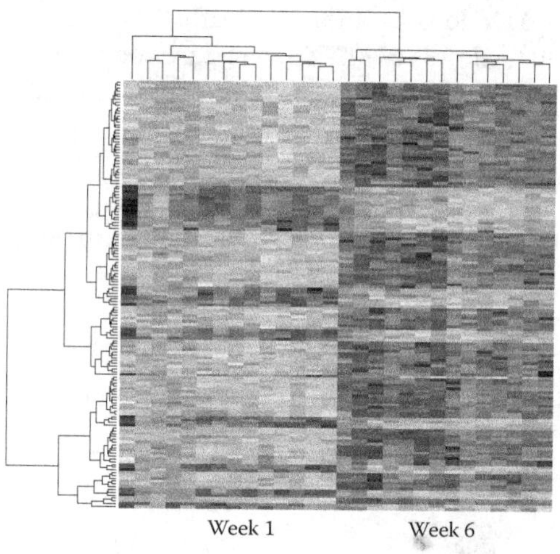

FIGURE 13.3 Differential expression of top 150 genes ($p < 10^{-8}$) before and after the high dietary intervention.

Based on analysis of before week 1 and after week 6 samples from the high-intervention diet, of the most significant ($p < 10^{-8}$) differentially expressed transcripts, we can see that transcript expression is changed over time. Expression has both increased and decreased showing that our high-intervention diet has had a highly significant effect on altering gene expression in just 6 weeks. It is also evident that this method gives very much more sensitive differentiation between the situation before and after the study, as compared with the more standard biomarkers previously shown (Figures 13.1 and 13.2).

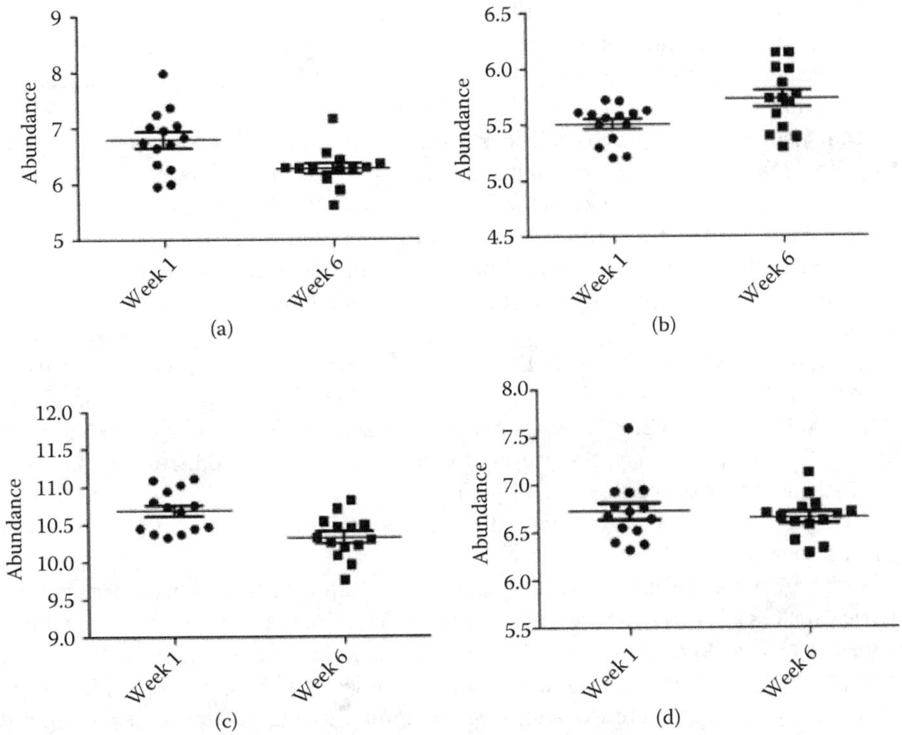

FIGURE 13.4 Examples of changes in transcript abundance of some key genes known to affect the expression of inflammatory bowel disease (IBD). *p*-values are adjusted using the Benjamini–Hochberg false-discovery rate correction to account for multiple testing. The examples above provide reason to believe that the diet will benefit IBD subjects since *JAK2, TLR2*, and *TLR4* are commonly upregulated while *IL10* is downregulated in this disease. These are recognized IBD susceptibility gene. (a) Probe ID: 11733373_at (*JAK2*), $p = 0.000{,}429$; (b) Probe ID: 11734307_at (*IL10*), $p = 0.026{,}081$; (c) Probe ID: 11754833_a_at (*TLR2*), $p = 0.008{,}111$; (d) Probe ID: 11743197_at (*TLR4*), $p = 0.002{,}62$.

The nature of the gene expression changes is of considerable significance. Since we had designed this diet as a potential resource for our IBD cohort, we were particularly concerned to ask the question as to whether any of the affected genes are among those known to be important in IBD risk in New Zealand [22–25]. This was indeed the case. Changes in gene expression for four key IBD genes are shown in Figure 13.4.

DISCUSSION

Our aim for this pilot study was to compare the relative performance of standard biomarkers of inflammation with the increased sensitivity offered by transcriptomics approaches. The GeneChip® PrimeView™ Human Gene Expression arrays were used as they provide complete coverage of the annotated genome enabling comprehensive whole-genome gene expression analysis. We were impressed by the orders of magnitude increase in sensitivity provided by these arrays, as compared with the more traditional technologies. The present data imply that short-term studies with small study numbers are now a possible approach. This has major implications for the cost and sensitivity of human clinical trials.

Our secondary aim was to consider if inflammation could be reduced in healthy New Zealanders with a dietary change and to gauge how much interaction and intervention would be needed to keep these volunteers on the diet for 6 weeks. In receiving feedback forms, we estimated an overall compliance of 70% in relation to a sustained change in dietary intake. The main comment was that compliance would have been increased if participants had direct contact with a dietician throughout the whole 6 weeks.

Compliance was also evaluated from the food diaries filled out on the last week of the diet. From the food diaries, we could see that the average vegetable intake increased from 1.48 to 2.11 servings per day, the average fruit intake increased from 1.3 to 1.8 servings per day, the average seafood intake increased from 0.40 to 0.78 servings per day, the average "healthy fats" intake increased from 0.47 to 1.15 servings per day, and the average "unhealthy food" intake decreased from 1.06 to 0.47 servings per day.

Although it may be easy for participants to exaggerate the truth when filling in food diaries, the CRP levels from their plasma collections and the gene expression patterns from the arrays both corroborated what the volunteers were saying in their food records. We found that the CRP levels, a good indicator of inflammation [7,8], were significantly reduced within 6 weeks, showing us that our Mediterranean-inspired diet held many anti-inflammatory properties. CRPs are produced in the liver and are released in direct response to injury, inflammatory diseases, infection, tissue damage, pregnancy, and many other inflammatory conditions [7,8]. These reinforce the information from the microarrays.

MN analysis is a slower process than examining the CRP levels, but it is a comprehensive technique for measuring DNA damage, which can be a good indicator of inflammation, and has been validated as a biomarker of cancer risk [9]. Micronuclei assays were found to be insensitive for determining the efficacy of our dietary intervention with this small number of subjects, within our short 6 week time frame. Because of the nature of lymphocytes being produced in bone marrow and maturing before entering circulation, and the short time frame of our intervention, we cannot be certain that the lymphocytes we cultured were produced after the intervention.

CONCLUSIONS

Inflammation can cause significant health problems and can lead to various diseases including Alzheimer's, CD, cardiovascular diseases, some cancers, autoimmune diseases, arthritis, and type II diabetes. It is therefore important to find ways for sufferers of inflammation to reduce these levels. The elegance of the current microarray technology used, on PBMCs as a surrogate biomarker, can be described as impressive. Although we had a starting hypothesis, which we confirmed here, one of the most useful aspects of the technology used is that the study can be hypothesis-free.

This means that food companies could use such an approach to discover what their food products or diets are actually doing at a genetic level, which may not necessarily be what they were designed to be doing and could lead to insights into the mechanism of action of a modified diet. Thus, ushers in a new phase of sensitivity in dietary intervention studies, negating a need for testing a wide range of endpoints, which is both expensive and time-consuming.

ACKNOWLEDGMENTS

We acknowledge contributions to the trial from the following companies: New Zealand King Salmon, Venerdi, Red Seal Natural Health, Plant & Food Research, Cereal Partners Worldwide, Nestle & General Mills, Fonterra, New Zealand Avocado, Matiatia Grove, Vegetables.co.nz, The New Zealand Merino Company.

REFERENCES

1. Castro-Puyana M, Garcia-Canas V, Simo C, Cifuentes A: Recent advances in the application of capillary electromigration methods for food analysis and Foodomics. *Electrophoresis* 2012, 33(1):147–167.
2. Calder PC: Fatty acids and inflammation: the cutting edge between food and pharma. *Eur J Pharmacol* 2011, 668 Suppl 1:S50–S58.
3. Corfield AP, Wallace HM, Probert CSJ: The molecular biology of inflammatory bowel diseases. *Biochem Soc Trans* 2011, 39(4):1057–1060.
4. Serhan CN: The resolution of inflammation: the devil in the flask and in the details. *Faseb J* 2011, 25(5):1441–1448.
5. Bannenberg G, Serhan CN: Specialized pro-resolving lipid mediators in the inflammatory response: an update. *Biochim Biophys Acta* 2010, 1801(12):1260–1273.
6. Bakker GC, van Erk MJ, Pellis L, Wopereis S, Rubingh CM, Cnubben NH, Kooistra T, van Ommen B, Hendriks HF: An anti-inflammatory dietary mix modulates inflammation and oxidative and metabolic stress in overweight men: a nutrigenomics approach. *Am J Clin Nutr* 2010, 91(4):1044–1059.
7. Bisoendial RJ, Boekholdt SM, Vergeer M, Stroes ESG, Kastelein JJP: C-reactive protein is a mediator of cardiovascular disease. *Eur Heart J* 2010, 31(17):2087–2091.
8. Karadag F, Kirdar S, Karul AB, Ceylan E: The value of C-reactive protein as a marker of systemic inflammation in stable chronic obstructive pulmonary disease. *Eur J Intern Med* 2008, 19(2):104–108.
9. Thomas P, Fenech M: Cytokinesis-block micronucleus cytome assay in lymphocytes. *Methods Mol Biol* 2011, 682:217–234.
10. de Graaf AA, Freidig AP, De Roos B, Jamshidi N, Heinemann M, Rullmann JAC, Hall KD, Adiels M, van Ommen B: Nutritional systems biology modeling: from molecular mechanisms to physiology. *PLoS Comput Biol* 2009, 5(11):e1000554.
11. Puiggros F, Sola R, Blade C, Salvado M-J, Arola L: Nutritional biomarkers and foodomic methodologies for qualitative and quantitative analysis of bioactive ingredients in dietary intervention studies. *J Chromatogr A* 2011, 1218(42):7399–7414.
12. Luciano M, Mottus R, Starr JM, McNeill G, Jia X, Craig LCA, Deary IJ: Depressive symptoms and diet: their effects on prospective inflammation levels in the elderly. *Brain Behav Immun* 2012, 26(5):717–720.
13. Esposito K, Di Palo C, Maiorino MI, Petrizzo M, Bellastella G, Siniscalchi I, Giugliano D: Long-term effect of Mediterranean-style diet and calorie restriction on biomarkers of longevity and oxidative stress in overweight men. *Cardiol Res Pract* 2011, 2011:293916.

14. Kastorini C-M, Milionis HJ, Esposito K, Giugliano D, Goudevenos JA, Panagiotakos DB: The effect of Mediterranean diet on metabolic syndrome and its components: a meta-analysis of 50 studies and 534,906 individuals. *J Am Coll Cardiol* 2011, 57(11):1299–1313.
15. Sola R, Fito M, Estruch R, Salas-Salvado J, Corella D, de La Torre R, Munoz MA et al.: Effect of a traditional Mediterranean diet on apolipoproteins B, A-I, and their ratio: a randomized, controlled trial. *Atherosclerosis* 2011, 218(1):174–180.
16. Triggs CM, Munday K, Hu R, Fraser AG, Gearry RB, Barclay ML, Ferguson LR: Dietary factors in chronic inflammation: food tolerances and intolerances of a New Zealand Caucasian Crohn's disease population. *Mutat Res* 2010, 690(1–2):123–138.
17. Rudkowska I, Ponton A, Jacques H, Lavigne C, Holub BJ, Marette A, Vohl M-C: Effects of a supplementation of n-3 polyunsaturated fatty acids with or without fish gelatin on gene expression in peripheral blood mononuclear cells in obese, insulin-resistant subjects. *J Nutrigenet Nutrigenomics* 2011, 4(4):192–202.
18. Rudkowska I, Raymond C, Ponton A, Jacques H, Lavigne C, Holub BJ, Marette A, Vohl M-C: Validation of the use of peripheral blood mononuclear cells as surrogate model for skeletal muscle tissue in nutrigenomic studies. *Omics* 2011, 15(1–2):1–7.
19. Bouwens M, van de Rest O, Dellschaft N, Bromhaar MG, de Groot LCPGM, Geleijnse JM, Muller M, Afman LA: Fish-oil supplementation induces antiinflammatory gene expression profiles in human blood mononuclear cells. *Am J Clin Nutr* 2009, 90(2):415–424.
20. Theuwissen E, Plat J, Mensink RP: Consumption of oat beta-glucan with or without plant stanols did not influence inflammatory markers in hypercholesterolemic subjects. *Mol Nutr Food Res* 2009, 53(3):370–376.
21. Alberti-Fidanza A, Fidanza F: Mediterranean Adequacy Index of Italian diets. *Public Health Nutr* 2004, 7(7):937–941.
22. Ferguson LR, Han DY, Fraser AG, Huebner C, Lam WJ, Morgan AR, Duan H, Karunasinghe N: Genetic factors in chronic inflammation: single nucleotide polymorphisms in the STAT-JAK pathway, susceptibility to DNA damage and Crohn's disease in a New Zealand population. *Mutat Res* 2010, 690(1–2):108–115.
23. Wang AH, Lam W-J, Han D-Y, Ding Y, Hu R, Fraser AG, Ferguson LR, Morgan AR: The effect of IL-10 genetic variation and interleukin 10 serum levels on Crohn's disease susceptibility in a New Zealand population. *Hum Immunol* 2011, 72(5):431–435.
24. Ferwerda G, Kullberg BJ, de Jong DJ, Girardin SE, Langenberg DML, van Crevel R, Ottenhoff THM, Van der Meer JWM, Netea MG: Mycobacterium paratuberculosis is recognized by Toll-like receptors and NOD2. *J Leukoc Biol* 2007, 82(4):1011–1018.
25. Browning BL, Huebner C, Petermann I, Gearry RB, Barclay ML, Shelling AN, Ferguson LR: Has toll-like receptor 4 been prematurely dismissed as an inflammatory bowel disease gene? Association study combined with meta-analysis shows strong evidence for association. *Am J Gastroenterol* 2007, 102(11):2504–2512.

14 Considerations in Estimating Genotype in Nutrigenetic Studies

Angharad R. Morgan

CONTENTS

INTRODUCTION

Nutrigenetic studies investigate relationships between diet and genotype with the aim that in the future genotyping will be used to make dietary recommendations on an individual basis to promote a healthier lifestyle and reduce the risk of disease. Using genotypes is preferable to other potential biomarkers as genotypes are fixed from birth, allowing early risk prediction and subsequent dietary intervention. Also, genotypes can be easily obtained from a simple buccal swab, which is quick, painless, and inexpensive. Furthermore, genotypes can be determined relatively quickly with minimal measurement error and minimal cost.

The genotype is obtained from some type of polymorphic marker, most commonly single-nucleotide polymorphisms (SNPs), as they are the most common and subsequently are also the easiest and cheapest to genotype, but microsatellite markers, insertion/deletions, variable number tandem repeats, and copy-number variants (CNVs) may also be used. In recent years there have been huge technological advances in the

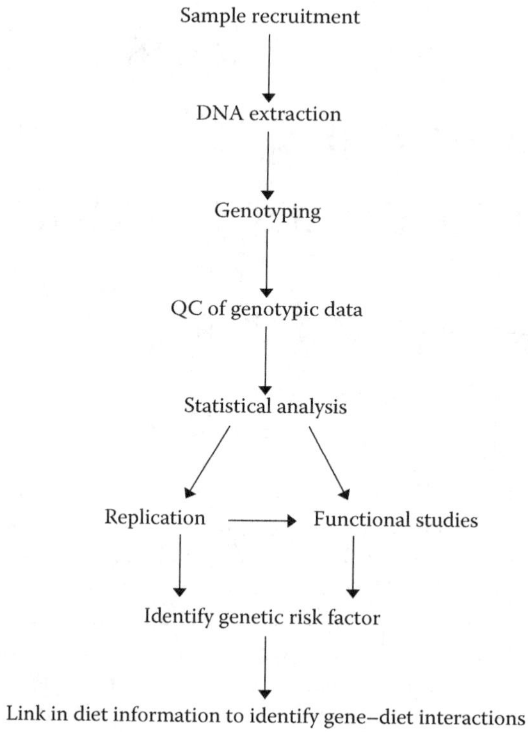

FIGURE 14.1 Schematic workflow for identifying genetic risk factors in nutrigenetic studies.

field of genotyping, and subsequently tremendous progress has been made in identifying genetic risk factors for a wide spectrum of complex diseases and traits.

The process of identifying genetic risk factors for a particular disease or trait involves a number of important steps (Figure 14.1), each of which is discussed in this chapter.

SAMPLE RECRUITMENT

A good genetic association study will start with a solid study design. The first step is to define the disease or phenotype of interest as accurately and specifically as possible and subsequently begin to recruit suitable individuals into the study. Blood, buccal, or tissue samples will be collected for DNA extraction and relevant phenotypic information recorded. At the same time as recruiting individuals with the disease or phenotype of interest, it is necessary to enroll individuals free of the disease or phenotype under investigation as controls. It is critical that cases and controls are from the same population to avoid confounding and spurious associations. Also, controls should be ideally matched for age and gender. Matching of samples will help to avoid biases that will inflate the overall type 1 error rate and lead to the reporting of false positive associations. For potential confounders for which matching may not be possible, posthoc adjustments can be performed during statistical analysis.

It is advisable to collect the largest sample set as possible so as to maximize the power of the study to detect true susceptibility genes. This need for large studies is encouraging research groups to join together and share their resources in collaborative efforts.

DNA EXTRACTION

Sample ID, receipt date, sample type, and storage location, together with any other available information, should be electronically logged into a secure database. DNA can be extracted from the sample (usually blood, buccal swab, or tissue sample) relatively easily—nowadays there are many commercial kits for DNA extraction and even automated DNA extraction using a high-throughput robotic platform.

Following DNA isolation, the quality and quantity of the genetic material should be assessed using standard methods. It is then ready for use in genotyping.

GENOTYPING METHODS

Candidate gene studies involve investigating specific genes, which are selected based on a prior hypothesis about their potential role in the disease/trait being studied. They can be conducted in either family cohorts by comparing transmission of disease alleles from parents to affected and unaffected offspring or in case–control cohorts of nonrelated individuals with disease and controls without disease. Association exists when the allele frequencies differ between cases and controls.

There are many different genotyping technologies available for carrying out candidate gene studies with each approach differing widely in cost, ease of use, and performance (as measured by throughput, efficiency, reproducibility, and accuracy). The basic principle for each genotyping method is the same and typically involves the generation and subsequent detection of allele-specific products for the SNP of interest. In most methods, PCR amplification of a short DNA sequence containing the SNP is performed to introduce specificity and increase the number of molecules for detection following allelic discrimination. Allele discrimination is achieved with allele-specific biochemical reactions such as enzymatic cleavage, ligation, primer extension, or hybridization.

In recent years, genetic association studies have progressed from genotyping 1–40 markers at a time to genotyping hundreds of thousands of markers in a single experiment. The first genome-wide association study (GWAS) was reported in 2005 and compared 96 patients with age-related macular degeneration with 50 healthy controls [1]. Today, thousands of individuals are tested in each GWAS (providing greater power to be able to detect SNP associations), and the number of SNPs per array has dramatically increased with now in excess of a million markers. GWAS has proven such a powerful and successful strategy that it is fast becoming the default study design for the identification of genetic risk factors.

There are two main companies that lead the production and development of GWAS arrays and both are widely used: Affymetrix and Illumina. There are differences between the two platforms in design, SNP selection, added value content (such as mitochondrial SNPs, nonsynonymous SNPs, and CNVs), amount of target DNA required, protocol complexity, chip throughput, scanner expense, and of course cost, but overall data quality and coverage appear similar. Both platforms give excellent genome-wide coverage in European populations, but there are also known to be significant gaps in both. However, these gaps are decreasing as the content of the GWAS arrays is improved in more recently designed GWAS chips.

QUALITY CONTROL OF GENOTYPIC DATA

Quality control (QC) of all genotypic data, whether it is from a single SNP in a candidate gene study or thousands of SNPs in a GWAS, is very important and is essential before analysis. QC is performed in two stages: firstly at the sample level and subsequently at the SNP level.

SAMPLE QC

DNA quality is one of the most important factors in achieving high genotyping accuracy. Thus, it is essential that the DNA quantity and quality is checked before it is used in a genotyping experiment. As genotyping becomes more highly multiplexed, the quality of DNA is becoming more and more important and starting with poor quality DNA samples is going to result in poor quality results. Once an assay has been completed, poor quality samples can still be detected, with low genotype call rates, and removed from analysis. The acceptable call rate depends on the nature of the study but generally should not be less than 95%. Differential rates of missingness between cases and controls may also be a problem. Standard laboratory practice of DNA extraction and storage should be consistent for the whole sample set—both case and control samples—and assigning both cases and controls to each plate and checking for differences in genotype frequency across plates can help eliminate systematic errors.

Samples with heterozygosity that is too high or too low compared with others in the population are also not reliable and could reflect mixed samples containing DNA from more than one individual. Contamination of DNA samples can be checked by having negative template controls on the sample plate. It is also advisable to include a few duplicate samples and to ensure that the genotypes for such duplicate samples match.

SNP QC

After sample QC, SNP QC is needed. In many studies, SNPs with a low minor allele frequency (less than 1% for large studies, or less than 5% for smaller studies) are not analyzed as calling rare genotypes is subject to more errors. SNPs for which many samples do not give genotypes are unreliable and are usually removed from analysis. The acceptable call rate depends on the nature of the study, but usually is set in the region of 95% or higher. Tests of Hardy–Weinberg equilibrium are useful in flagging SNPs with nonrandom dropping out of a genotype. To ensure accuracy of the genotype calls, it is a good idea to include some HapMap samples on the sample plates so that if the SNP is in the HapMap database (http://hapmap.ncbi.nlm.nih.gov/), concordance of the SNP genotype with that in the database can be checked. Many genotyping methods use Cartesian or polar plots that illustrate the clustering of the three genotypes for each SNP (Figure 14.2). This is a useful tool to determine the quality of the SNP data. Good-quality SNPs show three clearly defined and tight clusters, with the homozygotes falling along the vertical or horizontal axis and the heterozygotes along the diagonal. Any plots showing a deviation from this, for example, overlapping of the clusters, or more than three clusters, indicates a problem with the accuracy and reliability of the genotypes for that particular SNP. The huge number of SNPs in a GWAS makes it impossible to look at intensity plots of all of the SNPs, but it is recommended that the cluster plots of the most significant SNPs be examined.

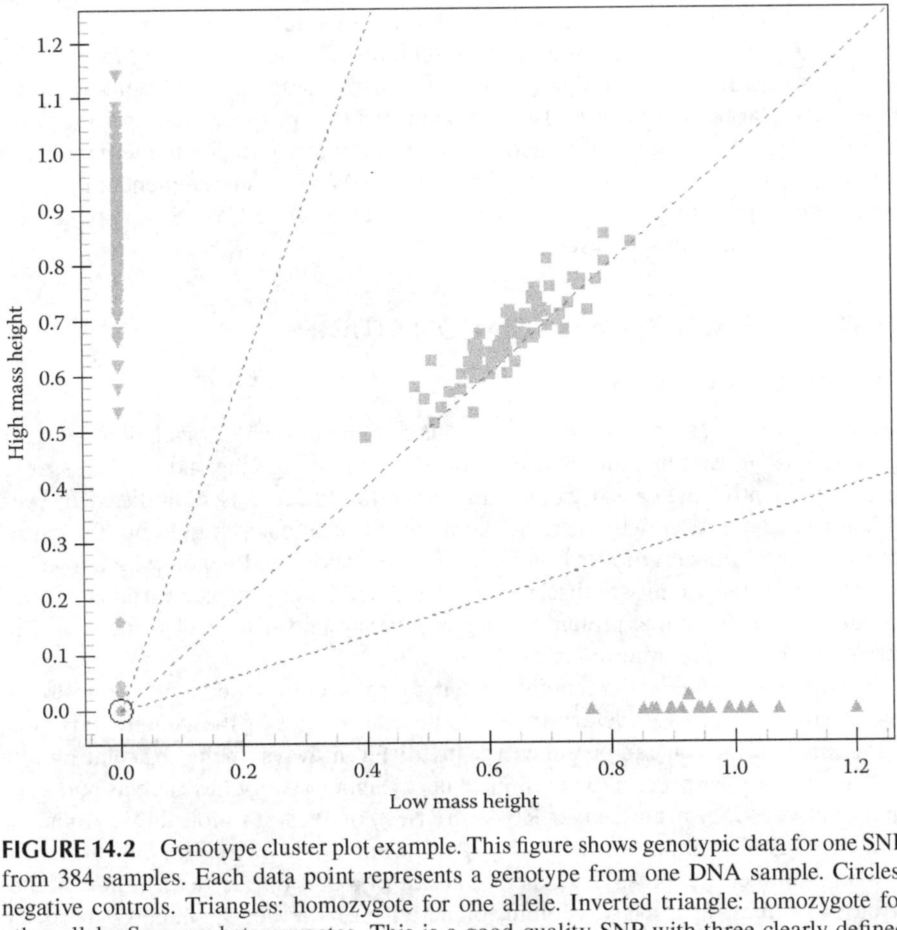

FIGURE 14.2 Genotype cluster plot example. This figure shows genotypic data for one SNP from 384 samples. Each data point represents a genotype from one DNA sample. Circles: negative controls. Triangles: homozygote for one allele. Inverted triangle: homozygote for other allele. Squares: heterozygotes. This is a good-quality SNP with three clearly defined and tight clusters.

STATISTICAL ISSUES

Methods for testing association between a genotype and phenotype are partly dependent on the type of sample being analyzed. When investigating association with disease status, it is determined if the frequency of a genotype is significantly different between cases and controls. Such comparisons can be made using chi-square analysis. However, such analysis does not allow adjustment for potential confounders. This can be achieved using the logistic regression framework. There are many other different statistical methods available for analyzing genotype data each with advantages and disadvantages, but these are beyond the scope of this book. One statistical issue that should be mentioned briefly is that of multiple testing, which is one of the most important, yet often misunderstood, statistical issues in genetic association analysis. The basic premise of multiple testing is that if the same hypothesis is examined multiple times, a number of positive associations will be observed due to random chance alone. Thus, using GWAS as an example, by genotyping several hundred thousand SNPs across the genome and then testing each SNP for association with the disease of interest, by chance we would expect to find a number of significant associations. Thus, correcting for multiple testing is very important to distinguish true positive associations from false negatives. Replication studies are also important for this purpose. Replication of the top SNPs can be performed in another population (using a candidate gene study approach) or it is possible to undertake another GWAS on an independent population. If multiple independent sample sets have undergone GWAS, it may be possible to perform meta-analyses.

FUTURE OF GENETIC ASSOCIATION STUDIES

Identifying the Causal Variant

Over the past decade, genetic studies have identified numerous associations between genetic variants and human diseases. Now the aim is to go beyond simple associations and identify the causal variants that underlie disease susceptibility. However, this is not easy (hence why there are so many associations reported but the causal variants remain uncertain) and typically involves additional genotyping as well as sequencing in the vicinity of disease-associated SNPs for sequence variants in functional elements including protein coding, regulatory, and structural sequences. This strategy is commonly referred to as fine mapping.

Findings of genetic associations need to be accompanied with or followed by functional studies to determine the potential impact of the genetic variation. Functional validation can be done in many different ways, including relating it to changes in gene or protein expression levels by using techniques such as real-time quantitative PCR for messenger RNA (mRNA), or Western blot, flow cytometry, enzyme-linked immunosorbent assay, and immunohistochemistry for protein. It is also possible to express the genetic variant in a cell line to determine whether it has an effect on mRNA, protein, or activity of the gene compared with the wild type.

Identifying the Missing Heritability

Although genotyping methods such as candidate gene studies and in particular GWAS have helped to advance the field of human genetics, it is evident that much of the genetic risk for most complex diseases remains unexplained. This is now commonly referred to as the "missing heritability" [2,3]. Uncovering this missing heritability is essential to the progress of genetic studies.

It had been suggested that structural variation, including CNVs such as insertions and deletions, may account for some of the unexplained heritability. However, there is little evidence that such CNVs contribute in a major way to disease risk beyond what has already been discovered by SNP arrays.

Common variants with small individual effects might contribute more substantially to disease risk through interactions with other genetic variants and/or environmental risk factors such as diet. Thus, the effects might be missed by examining single loci independently. In-depth post-GWAS analyses across multiple disciplines involving genetics, molecular biology, and bioinformatics for analyzing gene–gene interactions and gene pathways as well as gene–environment interactions are needed. Such studies are beginning to appear in the literature, and gene–diet interactions have been examined in a number of nutrigenetic studies. See Chapters 2 and 3.

There is a growing body of literature suggesting a role for epigenetic factors in the complex interplay between genes and the environment. Epigenetic effects are defined as chemical modifications of DNA and its associated proteins that can alter the expression of genes, and thus physical traits, without changing gene sequence. Unlike sequence changes, they can be reset or undone under certain conditions such as in early development. Mechanisms include changes in histone deacetylation and methylation of cytosines in CpG clusters. See Chapter 12 for a detailed discussion of epigenetics.

Rare variants are obvious contenders for the source of the missing heritability. It is now clear that new studies are needed to decipher these rare variants, using either arrays containing rare variants or high-throughput whole-genome sequencing methods.

SEQUENCING

The Human Genome Project, which was launched in 1990 with the primary goal of deciphering the DNA sequence of the human genome, took more than a decade to complete, even in a draft form, and cost close to 3 billion U.S. dollars [4,5]. Since that time, there has been considerable effort into developing new sequencing methodologies that will enable personal genomics. The new technologies are collectively referred to as next-generation sequencing and their application extends beyond DNA sequencing as the technology also allows the sequencing and analysis of the whole transcriptome (RNA-Seq), epigenetic modifications (Methyl-Seq), and transcription factor–binding sites (ChIP-Seq).

There are currently two routinely used platforms for next generation sequencing: the Illumina HiSeq [6], and the SOLiD system of Applied Biosystems [7]. The platforms differ with respect to template preparation, sequencing chemistry, imaging, read length, and quantity per run. Most of the high-speed instruments sequence DNA in very short segments (or "reads") of less than 100 base pairs at a time. This is significantly shorter than the reads produced by the first-generation Sanger instruments, which managed 800–900 base pairs per read, or the second-generation Roche 454 technology, whose reads approached 500 base pairs. Short reads make it difficult to assemble sequences into long stretches representing the chromosomes. Sequencing groups have tried to overcome these limitations by layering their results on one of the already published human genome sequences instead of trying to assemble the whole sequence from scratch. This gives a distorted view of any single genome, and despite all the advances in processing, the resulting data quality is still well below diagnostic standards. Also, analysis of such large amounts of data is not an easy task, and distinguishing disease-specific genetic variants from those that have no such effect remains a challenge.

The technology and sequencing output is improving and costs are decreasing every year. So, even though there will no doubt be GWAS chips with increasingly large numbers of markers, including rare variants, small insertions and deletions, and structural variation in the next year or two, as DNA sequencing technology becomes cheaper, it will likely become the method of choice for identifying novel genetic risk factors. There will be limited use in genotyping one, a hundred, a thousand, or even a million markers, when it is possible to get the sequence at every position in the genome for a sample set for a few thousand dollars. Yet, there is still some way to go before this capability can have a significant effect on medicine and health.

GENOTYPE–DIET INTERACTIONS

The generation of genotypic data will have little value without corresponding phenotypic information and computational tools for linking the two.

Although there are hundreds of genetic association studies reported in the literature, very few of these studies extend their investigations to diet–genotype interactions, as most of them have not captured information on the diet of the study participants. Collecting diet and other phenotype information presents a much greater challenge than genotypes because of the complexity of human biological and clinical information. The few nutrigenetic studies that have been undertaken are usually inconsistent in their findings, which is thought to be a result of inaccuracies and bias associated with the recording of dietary intake. The way forward may be to include the quantification of biomarkers of dietary exposure (e.g., micronutrients and specific fatty acids) as a dietary assessment tool.

Even if such detailed and standardized diet information was available for every person that was genotyped in a GWAS, it is unlikely we would be able to make use of it at the moment because we currently do not have the computational infrastructure to compare thousands of genotypes and phenotypes with each other. We need new computational approaches to deal with the considerably larger data sets and also people who are trained to use these methods and analyze/interpret the results. At the current rate of technological advancements, this is likely to happen in the very near future, and it is predicted that individualized dietary recommendations based on genotypes will revolutionize the way many of us make choices about the food we eat.

REFERENCES

1. Klein, R.J., Zeiss, C., Chew, E.Y. et al. (2005) Complement factor H polymorphism in age-related macular degeneration. *Science* 308(5720), 385–389.
2. Maher, B. (2008) The case of the missing heritability. *Nature* 456, 18–21.
3. Manolio, T.A., Collins, F.S., Cox, N.J. et al. (2009) Finding the missing heritability of complex diseases. *Nature* 461(7265), 747–753.
4. Lander, E.S., Linton, L.M., Birren, B. et al. (2001) Initial sequencing and analysis of the human genome. *Nature* 409(6822), 860–921.
5. Venter, J.C., Adams, M.D., Myers, E.W. et al. (2001) The sequence of the human genome. *Science* 291(5507), 1304–1351.
6. Bentley, D.R., Balasubramanian, S., Swerdlow, H.P. et al. (2008) Accurate whole human genome sequencing using reversible terminator chemistry. *Nature* 456, 53–59.
7. Valouev, A., Ichikawa, J., Tonthat, T. et al. (2008) A high resolution nucleosome position map of *C. elegans* reveals a lack of universal sequence-dictated positioning. *Genome Res.* 18, 1051–1063.

Section IV

Bringing Nutrigenomics to Industry, Health Professionals, and the Public

15 Bringing Nutrigenomics to the Food Industry

Industry–Academia Partnerships as an Important Challenge

Ralf C. Schlothauer and Joerg Kistler

CONTENTS

INTRODUCTION

Despite a wealth of knowledge and advice about the causative role of inadequate diet in chronic diseases, the incidence of diet-related chronic disease continues to rise in the Western world [1]. This has led to the concept of functional foods, defined as those which actively promote health and well-being and hence to the growth of a functional foods industry whose rationale is to identify the key components and increase accordingly the nutritional quality of individual foods.

Functional foods need a clear point of difference for added value in the eye of the consumer. That is why the industry's standard communication is developed around a single food [2–4], or a single molecule (e.g., sulforaphane) and a single benefit (cancer prevention). Although this makes it easier to convey the message to the consumer, it is too simplistic to gather meaningful scientific support [2,5] or to be sufficient to lead to a sustainable health claim. Traditionally, a consumer is primed with communications from the pharmaceutical or traditional food industry. A drug will contain one active molecule for one medical target. Neither the molecule nor the target needs to be fully comprehensible to the patient, as a health professional takes the responsibility.

Even a single food with known health benefits is likely to contain a range of beneficial components. For example, Ferguson and Schlothauer [5] concluded that broccoli alone contains four to—five classes of bioactive molecules, so that the nutritional value of broccoli is simply not captured by the measure of one single concentration of a bioactive component. Human dietary intervention studies have revealed multiple benefits of a broccoli enriched diet, including anti-inflammatory effects, effects on signal transduction, epigenetic effects, and modulation of the microbiota.

Systems biology approaches are increasingly used to study the complexity of events described earlier. The technologies applied to nutrigenomics comprise transcript-, proteome-, and metabolome-profiling techniques, in which responses to diets or individual ingredients are assessed in biological samples. Rather than making assumptions about genes and metabolites, and their interactions in response to foods, studying effects on gene expression pathways in a quantitative manner will be more informative. Already, microarray approaches have showed the complexity of mechanisms modulated by various foods or their combinations in animals. We seek to develop a rationale that an increasing emphasis on gaining more nutrigenomic data and unraveling the effects of food bioactives has the potential to change the current health perspective for functional foods.

HEALTH AND HOMEOSTASIS ARE INTRINSICALLY LINKED

The concept of maintaining good health is nothing new. "Homeostasis" describes the property of a living system that regulates its internal environment to maintain stable life-enabling conditions such as the right pH, temperature, nutrient concentration, and so on. Some scientists would argue that the entire evolution of life is centered around the ability to detect any deviation from the optimal settings of an internal milieu that is conducive to life, and quickly enables the body to act to remedy that situation [6].

Although humans are the most sophisticated living beings on the planet, we seem to have distanced ourselves from this most basic ability to maintain life within healthy boundaries, which seems to be mastered well by all life forms down to the most primitive single cell organisms. Our systems are functional on acute deviations from homeostasis, but we do not seem to have developed a response system for long-term gradual decay of homeostasis. This is especially true if that decay was generated by overfeeding and underexercising, which is unprecedented in animal or previous human history. Evolution has selected for acute short-term deviations from homeostasis, such as injury or short supply of nutrients, to be quickly noticed by an individual, but our modern slow creep away from homeostasis is mostly painless and goes unnoticed [6]. There is often a tendency to ignore gradual decay until it triggers symptoms, and then we find ourselves diagnosed with a degenerative disease, sometimes at that stage already with nonreversible effects on our health.

In terms of homeostasis, we are not so much one entity but composite of a few trillion entities stitched together—our cells. To be well, our cells have to be well and keep being well. It is clear that the right amount of nutrients and energy going into the cell, the right wastes being excreted from the cell, the right pH and temperature maintained in the cell is inextricably linked to the food we eat. In short, homeostasis has got a lot to do with what we eat.

Cellular systems have evolved to regulate the in-and-out flow of material, to activate different cellular states, to communicate with other cells, to shut down and multiply cells—all with the outcome to maintain long-term homeostasis within the ecosystem of cells we call organism. Post-digestion food-derived molecules enter the bloodstream and most of them will feed our energy demands and will be consumed in the process, some will be used as building blocks and others will feature as cofactors in cellular regulation. Thus, it is no surprise that dramatic changes in the food intake would result in big changes to the homeostatic stability of individual cells and, of course, in the well-being of the whole organisms as an ecosystem of trillions of cells. Maintaining this balance effectively is a major challenge of modern nutrition [7].

PREVENTATIVE AND REMEDIAL HEALTH CARE ARE VERY DIFFERENT PARADIGMS

The previous paragraphs set the scene for the two main paradigms prevalent in health care, "preventative" and "remedial." These are very contrasting paradigms. "Preventative" health care is based on keeping the organism "well," meaning in effect, within the homeostatic parameters. "Remedial" health care is focused on either slowing the progression or the reversal of an adverse condition that might have progressed over a number of years. Preventative health care is often a low priority for people on a low budget. In contrast, remedial health care post diagnosis takes a no-holds-barred approach for cost and attention, as the patient is faced with severe limitations of life quality or even death. Ironically, many issues of deviation from homeostatic balance, or in other words wellness balance that leads to degenerative disease, have a long period of reversibility. With appropriate willingness and management, severe disease can often be prevented even on a low budget, with little effort for the individual.

Although there are genetic and environmental stressors that we may have little or no control of, it is essential to understand the role of food in health, for either preventive or remedial health care [8]. An increasing number of nutrition practitioners are now prescribing "functional nutrition," for both the prevention and management of chronic disease. Such chronic diseases include obesity, diabetes, heart disease, stroke, hypertension, cancer, osteoporosis, pulmonary conditions, and mental disorders, and are currently leading to unsustainable economic and human costs in most countries. For example, in the United States alone, the direct and indirect costs of chronic disease, in terms of treatment and lost productivity, are currently estimated to exceed US$1 trillion annually [1].

The current medical dogma for chronic disease tends to focus on organ dysfunctions, rather than considering the whole person. We suggest that a desirable alternative would focus on the "health" component, with maintenance of homeostasis, promoting optimal health, and preventing diet- and lifestyle-related disease as important goals. This would be achieved through the concept of "functional nutrition," which includes the practice of personalized nutrition assessment, diagnosis, intervention, and monitoring [8]. The authors suggest that this practice will bridge nutrition and medicine in the 21st century.

REMEDIAL HEALTH CARE USING FOOD CREATES NEW CHALLENGES

A primary goal of nutrition research must be to optimize health, while preventing and/or delaying disease. Thus, it is necessary to characterize homeostasis with a new set of biomarkers that quantify optimal health, since most biomarkers are usually developed to measure susceptibility to or progression of disease. Developing novel validated biomarkers of health, or quantifying "normal homeostasis" are very challenging tasks.

There is no question that it is easier to monitor the effects of remedial than preventative health care. The effects of a remedial diet can be monitored by following reductions in known disease biomarkers, such as serum lipid profiles or insulin resistance [9,10]. For example, the latter authors studied the associations between cholesterol metabolism and liver or visceral fat content in healthy humans. They considered a cohort of 12 men and 8 women, aged around 30 years, following a 4 week dietary intervention study. Using some specific dietary regimes, they found that both visceral and liver fat contents of healthy humans were associated with cholesterol synthesis, and with dietary regime. A large number of similar examples can be found in the literature.

Much more difficult than remedial health care, is to convincingly prove the effect of dietary or other influences on homeostasis, an essential endpoint for preventative health care. The European-based Nutrigenomics Organization (www.nugo.org) has recognized the importance of, and focused a considerable resource on, developing the methods to measure this [7]. In effect, homeostasis is measured by the ability to maintain biochemical stability following some sort of physiological challenge. An often used approach to this uses either a high fat or high glucose challenge, and shows maintenance of homeostasis (measured in various ways) thereafter. The studies provide an important approach to identify suitable biomarkers for nutrition related health.

van Ommen et al. consider the following to be central in defining the physiology of a healthy individual [7].

1. A challenge to homeostasis may prove informative.
2. The processes involved in maintaining homeostasis require quantitative analyses of the many individual components involved.
3. "Health" covers a wide spectrum of response to nutritional interventions, and the effects of such interventions need to be comprehensively analyzed. Perturbation tests that quantify effects such as metabolism, oxidation, inflammation, and psychological stress may be informative.

HUMANS DIFFER IN THEIR RESPONSE TO FOODS, DIET, AND EXERCISE

Another problem in measuring optimum health relates to interindividual diversity. It has been repeatedly observed that individuals differ in their response to environment, including diet. The Masai, pastoralist tribes in Tanzania, have been traditionally used as an example of a race that appears genetically lean and fit, despite a diet high in saturated fat [11,12]. Their lipid profiles and cardiovascular risk factors appear to be distinctively different from other races or tribes living in the same territories [13], and it has been suggested that they may be genetically protected in some way. This has been proven correct through a comparative cross-sectional study published in 2010 that compared energy expenditure and cardiovascular risk of Masai, in comparison with rural or urban Bantu Tanzanians [14]. The study revealed that, despite a potentially artherogenic diet among the Masai, they are not only genetically distinct but also show very high energy expenditure. Thus, the study suggested complex interrelationships between genetics, diet, and lifestyle.

When diet and lifestyle patterns change, the prevalence of chronic disease may change. This has been documented for Japanese migrants to Hawaii [15]. After only one generation, the prevalence of degenerative disease had changed. However, even after several generations, despite most people of Japanese origin taking up a predominantly American diet lifestyle, the incidences and nature of chronic diseases are still somewhat different to those of the people of American heritage. This again provides a very good example of gene–diet interactions [15,16]. The very same diet and lifestyle may have much less of an effect on a more resilient genotype.

As the focus of nutrition research increasingly shifts to how we should be defining optimal human health and how to achieve it, interest in nutritional genomics is growing. It is becoming increasingly possible to match foods to an individual's genetically determined ability to digest, absorb, metabolize, and utilize the nutrients within those foods [17,18]. Whether this is achieved by genotyping, phenotyping, metabotyping, or other methods is discussed elsewhere [19–22]. In relation to the industry, the key question is: "what will this information mean to the consumer?"

NUTRIGENOMICS CREATES NEW OPPORTUNITIES FOR THE FOOD INDUSTRY

How can the industry benefit from the emerging findings of a nutrigenomics research program? It may be important to look at the key players separately: the food industry, the pharmaceutical industry and the emerging "functional food or nutrigenomic food" industry.

As discussed, there are two avenues for a health product or service to be offered to a consumer: the preventative and the remedial routes. The remedial work is usually the prerogative of the government-endorsed health care system, involving the prescription of pharmaceutical drugs. Pharmaceutical drugs are highly regulated, for very obvious and good reasons. Pharmaceutical companies develop drugs not only on a high risk, but also on a high-returns basis. They are predominantly based on single active compounds that are novel and can be patented. This provides an incentive for the company to tackle the high costs of research and development. This model is increasingly utilizing genetic and phenotypic data from patients (pharmacogenomics) to select the optimal therapy and to prevent unwanted side effects of the drug.

Recently, fish oils with eicosapentaenoic acid and docosahexaenoic acid as active compounds were one of the first bioactive foods that are now also available as prescription drugs, for example, Lovaza from GSK. Prescribing food bioactives as opposed to traditional drugs is an interesting trend, but the intent is curative, not preventative.

In contrast to the remedial model, the preventative model is based on the consumers' own choice from widely available products and information. The economic model of the food industry is in stark contrast to the pharmaceutical industry. Many food items are commodities; there are low hurdles to entry and the market features fierce competition, with intellectual property (IP) often being difficult to protect. Achieving economy of scale and strong branding are priorities in the food industry. Coke and McDonalds are common household names, penetrating the last remote niches on the globe. They have mastered a very refined low cost model on offering a standardized food experience to a consumer, anywhere in the world. Their brands are amongst the most 10 valuable global brands.

The development of new tools is emerging as an opportunity for industry and academia to work in conjunction. The science tools to keep a body in homeostasis, and the science tools to assess "wellness" for an individual, are very different from the science tools for remedial health care. Remedial health care looks at one issue at the time, for example, you see a cardiologist for cardiovascular disease, and he treats one symptom at the time, for example, by prescription of a drug to lower blood pressure. In preventative or wellness health care, the focus has to be on all body systems working well together. Preventative health care cannot afford to look at only one issue at the time as the focus has to be the synergistic workings of all body systems simultaneously. The science will have to be more wholesome as it will have to monitor the complex interactions of a "wholesome" food with a "wholesome" body. The science will have to be less reductionist and more complex. We would argue that we need to develop better science models and better communication models to overcome these problems.

Nutrigenomics knowledge will have very promising applications for the health food industry. Our genetic set is given to us irreversibly but we are starting to understand that we are not necessarily doomed by our genes. As our epigenetic understanding increases, we begin to understand that our parents had other ways than only their genes to influence how those genes are read and expressed [23–25]. We begin to appreciate that our parents' choices of food and lifestyle have very clear ramifications to our start in life, in addition to the genes they pass on to us.

In addition, our own choices of food and exercise have very clear consequences on us individually. Even monozygotic twins can turn out as very different phenotypes with very different health prospects by the time they are middle aged, depending on which of their genes are expressed or silenced differently through interactions with different diets. The important point for the consumer or even the patient may be that nutritional genomics may not be so much a science of how doomed we are with our genetic predispositions, but in fact how much control we still have with the food choices we make that will make the best out of our genes.

Researchers are now finding that even with major adverse health events, for example, cardiovascular disease or cancer, patients can make lifestyle changes that change their genetic read out and consequently on their quality of life and life expectancy [26–28]. Nutrigenomics may become an extremely useful tool to measure a huge set of activities, represented by the genetic expression changes that are based on better dietary choices. Instead of measuring a large range of very costly biomarkers and instead of looking at one food bioactive at the time, nutrigenomics could assess a whole set of foods with a whole set of bioactives each that are resulting in a complex set of expression changes in one hit.

Although we could argue that a gene regulation effect based on food intake can already be measurable after even one single meal, epidemiological data on dietary questionnaires may suggest we still need years of intake to make a significant difference big enough for general population health. The point here is that the choice to keep the body in homeostasis has to be a long-term sustainable one, a choice that needs to become a daily need and routine of an individual, requiring an intelligent selection of mixes of foods.

Would a consumer understand the claim: "this product helps to maintain wellness"? There is indeed a confusing variety of products already on the market with that very claim. Is the consumer in the position to verify this? Instead, the industry should focus on combinations, not individual foods, and nutrigenomics provides the tools to test this.

A better understanding of homeostasis or wellness can only be achieved through a more effective relationship between science and industry. The claim of enhanced wellness may look simple but the science of wellness is overwhelmingly complex. It is crucial for the industry to close the feedback loop to the customer. This is different from remedial health care which has closed this loop through the health professional. It is due diligence for a doctor to see the patient again and make sure the blood pressure has dropped and no adverse reaction has occurred.

In contrast, the functional food industry will need to invent new and creative feedback loops to establish their products and service have actually made a difference. It needs to show that even if the science is complex, the industry needs to find meaningful ways of engaging the consumer in that science and explain it to a general audience. This may change if a "branded food combination" will emerge to be a reliable partner for consumers to be well and stay well. A brand could be developed for a business model that will establish novel lifestyle or wellness partnerships with consumers. These partnerships will bring not only a functional food product to a consumer but also follow up on the efficacy of the offer. The partnership will be closing the kind of feedback loop that the remedial health care system already has. In our view, a business model and brand for such partnerships has the potential to grow to global scale.

WHY NUTRIGENOMICS METHODOLOGIES COULD BE IMPORTANT FOR TAKING NOVEL HIGH HEALTH FOOD COMBINATIONS TO THE MARKETPLACE

Although nutrigenomics approaches are currently being successfully used to study the diversity of mechanisms associated with consumption of individual foods in mice, the important question is whether they are sufficiently mature for use in human populations. Wittwer et al. 2011 critically evaluated the use of nutrigenomics approaches in human intervention trials by comparing the advantages and limitations of the current methodologies. Their analysis emphasized the current constraints in data interpretation, including huge knowledge gaps, the need for improved study designs, and more comprehensive phenotyping of volunteers before selection for study participation. However, the authors also emphasized the potential powers of such methods, and drew attention to a growing trend toward systemic approaches in which different technologies are combined and applied to the same sample. This allows physiological changes to be assessed very robustly throughout the various molecular layers of mRNA, protein, and metabolite changes. They suggested that nutrigenomics is maturing as a branch of the life sciences, and is gaining significant recognition in the scientific community. International agreement on consistency of study designs, technologies, data analysis, and interpretation will help to ensure comparability of data across study populations.

Although the disease prevention potential of various foods makes them desirable from a health perspective, practice suggests that most consumers select foods for taste, cost, and convenience rather than potential health benefits. However, the situation changes dramatically in groups who have actually developed a disease. High disease risk individuals and/or disease survivors are significantly more willing to take up advanced health foods or herbal supplements which they believe could improve their survival prospects.

From work described earlier [5], it becomes apparent that one of the reasons broccoli has such a strong reputation both as a disease preventative and disease retarding agent may be because of not just one component, but the complex interactions of a range of agents, acting through a range of biochemical pathways. A mix of different foods would be even better. This makes chemical analysis of a single bioactive or even multiple bioactives difficult as a measure for market consistency. However, the overall effects of mixed food extracts could be initially assessed in tissue culture models, such as HT-20, Caco-2, or various disease cell lines, using gene expression profiling or other bioactivity-related endpoints [29–31]. We suggest that an industrial model could combine foods based on the successful outcomes of such studies (Table 15.1).

STRONG WORKING RELATIONSHIP BETWEEN ACADEMIA AND INDUSTRY WILL HELP TO CONVEY THE HEALTH MESSAGE FROM FOODS

Consumers that turn to healthy foods and lifestyle to improve their well-being or prevent disease are not looking for a quick fix but will be prepared for a long-term engagement, and will have to enjoy the process to gain maximum benefit. To market healthier lifestyles to a wide cross-section of the community, an industry–academia partnership must overcome the dichotomy between the precision of scientific methodology and the complexity of its accredited communication, with the necessary simplicity and clarity for consumer appeal in the market place.

The underlying research that feeds into the product development and marketing of functional foods requires a hi-tech infrastructure that is often only seen in leading

TABLE 15.1
Contrasts Relevant Aspects of Preventative and Remedial Health Care Concepts

Remedial	Preventative	Domain
Patient	Consumer	Public
Prescription	Choice	Delivery
Advice	Advertising	Information
Government	Industry	Source
Molecule (drug)	Food (complex)	Product
Exclusive	Commodity	Market
Patent	Brand	Value
Organ	Body	System Level
Disease	Maintenance	Purpose

The comparison highlights the necessity of major paradigm shifts to make health care sustainable into the future.

universities. The "low hanging fruit" have been picked and contemporary science increasingly relies on expensive equipment, specialized facilities, and cutting-edge expertise. Nutrigenomics and bioactives research requires access to DNA sequencers, gene chip assay systems, mass spectrometers, cell culture facilities, robotic workstations, and so on. Such equipment facilities often require specialized expert personnel thereby increasing cost to the point where a shared model based on academic–industry collaboration becomes compelling financially and foremost as best practice to accelerate innovation. The partnership is complementary—the academic partner brings wide-ranging and in-depth research capability; the industry partner has the experience in translating the research findings into product development and marketing strategy. It is a win-win situation based on complementarity and risk sharing. A well working partnership not only benefits from the combined knowledge and technology pool but also from new ideas spawning by bringing different work cultures together. The complexities of science and product development toward novel healthy consumer foods clearly demands such new partnership models.

CASE STUDY OF A SUCCESSFUL INDUSTRY–ACADEMIC PARTNERSHIP HIGHLIGHTS NEW OPPORTUNITIES

As a case study Comvita New Zealand Ltd. (www.comvita.com) is developing a new model for academic engagement that has the potential to bridge the gap. Rather than setting up a research laboratory in their own headquarter, Comvita took up the offer from the Institute of Innovation in Biotechnology (IIB, www.biotech.co.nz) at the University of Auckland to collocate its R&D division spun out as the wholly owned subsidiary Comvita Innovations Ltd. Through this collocation, Comvita gets laboratory and office space, as well as full access to world-class hi-tech equipment, facilities, and expertise. This greatly accelerates innovation pathways and creates opportunities for the development of new products. Comvita's scientists also supervise MSc and PhD projects, summer studentships, and engage in teaching.

The difference from previous models is that Comvita's projects are not run in a "research to order" fashion but the company's scientists are actively engaging with these student projects on a weekly if not daily basis. The academic footprint on a comparable budget to "research to order" projects is much larger and more high-quality publications result [5,32–34]. The real difference between this new mode of conducting functional food research and more conventional models is the more intense reciprocal exchange of information. Comvita informs the academic partners more openly about its needs, for example, making scientific results understandable and accessible for the consumer and layperson. In addition, Comvita gets molded into an academic code of conduct, whereby peer review is an element of ongoing quality control.

The collocation of Comvita on the city campus of the University of Auckland has been operating successfully for more than 2 years allowing some initial evaluations to be made. Apart from several scientific publications, there are a range of very notable outcomes. In 2010, Comvita organized the first science symposium hosted by the IIB and the University of Auckland. Researchers from Comvita's science network from all around the globe visited to discuss outcomes related to research commissioned by Comvita but also their own initiatives in the field of functional foods. Comvita staff from across a whole spectrum of functions in the organization were invited to listen and network, but even more importantly, to participate and engage, ask questions, and give feedback on the meaning of the research outcomes relevant to their perspective. It became evident that some of the results will have uses in quality assurance and marketing that the research team has never dreamed of. The point we wish to emphasize is that innovation is not limited to scientific research. Traditionally, this would start from an idea sparked by consumer insights that inform a research team to look for bioactives in a food that a consumer group loves, or from a new revolutionary finding of an unknown metabolic pathway that has no potential to actually inform a purchase decision. Rather, we see innovation as a continuum that goes all the way from an idea that enables to the scientific research to a product that finds a route to market and fills a consumer need.

As discussed earlier, the science of functional foods is complex and cannot be condensed down to one food, one bioactive, and one benefit, even though that would be much preferred from a product development and marketing perspective.

To address the translation of science in the area of foods, Comvita devised a science challenge to university students in New Zealand. The company awarded NZ$5000 for the best 3 minute movie, which could translate the complex health aspects of good foods into a clear take-away message for consumers without losing the scientific credibility. The best contributions were screened at the social networking function of the Comvita science symposium and are displayed on Comvita's website and YouTube. This challenge is growing in popularity, and some of the clips display an amazing creativity and talent of the students. Our marketing team is using those movies in some markets to educate interested consumers about the benefits of functional foods.

CONCLUSIONS

A key property of many self-organized systems is that of criticality: a state of a system in which, on average, perturbations are neither dampened nor amplified, but are propagated over long temporal or spatial scales. Criticality enables the coordination of complex macroscopic behaviors that strike an optimal balance between stability and adaptability. In other words—a state of cellular homeostasis is highly desirable. If we make the right set of food molecules available to a cellular network that has been deprived of the right molecules, it is theoretically possible to move the cell (or the whole organism) back to homeostasis. The elegance of the nutrigenomics tool kit is that we may be able to show this in vitro in cell studies, and in vivo in humans. Based on this concept, the researchers will be able to identify relevant bioactives and foods and determine their efficacy, and the industry to develop optimal consumer products for long-term sustained wellness.

REFERENCES

1. Erler, A. et al., Preparing primary care for the future—perspectives from the Netherlands, England, and USA. *Z Evid Fortbild Qual Gesundhwes*, 2011. 105(8): 571–80.
2. Kussmann, M., A. Panchaud, and M. Affolter, Proteomics in nutrition: status quo and outlook for biomarkers and bioactives. *J Proteome Res*, 2010. 9(10): 4876–87.
3. Crawford, K. and J. Mellentin, *Successful superfruit strategy: how to build a superfruit business*. 2008, London, England: New Nutrition Business/Woodhead Pub Limited.
4. Chankvetadze, B. and A. Cifuentes, Natural bioactive compounds and Nutrigenomics. *J Pharm Biomed Anal*, 2010. 51(2): 289.
5. Ferguson, L.R. and R.C. Schlothauer, The potential role of nutritional genomics tools in validating high health foods for cancer control: broccoli as example. *Mol Nutr Food Res*, 2012. 56(1): 126–46.
6. Garrett, W.S., J.I. Gordon, and L.H. Glimcher, Homeostasis and inflammation in the intestine. *Cell*, 2010. 140(6): 859–70.
7. van Ommen, B. et al., Challenging homeostasis to define biomarkers for nutrition related health. *Mol Nutr Food Res*, 2009. 53(7): 795–804.
8. DeBusk, R., V.S. Sierpina, and M.J. Kreitzer, Applying functional nutrition for chronic disease prevention and management: bridging nutrition and functional medicine in 21st century healthcare. *Explore* (NY), 2011. 7(1): 55–7.
9. Krumholz, H.M. et al., Report of the National Heart, Lung, and Blood Institute working group on outcomes research in cardiovascular disease. *Circulation*, 2005. 111(23): 3158–66.
10. Silbernagel, G. et al., Cholesterol synthesis is associated with hepatic lipid content and dependent on fructose/glucose intake in healthy humans. *Exp Diabetes Res*, 2012. 2012: 361863.
11. Biss, K. et al., Some unique biologic characteristics of the Masai of East Africa. *N Engl J Med*, 1971. 284(13): 694–9.
12. Ho, K.J. et al., The Masai of East Africa: some unique biological characteristics. *Arch Pathol*, 1971. 91(5): 387–410.
13. Biss, K. et al., Atherosclerosis and lipid metabolism in the Masai of East Africa. *Afr J Med* Sci, 1971. 2(3): 249–57.
14. Mbalilaki, J.A. et al., Daily energy expenditure and cardiovascular risk in Masai, rural and urban Bantu Tanzanians. *Br J Sports Med*, 2010. 44(2): 121–6.

15. Maskarinec, G. and J.J. Noh, The effect of migration on cancer incidence among Japanese in Hawaii. *Ethn Dis*, 2004. 14(3): 431–9.
16. Le Marchand, L. and L.N. Kolonel, Cancer in Japanese migrants to Hawaii: interaction between genes and environment. *Rev Epidemiol Sante Publique*, 1992. 40(6): 425–30.
17. DeBusk, R., The role of nutritional genomics in developing an optimal diet for humans. *Nutr Clin Pract*, 2010. 25(6): 627–33.
18. DeBusk, R., Diet-related disease, nutritional genomics, and food and nutrition professionals. *J Am Diet Assoc*, 2009. 109(3): 410–3.
19. Castle, D. and R. DeBusk, The electronic health record, genetic information, and patient privacy. *J Am Diet Assoc*, 2008. 108(8): 1372–4.
20. Daniel, H. et al., The challenges for molecular nutrition research 3: comparative nutrigenomics research as a basis for entering the systems level. *Genes Nutr*, 2008. 3(3–4): 101–6.
21. Fay, L.B. and J.B. German, Personalizing foods: is genotype necessary? *Curr Opin Biotechnol.*, 2008. 19(2): 121–8.
22. German, J.B. et al., Nutrigenomics and personalized diets: what will they mean for food? *Annu Rev Food Sci Technol*, 2011. 2: 97–123.
23. Haluskova, J., Epigenetic studies in human diseases. *Folia Biol (Praha)*, 2010. 56(3): 83–96.
24. Niculescu, M.D. and D.S. Lupu, Nutritional influence on epigenetics and effects on longevity. *Curr Opin Clin Nutr Metab Care*, 2011. 14(1): 35–40.
25. McKay, J.A. and J.C. Mathers, Diet induced epigenetic changes and their implications for health. *Acta Physiol*, 2011. 202(2): 103–18.
26. Corella, D. et al., APOA2, dietary fat, and body mass index: replication of a gene-diet interaction in 3 independent populations. *Arch Intern Med*, 2009. 169(20): 1897–906.
27. Davis, C.D. and J.A. Milner, Nutrigenomics, vitamin D and cancer prevention. *J Nutrigenet Nutrigenomics*, 2011. 4(1): 1–11.
28. Fenech, M. et al., Nutrigenetics and nutrigenomics: viewpoints on the current status and applications in nutrition research and practice. *J Nutrigenet Nutrigenomics*, 2011. 4(2): 69–89.
29. Afman, L. and M. Muller, Nutrigenomics: from molecular nutrition to prevention of disease. *J Am Diet Assoc*, 2006. 106(4): 569–76.
30. Bhamre, S. et al., Temporal changes in gene expression induced by sulforaphane in human prostate cancer cells. *Prostate*, 2009. 69(2): 181–90.
31. Kleemann, R. et al., Anti-inflammatory, anti-proliferative and anti-atherosclerotic effects of quercetin in human in vitro and in vivo models. *Atherosclerosis*, 2011. 218(1): 44–52.
32. Stephens, J.M. et al., Phenolic compounds and methylglyoxal in some New Zealand manuka and kanuka honeys. *Food Chem*, 2010. 120(1): 78–86.
33. Gannabathula, S. et al., Arabinogalactan proteins contribute to the immunostimulatory properties of New Zealand honeys. *Immunopharmacol Immunotoxicol*, 2012. 34(4): 598–607.
34. Steinhorn, G. et al., Isolation and characterisation of arabinogalactan-proteins from New Zealand kanuka honey. *Food Chem*, 2011. 128(4): 949–56.

16 Commercialization and Potential of Nutrigenetics and Nutrigenomics

Virginia Parslow and Lynnette R. Ferguson

CONTENTS

INTRODUCTION

The aim of this chapter is to background the rise of nutritional genomics, show some existing applications of this still-new science, and briefly visit current challenges and future possibilities. As detailed in previous chapters, nutrigenetics seeks to quantify differing nutrient requirements in relation to different genotypes, whereas nutrigenomics reflects the impact of nutrients on the expression of genes. These complementary fields have significant potential for personalizing nutrition to optimize health and wellness, as well as prevent disease, delay its onset, and/or progression. They are also finding increasing utility in the food industry, in revealing previously unexpected properties of new or novel foods or food components among numerous other roles.

Personalized nutrition is one key outcome of the field, comparable to personalized medicine. Genetics potentially allows scientists to unravel the unique genetic code that is the characteristic of each individual. The current sophistication of this field is beginning to enable a description of the effects of inheritance on the absorption, distribution, and metabolism of nutrients [1]. In turn, this should facilitate an understanding as to how an individual's genetic background will influence the risks and/or benefits of consuming different levels and combinations of nutrients, types of foods or dietary patterns, and inform their selection. This genetic profiling may be important for segregating those who will respond from those who will not respond to certain diets. Although early work in this field primarily used genotyping [2], it may now be more common to use metabolic profiling, using the much more sensitive methods now available [3,4]. As in their use in pharmacogenomics, these methods can help to differentiate likely responders from nonresponders to dietary interventions.

The complementary field of nutrigenomics describes the effects of foods or food components on the expression of genes. Various omics technologies work together in identifying molecular biomarkers [3]. These biomarkers allow very sensitive measures of early effects of a dietary intervention, which help maintain homeostasis, and/or retain optimal health with enhanced performance, and even reverse the onset of diet-related diseases. Prior to the development of omics technologies, a separatist approach in research was unavoidable, whereby facets of an organism were studied in isolation. It is increasingly apparent that a systems biology approach, in which whole interrelated biological systems are studied rather than isolated components, is crucial to fully understand the workings of any organism or group of organisms, particularly when environmental factors such as nutrition are involved [5]. Nutrigenomics effectively utilizes the various omics technologies that have arisen out of genome sequencing, including genomics, transcriptomics, proteomics, lipidomics, and metabolomics. The sensitivity and specificity of these technologies have greatly increased, accompanied by substantial decreases in price in recent years. Similarly, there have recently been striking increases in the sensitivity and specificity of bioinformatic approaches for studying and combining these data. A further advantage of these technologies is that they are not hypothesis driven, meaning they are unbiased and unrestrictive, unlike more traditional nutritional research strategies.

Foodomics is sometimes described as the application of nutrigenomic technologies to the identification of novel or unexpected properties of foods. This is taken from the food angle, rather more than the human angle. Thereby, it has an enormous analytical potential that can be applied to solving questions related to food safety, traceability, and quality, as well as hitherto unexpected properties of new foods, functional foods, nutraceuticals, and so on. *S*everal of the health benefits assigned to many dietary constituents are still controversial, as evidenced by the large number of applications rejected by the European Food Safety Authority regarding health claims of new foods and ingredients. More sound scientific evidence is needed to demonstrate (or not) the claimed beneficial effects of these new foods and constituents. In this sense, the advent of new postgenomic strategies that are non-hypothesis-directed seems to be essential to understand how bioactive compounds from the diet interact at the molecular and cellular level, as well as to provide better scientific evidence on their health benefits. In vitro methodologies may initially suggest a novel mechanism of action of new compounds, leading through to the more informed application of the most appropriate tools to a human clinical trial.

APPLICATIONS

For our current purposes, we have structured our focus in the following manner:

1. The marketing of nutrigenetic tests in the health food industry, including in clinical settings
2. The marketing of pet foods through health claims developed using nutrigenomics technologies
3. The adoption of nutrigenetics and nutrigenomics by the human food and beverage sector, including major partnerships between academia and industry

Due to the wide nature of this topic, there is no attempt to name every company or detail every activity occurring. Instead, we attempt to show the "big picture" through profiling some of the key players in the current uptake of this still-new science.

Nutrigenetic Testing Companies

A number of companies have entered the arena of nutrigenetic testing, in the hope of capitalizing on recent genomic advancements in numerous ways (examples are summarized in Table 16.1). They claim, with varying degrees of honesty, to provide gene-based personalized health and nutrition analysis. Their recommendations are generally based on genotype data, sometimes including some very highly preselected genes, ranging through to more detailed genetic profiles based on one of the various DNA array technologies now available. The question is also being asked as to whether genotyping is even necessary, given some of the successes of metabolic phenotyping [6,7]. This information is generally combined with questions on current diet and lifestyle, to provide recommendations on maintenance of health and prevention of disease through modifications of diet and lifestyle.

Some of the early players in this field have now shut down operations. Sciona is a well-publicized example of a company that attracted considerable attention. Their original claim was of a "body benefits" test, based on a lifestyle questionnaire and genetic testing, using DNA from a buccal swab, of 19 common genetic polymorphisms. The advice provided often recommended vitamin and mineral mixes. Such direct-to-consumer online marketing companies have attracted considerable public opposition by watchdog groups such as Genewatch (www.genewatch.org). Although these provide ongoing and sometimes useful comparative analyses of such companies, they seem to class all in the same group and argue against all of them on grounds such as "targeting of fear," "undermining public health," "creating a genetic underclass," and so on. What such claims ignore is the number of well-characterized examples where genetic or functional testing is essential to the subject being able to maintain good health (e.g., Table 16.2).

Those companies that are becoming increasingly successful involve provision of genetic tests through clinicians and/or dieticians rather than directly to consumers [8]. There are now numerous successful examples, such as The Institute for Functional Medicine (www.functionalmedicine.org).

TABLE 16.1
Nutrigenetic Testing Services. Code: Grey = DTC; Black = Associated with Health Professionals

Company	Product/Service/Research Involvement	Website
23andMe	Provide genetic testing for over 100 traits and diseases as well as DNA ancestry. They use the Illumina OmniExpress Plus Research Use Only Chip that has been customized for use in their products and services. Customer orders an online kit over the web. Once the kit is received, customer provides saliva sample. Company's lab analyses DNA in 6–8 weeks and comes back with recommendations.	https://www.23andme.com/pgs
Advanced Genomics	Canadian based. Offers a variety of tests for medical conditions. From website: "NOTE: All these tests are for information purposes only. These are only for overall assessment of health condition. By receiving this information, a person can take preventive measures, change diet, and make overall life style changes. It does not nor is it intended to provide medical advice, recommendations, diagnosis or treatment. Person should never disregard professional medical advice or delay seeking medical advice based on these tests. We provide total confidentiality and will never disclose to third party." Only offered through hospitals, research institutes, academics, pharmaceuticals, biotechnology, and other institutes.	http://www.advancedgenomics.ca
Alphagenics	Their company, Wellness Genetics, offer DTC genetic testing. Instead of identifying the risk of medical problems and disease, Wellness Genetics aims to give insight into how genes relate to behavior, personality, weight loss, sex, mental acuity, and athletics. Their "MyGene DaVinci" test has over 50 traits in its profile that cover a very wide range of characteristics, including caffeine metabolism, obesity, sugar intake, and weight control.	http://alpha-genics.com/index.html
BioIndex	University of Oslo campus company engaged in biochemical phenotyping through a postal system. Ascertains specific nutrient levels (via pinprick test). Then offers personalized advice on nutrition and lifestyle changes that can reduce risk for common diseases.	http://www.bioindex.no

Bio.Logis	Based in Frankfurt, Germany. Offers among other services a DTC "Personal Genomics Service," which it states can be useful for those who are conscious of their nutrition and who want to achieve a positive effect on their health by adjusting their diet to their genetic predisposition. They analyze 15 different genes to ascertain what vitamins or minerals might be important for a client's diet or what foods should be avoided. A range of feedback is given including whether someone is lactose intolerant and whether their body is able to degrade toxins rapidly enough, such as those that are produced by roasting meat.	https://www.biologis.com
Consumer Genetics	DTC. Offer a small range of "Lifestyle" DNA tests, which include CaffeineGEN™ and WineGEN™.	http://www.consumergenetics.com
Cygene Direct	Offers a wide range of DTC tests, including: The CyGene Metabolic Health Assessment DNA Analysis looks at: Cardiac health Type II Diabetes and Obesity Immune Efficiency Osteoporosis DNA Analysis: Osteoporosis Gene Test and Osteoporosis Genetic Testing	cygene.infinityarts.com
DecodeMe	Claims to be the most comprehensive genetic health scan available. Tests genetic risk for 47 diseases and traits ranging from Heart Attack and Diabetes to Alcohol Flush Reaction and Male Pattern Baldness. It is for informational purposes only; it is not a medical test. Cost of full test is US$1100.	http://www.decodeme.com
DecodeHealth	The tests offered through deCODEhealth are reference-laboratory tests that must be ordered by a physician and are reimbursable under many healthcare plans. The exact price of tests depends upon the physician, lab, or distributor they are ordered through. Offers the same range of tests as for DecodeMe.	http://www.decodehealth.com
DNA Diet	Based in the USA, created by nutritionist, Carolyn Katzina. DNA profiles from buccal swabs are combined with a questionnaire to ascertain which of three nutrition groups people fall into. A program is then suggested accordingly. Both weight loss and weight gain options are included. Although tests are DTC, the programs themselves include one-on-one conversations with Carolyn over the 6-week period; 30 minutes for the first and last week, 15 minutes during the intervening weeks. Once the 6-week program is complete, clients may join the DNA Diet Health and Wellness System, the first two weeks of which are free.	http://www.thednadiet.com

(Continued)

TABLE 16.1 (*Continued*)
Nutrigenetic Testing Services. Code: Grey = DTC; Black = Associated with Health Professionals

Company	Product/Service/Research Involvement	Website
Dnalysis Biotechnology	South African–based company that offers DTC testing: • DNA Diet—tests for eight genes that impact metabolism and fat loss. The results provide recommendations that include dietary changes and guidance as to the type and amount of exercise required. • DNA Health—aims to optimize health and wellness through gene-based personalized nutrition. It tests 20 genes involved in seven key biological processes. The results provide individual recommendations that include a gene-based healthy eating plan, dietary goals for relevant vitamins, minerals, phytochemicals and foods, and requirements for nutritional supplementation, where required.	http://www.dnadiet.co.za
EoCyte Pharma Care (Brazil)	Specializes in personalized medicine. Offers Genotest, a range of 40 biomolecular tests. All of them are related to nutrigenomics or inborn errors of metabolism. Only available through practitioners.	http://www.eocyte.net
Fitgenes	Fitgenes Certified Practitioners use individual DNA profiles from saliva sample to tailor a customized program of lifestyle choices for an individual's optimal health and well-being, focusing on fitness, health, and nutrition. Concentrates on areas such as weight management, diabetes, cardiovascular health, chronic inflammation, bone health, fitness, and exercise. Have developed patented systems and methodologies to deliver Nutrigenomic interventions. Partners with Oborne Health Supplies for products suggested to clients. Active in Australia and Malaysia.	www.fitgenes.com.au http://www.oborne.com.au
Flylife	Based in Italy. Although primarily a medical biotech company, they also offer DTC testing that includes "G-nutrition" aimed at predictive and preventive personalized medicine/lifestyle. Although clients can access reports direct, they have qualified assistance available for discussing and acting on results.	http://www.flylife.it
GeneCare	Practitioner-based genetic tests on limited number of SNPs, using DNA from a buccal swab or saliva. GeneCare's sister company Nutrition Care manufactures vitamins, herbal medicines, and food supplements to sectors of the nutritional care industry. The two companies work together with diagnosis and suggested products.	www.genecare.com.au http://www.nutritioncare.com.au

GenCounT	DTC genetic testing company that offers wide range of tests plus one hour of free genetic counseling. Tests are aimed at enabling individuals to make appropriate lifestyle changes and include cardiac, cancer, IBD, and obesity tests.	http://www.gencount.com
Genelex	Offer a wide range of tests, including tests for Celiac Disease and hemochromatosis. Also offer clinical trial genotyping services. Clients can order testing directly but only if they have a physician prescription, or their healthcare provider can request testing for them. Genelex sends a cheek swab collection kit with directions by mail.	http://www.healthanddna.com
GeneLink Biosciences	Have created a methodology for SNP-based genetic profiling (patents issued and pending) and are marketing and/or licensing these proprietary assessments to companies that manufacture or market to the nutraceutical, personal care, and skin care industries, as well as developing their own proprietary products for sale based on their profiling system.	http://genelinkbio.com
GeneWize Life Sciences	Wholly-owned subsidiary of GeneLink Biosciences. GeneWize Life Sciences, Inc. ("GeneWize") provides genetically customized products and services to the nutrition and skincare markets.	www.genewize.com
Gene Smart Diagnostics	Early stage personalized nutrition venture developing proprietary Gene Smart® Genetic Tests and related products to prevent and treat serious diseases and disorders in genetically susceptible individuals.	http://www.genesmartdiagnostics.com/index.html
	Works with the genetics and biochemistry of the omega-3 and omega-6 pathway, associated with numerous inflammatory diseases, autoimmune disorders, neurological disorders, and cognitive development.	
Gene Smart Wellness	Market an omega-3 test for people to check their Omega-3 Index and Omega-6 to Omega-3 Ratio through a home blood test kit; interaction through Gene Smart Diagnostics.	http://www.genesmart.com/
Genetic Health	A medical company run by doctors who claim to have an active interest in preventative health.	http://www.genetic-health.co.uk
	The New Nutrition Gene test examines polymorphisms that affect the body's ability to: • Detoxify environmental substances • Regulate potassium metabolism • Influence immune defence and the aging processes • Control lipid and glucose metabolism	http://www.genetic-health.co.uk/dna-test-services/nutritional-test.htm
Genicys	Singapore company that offers genetic tests either through a physician or DTC. Offer a Disease Susceptibility Genetic Test that covers susceptibility to 108 diseases; categories of diseases covered are respiratory, circulatory, digestive, urinary, reproductive, liver, cerebral/nervous/neuro, musculo-skeletal + skin, immune + sensory.	http://www.genicsys.com

(Continued)

TABLE 16.1 (*Continued*)
Nutrigenetic Testing Services. Code: Grey = DTC; Black = Associated with Health Professionals

Company	Product/Service/Research Involvement	Website
Genova Diagnostics UK	Offers genetic tests through licensed healthcare professionals.	www.gdx.uk.net
Genovations	A Genova Diagnostics subsidiary that sells tests DTC.	http://www.healthremedies.com/genomic_testing.html
Genovive	The GenoVive Weight Management DNA Test and Genetic Profile Report focus specifically on weight loss and weight management related genes and gene variants. Each SNP has specific implications for changes in diet and/or exercise that have been documented in clinical studies. DNA test results are used to determine an optimal balance of macronutrients (carbohydrates, fats, and proteins) for a customized meal program. The GenoVive Customized meal program also features the following: • A package of nutritional supplements: Gen-Multi, Gen-Omega, and Gen-Biotics • An online video exercise program • Monthly support call with a registered dietician plus online and phone support from Customer Service	http://www.genovive.com/index.php/how-genovive-works.html
Gent Source	New York–based company. Offers a variety of gene-based tests DTC, including a genetic report that they say gives clients the power to understand their metabolism, eating behaviors, response to exercise, and shows the best ways to reach and maintain a healthy weight and lifestyle.	http://www.gentsource.net
HealthCheckUSA	DTC. Test DNA (provided by cheek swab) for eight or more genetic illnesses, including Celiac disease (an intestinal disorder) and Hemochromatosis (an overload of iron).	http://www.healthcheckusa.com
Illumina	Offers individual genome sequencing, but only through doctors.	http://www.everygenome.com/test_process/index.ilmn
Infinite Health and Wellness Center	Based in Florida, USA. "A holistic health enterprise that includes Functional Medicine/Nutrition and—as part of that—genetic testing in its practices. These tests are only done through a qualified FM practitioner who requests and interprets the tests for/with a client."	http://www.infinitehealthandwellnesscenter.com

Interleukin Genetics: Inherent Health	"Inherent Health is a health and wellness brand of genetic tests from Interleukin Genetics that empower consumers to help prevent some of the chronic diseases of aging through diet and lifestyle recommendations uniquely based on insights from a trusted source of genetic research. Results from the Inherent Health line of genetic tests provide individuals with a clear understanding of their genetic profile as it relates to a particular health concern, a summary of the role those genes have on their present health, and steps to improve their future health outcomes." Inherent Health sells tests direct to consumers. Recommends talking with a genetic counselor if necessary, but this is not mandatory to receive the tests or their results.	http://www.inherenthealth.com
Karma Life	Canadian-based company that offers tests DTC. Offers a "DNA diet," which tests specific genes and related proteins. Also offers a DNA Fitness Test, DNA Supplement Test. Also offers supplements for purchase	http://www.karmalife.ca
Knome	Knome specializes in the interpretation of human whole genomes. Its platform group provides clinics with big data, enterprise-wide genome interpretation systems that (1) manage whole genome sequence data; (2) help clinicians interpret genomes to make better decisions; and (3) aid medical researchers in the identification of causal variants. In 2010, BioMérieux and Knome entered into a strategic agreement to collaborate in the development of next-generation, sequence-based in vitro diagnostics. Under the agreement, bioMérieux now has exclusive rights to license Knome's proprietary genome analysis platform for use in the in vitro diagnostics market. Furthermore, Knome gained access to bioMérieux's intellectual property in DNA extraction and sample preparation	http://www.knome.com/solutions/knomebase-2
KnowYourGenetics.com	"This comprehensive look at the methylation pathway enables us to assess an individual's genetic differences and develop an individualized nutritional wellness program to aid detoxification and support your genetic and cellular memory system- a personal roadmap for optimal health in today's toxic environment."	www.knowyourgenetics.com
Lumigenix	Offers gene-based tests for a fairly wide (and growing) number of diseases. Does not offer counseling/guidance, but addresses medical practitioners through the website regarding working with test results as an essential part of personalized health care. Based in USA and Australia.	https://www.lumigenix.com
Malaysian Genomics Resource Centre Berhad (MGRC)	Offers a wide range of services, available only through practitioners.	http://www.mgrc.com.my/genetic_screening.php

(*Continued*)

TABLE 16.1 (*Continued*)
Nutrigenetic Testing Services. Code: Grey = DTC; Black = Associated with Health Professionals

Company	Product/Service/Research Involvement	Website
Matrix Genomics	Sante Fe company that offers a variety of health-related tests DTC, including a Heart Attack Gene-Gene Panel (6 genes) and an Alzheimer's Disease Gene APOE test.	http://matrixgenomics.com
MedCan Clinic	Medical clinic in Toronto that offers wide range of integrated services, including Personal Genome Testing (PGT) using Navigenics® tests in conjunction with in-person counseling by a certified genetic counselor.	http://www.medcan.com
Metagenics	"Science-based" medical foods, nutritional formulas, and lifestyle therapy programs. Metagenics University aims to help healthcare professionals stay on the leading edge of lifestyle medicine and incorporate nutrition into their clinical practice.	www.metagenics.com
Mydietclinic (South Africa)	DNA HEALTH TEST: Anti-aging Nutrition. Dietician-based, testing 20 genes for 23 gene variations. The genes tested are involved in cholesterol metabolism, detoxification, b-vitamin metabolism, inflammation, anti-oxidant status, bone health, and insulin sensitivity. Supply an associated tailored eating plan. DNA DIET TEST: Ultimate Weight Loss Tool. Dietician-based, testing for SNPs in seven genes that govern weight loss and five genes involved in exercising potential.	http://www.mydietclinic.co.za
MyGene	An Australian Biotechnology Company specializing in genetic testing for various endpoints, through healthcare professionals.	www.mygene.com.au
MyGenomics	Spinout company from the Newcastle (UK) Science City Innovation Machine programme. Tests for genes relevant to weight loss, only available through qualified healthcare providers.	https://www.mygenomics.co.uk
Navigenics	Offers testing for the following: • Genetic predispositions for a variety of health conditions • Personalized pharmacogenetic information • Access to genetic counselors Can be ordered directly by consumers.	http://www.navigenics.com

NutraGenomics	NutraGenomics, Inc. offers healthcare services. The company researches and develops diagnostic tests and identifies therapies for treatment of Type 2 diabetes, obesity, atherosclerosis, and cancer. The company develops protein and genome sequence products and engages in gene expression profiling and analyses of nutraceuticals, pharmaceuticals, and nutrients. The company has a strategic alliance with Davis Bioscience Group. NutraGenomics, Inc. was founded in 2002 and is based in Chicago, Illinois. Its key executives are Dr Nancy Fogg-Johnson and Dr Jim Kaput.	http://investing.businessweek.com/research/stocks/private/snapshot.asp?privcapId=34187645
Nutrigenomix	Offer tests only available through registered dieticians. Test kit covers seven genes that affect response to vitamin C, folate, whole grains, omega-3 fat, saturated fat, sodium, and caffeine.	www.nutrigenomix.com
	Nutrigenomix is developing a research funding program to support university-based research programs and provide travel grants to students and scholars to attend conferences and workshops on nutrigenomics. They will also fund specific dietetics research projects that focus on personalized nutrition.	http://www.nutrigenomix.com/investing-in-research
NutriPATH	Offer a range of testing panels in the areas of Hormonal, GIT, Food Allergy, Nutritional, and Metabolic Assessments. Tests can be ordered DTC or through a practitioner.	http://nutripath.com.au
Pathway Genomics	Tests are only available through physicians. Pathway offers pre- and posttesting assistance and guidance to physicians and their patients at no charge, with genetic counselors and medical professionals available to physicians in a number of ways such as clinical information, report interpretation, or general client service. Tests available include the following: Drug response (including caffeine metabolism) Prepregnancy planning Health conditions (e.g., propensity for obesity, cancers, diabetes, and heart disease) Pathway Fit®: report provides personalized information and recommendations based on genetics and gives detailed information on the following: Matching diet Eating behavior traits Food reactions	https://www.pathway.com

(Continued)

TABLE 16.1 (*Continued*)
Nutrigenetic Testing Services. Code: Grey = DTC; Black = Associated with Health Professionals

Company	Product/Service/Research Involvement	Website
	Nutritional needs Exercise Your body and weight Metabolic health factors	
Philips	My Kitchen (a helping hand) Plasma screen records everything in your kitchen, including in your larder. Menu suggestions and recipes (including instructional videos) will be offered by the system. • Device worn on your belt that records exercise output, reports it back to Direct Live website, and subsequently sends updated/improved exercise programmes back, which are devised by real sports scientists. Noninvasive glucose sensor and a noninvasive ketone body sensor; measures ketones in your breath to indicate negative energy balance, and thus indicates a need for dietary/exercise adjustments. Philips has a major interest in personalized medicine and it is a partner in the UCD-led FP7 project, Food4Me. Also partners in TI Food and Nutrition. Through its molecular imaging capabilities, it can offer tools for molecular diagnostics (slide show downloaded from www.slideshare.net).	www.philips.co.uk/kitchen
Prime Lab	Headquartered in the Netherlands, profiles itself primarily as an "anti-aging" company. Run by a doctor who has decided to focus solely on anti-aging medicine because, in his opinion, traditional health care is too focused on curing disease rather than preventing it and optimizing health. He has completed Anti-Aging Medicine Specialization training organized by the World Society of Anti-Aging Medicine (WOSAAM) in the field of functional genomics at the European Institute of Personalized Prevention. Treatment includes a questionnaire and a blood sample for DNA analysis, correction of nutritional deficiencies (the website recommends and sells supplements), lifestyle advice based on analysis of your DNA and replenishing low hormone levels with bioidentical hormones.	http://www.primelab.nl

Reach100	Genome Health Clinics for personalized DNA damage prevention REACH100 DOCTORS • interact with clients to explain genome health test • provide nutritional and lifestyle advice based on baseline data • verify with second test that DNA damage is actually decreased • if not, further adjustments to recommendations are made CSIRO GENOME HEALTH NUTRIGENOMICS LABORATORY • performs CBMN assay test • interprets result for Reach100 • provides scientific updates on dietary, lifestyle, and genetic variables affecting DNA damage • builds deidentified genome health nutrigenomics database	www.reach100.com.au
Research Nutrition	Integrative/Functional Medicine perspective. Website offers two arms: consumer/retailer arm for ordering of omega oil products and practitioner arm for ordering tests. Tests offered include the following: • Nutritional: Urine amino acids, urine halide; pre- and postloading, urine iodine; pre- and postloading, urine toxic and essential elements, urine toxic metals • Gastrointestinal tests • Specialty testing	www.researchnutrition.com
SmartDNA	SmartDNA provides an exclusive nutritional genomic service to practitioners. There are nine unique Boutique Panels covering Lipid Metabolism, Phase I and II detox, Oxidative stress, Bone Health, Lactose Intolerance, Inflammation, Nutriagen, Weight Management, and Anti-aging. Screens analyse over 70 nutritionally modifiable gene changes. Practitioners using the service have access to scientific information, training documentation, client forms, and more.	www.smartdna.net.au
SmartGene	"SmartGene develops specific modules for defined applications of sequence-based testing and creates integrated suites of tools best adapted to the task. As part of SmartGene's personalized service, our modules can be configured to suit an organization's particular requirements and workflow."	http://www.smartgene.com

(*Continued*)

TABLE 16.1 (*Continued*)
Nutrigenetic Testing Services. Code: Grey = DTC; Black = Associated with Health Professionals

Company	Product/Service/Research Involvement	Website
SorgenteGenetica	Italian company offering wide range of tests DTC. Tests include "Diet+," which promises to help improve a client's fitness with the optimal dose of carbohydrates, fibre and fat, and "Full Health," which analyzes relevant genes in the following five areas: bone health, anti-aging, heart health, inflammation, insulin, and glucose.	www.sorgentegenetica.it
Tailor Medical	A Toronto-based medical clinic dedicated to an integrative medicine platform. Offers a wide variety of tests and programmes, including the "Genomics Personalized Services Program." Results Reports are conducted with the client, the client's physician, and members of the in-house Tailor Medical Team.	http://www.tailormedical.com
The Makings of Me	DTC company offering two main tests: • MyDNA Insights Kit: Includes hair loss, becoming overweight, responding to certain diet, smoking behavior, having tall children, memory performance, excelling in endurance sports, longevity. • My Child's DNA Insights: Includes height, athletic potential, weight and diet needs, memory performance, nearsightedness, morning/night person. Website states that "The test results report will include a list of markers (indicators) relevant to the test along with your matched results. This will be followed by a brief, user-friendly explanation on each marker result." Website carries the following rider: "TheMakingsofMe.com™ is for informational purposes only and should NOT be used for medical decision."	http://www.themakingsofme.com
The Risk MD	Medical practice run by Florida-based physician (with PhD), which uses Navigenics' technology to genetically test for a wide range of conditions including heart disease and gastrointestinal disorders. Although this is mostly DTC, it also offers a "Follow-Up Health Risk Review" by phone or video conferencing.	http://www.theriskmd.com

TABLE 16.2
Well-Characterized Examples of Genetically Determined Conditions Which Can Be Controlled by Avoidance of Certain Foods

Genetic Condition	Foods to Avoid
Celiac disease (allergy to gluten)	Gluten-containing cereals (mostly wheat, rye, and barley)
Defective aldehyde dehydrogenase enzyme	Alcohol
Galactosemia (lack of a liver enzyme to digest galactose)	Lactose or galactose, including all milk and milk products
Phenylketonuria (inability to metabolize the amino acid phenylalanine)	High-protein foods such as fish, chicken, eggs, milk, cheese, dried beans, nuts, and tofu

Where there is a very major gap at present is in communication between nutritional genomics experts and health professionals, including the public health sector and the public themselves. Good DNA-based [9] or even metabolic phenotyping-based nutritional advice [4,10] needs to have informed interpretation around it, and there is a great deal of confusion at present. The biggest question here is whether this sort of data will be properly explained and understood and will motivate individuals into a healthier lifestyle and diet? Although there are a limited number of genetic counsellors who are also dieticians, this combined skill base is still unusual and the number of health professionals qualified to interpret the data are relatively modest at present.

Animal Food and Beverage Companies

Nestlé has a strong interest in the use of nutrigenomics in pet foods, production animals, and equine applications, sponsoring a yearly symposium in animal nutrition among other activities. In particular, they use transcriptomics methods to provide early indicators of changes in gene expression relevant to particular health conditions and to show potential benefits (or other effects) of different nutritional interventions. http://www.purinavets.eu/home/canine/innovations/nutrigenomics.htm. Examples are summarized in Table 16.3

In the equine feeding area, Nestle is researching solutions to conditions such as Hyperkalemic Periodic Paralysis (HYPP), a genetic disorder that has huge implications and economic ramifications within the horse industry. Researchers have ascertained that in many cases, proper nutritional management can control the negative effects of HYPP, particularly a triple-strategy regime of the following: (1) limiting dietary intake of potassium, (2) promoting potassium intake into cells, and (3) eliminating excess extracellular potassium through the urine [21].

Other major players include Alltech and Hills [22].

TABLE 16.3
Animal Food and Beverage Companies

Company	Product/Service/Research Involvement	Website
Alltech	Using nutrigenomics to boost production per animal and provides a more nutritious product, particularly associating biomarkers with specific growth and production responses, improved production efficiencies, and improved fertility. Also working toward avoidance of feed contamination using genomic tools. Very active in equine nutrition, with products such as Actigen™ that is advertised as "a cost effective, safe and traceable new technology developed through nutrigenomics that helps animals of all species to thrive and reach their genetic potential."	http://www.alltech.com
Hill's	Have used nutrigenomics tools to create IP for several novel animal products. Generated 3,178,297 reads of the feline genome sequence using eight different cats. These data were then combined with the publicly available 2x sequence of the feline genome to identify 3 million SNPs. They then donated the data along with $1 million to the Morris Animal Foundation to help identify genetic differences between cats to determine the association between genetics and disease/health.	http://www.veterinarypracticenews.com/vet-dept/small-animal-dept/nutrigenomics-takes-you-are-what-you-eat-to-new-level.aspx
	Hill's launched its first product based in nutrigenomic principles in 2005. Eicosapentanoic acid (EPA), as used in Hill's® Prescription Diet® j/d™ Canine pet food for dogs with osteoarthritis, was proved efficacious through gene expression studies. They have also identified the key gene expression profiles in adipose tissue of obese versus lean dogs and found that some key ingredients in Hill's® Prescription Diet® r/d® Canine pet food are able to normalize the expression of those genes toward the lean state.	http://www.hillspet.com Also, The Proceedings of the Hill's Symposium on Nutrigenomics, presented at the AVMA Convention in 2008, accessed via http://veterinarybusiness.dvm360.com
Hemopet	A not-for-profit organization; has been granted US patents for a number of tests relating to nutrigenomics, including the use of an electronic database and software routine to determine the effect of nutrition on gene expression. Other patents include "Diagnostic system for selecting nutrition and pharmacological products for animals," "Method of analyzing nutrition for a canine or feline animal," "System and method for determining a nutritional diet for a canine or feline animal," and "Multistage nutrigenomic diagnostic food sensitivity testing in animals."	http://www.hemopet.org
Kemin	Kemin looked at linking diet with gene expression through a trace mineral nutrigenomics experiment, a noninvasive study with Beagles examining the effects on gene expression in white blood cells after supplementation with one of the company's products, KemTrace Zinc. Funded the first study to show that a specific nutrient could alter the expression of genes in the body fat of dairy cattle; this was done at Washington State University.	http://www.kemin.com

Mars	Mars is parent company to numerous pet food brands, such as PEDIGREE®, ROYAL CANIN®, WHISKAS®, KITEKAT®, BANFIELD®, CESAR®, NUTRO®, SHEBA®, CHAPPI®, GREENIES® and CATSAN®. Mars holds the most comprehensive canine genetic database in the world. Mars Veterinary has researched the genetic signatures of more than 190 dog breeds and used data to create two mixed-breed analyses: WISDOM PANEL™ Professional and WISDOM PANEL™ Insights. This information allows owners to understand the medical, behavioral, nutritional, and training needs for their mixed-breed dogs. WISDOM PANEL™ Insights is an over-the-counter cheek swab DNA test that provides the dog owner with the breed profile of their dog. WISDOM PANEL™ Professional is a blood-based DNA test that is available exclusively through veterinarians. It provides the veterinarian and client with a weight-prediction range based on the breeds identified and the chromosomes that each contributed, which allows the client to plan for training, exercise, and nutritional needs over the life of their dog. WISDOM PANEL™ Professional also prescreens for specific diseases associated with certain breeds. If an at-risk breed contributed chromosomes to the mixed-breed dog, the veterinarian is alerted to educate the owner on the clinical signs and consider testing the dog for the disease.	http://www.mars.com
MetaMorphix	Founded in 1994 and based in Calverton, Maryland, MetaMorphix®, Inc. is a privately held life sciences company. Its website states that: "uses the code of life, DNA, to improve the global food supply and human health. In livestock, we help our customers produce higher quality, nutritious meat more efficiently; and in health care, we discover and license targets to pharmaceutical companies that develop therapies for better management of metabolic and muscular degenerative diseases." The company is developing a pipeline of innovative products addressing all major livestock sectors including cattle, swine, poultry and aquaculture, as well as developing products that enhance the health of companion animals. MetaMorphix® is developing products based on three foundation technologies that it believes hold the promise of significantly impacting agriculture's global challenges. It has a strong patent position and research and development pipeline. Research draws on two broad technology platforms: growth differentiation factors and genomics. Through an agreement with Celera Genomics that provides exclusive access to unique genomic assets for livestock, MetaMorphix® is utilizing genomic information to develop advanced selection tools that detect desirable agronomic traits in addition to disease susceptibility in livestock species. These unique toolsets are expected to dramatically improve breeds and to provide powerful methods to select superior animals for feedlot management and certification of meat quality. With the exclusive access to these genomic databases, MetaMorphix® is able to rapidly and precisely generate tests to detect specific genetic traits for livestock that have been otherwise undetectable. For the longer term, MetaMorphix® states that it will use its expertise and livestock genomic assets to discover novel gene-based therapeutic and disease prevention strategies for livestock production and animal health. MMI Genomics, Inc., a wholly owned subsidiary of MetaMorphix®, Inc., was acquired from Celera Genomics in March of 2002. MMI Genomics is a diagnostic company applying genomics and proteomics technologies to develop and commercialize innovative livestock and companion animal products that enhance animal health and productivity. http://www.mmigenomics.com/about1.html	www.metamorphixinc.com

(Continued)

TABLE 16.3 (*Continued*)
Animal Food and Beverage Companies

Company	Product/Service/Research Involvement	Website
Monsanto	Together with Cargill, they have formed a 50/50 joint venture named Renessen, whose principal objective is to engineer and market quality nutritional traits for feeding animals. http://dmedia.ucsc.edu/~bsharris/film%20170a/proj3/monsanto/monsanto/layout/farmprogress/renessenMavera.html	http://www.feedinfo.com/Biotech.aspx
Newsham Choice Genetics	Part of Groupe Grimaud, they deliver performance breeding solutions to the swine breeding industry. Using its unique Gentel® selection technology, Newsham provides high performance, high health swine genetics.	www.newsham.com
Purina	Now "Nestle Purina," and extremely active in research that includes genomic insights for improved health and nutrition for companion animals. Brands include Friskies®, Fancy Feast®, Mighty Dog®, Alpo®, Dog Chow®, Cat Chow®, Purina One®, ProPlan®, Tidy Cat®, and Beggin'®. Run a yearly symposium focusing on the latest research and techniques in this field. The company prefers the term "molecular nutrition" to "nutrigenomics," saying molecular nutrition includes nutrigenomics but utilizes other molecular tools and biological systems such as pure genetics (heritable traits), metabolomics (study of metabolites), and epigenetics. "We employ the use of multiple omics platforms in our research," says Rondo P. Middleton, Ph.D., a senior research scientist for the company. "These platforms can measure tens or hundreds of thousands of measurements at a time. It allows the researcher to investigate what changes in biology are occurring by pushing the limits of detecting all within that system. An example is transcriptomics and microarrays. Microarrays have the ability to measure nearly all transcripts [mRNAs, copies of genes about to be translated into proteins] in a cell. This becomes very powerful to the researcher. We can now let the cell tell us what is going on. We use this to not only characterize a physical state—growth, health, disease, etc—but also as a means to study how nutrients have affected that issue in the cell. This is performed in a non-invasive way for the pets, utilizing in vitro techniques." When Middleton Nestlé Purina, he and the group developed a canine microarray to investigate molecular changes associated with canine osteoarthritis. "We then used this and the knowledge we obtained about the disease, along with other technologies, to develop the Purina Veterinary Diet JM. JM was the first diet to use omega-3 fatty acids to help manage osteoarthritis in dogs," Middleton says. "The JM diet utilizes the anti-inflammatory properties of omega-3 fatty acids to nutritionally address the inflammation associated with osteoarthritis. This includes the positive modulation of very specific molecular changes identified in our canine osteoarthritis research. This is just one example of many that we have performed or are currently in the process of researching."	http://nestlepurinacareers.com/AboutNestle/CompanyOverview.aspx http://www.veterinarypracticenews.com/vet-dept/small-animal-dept/nutrigenomics-takes-you-are-what-you-eat-to-new-level.aspx

Human Food and Beverage Companies

Many industry players have realized the advantage of adding nutrigenomics to their toolbox. Examples are summarized in Table 16.4.

Some Examples of the Potential of Nutrigenomics for the Food and Beverage Industry

Mechanism of Action of a Common Dietary Component by "FoodOmics"

The mechanism of chemopreventive polyphenols from rosemary was examined through measuring the total gene, protein, and metabolite expression in human HT29 colon cancer cells following exposure to graded doses [11]. Complementary information on the bioactivity of polyphenols against colon cancer cells, based on the results from each of the different platforms (transcriptomics, proteomics, or metabolomics), were compared with previous data from older approaches. This corroborated the interest of using a global integrative strategy such as Foodomics. Transcriptomics, proteomics, and metabolomics platforms were effectively put together to study the health benefits from a dietary bioactive ingredient against colon cancer cells at the gene, protein, and metabolite level.

Proof of Human Efficacy of Novel Foods or Diets

Chronic inflammation is thought to be a frequent underlying mechanism of several common, noncommunicable diseases, including cardiovascular disease, type II diabetes mellitus, cancer, inflammatory bowel disease, Alzheimer's disease, asthma, and rheumatoid arthritis. As such, products targeting inflammation are likely to engage high levels of consumer interest. Individuals respond to compounds such as long chain n-3 PUFA and n-6 PUFA based on which genetic pathway is unique to them [12]. In this example, what is beneficial for the majority can in fact be harmful for a genetically based minority. This is a field ripe for nutrigenomic intervention.

Different nutrients or phytochemicals may modulate processes leading to chronic inflammation and increased risk of disease. Among these, numerous macronutrients are emerging as important in the inflammatory process, including amino acids such as glutamine and arginine, lipids such as omega-3 polyunsaturated fatty acids (n-3 PUFA) and certain novel carbohydrates [13–18]. Vitamins C and E, along with minerals zinc and selenium, are also showing significant impact on the immune system, as are some plant- and fruit-derived chemical compounds plus probiotics and prebiotics [19]. Because each of the stages involved in inflammation is likely to respond to a different dietary intervention, a complementary approach may be necessary to reduce symptoms. It is likely that nutrigenomics could provide tools with which to target this complex area.

An example of one such intervention is a study combining numerous approaches carried out by Bakker and colleagues [20]. Thirty-six overweight, but otherwise healthy, men were given an anti-inflammatory mix containing vitamins, lipids, and particular food extracts as a supplement over 5 weeks. Although the usual measure of C-reactive protein showed no shift in status, a large number of subtle positive shifts were detected in other inflammation markers through use of integrated omics

TABLE 16.4
Food and Beverage Companies, Including Industry/Academic Partnerships

Company	Product/Service/Research Involvement	Website
Chr Hansen (ingredients manufacturers)	Partner in the Netherlands-based industry/research partnership TI Food and Nutrition, which has functional genomics as one of the two main platforms underpinning its activities (http://www.tifn.nl) "It is not at all farfetched to imagine that within some years you could download your personal genotype onto your mobile phone and use it to scan the barcodes in the supermarket and make sure that you only buy what is healthy for precisely your body," Dr. Johansen, Associate VP, Science, Chr. Hansen, in 2008. (http://www.chr-hansen.com/news-media/singlenews/the-importance-of-bacterial-behavior.html)	http://www.chr-hansen.com
Danone Group	Major involvement in MetaHIT. Also major involvement in TI Food and Nutrition, which has functional genomics as one of the two main platforms underpinning its activities. As Dr Hanno Cappon, Vice President R&D Medical Nutrition explained in October 2010, "We are at the forefront of innovation in specialized nutrition and being partner in TI Food and Nutrition fits our strategy to invest in expanding the role of nutrition in health and disease." Hanno Cappon continues, "The decisive factor in joining TI Food and Nutrition is the new approach and research structure which enables industry partners like ourselves to select the research themes in which to participate. TI Food and Nutrition has become an attractive proposition because we can invest in research topics we consider to be of strategic importance to our business."	MetaHITenterotype_press_release.pdf http://www.nature.com/nature/journal/v464/n7285/index.html http://www.merieux-alliance.com/uk/projetssante_secualimentaire-offreglobale.php http://www.tifn.nl/page/Newsletters/$file/INTOUCH%20NEXT%20OCTOBER.pdf
DSM	Used nutrigenomics to make a fundamental breakthrough in 2004, exploring the molecular mechanisms by which feeding vitamin E and lycopene, the red carotenoid from tomatoes, can reduce the risk of prostate cancer. Their analysis revealed that both nutrients affected gene expression directly in the tumours. (http://www.dsm.com/en_US/html/dnp/news_rel_2004_02.htm?DCSext) In 2006, DSM Venturing invested €2 million in IntegraGen, a French biotechnology company specializing in the development and delivery of genetic tests for rapid diagnosis and better (personalized) treatment of complex diseases. This investment was partly to further DSM's interest in personalized nutrition through genetic mapping and led to a collaboration program in the area of weight management. (Business Insights Report: "The Top 10 Food and Drinks Ingredients Companies" and http://www.dsm.com/en_US/cworld/public/media/pages/press-releases/51_06_integragen.jsp) Invested €2 million in Finnish genetic research company Jurilab Oy in 2007. Jurilab work in identifying genetic markers associated with metabolic syndrome; the long-term aim of the deal was to develop "innovative nutritional products" to fit individual consumers' genetic profiles. In 2006, DSM and Jurilab began a joint discovery program in the area of hypertension. (http://www.nutraingredients.com/Industry/DSM-increases-nutrigenomics-investment)	http://www.dsm.com

	Involved with Netherlands Metabolomics Centre (Netherlands Metabolomics Centre factsheet fact sheet downloaded from www.genomics.nl) Partner in the Netherlands-based industry/research partnership TI Food and Nutrition, which has functional genomics as one of the two main platforms underpinning its activities (http://www.tifn.nl)	
Fonterra	Fonterra has used genomics approaches in microbes, pasture plants, and cows to understand the genetic basis for the commercial/beneficial attributes of the target organisms and, potentially, to accentuate the desired features in future organisms. Invested in a proprietary vending or food service technology that delivers "fresh," dairy-based foods through point of sale manufacture, with BASF and a NZ research institute.	www.fonterra.com
Food4Me	Food4Me is an EU (FP7) funded project, in which an international group of experts seek to answer the question, "how can we best use our current understanding of food, genes, and physical traits to design healthier diets tailored for each individual?" Food4me is about personalized nutrition; it uses nutrigenetic testing and is attempting to validate the interactions between certain key genetic polymorphisms and specific foods. They are complementary—and on the opposite side of the coin—to NutriTech. Industry partners in Food4Me include Crème Software Ltd, DSM Nutritional Products, and Philips Electronics.	www.food4me.org
Friesland Campina	Partner in the Netherlands-based industry/research partnership TI Food and Nutrition, which has functional genomics as one of the two main platforms underpinning its activities (http://www.tifn.nl/page/Newsletters/$file/INTOUCH%20NEXT%20OCTOBER.pdf). Also active in the Food & Nutrition Delta which works to translate cutting-edge research into industrial innovation.	www.frieslandcampina.com
Metagenics	"Science-based" medical foods, nutritional formulas, and lifestyle therapy programs. Metagenics University aims to help healthcare professionals stay on the leading edge of lifestyle medicine and incorporate nutrition into their clinical practice. Website lists the following: • Help with implementing advanced nutrigenomic protocols • Modifying dietary signals with therapeutic lifestyle changes • Modifying dietary signals with medical foods • Modifying dietary signals with SKRMs • Added help with targeted nutritional support	www.metagenics.com

(Continued)

TABLE 16.4 (*Continued*)
Food and Beverage Companies, Including Industry/Academic Partnerships

Company	Product/Service/Research Involvement	Website
	Has a wholly-owned subsidiary, MetaProteomics Nutrigenomics Research Centre. Lists 80 peer-reviewed articles and more than 50 international or domestic patents.	http://www.metaproteomicslabs.com/index2.asp
	MetaProteomics is a proteomics lab focused on innovating nutraceutical development.	
	Have developed the "ExpresSyn Process" to demonstrate efficacy, bioavailability, and predicted safety for their line of ExpresSyn products. The ExpresSyn Process combines the following: • Cell proteomic research • Safety evaluations • Human ex vivo research • Human clinical research	
	Metagenics University includes certification programs for First Line Therapy (FLT), a personalized lifestyle program centered on therapeutic lifestyle change.	
Nestle	Involved in all the major European programs through the supply of food and/or the provision of resources, expertise, and knowledge.	http://www.nestle.com
	Nestlé is one company that has openly discussed its use of nutrigenomics. The Nestlé Institute of Health Sciences established in September 2010 is using metabolomics, next generation sequencing and functional genomics, small molecule biochemistry and proteomics and bringing all of the information together with bioinformatics. Their aim is then to use the information collected to develop disease phenotype models and pathways against which GRAS/Food molecules can be screened in a high throughput manner.	
Nutrigenomics New Zealand	Research-for-industry collaboration between the University of Auckland, Plant and Food Research and AgResearch. Published the first diet-gene interaction paper for Crohn's disease in the world [22].	www.nutrigenomics.org.nz
	Offers the tools and knowledge to aid the development of products that improve the well-being and health of consumers. Offers relevant science to support companies by providing validated research results for use in product development and marketing of new products. Works with commercial partners to ensure they deliver science that addresses their specific requirements, through an in-depth consultation process. They then design projects to meet these needs.	

	Scientific expertise of Nutrigenomics New Zealand assists companies with • Scientific validation of the effects of ingredients or foods • Identification of novel functionality of ingredients or foods • Scientific data to support health or marketing claims on products • Identification of points of differentiation between new and existing products Current business partners include Comvita, King Salmon, and Fonterra.	
NutriTech	Funded under European Framework FP7-KBBE, NutriTech's focus is on Innovation and Technology Transfer. The project runs from 2012-01-01 to 2015-12-31. The consortium is comprised of 23 research organizations and universities from around the world, including Nutrigenomics New Zealand through The University of Auckland. A second consortium has been established with five major European food manufacturers contributing €4 million to accelerate application within the food industry. NutriTech are complementary to—and on the opposite side of the coin from—Food4Me. Nutritech utilizes nutrigenomics, including a variety of different endpoints, challenging homeostasis and looking at changes in gene expression profiles at set times thereafter. They will then put subjects on a diet for a certain time and will see whether their homeostasis capability has improved. Connected to NutriTech, a second project will work on the demonstration of Phenotypic Flexibility in human intervention studies, composed of major food industry partners.	http://cordis.europa.eu/projects/101663_en.html
TI Food and Nutrition	Superb example of academia and industry cooperating and collaborating. Has as its mantra "Industrial relevance, scientific excellence." More on this in body of chapter. TI Food and Nutrition industrial partner organizations: ACTA Dental Research, Cargill, CBL, Chr. Hansen, CRV, CSK food enrichment, CSM, Danone, DSM, Federatie Nederlandse Levensmiddelen Industrie (FNLI), Fromageries Bel, GlaxoSmithKline, Kellogg Company, Nestlé, Philips Research, Productschap Zuivel, Royal FrieslandCampina, Unilever, VION Food Group, Wrigley.	

methods and data. As a whole, these data showed improved endothelial function, lessened inflammation of adipose tissue and beneficial effects on oxidative stress.

How Industry and Academia Are Responding to the Opportunities and Challenges Created

Industry and academia are realizing the need to cooperate and collaborate on levels hitherto unknown to realize the full potential of nutrigenomics. This is leading to increased adoption of open innovation—combining internal and external ideas as well as internal and external paths to market to advance the development of new technologies and products. One such example of academia partnering with industry can be seen in the Top Institute (TI) Nutrition and Health based in the Netherlands. It has as its mantra "Industrial relevance, scientific excellence." TI boasts an impressive alliance between academia and industry and works closely with the Food and Nutrition Delta (FND). This is a partner to TI in the Dutch Innovation Programme Food and Nutrition, which ensures that small- and medium-sized enterprises (SMEs) are able to convert new findings into market-driven products. This has included SMEs gaining the assistance of multinational companies in their development of knowledge and products.

TI's research is organized into 11 themes, with two platforms of functional genomics (Nutrigenomics and Bio-IT) and knowledge management cutting across and contributing to all these themes to a lesser or greater degree. Industry partners have initiated and decided on these themes in conjunction with TI researchers. In the words of Jan Maat, Managing Director of TI, "By putting industry in the driver's seat, we ensure that the fundamental research we do is application-oriented, or 'need to have'. It's up to our research partners to come up with the ideas and creativity that will give answers for issues faced by the industry. Furthermore, I'm convinced that close interaction throughout the research process will lead to Intellectual Property rights that are of strategic value to the industry partners participating in the individual Research Themes." (Oct 2010 TI newsletter, downloaded from http://www .tifn.nl/tifn/website.nsf/xpPublications.xsp).

TI's new research structure, established for the period of 2011–2014, was credited with consolidating the commitment of TI's industry partners CSM, DSM, FrieslandCampina, Unilever, and Vion. It also attracted new partners who see the strategic advantage in joining forces for precompetitive research that would otherwise be extremely difficult, if not impossible, for many individual companies to do alone. These new partners were Christian Hansen, the Dutch Food Industry Federation (FNLI), the Dutch Food Retail Association (CBL), Danone, Fromageries Bel, Kellogg's, and Nestlé. Other industry partners include Cargill, GlaxoSmithKline, Philips, SmithKline Beecham, VION, and Wrigley. The research arm of TI includes ACTA Dental Research, Maastricht University/MUMC, NIZO food research, NZO, TNO, University of Groningen/UMCG, and Wageningen UR.

As well as being a partner with TI and other research parties, Nestle announced two major initiatives of its own in late 2010 that have been operational since the beginning of 2011 (http://www.Nestlé.com/NHW/Pages/Brands-services.aspx):

Nestlé Health Science Company, a Fully-Owned Subsidiary of Nestlé

Building on its existing Nestlé Health Care Nutrition, Nestlé added infant nutrition, weight management, and performance nutrition, thus consolidating these four key business areas under the stewardship of Nestlé Health Science company. Its focus is the creation of food-based products that assist with the prevention and amelioration of numerous medical conditions (http://www.Nestlé.com/NHW/Pages/Brands-services.aspx).

In a speech given in September 2010, Chairman of Nestlé S.A.'s Board of Directors Peter Brabeck-Letmathe described this new company as "a pioneer in a new industry that we are helping to shape in the space between a fast moving consumer goods company and a pharma company" (speech downloaded from www.Nestlé.com/Common/NestleDocuments/Documents/Library/). Brabeck-Letmathe's focus during said speech was on the burden of health care involved with chronic disease and the fact that "it is our strong conviction that disease prevention will have to play a much bigger role and, in this sense, personalized healthcare nutrition will become the first and most efficient step in an active prevention policy and for wellness and wellbeing."

Thus the company will produce nutritional solutions for diseases and conditions such as Alzheimer's disease, obesity, diabetes, and arteriosclerosis. This includes acquisition, in-licensing, and integration of companies that can assist Nestle with its goal of "modifying disease nutrition." An early example of such is Nestlé's 2010 acquisition of Vitaflo, a global provider of clinical nutritional products tailored to specific genetic conditions.

Nestle Institute of Health Sciences

Overseen by Nestlé Health Science Company, the Institute will provide much of the research behind Nestlé Health Science Company's products in the rapidly growing area between consumer goods and pharma solutions. The overall goal of the Nestlé Institute of Health Sciences is stated as being "to ensure the scientific base for personalized health science nutrition by developing a molecular understanding of disease processes with which to inform and design nutrition plans and products for individual prevention and maintenance of a healthier life" (speech downloaded from www.Nestlé.com/Common/NestleDocuments/Documents/Library).

Table 16.4 gives a "bigger picture" view of just some of the activities by some of the companies involved in bringing nutritional genomics to market.

CHALLENGES

Some of the numerous challenges in bringing nutritional genomics to market can be seen in Table 16.5.

TABLE 16.5
Some of the Serious Challenges to Commercializing Nutritional Genomics

- How to translate the science to the public in an affordable, ethical, workable way.
- How to be first and keep being first in such a hotly competitive environment.
- Pressure to commercialize too early by investors, funders, and so on.
- Misinformation by media.
- Ethical issues, particularly regarding privacy of people's genetic data.
- "Muddied water" left by those who started before the science was ready and jumped the gun.
- Educating the public, private, and professional sectors.

CONCLUSIONS

Nutritional genomics recognizes the extent to which the interaction of diet and genes can affect expression of genes and so impact health on many levels. As such it has numerous important contributions to offer to industry. Significant IP and point-of-difference opportunities will be created. In addition, the opportunity for consumers to determine whether they will uniquely benefit from health claims or not promises to be hugely attractive. Nutrigenomics has only just begun to show its full capabilities as the next real point of innovation for industry and consumers alike.

There are several ways in which this field can significantly enhance the industry potential of foods, diets, and/or dietary supplements. It is no longer a question of whether this evolving science and its many tools will be of use in commercial settings. It is a question of "how, when, and who." Awareness of ability to use genomic tools is already widely apparent and in growing use. Applications include increased ability to design, determine the mechanism of, and differentiate products; create and support health claims; improve plant, organism, and animal breeding and production; fine-tune personalized healthcare interventions and run clinical trials that cost less and offer far more in quality and quantity of data.

Newer developments are leading to the maturation of nutrigenomics and to its increasing recognition in the scientific community; similarly, nutrigenomics' appeal in the commercial world grows in parallel with its ability to fine-tune study designs in terms of participant selection, analytical methods, and interpretation of results. Industry looks likely to use combinations of these tools to design and implement "health packages" for consumers. One such package might include the use of diagnostic tools, personalized dietary and exercise advice and monitoring, and other relevant tools to support wellness and absence/amelioration of disease.

The lines between functional foods, dietary supplements, and medical foods are becoming increasingly blurred. As with public health, a great deal of communication and education is crucial so that industry can keep up with and help to bring to the public the fruits of nutrigenomics. Nutrigenomics advocates will need to use words and concepts that nonscientists can understand. Similarly, communication with people such as nutritionists, Research and Development managers, dieticians, and chefs will need to be clear and free from jargon. Business models will be needed that translate the relevant science into a commercial resource that companies can take advantage of.

REFERENCES

1. van Ommen B, El-Sohemy A, Hesketh J, Kaput J, Fenech M, Evelo CT, McArdle HJ et al.: The Micronutrient Genomics Project: a community-driven knowledge base for micronutrient research. *Genes Nutr* 2010, 5(4):285–296.
2. Joost H-G, Gibney MJ, Cashman KD, Gorman U, Hesketh JE, Mueller M, van Ommen B, Williams CM, Mathers JC: Personalized nutrition: status and perspectives. *Br J Nutr* 2007, 98(1):26–31.
3. Bictash M, Ebbels TM, Chan Q, Loo RL, Yap IKS, Brown IJ, de Iorio M et al.: Opening up the "Black Box": metabolic phenotyping and metabolome-wide association studies in epidemiology. *J Clin Epidemiol* 2010, 63(9):970–979.
4. O'Sullivan A, Gibney MJ, Connor AO, Mion B, Kaluskar S, Cashman KD, Flynn A, Shanahan F, Brennan L: Biochemical and metabolomic phenotyping in the identification

of a vitamin D responsive metabotype for markers of the metabolic syndrome. *Mol Nutr Food Res* 2011, 55(5):679–690.
5. Omenn GS: Bioinformatics and systems biology of cancers. *Prog Mol Biol Transl Sci* 2010, 95:159–191.
6. Fay LB, German JB: Personalizing foods: is genotype necessary? *Curr Opin Biotechnol* 2008, 19(2):121–128.
7. Kussmann M, Affolter M, Nagy K, Holst B, Fay LB: Mass spectrometry in nutrition: understanding dietary health effects at the molecular level. *Mass Spectrom Rev* 2007, 26(6):727–750.
8. Ferguson LR, Barnett MPG: Research in Nutrigenomics and potential applications to practice. *Nutr diet* 2012, In press.
9. Petermann I, Triggs CM, Huebner C, Han DY, Gearry RB, Barclay ML, Demmers PS, McCulloch A, Ferguson LR: Mushroom intolerance: a novel diet-gene interaction in Crohn's disease. *Br J Nutr* 2009, 102(4):506–508.
10. Holmes E, Wilson ID, Nicholson JK: Metabolic phenotyping in health and disease. *Cell* 2008, 134(5):714–717.
11. Ibanez C, Valdes A, Garcia-Canas V, Simo C, Celebier M, Rocamora-Reverte L, Gomez-Martinez A et al: Global Foodomics strategy to investigate the health benefits of dietary constituents. *J Chromatogr* 2012, 1248:139–153.
12. Simopoulos AP: Genetic variants in the metabolism of omega-6 and omega-3 fatty acids: their role in the determination of nutritional requirements and chronic disease risk. *Exp Biol Med (Maywood)* 2010, 235(7):785–795.
13. Auvin S, Collet F, Gottrand F, Husson M-O, Leroy X, Beermann C, Guery BP: Long-chain polyunsaturated fatty acids modulate lung inflammatory response induced by Pseudomonas aeruginosa in mice. *Pediatr Res* 2005, 58(2):211–215.
14. Bassaganya-Riera J, Hontecillas R: CLA and n-3 PUFA differentially modulate clinical activity and colonic PPAR-responsive gene expression in a pig model of experimental IBD. *Clin Nutr* 2006, 25(3):454–465.
15. Bouwens M, van de Rest O, Dellschaft N, Bromhaar MG, de Groot LCPGM, Geleijnse JM, Muller M, Afman LA: Fish-oil supplementation induces antiinflammatory gene expression profiles in human blood mononuclear cells. *Am J Clin Nutr* 2009, 90(2):415–424.
16. Calder PC, Albers R, Antoine JM, Blum S, Bourdet-Sicard R, Ferns GA, Folkerts G et al.: Inflammatory disease processes and interactions with nutrition. *Br J Nutr* 2009, 101 Suppl 1:S1–45.
17. Calder PC: Fatty acids and inflammation: the cutting edge between food and pharma. *Eur J Pharmacol* 2011, 668 Suppl 1:S50–58.
18. Iwaya H, Kashiwaya M, Shinoki A, Lee J-S, Hayashi K, Hara H, Ishizuka S: Marginal zinc deficiency exacerbates experimental colitis induced by dextran sulfate sodium in rats. *J Nutr* 2011, 141(6):1077–1082.
19. Appleyard CB, Cruz ML, Isidro AA, Arthur JC, Jobin C, De Simone C: Pretreatment with the probiotic VSL#3 delays transition from inflammation to dysplasia in a rat model of colitis-associated cancer. *Am J Physiol Gastrointest Liver Physiol* 2011, 301(6):G1004–1013.
20. Bakker GC, van Erk MJ, Pellis L, Wopereis S, Rubingh CM, Cnubben NH, Kooistra T, van Ommen B, Hendriks HF: An antiinflammatory dietary mix modulates inflammation and oxidative and metabolic stress in overweight men: a nutrigenomics approach. *Am J Clin Nutr* 2010, 91(4):1044–1059.
21. National Research Council 2007: Nutrient Requirements of Horses, 6th revised edition. National Academy Press. National Research Council, Washington, DC [quoted in] Feeding and Management for Horses with HYPP (Hyperkalemic Periodic Paralysis) By Dr. Stacy Appleton, downloaded from http://horse.purinamills.com.
22. Yamka RM, Friesen KG, Xiangming G, Al-Murrani S: Identification of genes related to obesity in dogs. *FASEB J* 2007, 21:28.4.

17 Bringing Nutrigenomics to the Public

Is Direct-to-Consumer Testing the Future of Nutritional Genomics?

David Castle

CONTENTS

INTRODUCTION

A little more than a decade ago, the California-based Institute for the Future (IFTF) undertook a horizon scanning and futures analysis of the emerging field of nutritional genomics [1]. Their report is premised on the idea that our knowledge about the relationships between food and health will be greatly clarified through human genetics and genomics. With this enhanced understanding, prospects will arise to exploit this knowledge through new products and services, and new types of commercial opportunities will develop. At the heart of the narrative about nutrigenomics is a key driver of change—the empowered consumer. This is the type of person who actively seeks information, particularly nutritional, health, and lifestyle information, from a variety of sources including consumer media, the health care system, and the food industry. These consumers are described by the IFTF as wealthy, educated, and motivated; they want information from a variety of sources so they, as masters of their own destiny, can make informed, highly individualized, decisions. "Sophisticated consumers" are above-average educated people who will canvass a wide variety of information sources in their searches, and they are also willing to consider a mix of traditional and untraditional sources of information [2]. For example, as trust in doctors as univocal sources of information declines overall, online access of information proliferates, ranging from peer-to-peer discussion groups to academic medical journals. Sophisticated consumers are not just information addicts, otherwise they would not be important drivers of change in the narrative around nutrigenomics. Rather, the interest in seeking information and the ability to get information are conjoined with a view about sophisticated consumers' motivation and capacity to act on new information in self-interested ways.

The IFTF suggested that consumers would move "upstream" in the flow of information, bypassing retailers, and other intermediaries to find original and what they perceive to be trusted sources of information. At the same time, the IFTF suggested that companies might provide information more immediately to consumers if they adopt approaches similar to pharmaceutical advertising in the United States—direct to the consumer. This new business model would mature over the coming decade, such that "about 33% of the consumer population will be gathering information derived from advances in nutrigenomics—and because they will see the real value of this information to their own lives, they will be willing to pay more for the products derived from this information" [1]. The business opportunity presented by the advent of direct-to-consumer (DTC) provision of nutrigenomic information to sophisticated consumers is explosive growth in traditional markets of nutritional supplements, health foods, and also new foods and bioactive compounds that become constitutive of tailor-made diets for individuals, based on genomics and individual genetics analysis.

This chapter addresses the question of whether DTC testing is (or continues to be in light of the IFTF predictions) the future of nutrigenomics, by examining how consumers and companies are currently engaged in DTC interactions. The first section will consider the primary justification for adopting DTC, namely that people want and will use the information and associated services in ways that will improve health outcomes. The second section will examine whether companies have been able to create the markets for providing information, products, and other services by using DTC. The above reference to the IFTF's figure in which one-third of the Americans use nutrigenomic information by 2010 is obviously meant to imply that DTC nutrigenomics has not reached that level. Indeed, it is doubtful that the potential for the market is as high as the US$730 million with 20% annual growth, as has been suggested [3]. As the evidence considered in this chapter indicates, consumer demand has yet to rise sharply and in ways predicted, and the business environment for nutrigenomics companies is more restricted than anticipated originally. Given what we now know, after more than a decade's experience with DTC, the question is not so much whether DTC testing represents nutrigenomics' future, but what kind of DTC testing looks likely to be a part of nutrigenomics' future?

Empowered Consumer

The empowered consumer, according to conception underpinning DTC nutrigenetic testing, is one who seeks information and acts on it. The informational dimension and the motivational dimension can be taken in turn for the purposes of discussion, although in actuality they are not really separable. As this section will discuss, DTC provision of nutrigenomic tests can mean that individuals who are probably not experts in genetics and nutrition will receive a considerable amount of unfamiliar information. On its own, this information might have novelty value, pique curiosity, or prompt further and more aggressive information searching. The motivation to act on the information, and ability to do so, however, comes when information is assimilated and becomes the basis of decision-making processes.

Information and Empowerment

What information would consumers want, or would need, to know if they are receiving information directly from nutrigenomics companies? First, it would be useful to have a basic understanding of what it means to say that a person's genetics and various factors, such as drugs, toxins, and nutrients, can interact. Essentially, this means having a lay understanding that "gene–environment interaction refers to the differential phenotypic effects of diverse environments on individuals with the same genotype or to the discrepant effects of the same environment on individuals with different genotypes" [4]. Further, it would be useful to contextualize the state of this knowledge in terms of our current understanding of gene–environment interaction. While the Human Genome Project (HGP) and subsequent investments in more specialized fields of genomics and genetics might have been based on the idea that gene discovery could disclose biological function and the aetiology of disease, a small fraction of our knowledge about genetics adheres to this paradigm. Instead, many alleles "not yet been identified have modest or weak effects and contribute to disease through interaction with other alleles and environmental factors, the environmental factors often conferring the greater relative risk. Thus, clearly, traversing the path to improved understanding of inherited contributions to complex disease will require other, non-genetic kinds of information." [5]. This nuance is important for dispelling deterministic conceptions of genetics and for putting the extent of our causal knowledge about genetics and genomics into realistic perspective [6].

Second, an easy appeal can be made to the complexity of genetic diversity by thinking through a few illustrative examples that draw on intuitions about phenotypes but have deeper genetic significance. In the year of an Olympiad, the point about human phenotypic diversity is easily made by drawing contrasts between members of national teams, between teams, and between the teams and the inert audiences enjoying televised coverage. Other contrasts can be drawn between athletes competing in London, and Winston Churchill, penchant for Pol Roger champagne and cigars as the antithesis of healthy behavior, and made his long life all the more remarkable. Deeper significance can be attached to phenotypic diversity beyond these kinds of mundane examples. Take, for instance, the effects of dietary pattern changes in the case of isolated groups such as the Pima Indians, who have a nearly 20-fold higher incidence of type II diabetes than elsewhere in the United States [7]. The contrasts between the health outcomes of the current generation compared with their forebears are striking.

The third type of information focuses on nutrigenomics itself. An appreciation for the limits of genetic and genomic knowledge, and a sense of the complexity of the phenomena that need to be explained, help to situate the main objectives of nutrigenomics, at least in broad outline. When interacting with the public, who generally show very low levels of awareness of nutrigenomics, a low level (grade 8–10) of scientific knowledge is generally presumed in definitions used with the public. For example, "Nutrigenomics is about how our genetic makeup affects how we respond to what we eat and drink, and how we can change our diet to help promote health and reduce our genetic risks of disease" [8]. More detail about the underlying goals of nutrigenomics can be added once the initial concept is absorbed, for example, nutrigenomics is "a new, developing science that studies the way our genetic make-up affects how our bodies respond to what we eat and drink, where testing is often done by taking a sample of saliva, examining people's genetic make-up and then providing them with nutrition and diet-related information—a kind of personalized nutrition plan—to potentially help them improve their health and reduce their risk of certain diseases" [9].

People also benefit from having a fourth body of knowledge, which is about the kinds of applications that nutrigenomics might have for them. In work undertaken by the author with the Public Health Agency of Canada, cited above, an example of nutrigenomics that has immediate relevance to many people was chosen. Canadians rank in the top 10 global consumers of coffee *per capita*, so different rates of caffeine metabolism and the influence it has on the risk of myocardial infarction is relevant and interesting to them [10]. A single nutrient such as caffeine is familiar enough, but consumers are also aware of differences within a class of nutrients, such as fats. Variation in the *APOA5* gene caused by a single base substitution can protect against obesity and overweight in cases where, remarkably, greater than 30 of a persons' caloric intake is from fats, especially monounsaturated fats [4]. In addition to avoiding certain fats and amounts of fat in their diet, other applications for nutrigenomics that would orient people to the field's potential could include weight loss [11], celiac disease [12], vitamin metabolism and deficiencies [13], and the relationship between vitamins and disease [14]. Each of these examples illustrates applications of nutrigenomics based on familiar subject matter, thereby building a pathway for assimilating new information based on antecedent knowledge.

Motivation

The nutrigenomics firm Sciona formed in the United Kingdom in 2000 and launched its first products in May 2001. Its CEO and co-founder, Chris Martin, recognized the potential of nutrigenomic science, and also saw commercial potential in the same way described by the IFTF. Bypassing intermediaries in the health system means that companies could provide genetic information direct to individuals. According to Martin, this meant being able to "put the power of gene technology directly in the hands of individuals" [15]. Sciona attempted to do just that, launching DTC products in the spring of 2001. The product format has become the convention in DTC genetic testing services—a DNA sample is collected from a customer, usually by a buccal swab, and it is sent to the firm along with the questionnaire. Questionnaires for nutrigenomic tests are typically focused on basic demographic information, health status, nutritional patterns, and lifestyle. In return for the fee, the firm analyzes the customer's DNA from a preset panel of genetic variants, and returns the analysis with some combination of dietary recommendations, specific advice about exposure to nutrients, and in some cases, discussion about what their nutrigenetic profile reveals about their susceptibility to certain diseases.

What would motivate someone to order a DTC test? This is a difficult question to answer in a direct way, since the companies offering DTC are privately held, thus making direct access to their clients a remote possibility. In fact, it is difficult to gauge how large the DTC market is for the same reason. This ought to be surprising, given the amount of concern expressed in print that DTC testing is potentially misleading, a possible source of stigmatizing information, potentially harmful to individuals, a threat to health care systems, and so forth—one would reasonably expect that theorizing about the risks of DTC would take into consideration the number of people exposed. One study attempted to analyze the structure and size of the DTC industry by using market share analytics from website hits, and then combining this data with the reported number of genomes or customer data two companies. For 2009, the estimated gross volume of sales for 23andme, Navigenics, and deCODEme was US$10 through 20 million, which the authors consider "fairly small" [16]. Since these companies test for genes primarily outside of the field of nutrigenomics, the nutrigenomic market is obviously much smaller.

Some prospective work with *potential* consumers of DTC nutrigenomics testing has been undertaken, for example, in a representative sample of nearly 6000 Europeans in 2005 [17]. Two thirds of respondents said that they would be willing to take a genetic test focused on nutrition, and nearly one-third said that they would be likely to follow a personalized diet. These individuals might be motivated by what we found in work supported by the Canadian Network of Centers of Excellence for Advanced Food and Materials Network (AFMNet) in partnership with the Public Health Agency of Canada in which 827 telephone survey respondents indicated 45% of the time that food and nutrition is the most important factor in personal health [8]. Over 90% of respondents in our survey indicated that genetic factors played a "big" or "moderate" role in health, although 64% indicated that on balance, environmental factors were more important. It must be noted, however, that focus groups held in parallel to the phone survey revealed that very few Canadians knew of nutrigenomics [18]. How these prospective numbers could translate into actual DTC purchases is unknown.

To summarize these points, people do express interest in having access to their genetic information in the way that Chris Martin anticipated. This is evident from the existence of a small DTC testing market that includes nutrigenomic testing, and some public engagement work in Europe and Canada reveals the same. The awareness of nutrigenomics remains low, however, and the market for DTC testing is also smaller—certainly much smaller than predicted by the IFTF. Yet, if these are factors related to creating public awareness and inducing people to buy DTC nutrigenetic tests, there is also the question about whether they would be motivated to follow through with the results and change their behavior. The sophisticated consumer envisaged for DTC markets is supposed to aggregate evidence from disparate sources and then act on it—do they?

As with the awareness and personal incentive that would motivate individuals to buy DTC tests, the evidence that they are motivated to act on the results is thin. Again, it should be pointed out that many of the concerns raised about nutrigenomics in the marketplace are focused on what would happen if consumers acted on the advice they are given without any decision support from health care professionals. Although there is much speculation about the severity of potential harms to individuals, evidence of harm, and the frequency of individuals being harmed have not been forthcoming. In fact, there is evidence to the contrary that suggests that people do not have a deterministic outlook about the contribution of genetics to their health [18], they do not endure psychological harm, and in the context of disease risk, they might be spurned on to have specific clinical screening tests [19,20]. Even in cases of potentially concerning distressing information concerning susceptibility for Alzheimer's disease, there is evidence that people can integrate new information and adapt to it [21].

In a review article of genetic predisposition tests, which are the type of tests used in DTC nutrigenetic disease susceptibility testing, it was found that "overall, predispositional genetic testing has no significant impact on psychological outcomes, little effect on behavior, and did not change perceived risk" [22]. The lack of impact on behavior might be a welcome thing if it means that people have not acted in ways contrary to interests if they have received misleading or false information from unscrupulous companies. On the other hand, DTC nutrigenetics testing companies depend on the use of its products to build the market; by analogy, would it contribute to the use of the Internet if people acquired email and Internet browser software but never used either? Here lies a serious conundrum around nutrigenetics and other testing services. While there are theories about how people are, or can be motivated to use genetic information coupled with nutritional advice [23], there is evidence that even in serious situations such as the risk of second heart attack [24], genetic information contributes little if anything to behavior change, let alone situations involving DTC genetic tests where new risk information is supposed to trigger behavior change [19]. If systematic reviews do not provide evidence that testing changes behavior [25], belief in the existence of sophisticated consumers aggressively seeking out and acting on this information is jeopardized.

DTC Marketplace

With the 10th anniversary of HGP now just past, we inevitably find ourselves in a period of questioning about the value of investments in human genomics. In terms of macroeconomics, it is fairly obvious that large-scale investments of public funds in science will have some kind of economic stimulus effect. A recent report claimed a return on investment (ROI) of 141:1 in stimulated economic activity [26], although the aggregated data and the input/output model makes it difficult to pinpoint the exact contributions attributable to the HGP [27]. Another report from the same period stated an ROI figure closer to 2:1 and suggested that nearly half a million jobs were created in the United States as a result of HGP investments [28]. Despite these positive accounts, questions remain about what new value is attributable to the HGP. One critical account suggests that the HGP has yet to prove its mettle in broad areas including: the clinical utility of genomics-based interventions; contributions to more nuanced understanding of risk and the communication of risk information; and the inducing enduring behavior change [29].

The question of the value of human genomics has arisen acutely in the context of nutrigenomics. As suggested above, it is difficult to assess the size and value of the DTC testing market overall, and for nutrigenomics, in particular. When Sciona was based in the United Kingdom, their DTC offerings attracted immediate attention of GeneWatch, the Human Genomics Commission, and some of the disputes about the wisdom and value of DTC nutrigenetic testing was played out in national papers such as *The Guardian* [15]. Controversy continued in the mid-2000s in the United States with warnings from the Federal Trade Commission warning consumers to be skeptical about DTC tests [30], with some academic commentators raising similar points [31]. Around the same time, the Food and Drug Administration issued guidance about so-called home brew genetic tests used by DTC companies [32]. The issue was the development and use of in vitro diagnostic multivariate index assays (IVDMIAs), which are the basic assays used in nutrigenomic testing. It became clear that tests would soon need to comply with the 1988 Clinical Laboratory Improvement Amendments standards for medical devices if sold in the United States. Statements were also made about the quality of DTC tests and the need to provide consumers with tests that were underpinned by evidence [33]. The State of California's Department of Public Health issued cease-and-desist letters in 2008 to DTC test providers on the grounds that companies were not providing the services under the auspices of a doctor, as required by state law. In addition to these regulatory actions, a chorus of sometimes overly zealous academic commentators published on the perils of DTC testing. These "highlights of the response to DTC genetic testing" are part of a broader story that has been discussed at length elsewhere [34].

The foundation of DTC nutrigenetic testing is the nutrient–gene association study, and there have been good scientific reviews raising questions about the strength of these associations [35,36]. Without strong empirical evidence linking nutrients and genes to health outcomes, DTC nutrigenetic testing is not likely to offer much to consumers, so the onus is on companies to make use of the best available science. That said, in the absence of evidence that consumers are being harmed by DTC testing, a balancing consideration is that these tests might have value to consumers for educational or perhaps even novelty value. If there is any merit to this point, it would suggest that policies and regulations holding DTC tests to the highest possible clinical standards would be well intentioned but might exceed the needs of the public [37]. Indeed, the Human Genetics Commission changed its perspective somewhat between 2003 and 2008: at first, the HGC suggested that genetic tests should be offered only through physicians or on a prescription basis, but later the view was that some of the lifestyle tests were "relatively innocuous" and could be offered on the basis of *caveat emptor* [38,39].

The other consequence is that regulating to a high standard, particularly in light of academic commentary describing potential (but not actual) risks of DTC tests, might unnecessarily drive companies out of the market. If in the long term DTC testing has the kind of future predicted by the IFTF and Forbes, and some value to consumers, it might be regretted in years to come if over-regulation stifles innovation [40].

There is evidence that this stifling has happened. For example, of the 26 companies mentioned in Ref. [41], eight no longer have an Internet presence. The Genetics and Public Policy Centre's (GPPC) update on DTC companies lists 20 companies currently offering DTC genetic tests in the United States [42]. Of the 19 providers of genetic testing test who received letters of warning from the FDA in 2010 [43], seven are still in business as DTC companies according to the GPPC, and two others have switched to offering tests through physicians. Many of the companies on the GPPC list offer tests that relate to nutrient–gene expression, but the GPPC categorizes just two companies as explicitly nutrition focused. Notably, the GPPC criteria for inclusion in their list are restricted to companies operating in the United States. Another study, however, indicated that 23 of 69 DTC companies including the United States and other countries stopped offering online services in the period 2008 through 2010, and the change is attributed to the impact of regulation [44].

The DTC genetic testing market has shrunk in the last 5 years in terms of the number of companies, and it remains difficult to estimate the value of the DTC market. Whether all of the volatility in the market is attributable to the actions of the FDA and FTC, as well as some individual states like California, is an open question. A contributing cause, if not the cause, of the volatility is surely the global economic crisis that is coincident with the main regulatory actions. Many DTC testing companies are small and medium enterprises that require multiple grounds of investment funding to stay afloat, and venture capital for enterprises that are perceived to be risky in the face of increased regulatory scrutiny will lose funding quickly. The first 10 years of DTC genetic testing have certainly been controversial and attempts to bring the applications of human genomics to the public, who paid for the initial investments, have slowed and in some cases stopped.

Empowerment and the DTC Business Model

Apart from considering DTC business and consumer trends, another issue persists about the future of DTC nutrigenomic testing. At the heart of the business strategy for DTC lies a conception of what interests and motivates consumers. What makes people "sophisticated consumers" in an information-rich environment where the appetite for personalized information is rewarded with promises of controlled destiny and self-improvement? These consumers are portrayed as savvy and autonomous economic agents, using their intellectual and financial resources in pursuit of their narrow self-interest. The sophisticated consumer is empowered; they are willing and able to make decisions for themselves. In addition to the buccal swab, the questionnaire, the DNA analysis, and the advice, selling people a conception of empowerment is the highest value proposition contained in DTC tests. The suggestion that DTC tests are actually about selling self-empowerment in a box, however, inverts the customary narrative in which DTC nutrigenomics is portrayed as catching the wave of genetics meeting nutrition in a pre-existing sea of pent-up, self-empowered consumer demand for DTC nutrigenetic testing. Which version is correct?

Pivotal to the idea of consumer empowerment is the view that people will embrace new science and technology as consumers, rather than as indifferent or perhaps even apprehensive citizens who are unconvinced by marketing and wary of new science and technology. While market research might disclose the presence of a cohort of individuals who will respond as consumers, the "early adopters," the presence of that cohort does not by itself suggest that other people have the same disposition to become consumers. It also does not suggest that the challenge for DTC marketing is to make manifest in people their inner, latent appetite to be consumers of new technology by raising their awareness. Empowered consumers might not exist all along, only waiting to be disclosed by market research. Rather, they are part of a narrative of how people might respond to genetics and genomics, and it is this narrative that is developed and projected into the marketplace. The job of the IFTF, and other horizon scanning and futures-oriented firms, is to create a vision of a future in which sophisticated consumers are common. Developing and projecting a plausible scenario enables strategic decision making by innovators, venture capitalists, and companies to create new markets for new products and services. The idea of sophisticated consumers empowered to aggressively seek information and act on it is less a matter of discovering who is already out there, and more a matter of projecting a vision of who could be there.

What people can control, and how they use information, raises some interesting challenges for consumer empowerment. Full control over one's genome is not possible since it is more or less a given—for each individual, their genome is context. What one is being empowered to do in this context is take information about genetics, lifestyle, and disease susceptibility and act in ways that mitigate risk. Such advice is actually very complicated, since it involves thinking about causal chains of events, and reflecting on connections between events in different time frames. That is, one is being asked to think about future states arising from present actions in light of past events over which one had no control. These temporal framings are made all the more complex since the causal connections do not involve causal connections that lead to definite health outcomes in a deterministic manner. Instead, inherited genomes are to be proactively managed in the present by controlling gene expression to address susceptibility of disease in the future.

Given that most people's understanding of genetics, nutrition, and susceptibility are insufficiently robust to understand the meaning of temporally complex information as full of uncertainties [45], most commentators want to reframe information provision in the terms of clinical encounters, rather than market exchanges. One solution that is widely advocated is to dispense with DTC testing altogether, since it does not uphold clinical genetics' values of informed consent, confidentiality, and non-directional counseling [41]. Another suggested solution is to shore up people's ability to apply statistical reasoning to personal genetics, thereby making them more responsive to genetic counseling [46]. The former is a recasting of the central differences in DTC and clinical paradigms that does not consider whether DTC testing can overcome the informational challenges just described, and the latter raises the obvious point about expertise but does not address how to set the boundary between lay understanding and professional expertise. Since health care professionals, who are not the only people who can possess expertise, are nevertheless notably deficient in genetics and nutritional training [47,48], they are not likely to meet people's needs in the near future.

A final point can be made about empowering people to become sophisticated consumers. Describing citizens as individuals acting in their narrow self-interest with easy access to a variety of information sources and the resources to carry out decisions is just one conception of what people are like and how they behave, and it is a conception of individuals that most would describe as strongly neoliberal. In retrospect, it typifies the ethos of the early 2000s—people as economic actors, fundamentally, constantly negotiating with everyone around them including their children, parents, at work with colleagues, in the marketplace, and with their governments. Implicit in this neoliberal description of individuals is a conception of autonomy in which people are rational agents, able to act in reasons-responsive ways to a variety of information sources, and who not only act in their own self-interest, but do so in a way that is consistent across types of decisions and times.

The above discussion about the informational uncertainties and their effects on empowerment might not seem, on the face of it, to present a direct challenge to this conception of citizens. There is, however, a problem lurking in descriptions of individuals presumed to be autonomous in the way just described, suddenly finding themselves unable to manage uncertainties from within the informed, autonomous agent conception of consumer empowerment. As Korthals and Komduur [49] have discussed, nutrigenomics presents a number of cognitive and social uncertainties, yet a well-established ethical framework that guides people through a selection process for choosing between uncertainties and resolving associated tensions does not exist. Faced with too many choices and too many uncertainties, autonomous individuals can become decisionally incapacitated; rational agency might have overarching goals, such as health, but the mechanics of decision making generally require more contextualized knowledge and situated clues about the best course of action. At issue, then, is not whether individuals ought to be getting DTC nutrigenetic tests in the context of the market, or whether the context should be changed to clinical encounters. Equally, it is not a political point about whether paternalistic interventions are warranted to control DTC nutrigenomics, as opposed to accepting that we live in a risk society in which the management of uncertainties is an endemic condition of modern life. Was it ever reasonable to think that ordinary people are capable of navigating the uncertainties they will confront, in an autonomous and consistent way and across different situations, or it is doubtful that ordinary people can meet the conditions of empowered, sophisticated consumerism—taken on its own terms?

Conclusion: Is DTC Testing the Future of Nutritional Genomics?

The period between 2001 and 2011 did not show flourishing of the DTC nutrigenomic market. Sophisticated consumers did not arrive in droves, and significant financial and regulatory impediments over the past 5 years pushed some companies out of the market and have put barriers before would-be entrants. These conditions are unlikely to change in the short term, and companies might have to try different strategies. These could include selling via the Internet from one country to the next to pick the most favorable jurisdictions from which to do business, fine-tuning claims associated with tests to comply with regulations, developing effective social media campaigns, or bundling nutrigenetic tests with other products and services. Perhaps, the ultimate salvation for DTC testing is to bow to pressure from various quarters to involve intermediaries such as dietitians to help consumers interpret information and integrate it into their decision making. In thinking through the ethical issues raised more than a decade ago in the IFTF horizon scanning and futures exercises, we came to the conclusion that a type of paramedical model was the only viable pathway toward the three-way optimization of access, responsible delivery of personal information, and minimization of regulatory scrutiny [50]. This is the kind of DTC testing that looks likely to be part of nutrigenomics' future, although with the near disappearance of the DTC nutrigenetic testing market, the products and services needing intermediaries might be gone before health care professionals will have caught up [51].

REFERENCES

1. Institute for the Future. 2001. *The Future of Nutrition: Consumers Engage with Science*. Cupertino, CA: IFTF.
2. Institute for the Future. 2003. *From Nutrigenomic Science to Personalized Nutrition: The Market in 2010*. Cupertino, CA: IFTF.
3. Herper, M., and R. Langreth. 2007. Will you get cancer? *Forbes* 179:52–68.
4. Corella, D., C.-Q. Lai, S. Demissie, L. Cupples, A. Manning, K. Tucker, and J. Ordovas. 2007. *APOA5* gene variation modulates the effects of dietary fat intake on body mass index and obesity risk in the Framingham Heart Study. *Journal of Molecular Medicine* 85 (2):119–128.
5. Foster, M. W., C. D. M. Royal, and R. R. Sharp. 2006. The routinisation of genomics and genetics: implications for ethical practice. *Journal of Medical Ethics* 32:635–638.
6. Dupré, J., and S. B. Barnes. 2008. *Genomes and What to Make of Them*. Chicago, IL: University of Chicago Press.
7. Knowler, W. C., P. H. Bennet, R. F. Hamman, and M. Miller. 1978. Diabetes incidence and prevalance in Pima Indians: a 19-fold greater incidence than in Roachester, Minnesota. *American Journal of Epidemiology* 108 (6):497–505.
8. Public Health Agency of Canada. 2007. Exploring how Canadians understand nutrigenomics. http://epe.lac-bac.gc.ca/100/200/301/pwgsc-tpsgc/por-ef/public_health_agency_canada/2008/184-07-a/report.pdf.
9. Weir, M., K. Morin, N. Ries, and D. Castle. 2010. Canadian health care professionals' knowledge, attitudes and perceptions of nutritional genomics. *British Journal of Nutrition* 104 (08):1112–1119.
10. Cornelis, M. C., A. El-Sohemy, E. K. Kabagambe, and H. Campos. 2006. Coffee, CYP1A2 genotype, and risk of myocardial infarction. *Journal of the American Medical Association* 8 (295):1135–1141.
11. Arkadianos, I., A. M. Valdes, E. Marinos, A. Florou, R. D. Gill, and K. A. Grimaldi. 2007. Improved weight management using genetic information to personalize a calorie controlled diet. *Nutrition Journal* 6:29.
12. Romanos, J., C. C. van Diemen, I. M. Nolte, G. Trynka, A. Zhernakova, J. Fu, M. T. Bardella et al. 2009. Analysis of HLA and non-HLA alleles can identify individuals at high risk for celiac disease. *Gastroenterology* 137 (3):834–840, 840 e1–840 e3.
13. Cahill, L. E., B. Fontaine-Bisson, and A. El-Sohemy. 2009. Functional genetic variants of glutathione S-transferase protect against serum ascorbic acid deficiency. *American Journal of Clinical Nutrition* 90 (5):1411–1417.
14. Davis, C. D., and J. A. Milner. 2011. Nutrigenomics, vitamin D and cancer prevention. *Journal of Nutrigenetics and Nutrigenomics* 4 (1):1–11.
15. Bensimon, C. M. 2001. Sciona Ltd.: A pioneer in nutrigenomics: The path to consumer acceptance. In *The Concise Encyclopedia of the Ethics of New Technologies*, edited by R. Chadwick. London: Elsevier Academic Press.

16. Wright, C. F., and S. Gregory-Jones. 2010. Size of the direct-to-consumer genomic testing market. *Genetics in Medicine* 12 (9):594.
17. Stewart-Knox, B. J., B. P. Bunting, S. Gilpin, H. J. Parr, S. Pinhao, J. J. Strain, M. D. de Almeida, and M. Gibney. 2009. Attitudes toward genetic testing and personalized nutrition in a representative sample of European consumers. *The British Journal of Nutrition* 101 (7):982–989.
18. Cassels, A. 2009. Understanding hopes and concerns about nutrigenomics: Canadian public opinion research involving health care professionals and the public. In *Nutrition and Genomics: Issues of Ethics, Law, Regulation and Communication*, edited by D. Castle and N. M. Ries. Amsterdam: Academic Press.
19. Bloss, C. S., L. Ornowski, E. Silver, M. Cargill, V. Vanier, N. J. Schork, and E. J. Topol. 2010. Consumer perceptions of direct-to-consumer personalized genomic risk assessments. *Genetics in Medicine* 12 (9):556–566.
20. Bloss, C. S., N. J. Schork, and E. J. Topol. 2011. Effect of direct-to-consumer genome-wide profiling to assess disease risk. *New England Journal of Medicine* 364 (6):524–534.
21. Green, R. C., J. S. Roberts, L. A. Cupples, N. R. Relkin, P. J. Whitehouse, T. Brown, S. L. Eckert et al. 2009. Disclosure of APOE genotype for risk of Alzheimer's disease. *New England Journal of Medicine* 361 (3):245–254.
22. Heshka, J. T., C. Palleschi, H. Howley, B. Wilson, and P. S. Wells. 2008. A systematic review of perceived risks, psychological and behavioral impacts of genetic testing. *Genetics in Medicine* 10 (1):19–32.
23. Bouwman, L. I., G. J. Hiddink, M. A. Koelen, M. Korthals, P. van't Veer, and C. van Woerkum. 2005. Personalized nurition communication through ICT application: how to overcome the gap between potential effectiveness and reality. *European Journal of Clinical Nutrition* 59:S108–S116.
24. Marteau, T. M., V. Senior, S. E. Humphries, M. Bobrow, T. Cranston, M. A. Crook, L. Day et al. 2004. Psychological impact of genetic testing for familial hypercholesterolemia within a previously aware population: a randomized controlled trial. *American Journal of Medical Genetics* 128:285–293.
25. Marteau, T. M., D. P. French, S. J. Griffin, A. T. Prevost, S. Sutton, C. Watkinson, S. Attwood, and G. J. Hollands. 2010. Effects of communicating DNA-based disease risk estimates on risk-reducing behaviours. *Cochrane Database of Systematic Reviews* (10):CD007275.
26. Battelle Technology Partnership Practice. 2011. *Economic Impact of the Human Genome Project*. Columbus, OH: Batelle Technology Partnership Practice.
27. Nature Editorial. 2011. What is the human genome worth? *Nature*, http://www.nature.com/news/2011/110511/full/news.2011.281.html.
28. United Medical for Research. 2011. *An Economic Engine: NIH Research, Employment and the Future of the Medical Innovation Sector*. Washington DC: United Medical for Research.
29. Evans, J. P., E. M. Meslin, T. M. Marteau, and T. Caulfield. 2011. Deflating the genomic bubble. *Science* 331 (6019):861–862.
30. Federal Trade Commission. 2006. *At-Home Genetic Tests: A Healthy Dose of Skepticism May Be the Best Prescription*. Facts for Consumers, http://www.ftc.gov/bcp/edu/pubs/consumer/health/hea02.shtm.
31. Geransar, R., and E. Einsiedel. 2008. Evaluating online direct-to-consumer marketing of genetic tests: informed choices or buyers beware? *Genetic Testing* 12 (1):13–23.
32. Food and Drug Administration. 2006. *Draft Guidance for Industry, Clinical Laboratories and FDA Staff: In Vitro Diagnostic Multivariate Index Assays*. U.S. Department of Health and Human Services.
33. American College of Medical Genetics. 2004. ACMG statement on direct-to-consumer genetic testing. *Genetics in Medicine* 6:60.

34. Ries, N. M., and D. Castle. 2008. Nutrigenomics and ethics interface: direct-to-consumer services and commercial aspects. *OMICS: A Journal of Integrative Biology*. 12 (4):245–250.
35. Janssens, A. C., M. Gwinn, L. A. Bradley, B. A. Oostra, C. M. van Duijn, and M. J. Khoury. 2008. A critical appraisal of the scientific basis of commercial genomic profiles used to assess health risks and personalize health interventions. *American Journal of Human Genetics* 82 (3):593–599.
36. Fenech, M., A. El-Sohemy, L. Cahill, L. R. Ferguson, T. A. French, E. S. Tai, J. Milner et al. 2011. Nutrigenetics and nutrigenomics: viewpoints on the current status and applications in nutrition research and practice. *Journal of Nutrigenetics and Nutrigenomics* 4 (2):69–89.
37. Caulfield, T. 2011. Direct-to-consumer testing: if consumers are not anxious, why are policymakers? *Human Genetics* 130 (1):23–25.
38. Human Genetics Commission. 2003. *Genes Direct: Ensuring the Effective Oversight of Genetic Tests Supplied Directly to the Public*. London: Human Genetics Commission.
39. Human Genetics Commission. 2007. *More Genes Direct: A Report on Developments in the Availability, Marketing and Regulation of Genetic Tests Supplied Directly to the Public*. London: Human Genetics Commission.
40. Castle, D. 2009. Applied human genomics from an innovation systems perspective. *Journal of Nutrigenetics and Nutrigenomics* 2 (2):103–110.
41. Hogarth, S., G. Javitt, and D. Melzer. 2008. The current landscape for direct-to-consumer genetic testing: legal, ethical, and policy issues. *Annual Review of Genomics and Human Genetics* 9:161–182.
42. Genetics and Public Policy Center. 2011. *GPPC releases updated list of DTC genetic testing companies*. http://www.dnapolicy.org/news.release.php?action=detail&pressrelease_id=145.
43. Genomics Law Report. 2010. *While you were meeting: FDA mails letters to 14 more genetic test providers*. http://www.genomicslawreport.com/index.php/2010/07/21/14-more-fda-letters/.
44. Cesagen. 2010. Report on the direct-to-consumer genetic testing industry. http://www.google.co.uk/url?sa=t&rct=j&q=&esrc=s&source=web&cd=1&ved=0CEUQFjAA&url=http%3A%2F%2Fwww.genomicsnetwork.ac.uk%2Fmedia%2FT1%2520-%2520Personal%2520Genomics%2520Link%2520PDF.pdf&ei=ToMuUJ2nFOST0QXD9YH4DA&usg=AFQjCNHljAOJ0u4pcGJfNagke_wGneIVOw&cad=rja.
45. Lachance, C. R., L. A. Erby, B. M. Ford, V. C. Allen, Jr., and K. A. Kaphingst. 2010. Informational content, literacy demands, and usability of websites offering health-related genetic tests directly to consumers. *Genetics in Medicine* 12 (5):304–312.
46. Kurzenhauser, S., and R. Hertwig. 2006. How to foster citizens' statistical reasoning: implications for genetic counseling. *Community Genetics* 9 (3):197–203.
47. Guttmacher, A. E., M. E. Porteous, and J. D. McInerney. 2007. Educating health-care professionals about genetics and genomics. *Nature Review. Genetics* 8 (2):151–157.
48. Farrell, J. 2009. Health care provider capacity in nutrition and genetics: a Canadian case study. In *Nutrition and Genomics: Issues of Ethics, Law, Regulation and Communication*, edited by D. Castle and N. M. Ries. Amsterdam: Academic Press.
49. Korthals, M., and R. Komduur. 2010. Uncertainties of nutrigenomics and their ethical meaning. *Journal of Agricultural and Environmental Ethics* 23 (5):435–454.
50. Castle, D., C. Cline, A. S. Daar, C. Tsamis, and P. A. Singer. 2006. *Science, Society, and the Supermarket: The Opportunities and Challenges of Nutrigenomics*. Hoboken, NJ: John Wiley and Sons.
51. Castle, D., and N. M. Ries. 2007. Ethical, legal and social issues in nutrigenomics: the challenges of regulating service delivery and building health professional capacity. *Mutation Research* 622 (1–2):138–143.

18 Nutritional Genomics in Practice

Interaction with Health Professionals in Bringing Nutritional Genomics to the Public

Colleen Fogarty Draper

CONTENTS

INTRODUCTION

Nutritional genomics is the scientific study of the impact of gene polymorphisms on the body's propensity for disease and functional imbalances and nutritional requirements; and the impact of food, nutrients, and related holistic aspects of human lifestyle on gene expression; which also effects gene regulation, transcription, early phase protein production, and intermediary markers of metabolism expressed by the metabolome. As this informative area of science progresses, the nutritional genomics term will increasingly encompass nutritional systems biology, including all of the "omics" sciences as they relate to nutrition, lifestyle, life experiences, and other related aspects of the environment that contribute to an individual's well-being. This exciting science has tantalized many of us for the last decade providing mechanistic insights that help us better understand impactful nutrition therapies and help scientists do better research. However, who will translate this new science for the public? In what paradigm can the science be applied best to optimize health? This chapter will provide an overview of the field for the practitioner with examples of scientific research that have a potential fit for practice and seek to evaluate the opportunity for the dietetics practitioners to integrate their nutritional science in practice knowledge with the growing, burgeoning field of nutritional genomics. This area of science is still maturing; however, it is important for the practitioner to start the education process now, to be prepared for a future in which holistic practice is synonymous with nutritional genomics.

Dr. Roger Williams taught us about biochemical individuality, long before we knew about the interactions between our genes, nutrients, and our environment. He published research data showing that children of the same family had significantly different nutritional needs; and adults of the same age and size with similar environmental settings and several-fold differences in nutritional requirements [1]. We now know that in every one of the 100 trillion cells in the body, except red blood cells, we house 25,000 genes whose variations govern our unique differences in body functioning, disease risk, nutrient requirements, and response to environmental factors, such as toxins or pharmaceutical agents. These variations are very small changes in our DNA, which can account for large differences in the body's response to and requirements for the food and nutrients we eat. Understanding the genetic association with human biochemical function and connection with food and nutrition offers health professionals, such as dietitians, an opportunity to add new tools to practice.

The optimal utilization of nutritional genomic research in practice forces a need to redefine goals. If the goal is to optimize the health of the individual, then what is health? According to the World Health Organization in 1938, "Health is a state of complete physical, mental and social well-being and not merely the absence of disease or infirmity" [2]. However, health is really a dynamic state of phenotypic plasticity or resilience and attaining complete wellness is likely unrealistic for many. Thus, health has been described as more of a concept that reflects, "the ability to adapt and self-manage in the face of physical, emotional and social challenges" [3]. In fact, salutogenesis is the study of the origin and cause of health that looks at how to strengthen homeostatic resiliency through creating, enhancing, and improving physical, mental, and social well-being [4].

In order to understand this salutogenic state of stress resilience and adaptability, it becomes important for scientists, researchers, and clinicians to be able to assess multiple components of the equation. The first component is genetic susceptibility. Although we know gene polymorphisms, such as single nucleotide polymorphisms (SNPs), only contribute 1% to our knowledge of heritability; and the large number of variants (including approximately 2 million SNPs) identified through genome-wide association studies (GWAS) on large numbers of people (as much as 250,000 in some studies) so far explain only 5%–10% of heritability for common chronic health issues, such as dyslipidemia, obesity, and diabetes; this offers us a place to start [5]. Although it takes millions of years for our genes to change from natural selection, as proposed by Charles Darwin, it takes far less time to impact their expression, either with epigenetic effects that last through generations or accrue over a lifetime, or changes in gene expression that are affected on a daily basis by transcriptional regulation in response to environmental influence. The strongest environmental influence is diet; however, there are many environmental factors to consider from exercise to stress management to weather and geographic location. So the first component of the equation is to know an individual's genetic susceptibility.

The next step is to understand the mechanistic interactions between this susceptibility, environmental choices (such as diet and lifestyle), and health plasticity. It is also important to know the limitations of this information. The "missing heritability" in relation to disease risk has not been fully explained due to the need for a better understanding of epistasis (gene × gene interactions—including the newly recognized impact of copy number variants), impact of rare variants, epigenomics interactions, and environmental interactions not yet identified [6].

Ultimately, the outcomes of this equation need to be measured and monitored, which can be done through gene expression analyses (mRNA microarrays), proteomic, and metabolomic analyses. For example, urinary metabolite testing is already used by early adopters in nutrition practice to conduct a functional nutrition assessment that identifies early phase markers of metabolic dysfunction that, if left unchecked, will eventually result in a loss of health plasticity and disease will ensue. Recently, researchers have been evaluating the interaction between genes and metabolites. Suhre et al. identified 25 genetic loci associated with blood metabolite concentrations, accounting for 10%–60% of differences in metabolite levels per allele. Disease target associations included cardiovascular disease, diabetes, kidney disorders, gout, and Crohn's disease. Although those associations discovered were not specifically targeted to particular mechanisms, many new hypotheses for influence of genotype on human metabolic individuality were generated, which hold the potential for future research translatable into practice [7].

NUTRITIONAL GENETIC TESTING

The clinical and personal utility of gene–diet/nutrient interactions that leads to optimal health fall into one of the three categories: (1) a need to increase the intake of a nutrient or bioactive food component, such as a B vitamin; (2) a need to decrease the intake of a nutrient or bioactive food component, such as gluten; or (3) a need to modify a standard nutrition therapy approach, such as increasing PUFA intake to optimize cholesterol ratio.

Nutritional genetic susceptibility testing has been available commercially, although sporadically, for the last decade. The testing can be purchased directly by the consumer or through a practitioner. Topics include detoxification, B vitamin metabolism, antioxidant function, bone health, heart health, salt sensitivity, inflammatory response, alcohol metabolism, cholesterol metabolism, estrogen metabolism, and weight management. The majority of testing is based on single nucleotide polymorphisms (SNPs) and individual interpretations are found in anywhere from one to six SNPs bucketed into a particular category. However, telomere length testing is also available that depicts telomere shortening with respect to age. Also, DNA damage testing is available as 8-hydroxy-2′-deoxyguanosine (8-OHdG).

In the United States, commercial genotyping laboratories fall under the Clinical Laboratory Improvement Amendments Act of 1998 (CLIA) to ensure quality laboratory testing, enforced by the US government. In addition, these companies ensure their test panels are not perceived as being diagnostic of a disease, requiring compliance with in vitro diagnostic testing regulations enforced by the Food and Drug Administration (FDA), costly and time consumptive regulations unrealistic for successful commercialization of genetic susceptibility testing. Like the US, Europe faces similar regulatory challenges. The European framework does not cover an independent evaluation procedure for genetic susceptibility tests prior to commercialization and postmarketing surveillance is, also, lacking [8].

Although single SNP testing offers some clues to the root cause of health imbalances and resulting nutritional requirements, there are limitations to information we know and utilize at present. When a positive SNP result suggests health risk and nutrition and lifestyle change, a negative result does not imply the absence of risk. SNPs only contribute 1% to our knowledge of heritability. Therefore, there are a myriad of other factors, such as, gene × gene interactions and lifestyle considerations, which require further exploration. Also, while a SNP panel test might look at 40 to 60 SNPs that relate to nutrition and health, 2 million SNPs have been identified through GWAS. Although we do not know the definitive risk and environmental associations with each of these SNPs discovered, the additional loci associated with many of the topics of commercial nutritional genetic testing suggest we are getting closer to understanding clusters of genes associated with health imbalances, as opposed to single genes. Gene clusters will provide more information on gene × gene and lifestyle interactions to further elucidate the presence of compensatory, collaborative, and inhibitory mechanisms that may alter the impact of individual SNPs. A great deal of genetics research has been done on Northern Europeans. Efforts are underway to extend this effort globally, such as, the Human Variome Project (HVP). However, ethnicity and geographic environment will effect whether a SNP is considered a risk allele. This adds to the complexity of using this testing in a variety of populations and is an important consideration for the practitioner's integration of genetic information in the overall assessment paradigm.

Circadian rhythmicity, fatty acid metabolism, and the brain–gluten connection are three interest areas, which hold promise for the future of nutrition therapy in practice. Therefore, these areas of research focus will be highlighted to give the reader a "taste" of the future potential for scientific applications of nutritional genomics.

CIRCADIAN RHYTHMICITY

The human circadian rhythm defines a 24-hour physiological, biochemical, behavioral cycle affected by availability of light, stress level, eating and sleeping times, temperature, and exercise. A greater biological understanding of circadian rhythmicity holds the potential of translatability into clinical practice. However, scientific research is necessary to understand unique, individual, and biochemically different responses to circadian challenges, such as night shift work or travelling over multiple time zones. These individual differences in response become clear among international travelers who seem to vary in their adaptation (i.e., phenotypic resilience) to changes in light, timing of food intake, and geographic location; and shift workers who develop problems with metabolic syndrome and obesity from night eating and excessive caloric intake [9].

The human master clock resides in the suprachiasmatic nuclei (SCN) located in the anterior part of the hypothalamus in the brain. Every organ/tissue of the body has its own biological clock; and all of these clocks need to be synchronized. In fact, lack of synchronization will decrease physiologic adaptability to stress (salutogenesis). The parallel to this would be interconnected train cars that are not moving at the same pace. If this is not corrected, the train will eventually cease to function. In this case, the body can be envisioned as a series of interconnected, synchronized train cars.

The United States and many other Westernized countries are now harnessing the power of light 24 hours/day and this could be the cause of some chronic disease, particularly in those individuals who are more genetically susceptible to the negative effects of rhythmicity stress.

Major acute health events seem to occur at common times of the day and during particular seasons. For example, according to a study in the Beijing metropolitan area, myocardial infarctions (MI) were found to occur frequently between 8 AM and 10 AM or 10 PM and 12 PM [10]. The Second International Study of Infarct Survival (ISIS-2) trial looked at five different geographic regions and found MI incidence increased between 6 AM and 8 AM and peaked between 8 AM and 11 AM [11]. The triggers and mechanisms of myocardial infarction (TRIMM) study group found MIs most commonly occurred within 3 hours of waking, between 6 AM and 9 AM [12]. Another study of medical records from the Beijing Emergency Medical Service found cases of Upper Gastrointestinal bleeding occurred more frequently during the cold months of the year and in the night time hours [13].

Some research suggests insufficient sleep time and shift work negatively affect our circadian rhythms and increase our risk of developing metabolic syndrome, diabetes, heart disease, and obesity [14–16]. In addition, some people are more biochemically sensitive to alterations in their circadian clock than others. The Circadian Locomotor Output Cycles Kaput (CLOCK) gene encodes a transcription factor responsible for modulating human circadian rhythms that affect metabolic alterations. Variations in the CLOCK gene have been linked to binge eating, reduced weight loss success, and the propensity to be a short time sleeper (> 6 hours/day) [17,18]. The TT genotype of the CLOCK 3111TC variant tends to be more obese and sleepless, with a high saturated fat diet; however, this effect is not seen for those who do not consume a diet high in saturated fat. Also, TT individuals lose less weight than the alternate genotype [18]. This is related to high ghrelin levels, which seem to translate to excessive food intake during the evening, lethargy in the morning, and lower overall physical activity [19]. A sample of 3311 adolescents from nine European countries reveals adolescents with short sleep duration (less than 8 hours) have higher body mass index values, body fat, waist and hip circumference, and fat mass index. In addition, these adolescents with short sleep duration are more sedentary and watch more TV. Finally, they eat less fish, vegetables, and fruits. Although it is difficult to say which issue comes first in the equation, it is interesting that sleep is also playing a role in the overall biochemical well-being of the adolescent community [20].

Gastrointestinal motility is, also, rhythmic with most people having bowel movements in the early morning and rarely at night. Gastrointestinal disruptions are common in shift workers and time zone travelers. In fact, the CLOCK gene is expressed in the cells of the colon [21]. Individuals with certain CLOCK gene variations may be more susceptible to gastrointestinal dysfunction because of changes in sleep cycle.

This latest research on sleep calls attention to the importance and opportunity for the holistic practitioner to integrate sleep into the patient/client assessment and treatment plan. It is fundamentally important to understand harmony in the body and its association with nutrition and wellness and the circadian clock. Chronotherapy is an emerging area of personalized practice in which therapy is administered to readjust the circadian clock.

GENETICS OF FATTY ACID METABOLISM

The delta-5 (D5D) and delta-6 desaturase (D6D) enzymes play a significant role in the desaturation and elongation of omega-6 and omega-3 by the body. They facilitate the conversion of linoleic acid into arachidonic acid (AA) and alpha linolenic acid (ALA) into eicosapentaenoic acid (EPA). These enzymes are expressed in the liver, brain, heart, and lungs. The fatty acid desaturase 1 and 2 (FADS1 and FADS2) genes encode the D5D and D6D enzymes, respectively, and their polymorphisms are associated with differences in fatty acid composition in phospholipid membranes and atopic disease development, particularly allergic rhinitis and atopic eczema [22]. They are, also, associated with increased risk of atherosclerotic vascular disease and Attention-Deficit/Hyperactivity Disorder [23,24]. A reduction in desaturase activity can reduce the body's capacity for cellular metabolism and incorporation of essential fats into cellular membranes and increasing the rate of fatty acid oxidation, to account for the excess, unmetabolized fats that accumulate. A recently published study looking at Caucasian and Asian subjects demonstrated a reduction of desaturase activity from polymorphisms in both FADS1 and 2 and a significant interaction between the FADS1 SNP (rs174547) and n-3 plasma fatty acid levels. [25]. These gene polymorphisms may impact the amount of dietary PUFAs required to optimize the fatty acid composition in cellular membranes and minimize the chronic disease that can ensue [26].

Additional research is needed to understand the mechanisms and effects of polymorphisms in these genes with an emphasis on the need for gene x diet interaction studies to further understand their impact on PUFA requirements [27]. This need presents a wonderful opportunity for the practitioner or registered dietitian to take a lead in the field of nutrition and genetics to further research the link between omega 3 fatty acid metabolism and genotype.

BRAIN–GLUTEN CONNECTION

Celiac disease is an inflammatory, immune-mediated, inherited disorder classically considered to affect the small intestine and treated by complete and permanent removal of dietary gluten (found in wheat, rye, and barley). A myriad of health disorders are associated with celiac disease and sometimes are the only manifestation of the disease ("silent celiac"). These include depression, irritability, anxiety, mental apathy, nonalcoholic fatty liver disease, rheumatoid arthritis, diabetes, dermatitis herpetiformis, gastroesophageal reflux disease, anemia and other vitamin insufficiencies, weight loss, weight gain, constipation, premenstrual syndrome, migraines, failure to thrive, and a protruding abdomen [28]. Human leukocyte antigens (HLAs) are markers located on leukocytes to help discriminate between host and foreign cells. Ninety-five percent of individuals with celiac disease are positive for HLA DQ2 and/or eight gene markers [29–31]. HLA DQ1 is found in 20% of patients with gluten intolerance and ataxia [32]. Approximately 1% of the US population has been diagnosed with celiac disease, however, 40% of the population carries either HLA DQ2 or DQ8 [33]. Because celiac disease symptomatology varies with the individual, most affected individuals have not been diagnosed, and this 1% represents only the tip of the iceberg [29]. Alternate manifestations of disease or states of suboptimal gluten intolerance could be the effect of additional gene × gene interactions, environmental interactions, and/or epigenetic or posttranscriptional changes; and looking closer at these interactions will give a better understanding of the mechanisms of disease evolution, leading to development of earlier stage diagnostics. Earlier stage diagnostics will help identify effected individuals not yet diagnosed.

In integrative and functional nutrition practice, it is common to see individuals with severe gluten intolerance, negative antibody results, and positive HLA DQ 2,8, or 1 genotypes. Many of these individuals have depression, foggy thinking, and/or other neurologic development issues. Published case studies support silent celiac disease diagnosis in adults and adolescents with depression [34,35]. Also, children with celiac disease demonstrate decreased levels of plasma tryptophan, suggesting their ability to generate sufficient brain serotonin may be compromised and lead to the observed mood disorders and behavioral disturbances in some of these children [36]. Removal of gluten from the diet results in amelioration of depressive symptomatology and improvement in plasma tryptophan levels [34–36]. The need to understand the brain-gut connection in celiac disease is one piece of the whole-body system effects of gluten intolerance and/or celiac disease, which deserve better elucidation in the scientific literature. With this understanding may come the opportunity to detect celiac disease or gluten intolerance earlier in the pathogenic process and to have a greater positive impact on optimal human health. In the meantime, HLA genotyping offers some additional insight on the root cause of gluten intolerance for our nontraditional patients or clients, giving the practitioner mechanistic insight to move forward with practical recommendations for lifestyle change.

Because the HLA genotypes aforementioned do not determine definitive celiac phenotypes, additional, non-HLA genes have been researched and implicated in celiac disease. Genome-wide association scans have identified 27 significantly associated loci, so far [37]. Specific genetic polymorphism associations identified include but are not limited to inflammatory genes, IL-6, IL1-B, TNFA; genes that affect immune function, such as T-cells, including CTLA4, ICOS, CD28; and genes that influence intestinal barrier function, including MAG12, MY09B, and PARD3 [38–41].

Polymorphisms in serotonin and dopamine metabolism, transporter and receptor genes, such as COMT, BDNF, 5-HTTLPR, TPH2, HTR2A, and 5-HT2A, are associated with alterations in neurologic functioning (mood, behavior, and ADHD) [42–44]. These polymorphisms have not been researched specifically with regard to celiac disease. However, microRNAs and epigenetic changes have been implicated as causative factors effecting neuronal homeostasis [45]. Understanding the epigenetic mechanisms behind the behavioral and mood disorders associated with celiac disease is an area of needed exploration.

Epigenetic evaluation of individuals with celiac disease, the extreme phenotype of gluten intolerance, is a relatively untapped area that would give insight on the mechanistic effects of celiac disease pathogenesis. Research data suggest epigenetic regulation is implicated in gastrointestinal development [46]. Aberrant CpG island methylation has been shown to be significantly different in celiac-associated adenocarcinoma verses nonceliac-associated adenocarcinoma [47]. So we know there is an epigenetic effect of celiac disease on gastrointestinal mucosa. Of interest is which genes are methylated within the human gastrointestinal tissue affected by celiac disease. Because an epigenetic analysis of celiac diseased intestinal tissue has not been conducted, it would be most appropriate to look for consistencies in global DNA methylation patterns in patients with confirmed celiac disease. However, it would be sensible to pay close attention to methylation patterns in those genes associated with celiac disease risk including the alleles that comprise HLA genotypes, as well as the inflammatory, immunity, and intestinal barrier function genes whose polymorphisms have been associated with celiac disease. In addition, due to the experiences of integrative and functional medicine, practitioners providing therapies for individuals with neurologic conditions, such as mood disorders, who have gluten intolerances, it would be most interesting to evaluate the methylation of the genes already listed that effect serotonin and dopamine metabolism.

MicroRNA destroys messenger RNA so it cannot complete the transcriptional process necessary to fully translate a protein. MicroRNAs are detected in the blood and have recently been shown to be useful as a diagnostic tool for pediatric Crohn's disease [48]. In addition, microRNAs play a key role in the etiology of depression [49,50]. Individuals with celiac disease are at risk of multiple micronutrient deficiencies, such as zinc, folate, B_{12}, vitamin D, and iron [51]. Of interest is that microRNAs are responsive to changes in nutritional status [52,53]. In the near future, the practitioner may realize the opportunity to not only use nutritional genetic testing, and refined, early-phase biomarker testing, but microRNA testing to gain insight on epigenetic changes. In the case of individuals with negative reactions to gluten, epigenetic testing may offer some answers to the root cause of their issues.

DATABASE ACCESSIBILITY

Large data sets of genomics, metabolomics, transcriptomics, proteomics, and nutrient biomarker data that crossover ethnicities and geographic regions to account for natural differences in genotype prevalence and environmental influence are needed to continue to see scientific progress in nutritional genomics research, translatable to practice. GWAS that cross over continents have been conducted and more are in progress to account for this need. In addition, researchers are pushing for more international research nodes to participate in and harmonize research protocols to allow for ease of data sharing. The HVP is a worldwide effort to identify all gene variations in the human genome associated with phenotypic variability and human disease risk. Kaput et al. 2010 proposed a collaboration between the HVP and the nutritional genomics research community to harmonize and systematize their research efforts to ensure cross-benefit of novel data and results [54]. Advances in systems biology and genomics research are increasing the feasibility to assess the mechanistic effects of micronutrients on metabolism. As a result, a central repository of micronutrient data has been developed for scientific researchers to submit and access data that will aid in further harmonizing and advancing nutritional genomics research efforts [55]. The micronutrient project ensures the environmental impact of nutrition is accounted for consistently on an international level. This database is likely to be useful to the practitioner of the future.

In the near future, data access will change to meet the growing needs of nutritional genetics and systems biology research and may be partially fueled by the wants and needs of individuals with chronic disease, desiring the opportunity to get closer to an understanding of the root cause of their health issues. Enterprises that link genetic data with clinical phenotypes and interventions, such as Patients Like Me (www.patientslikeme.com), the Personal Genome Project (www.personalgenomes.org), DIY Genomics(www.DIYgenomics.org), and Genomera (www.genomera.com) utilizing patient driven research and mandatory data collection in clinical will become part of the health routine and experience for the researcher, clinician, and patient.

DIETETICS PRACTITIONER INTEGRATION AND COMMERCIAL TESTING

One of the challenges in the utilization of nutritional genetic susceptibility testing lies in designing accurate and reliable translations of the research literature. The European Society of Human Genetics reports there is an urgent need for the assessment of genetic susceptibility information that is of clinical use [8]. This is an opportunity for the healthcare practitioner to get involved in genetic test development to ensure the most appropriate and reliable translations are provided to the public. Genetic literacy of the healthcare practitioner is an important component of the equation to not only contribute to the translation of testing but to be relied upon as an information source on commercial testing for the public [8].

The dietetics practitioner is a food and nutrition expert who utilizes various nutrition assessment and therapy approaches in a variety of settings in the treatment and prevention of disease. Most dietitians complete a minimum of bachelor's level coursework required by an accrediting body that includes food and nutrition sciences, foodservice systems management, business, economics, computer science, sociology, biochemistry, physiology, microbiology, and chemistry. Approximately 50% of US dietitians have advanced degrees, as well. Coursework is followed by a supervised internship practice program, which will vary from 6 months to 2 years. Following the completion of the supervised internship practice program, a national, written examination is required to obtain the dietetics practitioner credentials. These requirements are somewhat variable around the globe and efforts are underway to harmonize requirements through the International Confederation of Dietetics Associations (ICDA) (http://www.internationaldietetics.org/) and the DIETS Thematic Network (www.thematicnetworkdietetics.eu).

With a strong background in the nutritional sciences, the dietetics practitioner is the most reliable practitioner to interpret the diet and lifestyle implications of nutritional genetic testing for the public [56]. However, the dietetics practitioner needs to bridge the gap between present training, limited to genetic associations with inborn errors of metabolism, and the requirements of this new field. The United Kingdom and Canada surveyed the knowledge, interests, and perceptions of the dietitian with regard to nutritional genomics in 2007 and 2008. These surveys identified the need to increase involvement, confidence, and knowledge of the dietitian though exposure to university education and continuing professional development [57,58]. Although it is a challenge to incorporate human genetics into dietetics curricula, genetics and nutritional systems biology focused education is essential and will eventually be a requirement to become a dietitian capable of utilizing sophisticated nutritional genomics tools in practice [59]. Prasad et al., Texas Women's University, USA, have identified seven learning objectives for undergraduate dietetic student curricula [60]. The time to do this is now, so the dietitians are advancing their professional education as the science progresses.

ACADEMY OF NUTRITION AND DIETETICS FOCUS ON GENETICS

The American Dietetic Association (ADA) assumed a new name in January 2012 as the Academy of Nutrition and Dietetics (Academy). In October 2008, the ADA House of Delegates conducted a dialog on nutritional genomics in order to: (1) Create a vision of future practice; (2) Identify how registered dietitians (RDs) can prepare themselves to incorporate nutritional genomics into practice; and (3) Identify what AND can do to support members in these efforts. Guiding principles identified for consideration in moving forward included the following: (1) Collaboration with outside organizations and institutions with nutritional genomics expertise; (2) Development of education opportunities for students and practitioners; (3) Promotion of and participation in research opportunities; (4) Utilization of expert assistance; and (5) Development of programs to prepare members for future practice. Presently, a position paper that outlines the needs for competency and potential impact on professional practice is being written and will be published in the *Journal of the American Dietetic Association* (ADA).

The Dietitians in Integrative and Functional Medicine (DIFM) is a Dietetic Practice Group (DPG) of the ADA. DIFM has a long-standing effort in place to educate and update dietetics members in the field of nutritional genomics. Efforts include quarterly newsletter articles, webinars, and an informational nutritional genomics section of the website (www.integrativeRD.org). As of October 21, 2011, a network relationship was developed between the DIFM and Research DPGs and the International Society of Nutrigenetics and Nutrigenomics (ISNN) to facilitate the provision of education opportunities for dietitians from an outside organization, as specified in the House of Delegates dialog; and increase interdisciplinary membership participation in the ISNN needed to foster and grow the field. Members of the DIFM Executive Committee recently published standards of practice and performance for registered dietitians in integrative and functional medicine in the *Journal of the American Dietetic Association* (JADA) to establish the standards for a sophisticated dietetics professional. Included in these standards is a focus on genomics and other "-omics" tools [61].

INTERNATIONAL EDUCATION AND DIETETICS

Health professionals interested in furthering their knowledge base in nutritional genomics can consider taking academic genetics courses and joining professional organizations, such as the International Society of Nutrigenetics and Nutrigenomics

(ISNN) (www.isnn.info/) and the European Nutrigenomics Organization (NuGO) (www.nugo.org) for journal access, membership, and annual meetings. Staying abreast of the latest scientific research on the genetics and biochemical basis of diseases or optimal health areas of interest is an important component of a lifelong commitment to learning and will broaden the practitioner's perspective on the opportunities in the field of nutritional genomics.

Nutritional genomics coursework is becoming more widely available at various universities around the globe; including Tufts University in Boston, MA, USA; University of California at Los Angeles (UCLA) in California, USA; the University of Stellenbosch in South Africa; Wageningen University, in the Netherlands; the University of Auckland in New Zealand; and many more. In association with Section 5.1 of the Australian Dietetic Association's Manual for Accreditation of Dietetics Programs, dated October 2011, coursework in genetics and nutrigenomics is required as part of the underlying knowledge taught in a dietetics program [62].

CONCLUSION

This chapter has introduced nutritional genomics for the healthcare practitioner, reviewed areas of research likely to positively impact practice and the achievement of salutogenesis, and highlighted global efforts to educate and ready the dietetics practitioner for nutritional genomics in practice. The evolution of nutritional genetics in research and practice offers some clues to the root cause understanding necessary to use nutrition therapies to heal. It will also fuel the research in practice necessary to design evidence-based intervention strategies.

We need a sophisticated nutritionist who can utilize evidence-based nutritional genomics tools in practice. The dietetics practitioner has the potential to be the practitioner of choice to maximize the beneficial utilization of these technologies. The dietetics practitioner can be positioned globally to help all populations realize the power of "-omics" technologies in practice to provide the information needed to make the best nutrition and lifestyle choices that promote healing. Dietitians can become the lead translators for members of the healthcare team.

REFERENCES

1. Williams, R.J., *Biochemical Individuality: The Basis for the Genetotrophic Concept.* 1998, New Canaan, CT: Keats Pub. xviii, p. 267.
2. WHO., *Definition of Health.* 1946 [cited 2011 9-29-2011]; Available from: http://www.who.int/suggestions/faq/en/index.html.
3. Huber, M. et al., How should we define health? *British Medical Journal*, 2011. **343**: p. d4163.
4. Antonovsky, A., *Health, Stress, and Coping*. 1st ed. 1985, San Francisco, CA: Jossey-Bass Publishers.
5. Simonson, M.A., A.G. Wills, M.C. Keller, and M.B. McQueen, Recent methods for polygenic analysis of genome-wide data implicate an important effect of common variants on cardiovascular disease risk. *BMC Medical Genetics*, 2011. **12**(1): p. 146.
6. Lupski, J.R., J.W. Belmont, E. Boerwinkle, and R.A. Gibbs, Clan genomics and the complex architecture of human disease. *Cell*, 2011. **147**(1): p. 32–43.

7. Suhre, K. et al., Human metabolic individuality in biomedical and pharmaceutical research. *Nature*, 2011. **477**(7362): p. 54–60.
8. van El, C.G. and M.C. Cornel, Genetic testing and common disorders in a public health framework. *European Journal of Human Genetics: EJHG*, 2011. **19**(4): p. 377–81.
9. Garaulet, M. et al., CLOCK genetic variation and metabolic syndrome risk: modulation by monounsaturated fatty acids. *The American Journal of Clinical Nutrition*, 2009. **90**(6): p. 1466–75.
10. Li, Y. et al., Circadian, day-of-week, and age patterns of the occurrence of acute coronary syndrome in Beijing's emergency medical services system. *The American Journal of Emergency Medicine*, 2010. **28**(6): p. 663–7.
11. Group, I.-S.I.S.o.I.S.C., Morning peak in the incidence of myocardial infarction: experience in the ISIS-2 trial. *European Heart Journal*, 1992. **13**: p. 594–8.
12. Willich, S.N. et al., Association of wake time and the onset of myocardial infarction. Triggers and mechanisms of myocardial infarction (TRIMM) pilot study. TRIMM Study Group. *Circulation*, 1991. **84**(6 Suppl): p. VI62–7.
13. Du, T. et al., Circadian and seasonal rhythms of acute upper gastrointestinal bleeding in Beijing. *Emergency Medicine Journal: EMJ*, 2010. **27**(7): p. 504–7.
14. Spiegel, K., K. Knutson, R. Leproult, E. Tasali, and E. Van Cauter, Sleep loss: a novel risk factor for insulin resistance and Type 2 diabetes. *Journal of Applied Physiology*, 2005. **99**(5): p. 2008–19.
15. Karlsson, B.H., A.K. Knutsson, B.O. Lindahl, and L.S. Alfredsson, Metabolic disturbances in male workers with rotating three-shift work. Results of the WOLF study. *International Archives of Occupational and Environmental Health*, 2003. **76**(6): p. 424–30.
16. Reilly, J.J. et al., Early life risk factors for obesity in childhood: cohort study. *British Medical Journal*, 2005. **330**(7504): p. 1357.
17. Garaulet, M. et al., CLOCK gene is implicated in weight reduction in obese patients participating in a dietary programme based on the Mediterranean diet. *International Journal of Obesity*, 2010. **34**(3): p. 516–23.
18. Garaulet, M. et al., Genetic variants in human CLOCK associate with total energy intake and cytokine sleep factors in overweight subjects (GOLDN population). *European Journal of Human Genetics: EJHG*, 2010. **18**(3): p. 364–9.
19. Garaulet, M. et al., Ghrelin, sleep reduction and evening preference: relationships to CLOCK 3111 T/C SNP and weight loss. *Public Library of Science One*, 2011. **6**(2): p. e17435.
20. Garaulet, M. et al., Short sleep duration is associated with increased obesity markers in European adolescents: effect of physical activity and dietary habits. The HELENA study. *International Journal of Obesity*, 2011. **35**(10): p. 1308–17.
21. Hoogerwerf, W.A., Role of clock genes in gastrointestinal motility. *American Journal of Physiology. Gastrointestinal and Liver Physiology*, 2010. **299**(3): p. G549–55.
22. Morales, E. et al., Genetic variants of the FADS gene cluster and ELOVL gene family, colostrums LC-PUFA levels, breastfeeding, and child cognition. *Public Library of Science One*, 2011. **6**(2): p. e17181.
23. Martinelli, N. et al., FADS genotypes and desaturase activity estimated by the ratio of arachidonic acid to linoleic acid are associated with inflammation and coronary artery disease. *The American Journal of Clinical Nutrition*, 2008. **88**(4): p. 941–9.
24. Brookes, K.J., W. Chen, X. Xu, E. Taylor, and P. Asherson, Association of fatty acid desaturase genes with attention-deficit/hyperactivity disorder. *Biological Psychiatry*, 2006. **60**(10): p. 1053–61.
25. Merino, D.M. et al., Polymorphisms in FADS1 and FADS2 alter desaturase activity in young Caucasian and Asian adults. *Molecular Genetics and Metabolism,* 2011. **103**(2): p. 171–8.

26. Kotetzko, B., H. Demmelmair, L. Schaeffer, T. Illig, and J. Heinrich, Genetically determined variation in polyunsaturated fatty acid metabolism may result in different dietary requirements. *Nestle Nutrition Workshop Series. Paediatric Programme*, 2008. **62**: p. 35–49.
27. Lattka, E., T. Illig, B. Koletzko, and J. Heinrich, Genetic variants of the FADS1 FADS2 gene cluster as related to essential fatty acid metabolism. *Current Opinion in Lipidology*, 2011. **21**(1): p. 64–9.
28. Libonati, C.J., *Recognizing Celiac Disease: Signs, Symptoms, Associated Disorders & Complications*. 2007, Fort Washington, PA: Gluten Free Works Pub. xii, 302 p.
29. Kagnoff, M.F., Celiac disease: pathogenesis of a model immunogenetic disease. *The Journal of Clinical Investigation*, 2007. **117**(1): p. 41–9.
30. Louka, A.S. et al., A collaborative European search for non-DQA1*05-DQB1*02 celiac disease loci on HLA-DR3 haplotypes: analysis of transmission from homozygous parents. *Human Immunology*, 2003. **64**(3): p. 350–8.
31. Mazzarella, G. et al., An immunodominant DQ8 restricted gliadin peptide activates small intestinal immune response in in vitro cultured mucosa from HLA-DQ8 positive but not HLA-DQ8 negative coeliac patients. *Gut*, 2003. **52**(1): p. 57–62.
32. Hadjivassiliou, M., R.A. Grunewald, and G.A. Davies-Jones, Gluten sensitivity as a neurological illness. *Journal of Neurology, Neurosurgery, and Psychiatry*, 2002. **72**(5): p. 560–3.
33. Fasano, A. et al., Prevalence of celiac disease in at-risk and not-at-risk groups in the United States: a large multicenter study. *Archives of Internal Medicine*, 2003. **163**(3): p. 286–92.
34. Pynnonen, P.A. et al., Gluten-free diet may alleviate depressive and behavioural symptoms in adolescents with coeliac disease: a prospective follow-up case-series study. *BMC Psychiatry*, 2005. **5**: p. 14.
35. Corvaglia, L., R. Catamo, G. Pepe, R. Lazzari, and E. Corvaglia, Depression in adult untreated celiac subjects: diagnosis by the pediatrician. *The American Journal of Gastroenterology*, 1999. **94**(3): p. 839–43.
36. Hernanz, A. and I. Polanco, Plasma precursor amino acids of central nervous system monoamines in children with coeliac disease. *Gut*, 1991. **32**(12): p. 1478–81.
37. Hrdlickova, B., H.J. Westra, L. Franke, and C. Wijmenga, Celiac disease: moving from genetic associations to causal variants. *Clinical Genetics*, 2011. **80**(3): p. 203–313.
38. Chernavsky, A.C. et al., The simultaneous presence of IL-1B and TNFA two-positions risk haplotypes enhances the susceptibility for celiac disease. *Cytokine*, 2008. **42**(1): p. 48–54.
39. Mysliwiec, M. et al., Interleukin 6 -174(G>C) gene polymorphism is related to celiac disease and autoimmune thyroiditis coincidence in diabetes type 1 children. *Diabetes Research and Clinical Practice*, 2008. **82**(1): p. 108–12.
40. Brophy, K. et al., Haplotypes in the CTLA4 region are associated with coeliac disease in the Irish population. *Genes and Immunity*, 2006. **7**(1): p. 19–26.
41. Wolters, V.M. et al., Intestinal barrier gene variants may not explain the increased levels of antigliadin antibodies, suggesting other mechanisms than altered permeability. *Human Immunology*, 2010. **71**(4): p. 392–6.
42. Dunlop, B.W. and C.B. Nemeroff, The role of dopamine in the pathophysiology of depression. *Archives of General Psychiatry*, 2007. **64**(3): p. 327–37.
43. Lopez Leon, S. et al., The dopamine D4 receptor gene 48-base-pair-repeat polymorphism and mood disorders: a meta-analysis. *Biological Psychiatry*, 2005. **57**(9): p. 999–1003.
44. aan het Rot, M., S.J. Mathew, and D.S. Charney, Neurobiological mechanisms in major depressive disorder. *CMAJ: Canadian Medical Association Journal = Journal de l'Association Medicale Canadienne*, 2009. **180**(3): p. 305–13.

45. Ramocki, M.B. and H.Y. Zoghbi, Failure of neuronal homeostasis results in common neuropsychiatric phenotypes. *Nature*, 2008. **455**(7215): p. 912–8.
46. Waterland, R.A., Epigenetic mechanisms and gastrointestinal development. *The Journal of Pediatrics*, 2006. **149**(5 Suppl): p. S137–42.
47. Bergmann, F. et al., Small bowel adenocarcinomas in celiac disease follow the CIM-MSI pathway. *Oncology Reports*, 2010. **24**(6): p. 1535–9.
48. Zahm, A.M. et al., Circulating microRNA is a biomarker of pediatric Crohn disease. *Journal of Pediatric Gastroenterology and Nutrition*, 2011. **53**(1): p. 26–33.
49. Dwivedi, Y., Evidence demonstrating role of microRNAs in the etiopathology of major depression. *Journal of Chemical Neuroanatomy*, 2011. **42**(2): p. 142–56.
50. Xu, Y. et al., A polymorphism in the microRNA-30e precursor associated with major depressive disorder risk and P300 waveform. *Journal of Affective Disorders*, 2010. **127**(1–3): p. 332–6.
51. Malterre, T., Digestive and nutritional considerations in celiac disease: could supplementation help? *Alternative Medicine Review: A Journal of Clinical Therapeutic*, 2009. **14**(3): p. 247–57.
52. Parasramka, M.A., E. Ho, D.E. Williams, and R.H. Dashwood, MicroRNAs, diet, and cancer: new mechanistic insights on the epigenetic actions of phytochemicals. *Molecular Carcinogenesis*, 2012. **51**(3): p. 213–30. Epub 2011 July 7.
53. Khanna, A., S. Muthusamy, R. Liang, H. Sarojini, and E. Wang, Gain of survival signaling by down-regulation of three key miRNAs in brain of calorie-restricted mice. *Aging*, 2011. **3**(3): p. 223–36.
54. Kaput, J., C.T. Evelo, G. Perozzi, B. van Ommen, and R. Cotton, Connecting the Human Variome Project to nutrigenomics. *Genes & Nutrition*, 2010. **5**(4): p. 275–283.
55. van Ommen, B. et al., The Micronutrient Genomics Project: a community-driven knowledge base for micronutrient research. *Genes & Nutrition*, 2010. **5**(4): p. 285–96.
56. DeBusk, R.M., C.P. Fogarty, J.M. Ordovas, and K.S. Kornman, Nutritional genomics in practice: where do we begin? *Journal of the American Dietetic Association*, 2005. **105**(4): p. 589–98.
57. Whelan, K., S. McCarthy, and M. Pufulete, Genetics and diet—gene interactions: involvement, confidence and knowledge of dietitians. *The British Journal of Nutrition*, 2008. **99**(1): p. 23–8.
58. McCarthy, S., M. Pufulete, and K. Whelan, Factors associated with knowledge of genetics and nutritional genomics among dietitians. *Journal of Human Nutrition and Dietetics: The Official Journal of the British Dietetic Association*, 2008. **21**(6): p. 547–54.
59. Vickery, C.E. and N. Cotugna, Incorporating human genetics into dietetics curricula remains a challenge. *Journal of the American Dietetic Association*, 2005. **105**(4): p. 583–8.
60. Prasad, C., V. Imrhan, and M. Rew, Introducing nutritional genomics teaching in undergraduate dietetic curricula. *Journal of Nutrigenetics and Nutrigenomics*, 2011. **4**(3): p. 165–72.
61. Ford, D. et al., American Dietetic Association: standards of practice and standards of professional performance for registered dietitians (competent, proficient, and expert) in integrative and functional medicine. *Journal of the American Dietetic Association*, 2011. **111**(6): p. 902–13 e1–23.
62. Association, A.D., *Australian Dietetic Association's Manual for Accreditation of Dietetics Programs*. 2011 October [cited 2011 12-21-11]; Available from: http://daa.asn.au/wp-content/uploads/2011/03/DAA-accreditation-manual_v1.2_Oct-2011.pdf.

19 Harvesting Normative Potential for Nutrigenomic Research

Bart Penders and Michiel Korthals

CONTENTS

INTRODUCTION

Innovating is hard. In the nutritional field, most innovations fail. For instance, already in 1992, Fredericks and MacLaughlin argued that at least 50% of all new consumer food product releases never make it beyond a year on supermarket shelves [1]. Such product launches include nearly everything, from a new wrapper to a new taste, as well new research-based innovations. Numbers may vary between types of product launches, but even products developed and supported by ample nutritional and marketing research may suffer the same fate [2].

A famous example is the development of "Golden Rice." This provitamin A–enriched rice variety was initially heavily critiqued because it did not contain a sufficient level of provitamin A to alleviate the health problems it was designed to [3]. Technically, it was improved and the levels of provitamin A were raised [4]. Despite such improvements, "Golden Rice" as an innovation remains a failure. The intentions of its creators are laudable, but the context of the innovation matters just as much as its technical characteristics. Golden rice was accompanied by debates on the rights of small farmers versus large seed companies. It was a genetic modification (GM) technology, heavily opposed by some, while just as heavily supported by others. Despite its technical ingenuity, its apparent connection to a societally prominent issue, and its research-based developmental trajectory, this nutritional innovation failed [5].

Nutrigenomics is not primarily about the making of new golden rices [6–9], although it might provide new knowledge bases for fortification of various kinds [10].

It is, however, a line of inquiry, a field, a community, a process, and potentially a set of products (broadly defined) with a highly technological origin. An innovative way to innovate, if you will. This confronts those engaged in nutrigenomic research and those who enlist nutrigenomics in the development of novel products, product claims, or claim evidence bases with a similar scenario: the best science and the best of intentions are not enough.

In this chapter, we aim to map two domains of normative aspects connected to nutrigenomic research and innovation. In the section on "Politics of doing nutrigenomic research," we critically examine the way nutrigenomics research is being conducted and highlight salient normative elements it contains. In the section on "Normative matching of nutrigenomic research and society," we compare dominant sets of norms and values, as they are present in nutrigenomic research practices on the one hand and in society on the other. We end with a general reflection on the status of the relationship between nutrigenomic research endeavors and food consumption and evaluation in society at large. In our chapter, and the societal evaluation of nutrigenomic innovation that we forward, we focus on the relationship between nutrigenomics and the *healthy* consumer. Perspectives, priorities, and relationships can and will change enormously as a result of (perceived) disease.

We draw our insights from two bodies of scholarly work. The first is the field of science and technology studies, focusing on the development of science, the ways theories and facts gather credibility, and the contexts that influence this path. Beyond being a heuristic in understanding how science works internally, it enables us to connect activities as they take place within laboratories and clinics to the world beyond these highly disciplined settings of knowledge creation. The "outside" world beyond the lab is not a world without expertise or knowledge, but a world in which (1) scientific knowledge, expertise, and authority play a different role and (2) other types of knowledge are present, which are equally important in the determination of whether an innovation becomes a success.

The second body of work is the field of applied ethics and philosophy of science, a tradition of critical engagement with the process, products, and claims of science, as well as its role in the world. Beyond examining the content of scientific claims and methodologies, it focuses on evaluations of moral decisions as they are implicitly and explicitly made in and around science. Through the mobilization of philosophy and ethics of science, we are able not only to discern norms and values as they are made, unmade, embodied, and disembodied in scientific settings but also to contribute to the ethical evaluation of one position over another.

The uptake of novel technological possibilities into the field of nutrition science, including, but not limited to, genomic and metabolomic technologies, has radically changed the descriptive and normative power wielded by the discipline. New technological possibilities, alongside the new scientific approaches and positions that accompany them, changed the way in which nutrition science is done, not only technically and scientifically, but also socially and morally.

The norms and values embedded in the "new" nutrition science differ from those embedded in the pre-nutrigenomics stage. Not radically, but significantly. With new descriptive power, so it was expected, would come new prescriptive power. But this particular brand of description and prescription appeared to be quite difficult—as we shall see in section on "Niches for Nutrigenomic Research: Promise and (Dis) connection"—in terms of its technical complexity, as well as with respect to the social and moral connotations that come along with it.

Let us move toward nutrigenomic practice to find out where such new, or old, social and moral connotations, issues, or aspects come from. Later, we highlight some of the most salient normative elements nutrigenomic (research) practices and trace them, in the section on "Normative matching of nutrigenomic research and society," into wider society, to find out where they match.

POLITICS OF DOING NUTRIGENOMIC RESEARCH

The organization of research cannot be disconnected from its object of inquiry [11,12]. Research organization and research content influence one another in many ways. For instance, complex problems are thought to require large, interdisciplinary teams of researchers [13]. These complex problems may include global warming, credit crises, or public distrust of scientific expertise. They also encompass complex health problems, including but not restricted to pandemic risks or the "obesity epidemic." The social penetration and the technical and technological wide-spanning character of these problems are generally suggested to require strategies that are equally wide-spanning. The dominant strategy is to draw together experts from a variety of specialties: collaboration and interdisciplinarity.*

Large-scale science differs from an idealized pure curiosity-driven view of research. The severity of the problem, economically or socially, is the main motivator for political actors to allocate resources to solving it. In that sense, the academic content of the problem is secondary at best. Painting with a broad brush, the main motivations for large expenses into nutritional science across the globe are either (1) to promote (public) health or (2) to build or improve the economic position of the food sector in a given region [14]. Strikingly, most public health motivations are often explained by the rationale that public health solutions ultimately will lower health-care expenses, against the backdrop of the *knowledge economy*. Nutrigenomics is no exception.

Collaboration and Human Health

Whether motivated by the desire to improve health for the sake of (public) health, or whether supported by an underlying rationale directed by health-care expenditure, the elusive target of human health seems to be a very good reason to organize large-scale interdisciplinary and international collaborations dealing with nutrigenomics. In Europe, such examples encompass the DIOGenes and NuGO [15] consortia and other examples include the Dutch Nutrigenomics Consortium, the Nutrigenomics New Zealand (NuNZ) collaboration, as well as large groups of scientists collaborating at the FDA and at UC Davis in the United States. The list is not endless, but it is very long.†

* This movement to involve more actors, more disciplines, and more sectors and the challenges that accompany this have been addressed in literature dealing with innovation before [14–18].

† For an annotated inventory, please see Annex 2 of Ref. [21].

Despite a common focus on molecular nutrition science or nutrigenomics, funding sources and types differ between such programs, as do the details of the objectives and the characteristics of management practices. However, a collaborative element on the one hand, and a more or less explicit goal of health, is something they all share [15,16].

How well does a central goal or master value of *health* match collaborative *research organization*? Let us first critically examine the notion of human health. Health is often used as a legitimation for large endeavors and large expenditures. It grants credibility to research and researchers through its apparent relevance. After all, our health, so it is often argued, is our most valued asset. To question this is a folly. As a value, health and well-being are important to us. We strive for them, we invest in them, and we work to reach or keep them. As a research goal, however, the notions of health, or public health, are quite elusive.

The value of health is a result of the context in which it appears. In the case of nutrigenomic research, this is a highly technological context with a preference for the molecular resolution of the processes of life. It is linked to nutrients on the one hand and molecular indicators on the other (indicators in general, since the focus on gene sequences and gene expressions has, as other chapters in this book clearly demonstrate, been widened significantly). Nutrigenomics' notion of health is embedded in a structure of doing science that is characterized by high specialization, thematically and technologically, and by an explicit collaborative working mode. However, from this connection of nutrigenomics with nutrients, it is also clear that in nutrigenomics a conception of food plays a role, that is, the conception that food's primary function is to enhance or restore the health of the eater. The concept of food is interpreted in as many ways as that of health; many would not consider food as a medicine but as something that gives pleasure or connects one with ones relatives and friends (see section on "Normative Matching Of Nutrigenomic Research And Society").

The focus on collaboration is not exclusive to nutrigenomic research. Well-studied examples of collaboration range from high-energy physics [17] and ecology [18] to synthetic biology [19]. Against this backdrop, Afman and Müller [20] argue for nutrition to become "big science" (p. 68) and call for the inclusion of nutrigenomic analysis in *every* nutritional study (p. 63).

In his analysis of two nutrigenomics consortia, Penders [13] has shown what happens when large-scale collaborative big science meets ambitious, but unstable, multi-interpretable research goals such as the value of health.* Penders describes how the "feasibility" or "doability" of research programs and problems is of primary importance to scientific practice. Doability is a state-of-affairs that is constantly pursued. It requires the availability of, for instance, research materials, skill, and resources to conduct a specific experiment. It also requires access to that laboratory, man power to do, institutional support, and access to all sorts of neighboring expertise. Finally, it also requires broader political and public support and an audience. The latter can be, for instance, a disciplinary group. *Constructing doability* is then

* Based on interviews with >35 nutrition scientists and nutrigenomicists, literature research as well as months of (laboratory) observations. For more details, see Ref. [13].

the process of making sure all those elements are available and accessible at the right time and place [21,22].

Large research problems are not considered to be feasible problems for single laboratories to solve [20]. They are too big and too complex, encompassing too many variables and unknowns. Where would one begin? Consortia, institutions, or networks dealing with such problems, for instance, NuGO or NuNZ, construct a doable research organization through the strategic division of problems into smaller bits: modules. These are handed over to the laboratories or departments that make up the consortium, based on, among many other things, their available expertise, skill, machinery, and access to biological material [23]. Some do protein work, other transcriptomic analyses, some do human experiments, others focus on animals or cell lines—but all do so within the institutional bounds of the nutrigenomic consortium, while referring to, and drawing legitimacy from, the overall research goal.

The modules of the research problem thus are also modules of the research organization. Each module is (supposedly) linked to neighboring modules, socially and materially, through the exchange of data, insights, expertise, and above all else research materials. However, the modular design of nutrigenomic research has consequences for the conception of the overall problem of health and food. The local "doability" of the modular problem is of prime importance to researchers. This problem and the research connected to it get them published, recognition, prestige, and ultimately enhanced credibility [24]. The overall problem is of prime importance for broader legitimation and for getting resources to compile consortia in the first place, but now that laboratory work has commenced, local doability overrules all others. A nutrigenomicist quoted in Penders [13] states this as follows: "I think everybody does his own thing, eventually [...]. I cannot say that people working in a different group add something to my subject" (p. 74).

The modularity of the research problem of health and food is subject to a significant risk of fragmentation. Penders and colleagues have argued before that upon entering research practice, science-in-action if you will, health and food in general are strikingly esoteric in most laboratories [13,25].

Current large-scale research, including large-scale nutrigenomic research, is confronted with a research situation in which problem modules take precedence over overall problems and the notions of health and food are framed and reframed based on the context in which they are used. Health and food, although esoteric in the laboratory context, are (re)framed based on the context in which it is present. This context is, on the one hand, laboratory-specific, thus creating a diversification, and on the other hand a number of characteristics can be recognized in many of the laboratories devoted to nutrigenomic inquiry: health and food seem to be accessible on the molecular level, they are above all else an individual characteristic and they can be maintained through careful and balanced intake of specific nutrients. Health and food are diverse, yes, but their core seems to be molecular, personal, and manageable.

Strikingly, these three elements of what health and food are exist in stark contrast to social and cultural framings of health and food as somatic, shared, collective, and cumbersome and in the case of food as (social) pleasure. We get to this in section "Normative Matching Of Nutrigenomic Research And Society".

Niches for Nutrigenomic Research: Promise and (Dis)connection

The large-scale character of nutrigenomics research is one of its defining features. Its collaborative and interdisciplinary character is one of the elements distinguishing it from prior nutrition research, granting, among other things, credibility to nutrition science in general. Hannelore Daniel argues that "For the first time now, nutrition science is being taken seriously" [quoted in Ref. 13, p. 13].

Nestled firmly within a genomic tradition, sharing technologies with other fields, including but not limited to pharmacogenomics and toxicogenomics, nutrigenomics developed an economy of promise. An economy of promise is a set of promises and expectations that is widely shared across a social group (in this case, nutrigenomicists). Economies of promise perform and project a desired future into the present—that is to say that they require work, orchestration, and have consequences: they create (social) realities and have the ability to gather support and momentum [26–29]. Such momentum consists of, for large-scale research, institutional structures and support as well as ample funding for research and coordination.

Looking back upon a decade of nutrigenomics research, we may conclude that nutrigenomics has performed its economy of promise well. Large research structures and consortia with budgets ranging up to the dozens of millions of euros or dollars have been set up. Why did it work out well? Some promises acquire more support than others. It is important for an economy of promise to align itself with existing dominant social and political trends (this can be read as a strategic approach toward opportunism).

For nutrigenomics, this has been the case. We highlight two of the most prominent sociopolitical trends. The first is the policy focus on the constant improvement of (national) economic competitiveness and the desire to triumph in the competitive market of bioeconomies [30]. Nutrigenomicists have linked in their promises, as argued in "Introduction", the lowering of health-care expenditure due to improved prevention as well as hinted at the support nutrigenomic research programs may offer for (local) food industries [31]. The second is the current political climate, which is increasingly neoliberal in nature. Nutrigenomicists have explicitly argued that through increased insight in one's personal genomic or metabolomic profile, individuals would be empowered to take (preemptive) action to remain healthy [32]. The sometimes implicit, but often explicit focus on personalization aligns with the neoliberal tendency to increasingly shift responsibility from the collective to the individual.

The alignment of nutrigenomic promises and expectations with existing neoliberal trends and movements brings together interests of policy-makers, public health officials, the food industry, and scientists. Together, they have been able to collect impressive amounts of funding and rally supporters to their side, meant to craft *nutrigenomic reality* from *nutrigenomic promise*. After a period of divergence, in which more traditional nutrition science and nutrigenomics developed more or less independently, a period of convergence has now started [20]. Most of the large funds devoted to nutrigenomics have depleted or are quickly reaching their end.

All economies of promise are temporary. Scientific realities change as science progresses. Individualization has been found not attractive for industry and given way to group-based intervention and nutrigenomics, which—despite impressive progress—has proven to be more complex than anticipated. Simultaneously, genomic technologies have become rather commonplace: their status apart, in terms of skill and expertise, has given way as well. However, key elements of the social reality crafted in the context of nutrigenomics' initial economy of promise remain in place: an economic, individual, neoliberal focus [14,33]. Molecular nutrition science, nutrigenomics, or nutrition science 2.0 deal with health on a programmatic level, but much more esoterically so on a practical level.

NORMATIVE MATCHING OF NUTRIGENOMIC RESEARCH AND SOCIETY

The organization of nutrigenomics research showed, at least initially, a focus on tech-development. Embedded in that technology, as well as in the context of application within nutrigenomic inquiry, we can discern a dominant set of norms and values. These do not necessarily match their counterpart in society.

Komduur et al. [34] explicated on the basis of an analysis of a selected set of scientific journal articles* three sets of normative assumptions embedded in the present nutrigenomics research covered by these articles. Together, these most salient normative assumptions on health and food, qualitatively identified and analyzed, comprise a prominent script in nutrigenomics.

As a result of their analysis, it turned out firstly that in the texts chosen, food is exclusively interpreted in terms of disease prevention. Health is therefore seen as a state preceding a sum of possible diseases and food has an intervening role in delaying these possible diseases. Secondly, it is assumed that health should be explained as a calculable interaction between food and genes. Health is minimized to quantifiable health risks and disease prevention through food–gene interactions by the "right" food choice. The third assumption is that disease prevention by minimization of risks through the right food choice is in the hands of the individual; through this individual responsibility either through finding out personal risks, revealed through personal tests, or through belonging to a risk group, the individual has to act and spend time to make the proper food choice. The individual has to play a large role in disease prevention by minimizing personal risks through tests or belonging to a risk group and eating the right stuff.

Together, these three concepts suggest that the *meaning of life* is interpreted as a healthy life, in which preventively risks should be calculated and balanced and in which the individual should have the prime responsibility to act in accordance to the outcome of tests by selecting the right type of food. Those people, who do not accept this task, do not act responsibly.

When we compare these assumptions to existing research on food styles as they exist in the plural societies that make up our world [35–39], a large gap appears. Only a few styles stress a direct link between eating and health and emphasize

---

* Komduur et al. draw upon a selection of papers, written by 10 nutrigenomics scientists (Ordovas, Mooser, Müller, Kersten, Afman, Milner, Dwyer, Wahli, Saguy, and Saris), four representatives of the food industry (German, Watzke, Mutch, and Moskowitz), and two nutritionists (Trujillo and Davis). For selection criteria and methodological details, see Ref. [40].

the view on food as prevention against diseases. Other food styles are less likely to adopt nutrigenomics, especially those that adopt a traditional, social, culinary, or slow food approach. Petrini [40], the founder of the Slow Food movement and a fierce defender of the social and cultural aspects of enjoying food, approvingly quotes Madame Sevigny: "Health is enjoying the other enjoyments. When the other enjoyments are taken away, we live longer, but we lose our health." The Slow Food movement, which is gaining considerable momentum in the western world, does not clearly subscribe to the narrow definition of health propagated by personalized nutrition and nutrigenomics.

In the same vein, traditional, natural, and cosmopolitan food styles have objections against the identification of food and prevention of diseases. Proponents of these styles would say that society is not a hospital, meaning that health should not be the all determining value in food choices. Food contributes to the values of society (a traditional food style) or to the conversation of mankind (a cosmopolitan style), and if food is only produced with a focus on health, or more specifically, with a focus on disease prevention, these other values will be lost [41]. The English Food Ethics Council views the exclusive orientation on health in food choices as a transformation of society into a hospital [42]. Seen from this perspective, it is no wonder that government campaigns to stop people (in particular adherents of traditional, natural, and cosmopolitan food styles) from living according to so-called unhealthy life styles are without avail [43,44].

The remark of the Food Ethics Council, however, does not exclude that for people that are diagnosed for a certain illness, are advised to look for a dietician, and do not feel healthy, nutrigenomics can play a (potentially large) role. In (pre)clinical treatments, the relation between diet and health (the subject matter of nutrigenomics) becomes progressively more urgent and potent [45].

Nutrigenomics may conflict with food styles by emphasizing the paramountcy of food as a means to achieve prevention of diseases. The conclusion is that there is a considerable mismatch between most of the concepts of food and health of current lifestyles and those of nutrigenomics. The mismatch between the normative concepts of nutrigenomics and those of various food styles cannot be corrected by producing information or new products, or more generally, by a one-sided informative offensive from the side of nutrigenomics and nutrigenomics-inspired innovation networks [43]. The concepts of food and health in (health and) not-health-dominated food styles are normative choices that are predominantly not based on information but on views of life. A more feasible innovation trajectory could include the uptake of alternative normative conceptualizations of food and health by nutrigenomics innovation networks and thereby to take more into account the complicated web of responsibilities with respect to the relationship between food and health.

SELLING SCIENCE TO SOCIETY: FROM RESEARCH TO MARKETING

The contrast between sets of norms and values becomes clear when scientific insights are to be marketed to the general public. After all, nutritional innovation, or food innovation, is about much more than establishing a proof-of-principle for any given health effect.

Food innovation and marketing strategies are not processes that will have to be invented anew, now that nutrigenomics is moving toward the market more and more. Existing functional foods—one of the potential outcomes for nutrigenomic innovation trajectories—the science that supports them, the regulatory bounds that govern them, and the marketing practices that assist in selling them, present a number of lessons for each and every attempt to produce and sell nutrigenomic foods. That is, provided existing proofs-of-principle can indeed be successfully up-scaled in terms of production (materially, economically, and logistically) and in terms of marketing (identifying audiences and issues) to cover a potential market share, which is interesting enough to cater to.

Two main observations can be drawn from literature on the history of dietetics and the context of food innovation. First, scientific claims and claims that carry meaning to potential consumers vary greatly in their content, form, medium for communication, and style of presentation [46]. Secondly, if claims accompanying novel foods exclusively focus on health and health effects, all potential consumers save those adhering to one food style (see section on "Normative Matching Of Nutrigenomic Research And Society") may be alienated [47].

Let us first turn to the presentation of claims to peers and public. Claiming a health effect and establishing that claim as probably, credible, valid, and/or true among scientific peers mean taking a route we are all quite familiar with: designing an experiment, generating data, building arguments, writing papers, having those papers reviewed and published, and allowing one's peers to continue assessing the data and arguments contained in those papers and the health claims such evidence is associated with. Whether that claim is *this food product normalizes gut activity for Crohn's disease patients* or *this food product will lower you risk for heart disease*, although addressed to totally different types of end users, the procedure for getting there is the same: validity, credibility, and truth are built through academic conventions such as peer review, methodological scrutiny, and above all else, a shared notion of proper science [48]. They are part and parcel of a scientists' repertoire, and the mobilization of each of them will help (firmly) establish a claim and a reputation [24,49,50].

For health claims to be perceived as relevant, significant, and valid in the public domain, they need to align themselves with a need or a demand. Issues in nutrition science can be "high cholesterol," "high blood pressure," or an inability to get up the stairs as a result of being obese. They tend not to include raised inflammatory biomarkers or other molecular claims because they are inaccessible to bodily, personal, or shared experience. Such issues will or will not easily align with a specific audience. The diversity of food styles we discussed in section "Normative Matching Of Nutrigenomic Research And Society" already showed that "health" as a general central issue will align with the priorities of few, while remaining on the background for most others. Furthermore, health has a distinct and different form of appearance in the public domain: free of molecular indicators and full of experiential indicators—what I can or cannot *do*, what I do, or do not *like* and what does or does not *agree* with me.

Issues do not only exist in the abstract—they come with a public [51]. The "issue" high cholesterol is accompanied by an audience that subscribes to this issue, people who care or worry about their cholesterol. This may be because they have had a medical diagnosis, or because others in their vicinity, in whom they recognize their own lifestyle, have had *cholesterol issues*. This recognition is called "metaphorical extension" and it encompasses the real and the virtual. Just like people can relate to their neighbors, they can also relate to virtual characters, for instance, in food commercials. Two key elements that distinguish scientific dissemination from metaphorical extension are, first, the contrast between universal and particular claims and, second, the willingness to openly articulate values.

Science speaks to abstract bodies in potential situations, whereas metaphorical extension relates to you and me and our current situation. In many cases, the best possible science cannot create a sense of relevance among consumers, whereas a single marketing message can. The selection of issues, their articulation, presentation and the voice, medium, and strategy to communicate about them, and taking into account the context of the end user, ultimately contributes as much to the credibility of any nutritional claim as science at least [46]. In addition, the reason certain foods and certain lifestyles (and thus certain individuals readily available for metaphorical extension) resonate with people is because they openly display a set of norms and values they subscribe to: ease, pleasure, enjoyment, taste, texture, quality, and much more.* Health can but does not have to be one of them.

CONCLUSION

Whether in the form of nutritional advice, or in the form of food products, nutrigenomic expertise has a different status within the compounds of the scientific community or in (pre)clinical settings than in society at large. In the first two, the value of health is prioritized over all others. In the latter, as we have shown in preceding sections, the normative picture is significantly more diverse.

The question "is society ready for nutrigenomics?"—which we were asked to write about for this book is a question that makes sense only from the perspective of a scientocratic point of view. Its mirror image "is nutrigenomics ready for society?" is equally valid and perhaps even more valuable as a starting point for discussion. Only when both questions are considered simultaneously, it becomes evident that a normative mismatch exists between science and society and between nutrigenomics and the eating public. As we have shown, the differences between the societal views on health and food and those assumed by nutrigenomics are considerable; they are currently not a happy match, at least outside the (pre)clinical context.

A usual strategy in such a case of misalignment is to mobilize resources for implementing the aspects necessary for accepting the foodstuffs and services that are associated with the molecular, personal, and manageable food style of nutrigenomics. This was Pasteur's strategy of implementation in the nineteenth century

* Ferguson and Schlothauer [55] conclude that marketing broccoli as a cancer-preventative food to healthy consumers is difficult to nearly impossible. We are not that pessimistic. Since health claims are often not the defining element in consumer choice [see, e.g., Refs 56,57], marketing broccoli as cancer-preventative may be hard, but aligning this particular vegetable to other prominent issues may very well be possible. Although it is not the most important value guiding consumer choice, health is part of the normative package [58,59]. Thus, to support cancer prevention, selling broccoli ought to be about something else than cancer prevention.

[52]. However, the social situation is currently fundamentally different from the nineteenth century, and parts of the lay public are much more knowledgeable. The relationship between science and society has changed. Indeed, "In modern times, science has always spoken to society … But society now speaks back" [53]. Both partners will have to take each other seriously. From the societal end (consumers, citizens, and representatives of both), one ought to invite a careful consideration of the innovation trajectories nutrigenomic scientists and research programs are embarking upon. From the scientific end, one ought to expect a serious effort to implement knowledge about their respective end users into the research programs that are developed (ask questions considered relevant not only for their scientific merit but also for social merit) and the ways in which they are organized—for instance, through the active inclusion of consumer panels (not just for show). Increasingly, such initiatives are taken. Consider, for instance, the EU Food4Me project, which was launched in early 2011. It includes consultations of nearly 8000 consumers about the topic of personalized nutrition, to develop novel business models to implement personalization (or to work toward a functional metaphorical extension, see section on "Selling science to society: From research to marketing").

The January 2012 NuGO newsletter opened with the statement that "Mechanistic research, genetics and transcriptomics, metabolomics and epigenetics are now routine in nutrition." In order for each of those to add to a body of nutritional knowledge that can be mobilized for the benefit of society at large, we would like to add broader consultation of the general public to the list. While most people may be very bad at self-reporting their nutritional intake [54], it is with great ease and detail that they can express their preferences.

These preferences are not, nor will they ever be, stable. The ratios of people adhering to certain food styles will change as the result of social, demographic, and cultural trends. They may shift the normative orientation of society toward the position nutrigenomic research agendas currently occupy. Until then, nutrigenomic researchers and nutrition researchers in general can start harvesting the potential contained in the normative preferences of all of us.

REFERENCES

1. Fredericks, P.J. and E.W. MacLaughlin, *New Product Procurement: A Summary of Buying Practices and Acceptance Criteria at U.S. Supermarket Chains* 1992, Ithaca, New York: Cornell University, Department of Agricultural Economics, College of Agriculture & Life Sciences.
2. Enzing, C.M. et al., Where innovation processes make a difference in products' short- and long-term market success. *British Food Journal*, 2011. 113(7): pp. 812–837.
3. Enserink, M., Tough lessons from golden rice. *Science*, 2008. 320: pp. 468–471.
4. Beyer, P., Golden rice and "golden" crops for human nutrition. *New Biotechnology*, 2010. 27(5): pp. 478–581.
5. Grünes, D., Why golden rice failed. Intellectual property and credibility in innovation, in *Governance of Health Care Innovation. Excursions into Politics, Science & Citizenship*, K. Horstman, E. Dow, and B. Penders, Editors. 2011, Lulu Academic: Raleigh, NC.
6. Mutch, D.M., W. Wahli, and G. Williamson, Nutrigenomics and nutrigenetics: the emerging faces of nutrition. *FASEB Journal*, 2005. 19: pp. 1602–1616.

7. Kaput, J., Nutrigenomics research for personalized nutrition and medicine. *Current Opinion in Biotechnology*, 2008. 19(2): pp. 110–120.
8. van Ommen, B., Nutrigenomics: exploiting systems biology in the nutrition and health arena. *Nutrition*, 2004. 20(1): pp. 4–8.
9. Müller, M. and S. Kersten, Nutrigenomics: goals and strategies. *Nature Reviews Genetics*, 2003. 4(4): pp. 315–322.
10. Mead, M.N., Nutrigenomics: the genomics-food interface. *Environmental Health Perspectives*, 2007. 115(12): pp. A582–A589.
11. Parker, J.N., N. Vermeulen, and B. Penders, eds. *Collaboration in the New Life Sciences* 2010, Farnham, UK: Ashgate.
12. Vermeulen, N., *Supersizing Science. On Building Large-Scale Research Projects in Biology* 2009, Maastricht: Maastricht University Press.
13. Penders, B., *The Diversification of Health. Politics of Large-Scale Cooperation in Nutrition Science* 2010, Bielefeld (D): Transcript Verlag.
14. Penders, B. and J. Goven, Nutrigenomics and the stewardship of scientific promises. *Biotechnology Journal*, 2010. 5(9): pp. 909–912.
15. NuGO, European nutrigenomics organisation: linking genomics, nutrition and health research, in *Network of Excellence Proposal*, 2003. p. 133. http://cordis.europa.eu/search/index.cfm?fuseaction=proj.document&PJ_RCN=7518508.
16. Bergmann, M. et al., Bioethics in human nutrigenomics research: European Nutrigenomics Organisation workshop report. *British Journal of Nutrition*, 2006. 95: pp. 1024–1027.
17. Shrum, W.M., J. Genuth, and I. Chompalov, *Structures of Scientific Collaboration* 2007, Cambridge MA: MIT Press.
18. Parker, J.N., Integrating the social into the ecological: organisational and research group challenges, in *Collaboration in the New Life Sciences*, J.N. Parker, N. Vermeulen, and B. Penders, Editors. 2010, Ashgate: Farnham, UK. pp. 85–110.
19. Calvert, J., Systems biology, interdisciplinarity and disciplinary identity, in *Collaboration in the New Life Sciences*, J.N. Parker, N. Vermeulen, and B. Penders, Editors. 2010, Ashgate: Farnham, UK. pp. 201–218.
20. Afman, L.A. and M. Müller, Human nutrigenomics of gene regulation by dietary fatty acids. *Progress in Lipid Research*, 2012. 51(1): pp. 63–70.
21. Fujimura, J.H., Constructing "do-able" problems in cancer research: articulating alignment. *Social Studies of Science*, 1987. 17: pp. 257–293.
22. Fujimura, J.H., *Crafting Science: A Sociohistory of the Quest for the Genetics of Cancer* 1996, Cambridge, MA: Harvard University Press. p. 322.
23. Penders, B., K. Horstman, and R. Vos, Large-scale research and the goal of health: an analysis of doable problem construction in "new" nutrition science. *Interdisciplinary Science Reviews*, 2009. 34(4): pp. 332–349.
24. Latour, B. and S. Woolgar, *Laboratory Life: The Construction of Scientific Facts* 1986 [1979], Princeton: Princeton University Press. p. 294.
25. Penders, B., R. Vos, and K. Horstman, Side effects of problem-solving strategies in large-scale nutrition science: towards a diversification of health. *British Journal of Nutrition*, 2009. 102(10): pp. 1400–1403.
26. Brown, N., Hope against hype—accountability in biopasts, presents and futures. *Science Studies*, 2003. 16(2): pp. 3–21.
27. Brown, N., B. Rappert, and A. Webster, eds. *Contested Futures* 2000, Aldershot: Ashgate. p. 277.
28. van Lente, H., *Promising Technology. The Dynamics of Expectations in Technological Developments* 1993, Delft: Eburon.

29. van Lente, H., Forceful futures: from promise to requirement, in *Contested Futures. A Sociology of Prospective Techno-Science*, N. Brown, B. Rappert, and A. Webster, Editors. 2000, Ashgate: London. pp. 43–64.
30. Expert Group on Science and Governance, *Taking European Knowledge Society Seriously. Report of the Expert Group on Science and Governance to the Science, Economy and Society Directorate, Directorate-General for Research; European Commission*, 2007, Office for Official Publications of the European Communities #291: Luxembourg.
31. Goven, J. and J.A. Heinemann, *Nutrigenomics and Public Engagement: An "Upstream" Inquiry*, Constructive Conversations/Korero Whakaaetanga Research Report. No. 17, Foundation for Research, Science and Technology, 2008, Wellington, New Zealand.
32. Penders, B. et al., From individuals to groups: a review of the meaning of "personalized" in nutrigenomics. *Trends in Food Science & Technology*, 2007. 18(6): pp. 333–338.
33. Bauer, S., Nutrigenomik: Technowissenschaftliches fine-tuning von nahrung und körper, in *Essen in Europa* [*Nutrigenomics: Technoscientific fine tuning of food and body*]. *Kulturelle Rückstände in Nahrung und Körper* [*Eating in Europe. Cultural Remnants in Food and Body*], S. Bauer et al., Editors. 2010, Transcript Verlag: Bielefeld (D).
34. Komduur, R., M. Korthals, and H. Te Molder, The good life: living for health and a life without risks? On a prominent script of nutrigenomics. *British Journal of Nutrition*, 2009. 101: pp. 307–316.
35. Douglas, M., *Natural Symbols* 1970, London: Barrie & Rockliff.
36. Rozin, P. et al., Attitudes to food and the role of food in life in the U.S.A., Japan, Flemish Belgium and France: possible implications for the diet-health debate. *Appetite*, 1999. 33: pp. 163–180.
37. Schulze, G., *Die Erlebnisgesellschaft. Kultursoziologie der Gegenwart* [*The Experiential Society: A Cultural Sociology of the Present*] 1992, Frankfurt: Campus.
38. Pollan, M., *The Omnivore's Dilemma: A Natural History of Four Meals* 2006, London: Bloomsbury.
39. Singer, P. and J. Mason, *The Way we Eat* 2006, London: Penguin.
40. Petrini, C., *The Pleasures of Slow Food: Celebrating Authentic Traditions, Flavors and Recipes* 2002, San Francisco: Chronicle Books.
41. Korthals, M., *Before Dinner: Philosophy and Ethics of Food* 2004, Dordrecht: Springer. p. 215.
42. Food Ethics Council, *Getting Personal: Shifting Responsibilities for Dietary Health* 2005, Brighton: Food Ethics Council.
43. Brunso, K., Development and testing of a cross-culturally valid instrument: food-related life style. *Consumer Research*, 1995. 22: pp. 475–480.
44. Korthals, M., Co-evolution of nutrigenomics and society: ethical considerations. *American Journal of Clinical Nutrition*, 2011. 94(6): pp. 2025S–2029S.
45. DeBusk, R., V.S. Sierpina, and M.J. Kreitzer, Applying functional nutrition for chronic disease prevention and management: bridging nutrition and functional medicine in 21st century healthcare. *Explore (New York, N.Y.)*, 2011. 7(1): pp. 55–57.
46. Penders, B. and A.P. Nelis, Credibility engineering in the food industry. Linking science, regulation and marketing in a corporate context. *Science in Context*, 2011. 29(4): pp. 487–515.
47. Menrad, K., Market and marketing of functional food in Europe. *Journal of Food Engineering*, 2003. 56: pp. 181–188.
48. Penders, B., K. Horstman, and R. Vos, Proper science in moist biology. *EMBO Reports*, 2007. 8(7): p. 613.
49. Latour, B., *Science in Action: How to Follow Scientists and Engineers through Society?* 1987, Cambridge, MA: Harvard University Press.

50. Hessels, L. and H. van Lente, Practical applications as a source of credibility: a comparison of three fields of Dutch academic chemistry. *Minerva*, 2011. 49: pp. 215–240.
51. Marres, N., The issues deserve more credit: pragmatist contributions to the study of public involvement in controversy. *Social Studies of Science*, 2007. 37: pp. 759–780.
52. Latour, B., *The Pasteurization of France* 1988, Cambridge, MA: President and Fellows of Harvard College. p. 273.
53. Nowotny, H., P. Scott, and M. Gibbons, *Re-thinking Science. Knowledge and the Public in an Age of Uncertainty* 2001, Oxford: Blackwell. p. 278.
54. Schaefer, E.J. et al., Lack of efficacy of a food-frequency questionnaire in assessing dietary macronutrient intakes in subjects consuming diets of known composition. *The American Journal of Clinical Nutrition*, 2000. 71(3): pp. 746–751.
55. Ferguson, L.R. and R.C. Schlothauer, The potential role of nutritional genomics tools in validating high health foods for cancer control: Broccoli as example. *Molecular Nutrition & Food Research*, 2012. 56(1): pp. 126–146.
56. Jaeger, S.R. et al., The food choice kaleidoscope. A framework for structured description of product, place and person as sources of variation in food choices. *Appetite*, 2011. 56(2): pp. 412–423.
57. Garretson, J.A. and S. Burton, Effects of nutrition facts panel values, nutrition claims, and health claims on consumer attitudes, perceptions of disease-related risks, and trust. *Journal of Public Policy & Marketing*, 2000. 19(2): pp. 213–227.
58. Roe, B., A.S. Levy, and B.M. Derby, The impact of health claims on consumer search and product evaluation outcomes: results from FDA experimental data. *Journal of Public Policy & Marketing*, 1999. 18(1): pp. 89–105.
59. Kozup, J.C., E.H. Creyer, and S. Burton, Making healthful food choices: the influence of health claims and nutrition information on consumers' evaluations of packaged food products and restaurant menu items. *The Journal of Marketing*, 2003. 67(2): pp. 19–34.

20 Public Health Context for Nutrigenomics and Personalized Nutrition

Elizabeth H. Marchlewicz, Karen E. Peterson, and Gilbert S. Omenn

CONTENTS

INTRODUCTION

Imagine that you arrive home to have dinner with your family and, instead of sharing common food dishes, each family member eats specific foods they have been advised to consume based on their individual genotypes to decrease their disease risks. Current food choices and decisions are uninformed regarding nutrigenetics and nutrigenomics; they may be based on individuals' food preferences, intolerances, allergies, or dietary guidelines to promote health and reduce risk of common conditions such as obesity, type 2 diabetes mellitus (T2DM), kidney disease, cardiovascular disease (CVD), and some cancers. In the future, nutritional genomics testing could make it possible for individuals to have dietary recommendations tailored both to their genotypes and to the environments where they live, work, and play. Despite the potential public health significance of reducing individuals' and population risk of nutrition-related diseases, this scenario also stimulates questions such as: How will school and work cafeterias provide daily access to foods that people of all genotypes will be able to consume? How will multiple health care providers ensure a unified set of recommendations based on nutritional genomics testing? How much of a difference will eating these recommended foods make on individual and population health?

This chapter addresses the integration of nutrigenomics into public health practice, providing background context, presenting benefits and challenges, reviewing current applications, and suggesting factors to consider before implementation. Nutrigenomics builds on a legacy of nutrition promotion in public health, long recognized for the health and societal benefits adequate nutrition provides. These benefits arose from evolutionary adaptations: interactions between individuals' genomes and their differing environments result in genomic variability between human subgroups. Understanding genomic variation benefits public health by increasing prediction power for disease risk in individuals and subgroups. Nutrigenomics can also be used to add a layer of mechanistic understanding to exposure and disease associations observed in epidemiologic studies. Methodological challenges with nutrigenomics research still exist; these challenges must be carefully contemplated to assess the quality of data and strength of evidence available to recommend the potential use of nutrigenomics in public health.

Current evidence supports nutrigenomics as a promising predictive tool for determining disease propensity and the potential to improve preventive and therapeutic interventions, thereby increasing health and quality of life of the general public. Implementation of nutrigenomics in public health practice should occur gradually, beginning in clinical, high-risk populations with well-characterized genome polymorphisms and disease phenotypes. As deeper knowledge of polymorphisms and their potential interactions accumulates, nutrigenomics will likely be applied to increasing numbers of health conditions across population subgroups.

PUBLIC HEALTH PERSPECTIVE

Nutrition has been recognized as a critical component of public health for centuries. Discoveries of essential nutrients near the start of the twentieth century spurred recognition of the societal benefit of healthy diets [1]. New knowledge of nutrient requirements informed the composition of World War II rations in Europe and the

United States [2] and supported the creation of the U.S. Recommended Dietary Allowances [3]. The Food and Agriculture Organization of the United Nations was established on the understanding that the public health impacts of nutrition extend beyond individuals' health to improved learning, greater physical capacity, and higher productivity [4,5]. Dietary guidelines frame the services provided by public health nutrition programs worldwide that aim to reduce food insecurity, increase diet quality, improve food safety, and prevent and manage nutritionally related diseases [6,7]. Emerging nutrigenomics research suggests that the same nutrient can affect individuals differently, based on their genotype and environmental context. Thus, public health nutrition guidelines may not confer equal benefit for individuals or population groups and could even increase disease risk. For example, the U.S. 2010 Dietary Guidelines for Americans recommended that adults consuming a 2000-calorie diet replace solid fat (saturated fatty acids [SFAs] and trans fatty acids [TFAs]) with 27 g of monounsaturated fatty acids (MUFAs) and polyunsaturated fatty acids (PUFAs) in the form of oils [7]. A polymorphism in *APOA1* gene encodes apolipoprotein A-1, a major protein component of high-density lipoprotein (HDL) in plasma. A high-PUFA diet benefits individuals with an A allele at the -75 G/A polymorphism but not those homozygous for the more common G allele. GG homozygotes have decreased HDL cholesterol (HDL-C) levels with higher PUFA intake [8], a risk not addressed in the guidelines. In contrast, nutrigenomics research did support a reevaluation of the recommendation of a low-fat, low-cholesterol diet to highlight its benefit specific to people with the apoE4 allele at the *APOE* gene [8].

EVOLUTIONARY CONTEXT

Human genetic variation (HGV) across different geographic locations is influenced by gene-specific (natural selection, mutation rates, and recombination) and demographic (population size, structure, founder effect, and admixtures) factors [9]. Ancient polymorphisms, shared by all human populations, account for approximately 90% of HGV [10], but new alleles arise at an estimated rate of 175 per diploid human genome per generation [11]. African populations, largely stable over the past 200,000 years, have comparatively more genetic variation than European and Asian populations, likely due to the greater linkage disequilibrium encountered by populations migrating out of Africa 50,000–60,000 years ago [10,12]. The environmental challenges of adaptation to new climates and resources for these populations likely caused populations to plummet, resulting in a significant reduction in genetic variation.

Research on HGV reveals how human populations are biologically related and how disease-risk allele frequency (AF) and variant location differs among people from disparate geographic regions. Population-specific HGV is crucial to understanding genetic components of disease, gene–nutrient, and gene–environment interactions to effectively address disease susceptibility. Mutations causing deleterious effects, especially on fertility, are infrequently transmitted to subsequent generations [10]. Some common genetic variants contribute to diseases, such as sickle cell anemia, thalassemias, autoimmune disorders, and Alzheimer's disease. Persistence of these common alleles reflects evolutionary forces that may have protected against geographic-associated infections, overcoming any reduction in reproductive fitness.

Environmental and cultural factors influence the dietary intake of human populations; these differences in turn have influenced HGV. Archeological evidence suggests that early human populations in the tropics consumed a largely plant-based diet, while humans migrating to temperate climates introduced more animal products into their diets [13]. With the development of agriculture and animal husbandry practices beginning about 10,000 years ago in the Middle East, food security and caloric density of diets increased, fueling exponential population growth and selecting for numerous new alleles. Since many human populations were already geographically separated, this resulted in population-specific HGV [10,13]. Understanding and characterizing these variations may explain differences in disease susceptibility, prevalence, and response to diet between individuals and populations.

Lactose tolerance is a well-studied phenotype resulting from genetic variants across human populations. The introduction of animal milk to the diets of people who domesticated animals around 6000 years ago was associated with the persistence of lactose tolerance after weaning and into adulthood, based on continued expression of the intestinal lactase enzyme for digestion [14,15]. Prevalence of the gene *LAC1* varies based on societal and historical dietary practices of different population groups and occurs in 90% of Northern Europeans; 50% of Middle Easterners, Mediterranean, and pastoral groups in Africa; <20% among many East Asian and sub-Saharan African peoples; and <5% of Native Americans [16]. Another example of dietary intake impacting gene expression is the difference in copy number variation (CNV) of the salivary amylase gene, *AMY1*. Starch consumption is greater in agricultural and arid hunter-gatherer societies than among rainforest and circumarctic hunter-gatherers and some pastoralists. Asian and African populations comprise both high and low starch consumption groups [17], suggesting that diet more strongly predicts *AMY1* CNV than geographic proximity. In addition to a greater efficiency of starch digestion, greater *AMY1* CNV may confer evolutionary advantage, protecting against intestinal diseases such as diarrhea [17].

Dramatic dietary changes over the past 200 years have strained human metabolism, which is based on a "stone-age" genome [18]. Humans evolved to have large stomachs, long small intestines, and enormous livers to digest and absorb very low-fat, high-fiber foods [18]. The "nutrition transition" worldwide is characterized by increased consumption of cereal grains, refined sugars, alcoholic beverages, dairy products, mammalian red meat, salt, and refined vegetable oils [19]. These changes have shifted the nutritional qualities of human diets: macronutrient composition, micronutrient density, fatty acid composition, glycemic load, fiber content, acid–base balance, and sodium–potassium ratio [20,21]. Adaptations to the metabolic stress of secular changes in diet can be related in part to increased prevalence of many chronic diseases including obesity, T2DM, metabolic syndrome (MetS), atherosclerosis, dyslipidemias, high blood pressure, bowel disorders, osteoporosis, inflammatory and autoimmune disorders, and certain types of cancers [15,16,20,21].

Leptin receptor (*LEPR*) polymorphisms are one example of the body's attempt to metabolically adapt to this new food environment. In the LIPGENE-SU.VI.MAX study of adults with MetS and matched controls, GG homozygotes at *LEPR* rs3790433 had an increased risk of MetS, compared to carriers of the minor A allele, with odds ratio (OR) of 1.65 [22]. GG homozygotes also had increased risk of elevated insulin concentrations (OR = 2.40) and insulin resistance (OR = 2.15) compared to carriers of the minor A allele [22]. The fact that the dominant allele predisposes to MetS, as well as elevated insulin concentrations and insulin resistance, suggests that efficient storage of excess calories was beneficial to ancestral humans. The minor A allele may be a more recent variant that has become an adaptive advantage in the current obesogenic environment.

Increased obesity rates are characteristic of countries' progress through the nutrition transition. The pace of adaptive genetic change is too slow to account for these trends, underscoring behavioral and environmental changes as fundamental drivers of the obesity epidemic. This is commonly illustrated by observing the impact of dietary and environmental change on two indigenous, genetically isolated populations: Western Pacific Islanders and Pima Indians. Western Pacific Islanders experienced a relatively long period of genetic isolation from other human populations until European explorers arrived in the sixteenth century and colonialism began in the eighteenth century. Pacific Islanders have the highest obesity rates in the world, with 70%–75% of the adult population obese. Unlike agricultural European populations, hunter-gatherer Western Pacific Islanders had few evolutionary pressures for genotypic adaptation to handle the increased fat content of an animal-based diet [23].

The Pima Indians of Northern Mexico and Arizona in the United States demonstrate the drastic impact that lifestyle and environment can play on genetically similar populations. Pimas living in the Sierra Madre Mountains of Northern Mexico continue to live by the subsistence practices of their ancestors, while Pimas in Arizona have rapidly westernized. Rates of obesity (7% men; 20% women) and T2DM (7% men and women) among Mexican Pimas are significantly lower than prevalence rates observed among American Pimas, with 38% T2DM, and obesity prevalence 10 times greater in men and three times greater in women. This stark contrast illustrates the extent to which phenotypic expression of genotype is tempered by the prevailing food environment and the extreme health consequences of rapid dietary change ahead of genetic adaptation [23–25].

Many aspects of obesity, diabetes, and CVDs, including genome-wide association studies (GWAS), are covered in Chapters 6 and 7 of this book.

BENEFITS OF NUTRIGENOMICS FOR PUBLIC HEALTH

Predictive Power of Nutrigenomics

The public health significance of nutrigenomic testing lies within its potential use as an early detection method to identify individual susceptibility and population subgroups propensities based on responses to various dietary components and genetic predisposition to a spectrum of diseases. This screening would affect clinical practice guidelines and would advance personalized medicine as the standard of care. Nutritional genomics could facilitate use of personalized nutrition as a preventive strategy to combat the rising tide of chronic and degenerative diseases. Nutrigenomics will also influence pharmaceutical therapy, by elucidating the underlying mechanisms of diet–drug interactions [26] and microbiome–metagenome interactions with diet. For example, a cross-sectional intervention study in 400 healthy Chinese adults found that *CYP3A5**3 and *MDR1* variants influenced the extent of cytochrome P450 inhibition by grapefruit juice [27]; knowing a patient's *CYP3A5**3 and *MDR1* genotypes could inform drug dosing. Nutritional advice could also be prescribed based on individual genetic test results.

GWAS and deep sequencing of RNA have revealed numerous genomic variants (usually not gene variants) for such phenotypes as blood glucose or cholesterol levels, blood pressure, height, body mass index, obesity, and diabetes types 1 and 2. However, even with up to 180 loci for height identified, the variants explain only about 10% of the variance for highly heritable traits [28]. Additional variants at a locus have been suggested as a partial explanation for this heritability [29]. However, it is certain that a large part of the "missing heritability" is due to nongenetic variables, especially diet, interacting with the genomic variants and gene regulatory phenomena [13,30,31]. Regulatory mechanisms may include promoters, enhancers, small RNAs, transposons, alternative splicing, epigenetics, and even endogenous retroviral sequences [16]. Such gene–environment interactions are counted toward heritability, h^2 = genetic component of the variance (G) + GxE, divided by total variance (including environmental/behavioral components) (E) [32]. The tremendous potential number of gene–nutrient interactions underscores the importance of having sufficient power to detect interaction terms in nutrigenetic and nutrigenomic analyses. Another potential layer of unexplained interaction includes nutrient–environment exposure interactions and the impact on genotypic expression. Some nutrients exert this therapeutic role through epigenetic modifications, namely, cytosine methylation in DNA and acetylation and methylation of histone proteins in chromosomes (see Chapter 12).

The role of epigenetics in personalized nutrition is discussed at length in Chapter 12. One example is shared here to illustrate the potential public health impact of epigenetic modification by nutrients. One-carbon metabolism nutrients, folate, vitamin B_{12}, vitamin B_6, riboflavin, methionine, choline, and betaine, can impact DNA methylation by regulating levels of methyl donors, S-adenosylmethionine and methyltransferase inhibitor S-adenosylhomocysteine. Methyl donors, such as folate, are necessary for establishing and maintaining DNA methylation. The developmental origins of health and disease theory suggests that altered epigenetic regulation of growth processes induced by periconceptional folic acid may contribute to both immediate effects and chronic disease associations later in life [33,34].

Folate has been demonstrated to be essential to fetal neural development since the 1980s [35]. The results of many randomized controlled trials (RCTs) prompted the current recommendation of 400 μg of folic acid per day through the first trimester of pregnancy [36]. Mandatory folic acid fortification of foods in many countries, including the United States and Canada, since 1998 has been a major public health success [37], with significantly decreased rates of neural tube defects, orofacial clefts, congenital heart defects, and diaphragmatic hernias [38–41]. Unfortunately, adverse effects of periconceptional folic acid use have also been reported, including an increased risk of pyloric stenosis, obstructive urinary tract defects, obesity, insulin resistance, colon cancer [38,42], and childhood asthma [43].

Folate's physiologic role as a methyl donor has created great interest in the health impacts of methyl tetrahydrofolate reductase (*MTHFR*) gene variants. Two common polymorphisms in the *MTHFR* gene, C677T and A1298C, reduce enzymatic activity.

In Early Life Exposure in Mexico to Environmental Toxicants, a longitudinal, birth cohort study, the maternal *MTHFR* C677T variant allele was associated with lower child cognitive development at 24 months of age. This suggests that maternal folate metabolism during pregnancy may program the child's neurodevelopmental trajectory [44]. *MTHFR* highlights the central role nutrients can play in moderating health impacts of environmental exposures. Epigenetic modifications impact physiologic adaptation from the prenatal period to old age, making personalized nutrition critical across the entire life course.

Addressing Epidemiologic Questions: Chemoprevention Trials

Nutrigenomics research can be a valuable tool in the exploration of the molecular mechanisms underlying diet and disease associations before testing in RCTs and potentially in explaining findings of RCTs. In the 1990s, reported inverse statistical associations of antioxidant vitamin intake with CVD mortality in large U.S. and European cohorts were not confirmed in RCT of supplements [45–49]. One of the most striking examples is the beta-Carotene and Retinol Efficacy Trial (CARET), in which 30 mg beta-carotene and 25,000 IU retinyl palmitate were given to adult men and women at high risk for lung cancer, smokers, former smokers, and asbestos-exposed workers. CARET was terminated before the scheduled completion due to compelling evidence that the participants in the active treatment arm of the trial had higher incidence of lung cancers and increased mortality from lung cancer, CVD, and all causes [50], an effect that persisted 5 years, after stopping the vitamins [51]. The CARET results confirmed similar findings in male smokers in Finland in the Alpha-Tocopherol, Beta-Carotene Trial [52]. The CARET results also stimulated laboratory research showing multiple mechanisms for carcinogenic action of these chemical agents [53].

Recent nutrigenomics studies on the interindividual variability in carotenoid absorption, metabolism, and status may provide insight into the unexpected health risk, heterogeneity of response to chemoprevention agents, and subsequent dilution of any beneficial effects observed in CARET. Retinoids are potent metabolic and signaling regulators, influencing at least 500 genes [54]. Beta-carotene absorption and conversion into retinal is extremely variable among individuals; recently, genetic variants in scavenger receptor class B type I, associated with beta-carotene influx and efflux in intestinal enterocytes, have been implicated in the heterogeneity of beta-carotene status [55]. Two common nonsynonymous SNPs within the beta-carotene 15,15'-monoxygenase 1 gene coding region were shown to have reduced catalytic activity and contribute to the low responder phenotype with four additional SNPs upstream also affecting carotenoid concentrations and beta-carotene conversion efficiency; frequencies varied across ethnic groups [56]. Additional variants have been reported by Borel et al. [57,58], Herberth et al. [59], and Mondul et al. [60].

Similar to the beta-carotene/retinoid results for lung cancer, a major chemoprevention trial of selenium plus vitamin E to reduce the incidence of prostate cancer (SELECT) not only failed to show any benefit but also showed adverse effects, with a statistically greater incidence of prostate cancers in healthy men [61].

Mendelian randomization, a technique for indirectly studying the relationship between a biomarker and disease by investigating the relationship of the biomarker and disease to a gene that influences the biomarker of interest, can be used in observational studies to more accurately predict the relationship between exposure and disease risk [31,32]. The genotype becomes an instrumental variable, with the null hypothesis that the gene has no effect on the disease independent of this instrumental phenotype. Identifying the likely causal path of a genetic variant on disease risk or the impact of an environmental exposure on gene regulation can facilitate the development and testing of targeted preventive or therapeutic interventions. When large numbers of genes are deployed in a molecular signature, special attention must be paid to avoid overfitting and to validate the test assay for specific clinical uses [62].

Results with the Mendelian randomization method have caused quite a controversy about the long-standing recognition of HDL-C as "good cholesterol" from observational epidemiology. Voight et al. [63] found no reduction in cardiovascular mortality associated with alleles causing higher HDL-C, while the method did confirm the adverse effects of high low-density lipoprotein cholesterol (LDL-C) [63]. Individuals with the 396Ser allele in the endothelial lipase gene, *LIPG*, had slightly higher HDL-C levels than noncarriers; however, this HDL-C increase was not associated with decreased risk of heart attack as expected based on epidemiologic studies. The authors concluded that HDL-C may serve as a biomarker for multiple physiological processes and that all genetic mechanisms that increase HDL-C cannot be expected to lower risk of heart attack [63]. This study demonstrates the need for greater understanding of the factors that influence HDL-C to improve and tailor cardiovascular therapeutics.

APPLICATIONS OF NUTRIGENOMICS

The GWAS era identified thousands of genetic variants that are potentially associated with altered risk for common diseases. Mechanistic studies linking genetic and genomic variants to biomarkers or physiological processes known to relate to the disease of interest are now under way to test these potential associations. After identifying a mechanistic link between variants and disease intermediates, human intervention trials are necessary to assess whether nutrigenomic therapies targeting these variants or pathways can reduce the increased risk of disease in selected populations. The epidemiologic/nutritional transition has increased the need for public health efforts to combat health care-intensive, chronic, and degenerative diseases in geographic locations where these conditions were not common as recently as one decade ago.

Developing countries already bear the burden of 80% of deaths worldwide due to CVD and diabetes. Within high-income countries, differences in disease risk and prevalence are common between subgroups of the population. Although cultural norms and values, educational attainment, socioeconomic status, and access to health care influence these health disparities, differences in genetic susceptibility form a foundation on which the environmental factors interact to cause or prevent disease.

Section III discusses the potential to characterize and modify multiple disease risks, such as CVD (Chapter 6), obesity and diabetes (Chapter 7), and inflammatory bowel diseases (Chapter 8). Here we highlight applications of nutrigenomics to two additional diseases with high global prevalence and public health concern: colon cancer and nonalcoholic fatty liver disease (NAFLD).

Colorectal Cancer

With a lifetime risk of developing colorectal cancer (CRC) of 5% (1 in 20), CRC is the third most common cancer diagnosed and the third leading cause of cancer deaths in both men and women in the United States. Dysregulation of energy homeostasis is associated with CRC risk and research in five Asian countries suggests that CRC mortality increases within a decade of the nutrition transition [64]. Many potential mechanistic pathways are being investigated, including body weight, circulating fatty acid levels and composition, serum insulin, and glucose levels, thus making it a good early target for nutrigenomic interventions. Current dietary recommendations to decrease risk of CRC include decreasing consumption of red and processed meats, not cooking meats at very high temperatures, and increasing fruit, vegetable, and whole grain intake. However, these recommendations are not equally effective for all individuals with CRC, depending on their genotype.

Mendelian randomization investigation methods have been employed in the study of the genetic basis for CRC. Many SNPs within *LIPC* are associated with changes in serum lipid levels, and increased circulating LDL and decreased HDL levels are linked to increased CRC risk. This suggests that genetic polymorphisms in genes controlling serum lipids may also directly impact CRC risk and that serum lipid levels can serve as an intermediary biomarker. Certain SNPs in *LIPC* were associated with increased CRC risk in the case–control Molecular Epidemiology of Colorectal Cancer study conducted in Israel. The G allele of *LIPC* rs9652472 was associated with increased risk of CRC, with a per-allele OR of 1.52. Structural equation modeling identified the relationships between *LIPC* rs9652472 to serum lipid levels and lipid levels to CRC risk to be direct effects, with the impact of dietary fat, energy intake, and BMI acting indirectly as modifiers of these associations [65].

A recent meta-analysis of epidemiologic studies investigating the relationship between 25(OH)D, a vitamin D metabolite, and CRC risk found adults with 25(OH)D concentrations ≥33 ng/mL had a 50% lower incidence of CRC than those with 25(OH)D ≤ 12 ng/mL. This suggests that consuming 1000–2000 IU/day of vitamin D_3 could reduce CRC incidence with low risk of toxicity [66]. Recent genotyping efforts of the vitamin D receptor (VDR) may explain this relationship. Variation in length of the coding region in the *Fok*I gene impacts VDR function, with the shorter form being more biologically active. Individuals with the *ff* genotype have lower serum 25(OH)D concentrations than those with FF genotype. Although no direct relationship between VDR *Fok*I genotype and CRC risk has been observed, lifestyle factors may mediate the relationship. A large case–control study found the *ff* genotype was associated with double the CRC risk (OR = 2.62) for obese individuals and triple the CRC risk (OR = 3.46) among individuals who are not physically active [67].

A smaller, case–control study among *ff* genotype Singapore Chinese adults found that individuals with calcium or fat intake below the median values of controls had about 2.5 times the risk of CRC compared to *FF* genotype individuals. VDR polymorphism did not impact CRC risk in individuals with fat or calcium intake above the mean. The mechanism for this difference is not well described, but it has been suggested that higher fat or calcium intakes are able to compensate for the decreased bioactivity of VDR in *ff* genotype individuals [68]. Caution should be exercised when applying these findings to all populations, due to significant ethnic variation in the occurrence of polymorphisms at the *VDR* gene locus. The *f* AF in *Fok*I, dependent on ancestry, is 51% in Asians, 34% in Europeans, and 24% in Africans [69].

Nonalcoholic Fatty Liver Disease

NAFLD encompasses a range of conditions from simple fat deposition (hepatic steatosis) to inflammation around the fat (steatohepatitis) and scarring of liver tissue (cirrhosis). NAFLD progresses to the development of liver failure in some individuals. The increasing trend of obesity worldwide, resulting from the impacts of the nutrition transition on evolutionarily unprepared genomes, correlates with increased fat deposits in the liver. Few data exist on the incidence of NAFLD, but one population-based cohort study, the Dallas Heart Study, found one in three adults in an ethnically diverse U.S. population had steatosis [70]. Prevalence among children is less documented, but some data suggests that 9% of children have NAFLD, increasing to 38% among obese children [71]. This trend is very concerning due to the increasing rates of overweight and obesity among children and adults worldwide. If these preliminary prevalence figures are accurate, it would seem that NAFLD develops in concert with obesity, affecting a large percentage of the population worldwide.

Genetic differences may be responsible for the fact that not all obese individuals develop NAFLD. An extensive meta-analysis of multiple population–based studies, including 7176 participants, identified SNPs related to NAFLD near five gene loci: *NCAN*, *GCKR*, *LYPLAL1*, *PNPLA3*, and *PPP1R3B*. Genotyping in almost 600 subjects with biopsy-proven NAFLD from the NASH Clinical Research Network identified two variants from the original meta-analysis that were also significantly associated with histologic NAFLD: rs738409 in *PNPLA3* (OR = 3.26) and rs2228603 in *NCAN* (OR = 1.65). Epidemiologic studies of NAFLD have shown an association between hepatic fat deposition and central obesity, higher LDL, lower HDL, impaired fasting glucose, and increased insulin resistance. However, this meta-analysis found the alleles associated with hepatic steatosis to have the following effects at each loci: *NCAN* was also associated with lower triglycerides and plasma LDL levels; *GCKR* was associated with higher plasma LDL and triglyceride, lower fasting insulin, and increased 2-hour glucose; *PPP1R3B* was associated with increased HDL-C and LDL-C and decreased fasting glucose [72].

Investigation into the genomic components of NAFLD is relatively new; most current research focuses on potential genomics through in vitro and animal models that will be used to inform future human studies. Recent animal studies are working to elucidate the metabolic mechanism by which some *PNPLA3* polymorphisms increase the risk of hepatic steatosis. *PNPLA3* encodes the enzyme palatin-like phospholipase domain-containing protein 3 (PNPLA3), which has nonspecific lipid acyl hydrolase activity. PNPLA3 levels are low in the adipose tissue of fasted mice, but levels rapidly increase in adipose and liver tissue with refeeding a high carbohydrate diet. Insulin appears to partially mediate the increase in PNPLA3 during refeeding, and PNPLA3 mRNA levels are elevated in insulin-resistant, obese murine models (*ob/ob* mice and *fa/fa* rats).

In addition to the nutritional regulation at the transcriptional level through insulin-stimulated upregulation, in vitro studies suggest posttranslational regulation of PNPLA3 by fatty acids occurs in the liver. PNPLA3 levels increased in cultured hepatocytes after the addition of SFAs (palmitate), MUFAs (oleate), and PUFAs (linoleic acid) but not very long chain PUFAs (arachidonic acid and eicosapentaenoic acid). Inhibition of degradation of PNPLA3 by oleate in vitro suggests this as the mechanism for elevated PNPLA3 levels in the presence of these selected fatty acids [73]. In vitro studies on HepG2 cells and Chinese hamster ovary (CHO) cell lines found *PNPLA3* promoter activity was upregulated by 4.7-fold in HepG2 cells and 2-fold in CHO cells when cultured in 25 mM glucose. In CHO cells expressing human insulin receptor (CHO-IR), the increase in *PNPLA3* promoter activity was concentration dependent by insulin in the presence of glucose [74]. These in vitro results support the potential for nutritional regulation of PNPLA3 expression and its upregulation through obesity in NAFLD in humans. *PNPLA3* gene expression was induced by insulin and glucose infusion and they had an additive effect in a glucose-insulin clamp study of 23 healthy lean human subjects, suggesting that these physiologic mechanisms may play a role in NAFLD [75].

A SNP in *PNPLA3* at rs738409 leads to increased fat deposition in the liver but not insulin resistance. The G risk allele impedes triglyceride hydrolysis in vitro and G allele carriers have an increased risk of developing severe liver disease. Since weight loss is currently one of the recommended treatments for NAFLD, a very small, human intervention trial in Finland investigated if genetic variation at *PNPLA3* impacted weight loss in humans. The trial placed 8 adults homozygous for the G risk allele and 10 adults homozygous for the C allele on a hypocaloric low-carbohydrate diet for 6 days. Despite no difference in total weight loss between participants with the two allelic profiles, individuals with the G risk allele lost significantly more liver fat over the 6 days than did CC individuals [76].

METHODOLOGICAL CHALLENGES IN PUBLIC HEALTH NUTRIGENOMICS

Investigators bringing nutrigenomics and nutrigenetics to population research need to become aware of the standard principles and caveats of epidemiologic research. Complete understanding of these principles will allow for the critical analysis of nutrigenomics and will lay the foundation for building the strongest possible evidence surrounding the use of nutrigenomics in public health.

Measurement Accuracy and Reliability

Environmental factors, and especially diet and nutrition, are complex to measure. The temporal variation of dietary intake and the complexity of the mixtures composing diet make accurate assessment of nutritional exposures challenging [32]. A paucity of studies collecting both detailed genomic and epidemiologic data poses another challenge. One potential solution is to conduct genomic analyses on archived biological specimens from large epidemiologic studies with extensive phenotypes, physiological, anthropometric, behavioral, biochemical, and chemical measurements, such as the National Health and Nutrition Exposure Study (NHANES) [77]. Detailed exposure data matched with physiologic and genomic measures is not common in large epidemiologic studies, but it is necessary to accurately estimate associations between dietary exposure and genomic variation.

Inaccuracies of exposure measurements introduce bias and make definitive conclusions about gene–nutrient interactions difficult. Numerous publications have addressed the intricacies of exposure measures in depth [78–81]; an overview is provided here. All current nutrition metrics rely on an individual's self-report or daily records of his/her dietary intake. Although these existing measures (24-hour food recalls, 3-day food diaries, and food frequency questionnaires) are validated in many populations, correlations between self-report measures and observed dietary intake are around 40% at best. Novel approaches to more accurately capture dietary intake include before and after photographs of food servings [82], web-enabled software that captures dietary intake in real-time [83], and omic analyses linking food exposure to defined biomarkers [84]. This imprecision will be a continuing limitation for gene–nutrient interaction studies.

Study Design

The limitations of imprecise exposure assessment can be partially recouped if investigators utilize an optimal study design for their association of interest. Sample size, power, method of genomic measurement, and recruitment design all impact the reproducibility and comparability of a study [30,32]. Thomas provides a detailed table of study design advantages, disadvantages, and suggestions for use with different gene–environment interactions [32]. Prospective, longitudinal studies that include repeated sampling and include more accurate phenotype assessment are optimal for better characterization of gene–nutrient interactions. Major challenges to developing personalized nutrition applications, even when study design is optimized include the genetic diversity of human populations, the complexity of diets and cultures, and the intricacies of physiology dependent on gene–nutrient interactions that differ between individuals.

Sample Size and Power

Gene–nutrient interaction studies require very large sample sizes, with thousands of cases typically needed for candidate gene studies and tens of thousands required for GWAS. GWAS requires much higher levels of significance than do candidate gene studies. Underpowered studies, either at the initial or at replicate stage, may be primarily responsible for the poor reproducibility of gene–nutrient interaction findings [16]. At least a fourfold larger sample size is required to detect gene–nutrient interactions than to find a main effect of comparable magnitude. Enriching the study sample with individuals likely to have the hypothesized gene–nutrient interaction, such as those with a positive family history or high exposure levels, will improve power [32]. Prevalence of exposure, AF, mode of inheritance, and the postulated or previously reported interaction OR are key determinants of sample size and power requirements [16].

GWAS versus Candidate Gene Analysis Studies

To gain the most complete picture of how genetic and epigenetic factors may influence disease outcomes in the shortest amount of time, multiple levels of genomic analyses should be used together in an iterative process.

Although GWAS are sometimes criticized as nonhypothesis-driven, "fishing expeditions," some important unpredicted associations have been found. GWAS have enabled the identification of hundreds of gene loci associated with complex phenotypes of chronic disease, which provide starting points for researchers to begin to investigate potential mechanistic links between genomic variants and health outcomes. The challenge of translating GWAS findings, from association signal to causal variant to cellular and molecular mechanisms, is addressed by McCarthy and Hirschhorn [85]. They suggest improved characterization of gene loci and causal variants (genetic and phenotypic refinement of association signals) and an integrated understanding of function and genetics (expression information, genome annotation, and functional experimentation) will improve the translation and application of GWAS findings in public health through the development of predictive, preventive, or therapeutic measures [85].

Interactions can sometimes be observed in GWAS when direct effects are marginal or not detectable, by testing for the interaction of genetic effect in an environmental subgroup. This approach has great public health implications and is currently being used in GWAS searching for dietary factors that impact susceptibility to CRC and for genes that impart susceptibility to radiation in second breast cancers or air pollution in childhood asthma. Identifying these interactions may explain some of the "missing heritability" that exists for these conditions [30].

A candidate gene approach can be used to study gene variants, identified by GWAS, in greater detail, thereby facilitating the translation of association signals to cellular mechanisms underlying common disease outcomes. Utilizing the most accurate, efficient method to identify causal variants is crucial to timely and cost-effective implementation of genomics findings in public health applications: individual SNPs complicate conclusions about gene–nutrient interactions because individual genes often have multiple variants, whereas identifying haplotypes is a more efficient method of performing candidate gene analysis [16,26]. Candidate gene analysis has already contributed to public health efforts through effective identification of genetic variants contributing to extreme HDL-C and LDL-C levels [86]. Although each rare recessive allele explained a small number of cases, the identified mutations and heterozygote status are responsible for a substantial portion of metabolic disease [13,87].

Rare coding variants (RCVs) could provide another layer of analysis that will contribute to the overall picture of linking genomics to disease phenotypes with public health relevance. Heterozygotes for the autosomal recessive monogenic disorders often caused by RCVs are not so rare. A homozygous disorder with prevalence 1 in 40,000 would have heterozygotes in 1 in 100 members of the general population. Recent, deep sequencing of individuals' genomes from multiple populations in large, international studies, like the 1000 Genomes Project and HapMap, suggests RCV, with AF less than 1%, are significantly more common than predicted by traditional population genetics [83,88,89]. Advances in deep sequencing technology will identify more RCVs, as well as CNVs (deletions and amplifications) [90]. Such genome variation could contribute to multifactorial conditions and therefore the public health potential of RCVs should not be overlooked.

Data Analysis and Management

The tremendous quantity of data generated by "omics" studies presents an ongoing challenge. Meticulous data storage and management is critical for high-quality nutrigenomics research. Epidemiologic data could be added to existing genomics databases, such as HuGENet [91], ENCODE Project [92], or the 1000 Genomes Project [93]; alternatively, as the cost of genotyping and of sequencing continues to decrease, genomic analyses could be added to large-scale nutritional epidemiology projects, such as NHANES. Collecting common, important variables in all genomics and large epidemiologic studies would improve comparisons between population subgroups and studies.

International consortia ideally composed of developed and economically emerging countries have been proposed as the most effective way to share standardized data collection and analysis protocols, best practices, and datasets. Differences in genomic variants or gene–exposure interactions between individuals in developing and emerging economy countries, at all stages of the epidemiologic transition, could help identify the genomic changes occurring in conjunction with the transition [90].

Capturing Human Heterogeneity and Diversity

The cost and technological resources required for nutrigenetic and nutrigenomic testing may be initial, prohibitive barriers to certain populations. However, to create a complete picture of human genotypes and their corresponding phenotypes, diverse study populations are optimal [32]. This may be challenging. Efforts to build rapport and educate population subgroups distrustful of research about the potential health and social benefits of participating in genomic testing should begin as soon as possible. The time investment to include these subgroups is critical to capture genomic variation between groups, such as the ethnic differences identified in *LIPC* gene polymorphisms. Sex-specific differences in the interaction of carbohydrate intake with HDL-C were modified by APOE genotype [94]. Stratification of effect by gender and ethnicity may partially explain the lack of success reproducing nutritional genomic findings in broad population-based studies.

The Wellcome Trust Case Control Consortium (WTCCC) demonstrated that a carefully selected control group of similar ancestry is an effective method for analyzing multiple disease phenotypes in GWAS. Data generated by the WTCCC suggests that if individuals of non-European ancestry are excluded, the extent of population stratification in the British population is generally modest. However, even within this relatively homogenous cohort of over 16,000 adults, substantial geographic variation in allele frequencies was observed across Britain, likely due to natural selection in ancestral populations [95]. The HapMap project is a valuable start to collecting rich genetic data from multiple different populations; however, due to the limited number of genomes included in HapMap, the database represents only a small fraction of the total genetic variation in humans. The Human Genome Diversity Project (http://www.stanford.edu/group/morrinst/hgdp.html) and Human Variome Project (http://www.variome.org) are expanding analyses of sequence variations by including individuals in many other human populations [84]. The Human Genome Epidemiology (HuGE) study surveyed uncommon variants (minor AF, ≤5%) that reached genome-wide significance ($P \leq 10^{-7}$) in GWAS. Findings suggest a possible confluence of rare and common genetic variation on the same genetic loci. Twenty-five uncommon variants are common in at least one of the four different ancestry samples of the HapMap [96]. This underscores the benefit of repeating GWAS in different human populations to identify disease risk alleles in individuals with various ancestries [9].

IMPLEMENTATION OF NUTRIGENOMICS IN PUBLIC HEALTH PRACTICE

PRACTICAL IMPACT

Before recommending widespread implementation of genotyping in clinical practice, it is important to assess the health impact of nutrigenetic and genomic screening. Genotypic variation impacts an individual's disease risk. Nutrigenomics and personalized nutrition provide an opportunity to implement preventive measures against these diseases. For conditions where current guidelines coincide with risk prevention, genotyping would not be a prudent use of resources. For example, current guidelines for maintaining or achieving a healthy weight include decreasing SFAs and TFAs to <10% total energy intake and completing at least 150 minutes of moderate to vigorous intensity physical activity weekly. *FTO* polymorphisms increase obesity risk in those with high SFA and TFA intakes and low physical activity levels; risk is not increased in those who consume low SFA and TFA diets and perform regular activity [97–99]. Therefore, genotyping individuals at the *FTO* allele would not be an efficient use of time and resources.

Identifying groups of individuals with similar metabolic profiles based on similar genetic profiles, effectively creating categories or "bins," will provide a rubric for the range of genotypes and phenotypes. This rubric could then be used by clinicians to more accurately estimate individual patients' disease risk [84,90].

Genomics will support evaluation of the success of existing health strategies (medications, social, behavioral, and policy interventions) across all segments of the population and will determine if modification by predicted individual susceptibility would be more effective. These evaluations will not only inform new preventive and therapeutic interventions based on nutrigenomics but could also identify environmental factors amenable to intervention at the policy level. Determining the maximum allowable exposure levels among the most susceptible population subgroups would support more efficient investments tailoring intensive environmental or behavioral interventions for the most susceptible groups [100].

Literacy and Training

Genetic and genomic testing was once only available in clinical health care facilities, but in the past decade, many direct-to-consumer testing options have emerged. Chapters 17 and 18 of this book have already discussed these avenues of testing and information dispersal in detail. The point is raised here only to comment on the public health significance of each venue.

Genomics literacy and training is needed among both health care professionals and the general public to ensure that test results are interpreted correctly and utilized to most effectively improve individual's health. Training of health care professionals on when to order genomics testing, how to analyze the test results, and what intervention to recommend as a result is necessary for successful implementation of nutritional genomics testing [101]. While research into the most effective methods of communicating nutrigenomic research to clinical and public audiences continues, health care professionals should be educated on nutrigenomics. As personalized nutrition becomes increasingly publicized, health care professionals will be expected to answer their patients' many questions.

Increasing genetic and genomic literacy of the general public is an important step toward responsibly implementing the use of nutrigenomics data to inform personalized nutrition recommendations. Information now travels at lightning speed through the Internet. Information propagated by news media and the general public is equally accessible to evidence-based scientific publications. Direct-to-consumer marketing of nutrigenomics testing kits already occurs. Educating the public on the general concept of nutrigenomics, its potential benefits, limitations, and current, evidence-based uses could help create not only an informed consumer market but also a public more shrewdly critical of ungrounded genomic claims. Genetic testing already occurs in clinical settings where it is guarded by health care privacy securities. Concerns for direct-to-consumer testing include the ethical and legal ramifications of individuals collecting genomic data on themselves. Privacy, security, and ownership (in addition to accurate interpretation) of results generated by direct-to-consumer testing are important considerations before recommending home testing for the general public's health.

Cost Efficacy of Nutrigenomics

Although the cost of chips and microarrays has decreased significantly in the past decade, the initial expense of genomic analysis is still significant. This raises the question: who would be able to afford this detailed health analysis? Currently, insurance companies do not cover most genomic tests, so expenses are incurred by research teams or wealthy individuals. Insurance reimbursement would help genomic testing become a routine part of clinical care. To make these analyses available to all people in the population, government insurance, such as Medicare and Medicaid in the United States, would have to approve coverage. Cost-benefit analysis or studies defining the potential return on investment of widespread use of nutrigenomic are likely necessary before insurance coverage will occur.

Potential for Behavior Change

Current public health efforts to modify health behaviors have generally been unsuccessful. More research is required to determine whether individuals would be willing to undergo genetic testing to identify the optimal nutrition regimen, personalized for them. Genetic testing could have the unintended negative consequence of undermining current healthy eating guidelines by implying that only individuals with high-risk genotypes need to eat healthfully [102].

Other Considerations

It is prudent to consider unintended consequences of implementing nutrigenetic screening and nutrigenomic therapeutics now, while the technology is relatively new and not yet widely used in regular clinical care. Questions regarding the potential scope of impact that personalized nutrition will have on decreasing chronic disease risk and prevalence suggest efforts should be focused on the food industry and built environment instead of personalized nutrition recommendations [103]. As people are increasingly given individualized diets to follow, strains on the agricultural system and environmental resources may occur. If all people consumed the recommended two to three servings of oily fish per week, there would not be enough wild and farmed fish to sustainably support this demand. Agricultural practices and the percentage of land devoted to grain compared to fruit, vegetable, nut, and other specialty crops should be reviewed to ensure the system can support the potential demand for foods recommended in personalized nutrition plans.

Nutrigenomics focuses on the physiologic interactions of individual nutrients and bioactive compounds, but if people were only to consume their individually prescribed nutrients in supplement form, "food" production would shift from agriculture to laboratory synthesis. This scenario would negatively impact the livelihood and therefore health of farmers and farming communities around the world. Due to their rural nature and potential for subsistence farming, these communities may have decreased access to health care, potentially exacerbating health disparities between socioeconomic groups.

EMERGING DIRECTIONS AND FUTURE PROGRESS

Introduction of nutrigenomic analyses in public health will likely begin in clinical settings with high-risk populations with well-characterized genomic polymorphisms and disease phenotypes. Clinical trials of preventive and therapeutic interventions based on nutrigenomic testing should be conducted, analyzed, and evaluated before recommending the use of nutrigenomics in all public health settings. Clinical implementation of personalized nutrition, under close supervision of health care professionals, will provide additional high-intensity monitoring and evaluation period. All research should undergo an intensive review process before widespread clinical and community health applications of nutrigenomics are recommended. Nutrigenomic testing could be prioritized based on novel health impact and greatest public health impact.

Genomic literacy and training of health care professionals should begin now. Provider understanding and comfort incorporating genetic and genomic testing into clinical care is necessary for effective implementation. Beginning to forge relationships with traditionally underrepresented communities to increase genomic literacy is a critical step in bringing genomic technology to the entire human population to improve the public's health without reinforcing or worsening existing health disparities.

Research across the continuum from basic genomic variation and gene–nutrient interactions to physiologic mechanisms, to clinical therapeutics, to population access, and to policy support should continue simultaneously as an iterative process. Basic nutrigenomics research should be evaluated for translation to the population as discoveries occur, since the process of discovering the full spectrum of heritability and environmental interaction is complex and likely to continue for years. Standardization of nutrigenomic research protocols will assist in comparability of study results and compilation into large, international databases. Longitudinal, prospective study design with sufficient sample size and power to detect gene–nutrient associations, including participants from diverse ancestral populations, is optimal for future research study design. Consideration of multiple nutrient–gene–environment interactions is imperative to provide accurate, personalized nutrition recommendations in the future. Extensive biorepositories and haplotype databases will facilitate a more complete understanding of potential nutrigenetic interactions.

ACKNOWLEDGMENTS

Gilbert S. Omenn acknowledges support from NIH cooperative agreement grants U54DA021519, UL1 RR024986, RM-08-029, and U54ES017885. Elizabeth H. Marchlewicz and Karen E. Peterson acknowledge support from NIEHS P20ES018171, EPA RD834800, and NIDDK P30 DK089503.

REFERENCES

1. Pollack, H., Eugene Floyd Dubois—a biographical sketch. *J Nutr*, 1961. **75**: pp. 3–6.
2. Huxley, R.R. et al., Nutritional research in World War 2: the Oxford Nutrition Survey and its research potential 50 years later. *Br J Nutr*, 2000. **84**(2): pp. 247–251.
3. Penland, J.G., *Dietary Reference Intakes (DRIs)—new dietary guidelines really are new!* http://www.ars.usda.gov/News/docs.htm?docid=10870, 2006. Accessed December 21, 2011.
4. FAO, Targeting for nutrition improvement. *Nutrition in Agriculture*, p. 115 http://www.fao.org/docrep/004/Y1329E/Y1329E00.HTM, 2001. Agriculture and Consumer Protection Department of FAO. Accessed May 18, 2013.
5. FAO, *Fighting hunger and obesity. Agriculture, biosecurity, nutrition and consumer protection department of FAO.* http://www.fao.org/ag/magazine/pdf/0602-1.pdf 2006 Accessed May 18, 2013.
6. Darnton-Hill, I., B. Margetts, and R. Deckelbaum, Public health nutrition and genetics: implications for nutrition policy and promotion. *Proc Nutr Soc*, 2004. **63**(1): pp. 173–185.
7. USDA, *Dietary Guidelines for Americans, 2010*, 2011, Center for Nutrition Policy and Promotion, United States Department of Agriculture: Washington, DC.
8. Ordovas, J.M., The quest for cardiovascular health in the genomic era: nutrigenetics and plasma lipoproteins. *Proc Nutr Soc*, 2004. **63**(1): pp. 145–152.

9. Bustamante, C.D., E.G. Burchard, and F.M. De la Vega, Genomics for the world. *Nature*, 2011. **475**(7355): pp. 163–165.
10. McEvoy, B.P. et al., Human population dispersal "Out of Africa" estimated from linkage disequilibrium and allele frequencies of SNPs. *Genome Res*, 2011. **21**(6): pp. 821–829.
11. Nachman, M.W. and S.L. Crowell, Estimate of the mutation rate per nucleotide in humans. *Genetics*, 2000. **156**: pp. 297–304.
12. Villa, P. et al., Cannibalism in the Neolithic. *Science*, 1986. **233**(4762): pp. 431–437.
13. McClellan, J. and M.C. King, Genetic heterogeneity in human disease. *Cell*, 2010. **141**(2): pp. 210–217.
14. Omenn, G.S., Overview of the symposium on public health significance of genomics and eco-genetics. *Annu Rev Public Health*, 2010. **31**: pp. 1–8.
15. Simopoulos, A.P., Nutrigenetics/nutrigenomics. *Annu Rev Public Health*, 2010. **31**: pp. 53–68.
16. Omenn, G.S., Gene-environment interactions: eco-genetics and toxicogenomics, In *Genomic and Personalized Medicine, 2nd Ed.*, G.S. Ginsburg and H. Willard, Editors. In Press, Academic Press: Burlington, MA.
17. Perry, G.H. et al., Diet and the evolution of human amylase gene copy number variation. *Nat Genet*, 2007. **39**: pp. 1256–1260.
18. Chavez, A. and M. Munoz de Chavez, Nutrigenomics in public health nutrition: short-term perspectives. *Eur J Clin Nutr*, 2003. **57**(Suppl 1): pp. S97–S100.
19. Popkin, B.M., The nutrition transition and obesity in the developing world. *J Nutr*, 2001. **131**(3): pp. 871S–873S.
20. Cordain, L. et al., Origins and evolution of the Western diet: health implications for the 21st century. *Am J Clin Nutr*, 2005. **81**(2): pp. 341–354.
21. Omenn, G.S., Evolution and public health. *Proc Natl Acad Sci USA*, 2010. **107**(Suppl 1): pp. 1702–1709.
22. Phillips, C.M. et al., Leptin receptor polymorphisms interact with polyunsaturated fatty acids to augment risk of insulin resistance and metabolic syndrome in adults. *J Nutr*, 2010. **140**(2): pp. 238–244.
23. Hetherington, M.M. and J.E. Cecil, Gene-environment interactions in obesity. *Forum Nutr*, 2010. **63**: pp. 195–203.
24. Pratley, R.E., Gene-environment interactions in the pathogenesis of type 2 diabetes mellitus: lessons learned from the Pima Indians. *Proc Nutr Soc*, 1998. **57**: pp. 175–181.
25. Schultz, L.O. et al., Effects of traditional and Western environments on prevalence of type 2 diabetes in Pima Indians in Mexico and the U.S. *Diabetes Care*, 2006. **29**: pp. 1866–1871.
26. McVean, G., C. Spencer, and R. Chaix, Perspectives on human genetic variation from the HapMap project. *PLos Genet*, 2005. **1**: p. e54.
27. Li, D. et al., Influence of CYP3A5 and MDR1 genetic polymorphisms on urinary 6 beta-hydroxycortisol/cortisol ratio after grapefruit juice intake in healthy Chinese. *J Clin Pharmacol*, 2010. **50**: pp. 775–784.
28. So, H.C. et al., Evaluating the heritability explained by known susceptibility variants: a survey of ten complex diseases. *Genet Epidemiol*, 2011. **35**: pp. 310–317.
29. Wood, A.R. et al., Allelic heterogeneity and more detailed analyses of known loci explain additional phenotypic variation and reveal complex patterns of association. *Hum Mol Genet*, 2011. **15**: pp. 4082–4092.
30. Davey Smith, G., Use of genetic markers and gene-diet interactions for interrogating population-level causal influences of diet on health. *Genes Nutr*, 2011. **6**: pp. 27–43.
31. Thomas, D., Methods for investigating gene-environment interactions in candidate pathway and genome-wide association studies. *Annu Rev Public Health*, 2010. **31**: pp. 21–36.

32. Thomas, D., Gene–environment-wide association studies: emerging approaches. *Nat Rev Genet*, 2010. **11**(4): pp. 259–272.
33. Smith, A.D., Y.I. Kim, and H. Refsum, Is folic acid good for everyone? *Am J Clin Nutr*, 2008. **87**: pp. 517–533.
34. Yajnik, C.S. and U.S. Deshmukh, Maternal nutrition, intrauterine programming and consequential risks in the offspring. *Rev Endocr Metab Disord*, 2008. **9**: pp. 203–211.
35. Lumley, J. et al., Modeling the potential impact of population-wide periconceptional folate/multivitamin supplementation on multiple births. *BJOG*, 2001. **108**: pp. 937–942.
36. CDC, Recommendations for the use of folic acid to reduce the number of cases of spina bifida and other neural tube defects. *MMWR Recomm Rep*, 1992. **41**: pp. 1–7.
37. Honein, M.A. et al., Impact of folic acid fortification of the US food supply on the occurrence of neural tube defects. *JAMA*, 2001. **285**: pp. 2981–2986.
38. De Wals, P. et al., Trend in prevalence of neural tube defects in Quebec. *Birth Defects Res A Clin Mol Teratol*, 2003. **67**: pp. 919–923.
39. Godwin, K.A. et al., Changes in frequencies of select congenital anomalies since the onset of folic acid fortification in a Canadian birth defect registry. *Can J Public Health*, 2008. **99**: pp. 271–275.
40. Ray, J.G. et al., Association between folic acid food fortification and congenital orofacial clefts. *J Pediatr*, 2003. **143**: pp. 805–807.
41. Sayed, A.R. et al., Decline in the prevalence of neural tube defects following folic acid fortification and its cost-benefit in South Africa. *Birth Defects Res A Clin Mol Teratol*, 2008. **82**: pp. 211–216.
42. Roberfroid, D. et al., Effects of maternal multiple micronutrient supplementation on fetal growth: a double-blind randomized controlled trial in rural Burkina Faso. *Am J Clin Nutr*, 2008. **88**: pp. 1330–1340.
43. Garantziotis, S. and D.A. Schwartz, Ecogenomics of respiratory diseases of public health significance. *Ann Rev Public Health*, 2010. **31**: pp. 37–51.
44. Pilsner, J.R. et al., Maternal MTHFR genotype and haplotype predict deficits in early cognitive development in a lead-exposed birth cohort in Mexico City. *Am J Clin Nutr*, 2010. **92**: pp. 226–234.
45. Eidelman, R. et al., Randomized trials of vitamin E in the treatment and prevention of cardiovascular disease. *Arch Intern Med*, 2004. **164**: pp. 1552–1556.
46. Group, H.P.S.C., MRC/BHF Heart Protection Study of antioxidant vitamin supplementation in 20536 high-risk individuals: a randomised placebo-controlled trial. *Lancet*, 2002. **360**(9326): pp. 23–33.
47. Khaw, K.T. et al., Relation between plasma ascorbic acid and morality in men and women in EPIC-Norfolk prospective study: a prospective population study. *Lancet*, 2001. **357**: pp. 657–663.
48. Rimm, E.B. et al., Vitamin E consumption and the risk of coronary disease in men. *N Engl J Med*, 1993. **328**: pp. 1450–1456.
49. Stampfer, M.J. et al., Vitamin E consumption and the risk of coronary disease in women. *N Engl J Med*, 1993. **328**: pp. 1444–1449.
50. Omenn, G.S. et al., Effects of a combination of beta carotene and vitamin A on lung cancer and cardiovascular disease. *N Engl J Med*, 1996. **334**: pp. 1150–1155.
51. Goodman, G.E. et al., The beta-carotene and retinol efficacy trial: incidence of lung cancer and cardiovascular disease mortality during 6-year follow-up after stopping beta-carotene and retinol supplements. *J Natl Cancer Inst*, 2004. **96**: pp. 1743–1750.
52. Group, A.-T.B.C.C.P.S., The effect of vitamin E and beta carotene on the incidence of lung cancer and other cancers in male smokers. *N Engl J Med*, 1994. **330**(15): pp. 1029–1035.
53. Omenn, G.S., Chemoprevention of lung cancer: the rise and demise of beta carotene. *Ann Rev Public Health*, 1998. **19**: pp. 73–99.

54. D'Ambrosio, D., R. Clugston, and W. Blaner, Vitamin A metabolism: an update. *Nutrients*, 2011. **3**: pp. 63–103.
55. Borel, P., Genetic variations involved in interindividual variability in carotenoid status. *Mol Nutr Food Res*, 2012. **56**: pp. 228–240.
56. Lietz, G. et al., Single nucleotide polymorphisms upstream from the beta-carotene 15,15'-monoxygenase gene influence provitamin A conversion efficiency in female volunteers. *J Nutr*, 2012. **142**(1): pp. 161S–165S.
57. Borel, P. et al., Human fasting plasma concentrations of vitamin E and carotenoids, and their association with genetic variants in apo C-III, cholesteryl ester transfer protein, hepatic lipase, intestinal fatty acid binding protein and microsomal triacylglycerol transfer protein. *Br J Nutr*, 2009. **101**(5): pp. 680–687.
58. Borel, P. et al., Human plasma levels of vitamin E and carotenoids are associated with genetic polymorphisms in genes involved in lipid metabolism. *J Nutr*, 2007. **137**(12): pp. 2653–2659.
59. Herberth, B. et al., The lipoprotein lipase serine 447 stop polymorphism is associated with altered serum carotenoid concentrations in the Stanislas Family Study. *J Am Coll Nutr*, 2007. **26**: pp. 655–662.
60. Mondul, A.M. et al., Genome-wide association study of circulating retinol levels. *Hum Mol Genet*, 2011. **20**(23): pp. 4724–4731.
61. Klein, E.A. et al., Vitamin E and the risk of prostate cancer: the Selenium and Vitamin E Cancer Prevention Trial (SELECT). *JAMA*, 2011. **306**(14): pp. 1549–1556.
62. Micheel, C., S. Nass, and G.S. Omenn, *Evolution of translational omics: Lessons learned and path forward.* http://www.iom.edu/Reports/2012/Evolution-of-Translational-Omics.aspx, 2012, National Academy Press: Washington, DC Accessed December 21, 2012.
63. Voight, B.F. et al., Plasma HDL cholesterol and risk of myocardial infarction: a Mendelian randomization study. *Lancet*, 2012. **380**(9841): pp. 572–580.
64. Zhang, J. et al., Trends in mortality from cancers of the breast, colon, prostate, esophagus, and stomach in East Asia: role of nutrition transition. *Eur J Cancer Prev*, 2012. **21**(5): pp. 480–489.
65. Crous-Bou, M. et al., Genetic polymorphisms in fatty acid metabolism genes and colorectal cancer. *Mutagenesis*, 2012. **27**: pp. 169–176.
66. Gorham, E.D. et al., Optimal vitamin D status for colorectal cancer prevention: a quantitative meta-analysis. *Am J Prev Med*, 2007. **32**: pp. 210–216.
67. Slattery, M.L. et al., Associations between BMI, energy intake, energy expenditure, VDR genotype and colon and rectal cancers (United States). *Cancer Causes Control*, 2004. **15**: pp. 863–872.
68. Wong, H.L. et al., Vitamin D receptor start codon polymorphism and colorectal cancer risk: modification by dietary calcium and fat in Singapore Chinese. *Carcinogenesis*, 2003. **24**: pp. 1091–1095.
69. Davis, C. and J. Milner, Nutrigenomics, vitamin D, and cancer prevention. *J Nutrigenet Nutrigenomics*, 2011. **4**: pp. 1–11.
70. Powell, E.E., J.R. Jonsson, and A.D. Clouston, Steatosis: co-factor in other liver diseases. *Hepatology*, 2005. **42**: pp. 5–13.
71. Schwimmer, J.B. et al., Prevalence of fatty liver in children and adolescents. *Pediatrics*, 2006. **118**: pp. 1388–1393.
72. Speliotes, E.K. et al., Genome-wide association analysis identifies variants associated with nonalcoholic fatty liver disease that have distinct effects on metabolic traits. *PLOS Genet*, 2011. **7**: p. e1001324.
73. Huang, Y. et al., A feed-forward loop amplifies nutritional regulation of PNPLA3. *Proc Natl Acad Sci USA*, 2010. **107**: pp. 7892–7897.
74. Rae-Whitcombe, S.M. et al., Regulation of the promoter region of the human adiponectin/PNPLA3 gene by glucose and insulin. *Biochem Biophys Res Commun*, 2010. **402**: pp. 767–772.

75. Moldes, M. et al., Adiponutrin gene is regulated by insulin and glucose in human adipose tissue. *Eur J Endocrinol*, 2006. **155**: pp. 461–468.
76. Sevastianova, K. et al., Genetic variation in PNPLA3 (adiponectin) confers sensitivity to weight loss-induced decrease in liver fat in humans. *Am J Clin Nutr*, 2011. **94**: pp. 104–111.
77. CDC. *National Health and Nutrition Examination Survey (NHANES): Questionnaires, datasets, and related documentation*. http://www.cdc.gov/nchs/nhanes/nhanes_questionnaires.htm, 2011. Accessed January 26, 2012.
78. Bennett, D. et al., Study protocol: the empirical investigation of methods to correct for measurement error in biobanks with dietary assessment. *BMC Med Res Methodol*, 2011. **11**: pp. 135–139.
79. Freedman, L.S. et al., Dealing with dietary measurement error in nutritional cohort studies. *J Natl Cancer Inst*, 2011. **103**: pp. 1086–1092.
80. Preis, S.R. et al., Application of a repeat-measure biomarker measurement error model to 2 validation studies: examination of the effect of within-person variation in biomarker measurements. *Am J Epidemiol*, 2011. **173**: pp. 683–694.
81. Souverein, O.W. et al., Comparing four methods to estimate usual intake distributions. *Euro J Clin Nutr*, 2011. **65**: pp. S92–S101.
82. Kikunaga, S. et al., The application of a handheld personal digital assistant with camera and mobile phone card (Wellnavi) to the general population in a dietary survey. *J Nutr Sci Vitaminol (Tokyo)*, 2007. **53**: pp. 109–116.
83. Gravel, S. et al., Demographic history and rare allele sharing among human populations. *Proc Natl Acad Sci USA*, 2011. **108**(29): pp. 11983–11988.
84. McCabe-Sellers, B. et al., Personalizing nutrigenomics research through community based participatory research and omics technologies. *OMICS*, 2008. **12**(4): pp. 263–272.
85. McCarthy, M.I. and J.N. Hirschhorn, Genome-wide association studies: potential next steps on a genetic journey. *Hum Mol Genet*, 2010. **17**: pp. R156–R165.
86. Cohen, J. et al., Multiple rare variants in NPC1L1 associated with reduced sterol absorption and plasma low-density lipoprotein levels. *Proc Natl Acad Sci USA*, 2006. **103**: pp. 1810–1815.
87. Fahmi, S. et al., Functional characterization of genetic variants in NPC1L1 supports the sequencing extremes strategy to identify complex trait genes. *Hum Mol Genet*, 2008. **17**: pp. 2101–2107.
88. Coventry, A. et al., Deep resequencing reveals excess rare recent variants consistent with explosive population growth. *Nat Commun*, 2010. **1**: p. 131.
89. Marth, G.T. et al., The functional spectrum of low-frequency coding variation. *Genome Biol*, 2011. **12**(9): p. R84.
90. Kaput, J. et al., The case for strategic international alliances to harness nutritional genomics for public and personal health. *Br J Nutr*, 2005. **94**(5): pp. 623–632.
91. CDC. *Human Genome Epidemiology Network (HuGE Net)*. http://www.cdc.gov/genomics/hugenet/, 2011. Accessed January 18, 2012.
92. NHGRI. *The ENCODE Project: ENCyclopedia Of DNA Elements*. http://www.genome.gov/10005107, 2011 Accessed January 18, 2012.
93. *1000 Genomes: A deep catalog of human genetic variation*. http://www.1000genomes.org/home, 2010. Accessed January 18, 2012.
94. Mosher, M.J. et al. Sex-specific interaction between APOE genotype and carbohydrate intake affects plasma HDL-C levels: the Strong Heart Family Study. *Genes Nutr*, 2008. **3**(2): pp. 87–97.
95. Consortium, W.T.C.C., Genome-wide association study of 14,000 cases of seven common diseases and 3,000 shared controls. *Nature*, 2007. **447**(7145): pp. 661–678.

96. Panagiotou, O.A., E. Evangelou, and J.P. Ioannidis, Genome-wide significant associations for variants with minor allele frequency of 5% or less—an overview: a HuGE review. *Am J Epidemiol*, 2010. **172**(8): pp. 869–889.
97. Fischer, J. et al., Inactivation of the FTO gene protects from obesity. *Nature*, 2009. **458**: pp. 894–898.
98. Frayling, T. et al., A common variant in the FTO gene is associated with body mass index and predisposes to childhood and adult obesity. *Science*, 2007. **316**: pp. 889–894.
99. Speakman, J., D.M. Jackson, and A.M. Johnstone, Polymorphisms of the FTO gene are associated with variation in energy intake but not energy expenditure. *Obesity*, 2008. **16**: pp. 1961–1965.
100. Khoury, M.J. et al., Beyond base pairs to bedside: a population perspective on how genomics can improve health. *Am J Public Health*, 2011. **102**: pp. 34–37.
101. Feero, W., A. Guttmacher, and F. Collins, The genome gets personal—almost. *JAMA*, 2008. **299**: pp. 1351–1352.
102. McBride, C.M. et al., The behavioral response to personalized genetic information: will genetic risk profiles motivate individuals and families to choose more healthful behaviors? *Annu Rev Public Health*, 2010. **31**: pp. 89–103.
103. Lovegrove, J.A. and R. Gitau, Nutrigenetics and CVD: what does the future hold? *Proc Nutr Soc*, 2008. **67**(2): pp. 206–213.

21 Nutrigenomics and Public Health

Maria Agelli and John A. Milner

CONTENTS

INTRODUCTION

People throughout the world are increasingly questioning their diets in terms of quality and safety and of its overall influence on their health. This interest stems from mounting evidence indicating that numerous bioactive food components influence the ability to achieve one's genetic potential, influence our quality of life in terms of both physical and cognitive performance, and modify the risk and/or severity of a variety of diseases in each individual. A wealth of evidence points to the association of dietary habits with premature death and with many diseases, for example, cardiovascular diseases, stroke, diabetes, liver disease, and certain cancers (Gonzalez and Riboli, 2010; Tourlouki et al., 2009). Nevertheless, a considerable individual variability exists in the response to foods and their components. This variability is due to individual differences in the genetic and epigenetic regulation of cellular events critical for shifting from health to disease (Burdge et al., 2007; Burdge and Lillycrop, 2010; Jackson et al., 2010; Lillycrop and Burdge, 2011b). This interrelationship between foods and their components with an individual's genome is briefly reviewed.

The fact that foods and nutrition are environmental factors of major importance for the health of individuals and populations is undisputable. Nutrigenetics and nutrigenomics hold promise for providing to public health important information for improving the health of the public at all levels and this promise is discussed.

This chapter briefly reviews (1) the conceptual tenets for nutrigenomics, (2) the basic principles guiding public health practice, (3) emerging indications that the knowledge gained by nutrigenomics might be applied to improve the public's health, (4) availability of technologies for the public, and (5) challenges and opportunities to consider for bringing nutrigenomics closer to public health applications.

DEFINITIONS

Nutrigenomics is the study of the effects of foods and of their components on gene expression. It focuses on the transcription of DNA into mRNA in response to nutrients and on their ultimate impact on an individual's health taking into account the entire genetic makeup, or genome, of an individual. It encompasses nutrigenetics, which studies the effect of the genetic variations occurring because of single-nucleotide polymorphisms (SNPs), enhanced copy number, deletions, and so forth on the digestion, absorption, and metabolism of bioactive food components. Thus, nutrigenomics provides a biological basis for evaluating the needs for specific foods or food components to optimize health. Epigenetic events are other critical factors in determining which functions of genes are activated or suppressed (Dolinoy et al., 2006; Kaati et al., 2002; Kaati et al., 2007; Lillycrop and Burdge, 2011a; Ng et al., 2010). For example, the degree of methylation depends on the availability of methyl donors, on the activity of methyltransferase, and, potentially, on demethylation activity (Hardy and Tollefsbol, 2011; Ross, 2010). Likewise, certain foods can markedly influence histone homeostasis (Rajendran et al., 2011), another epigenetic regulator. Even the formation of microRNA, a posttranscriptional regulator, appears to be influenced by certain food (Chartoumpekis et al., 2012; Joven et al., 2012). Furthermore, many nutrients can alter atomic valances and therefore influence the formation of polycomb-group proteins, which can dictate epigenetic gene expression patterns (Balasubramanian et al., 2008). Thus, diet can have a profound impact on epigenetics and by multiple mechanisms. Since these epigenetic processes are occurring simultaneously in a cell and are sometimes influenced by the same food component, determining which of these effects is most important for producing a specific biological response it is likely to be difficult.

Public health is "the science and art of preventing disease, prolonging life and promoting health through the organized efforts and informed choices of society, public and private organizations, communities and individuals" (Winslow, 1920). It identifies threats to the health of the population of interest through population health analysis. Its scope changes with the socioeconomic status of the population ranging, for example, from preventing the spread of acute infective diseases to addressing the obstacles that prevent the achievement of health as "a state of complete physical, mental, and social well-being and not merely the absence of disease or infirmity" (World Health Organization, 1946). It incorporates an interdisciplinary approach that builds on epidemiology, biostatistics, and health services. Nutrition is critical to the well-being of individuals and populations; thus, it is fundamental to public health strategies. Topics span multiple areas including those associated with food insecurity, food supply inadequacies and excesses, human ecology, as well as the prevention and/or the management of obesity (Beaglehole et al., 2011; Davis and Milner, 2011; Glanz et al., 2012; Last, 1998; Li and Heber, 2012).

NUTRIGENOMICS AND PUBLIC HEALTH OPERATE AT DIFFERENT LEVELS

Much of what has been written about nutrigenomics and public health deals with the differences between these two disciplines and discusses their incompatibility. This often equates nutrigenomics and genetics to individuals' rights and freedom of choice and public health to a paternalistic and utilitarian discipline where the benefit to society as a whole outweighs the rights of individuals (Castle, 2009; Penders et al., 2007). However, nutrigenomics and public health do not need to be in a conflict either now or in the future; rather, nutrigenomics should provide important information for improving the health of the public at all levels. However, it must be recognized that nutrigenomics is in its infancy and its public health applications lie in the future.

Discussions about the incompatibility of nutrigenomics and public health are also blurred by the failure to distinguish between research and practice (Childress and Bemheim, 2003). Nutrigenomics is a science in its initial stages and far from the stage of applicability to improve human health because of its proven benefits to large groups of individuals. Nutritional genomics emerged in the wake of the powerful development of genetic research and of the demonstration of genetic variability in humans. Genetic and epigenetic differences may affect how individuals respond to environmental factors (nutrients/diet) (Simopoulos et al., 1999). The final goal of nutrigenomics is to develop means to optimize nutrition based on an individual's genotype. Because of this, nutrigenomics has been receiving increasing attention for its potential for preventing chronic diseases in individuals whose genotype put them at increased risk for these diseases (Kaput, 2008).

The conceptual basis of nutrigenomics is usually summarized by what are known as the five tenets of nutrigenomics: (1) under certain circumstances and in some individuals, diet can be a serious risk factor for a number of diseases; (2) common dietary chemicals can act on the human genome, either directly or indirectly, to alter gene expression or structure; (3) the degree to which diet influences the balance between healthy and disease states may depend on an individual's genetic makeup; (4) some diet-regulated genes (and their normal, common variants) are likely to play a role in the onset, incidence, progression, and/or severity of chronic diseases; and (5) dietary intervention based on knowledge of nutritional requirement, nutritional status, and genotype (i.e., "personalized nutrition") can be used to prevent, mitigate, or cure chronic disease. The promise of nutritional genomics is the achievement of health—or of better health—through personalized nutrition based on the understanding of individuals' nutritional needs in relation to their specific genotype. While there is hope and even a strong belief that nutritional genomics will ultimately make possible such personalized dietary advice, nutrigenomics is still in its infancy.

GENOMIC ANALYSIS

Genetic variation is also associated with different susceptibility to diseases and different sensitivity to drugs (Mocchegiani et al., 2011; Silverton et al., 2011). This finding together with the sequencing of the human genome and the efforts to attempt mapping the extent of human genetic variation (e.g., the HapMap Project; Lin et al., 2005; Liu et al., 2004) significantly increased the interest and the expectations in personalized medicine, that is, in prevention and treatment interventions based on a person's genotype. However, it soon became apparent that the susceptibility to common chronic complex diseases, such as diabetes, cardiovascular diseases, arthritis, cancer, asthma, and autoimmune diseases, is associated with multiple genes and possibly with thousands of polymorphisms (genetic variation) and that the development and progression of chronic complex diseases are the result of the interactions of all this genetic variation with the environment and with constitutional factors (e.g., age and sex). Thus, when genomic research moved from single-gene diseases (e.g., Huntington's chorea, phenylketonuria, and hemophilia) to polygenic complex diseases, the apparent unstoppable advancement of genetic-based (personalized) medicine came, instead, almost to a halt because of the difficulties—both technical and financial—of studying the interactions of thousands of genetic polymorphisms with thousands of environmental factors. Publication of the draft sequences of the human genome (Lander et al., 2001; Venter et al., 2001) raised the hopes for rapid translation of genomic science into applications for the treatment and prevention of diseases and transition into a new era of personalized medicine. A biohype on personalized medicine has been building during the years of sequencing of the human genome (Gerard et al., 2002) and it is yet to be fulfilled (Agelli, 2010; Bell, 2004; Khoury and Mensah, 2005).

Genomics—and nutrigenomics and pharmacogenomics—has still to identify an approach that may successfully resolve the dilemma of how to study, identify, and eventually correct the susceptibility for chronic complex diseases. Multiple low-penetrance high-prevalence genes and thousands of polymorphisms play a role in the development and progression of common complex diseases and in the individual's response to pharmacological agents. The complexity of the genetic variations associated with an increased susceptibility for these diseases has prompted studies that focus on the sequencing of entire genomes, despite their high costs, to compare, gene by gene and polymorphism by polymorphism, the genomes of individuals with and without the disease. Despite the technical difficulties and the high financial costs, genome-wide association studies hold the promise to identifying the genetic variations most frequently associated with an increased risk for complex chronic multifactorial diseases including cancer. What has become increasing clear is that biological systems have multiple redundant processes and thus a battery of genes will likely be needed to identify vulnerable people within a population and those who will benefit most from a dietary intervention.

Genome-wide association studies to identify genetic variation associated with common complex diseases have been initiated by public–private partnerships. The Wellcome Trust Case Control Consortium (WTCCC) was established in the United Kingdom in 2005 to explore the feasibility of genome-wide association studies. To capitalize on its success, further rounds of Genome Wide Association (GWA) studies were funded in 2008 (WTCCC2) and in 2009 (WTCCC3), both international partnerships. Overall, the WTCCC conducts genome-wide association studies for several complex diseases (ankylosing spondylitis, Barrett's esophagus and esophageal adenocarcinoma, glaucoma, ischemic stroke, multiple sclerosis, preeclampsia,

Parkinson's disease, psychosis endophenotypes, psoriasis, schizophrenia, ulcerative colitis, visceral leishmaniasis, primary biliary cirrhosis, and anorexia nervosa) (Wellcome Trust Case Control Consortium, 2007, 2013). Similarly, in the United States, a public–private partnership managed by the Foundation for the National Institutes of Health, the Genetic Association Information Network (GAIN), was founded in 2006 to perform genome-wide association studies for five common diseases (attention deficit disorder, diabetic nephropathy in type I diabetes, major depression, psoriasis, schizophrenia, and bipolar disorder) (Genetic Association Information Network [GAIN], 2006). The results obtained by GAIN are being deposited in a database located within the National Library of Medicine and are readily accessible by the scientific community. Similarly, the results obtained by the WTCCC are also readily accessible. The intention clearly being that of facilitating the use of these data by the scientific community and expanding the number of genome-wide association studies.

GENES, DIET, AND RISK

From the perspective of nutrigenomics, each of these polymorphisms may result in deviations in nutritional biochemistry. The rationale behind nutrigenomics is that nutrients act as cellular signals providing to the cells information about their environment, that is, the diet. The interaction with a nutrient is then followed by changes in gene expression, that is, in the transcription of DNA into mRNA and, consequently, by changes in the proteins being translated by the mRNA. Thus, the interaction of a person's genome with a nutrient changes both protein expression and metabolite production in that person. Nutrigenomics encompasses not only the study of gene–nutrient interaction but also of protein expression (proteomics) and metabolite production (metabolomics) or, in other words, it studies how dietary exposures influence entire cascades of complex cell signaling (Figure 21.1). However, appropriate intake of bioactive food components must also be considered in the context of other cellular stressors including, for example, environmental toxins, free radical generation resulting from excess calories, and metabolic shifts due to exposures to microbes and viruses, as indicated in Figure 21.1.

Foods and their components have both positive and negative effects on human health. These effects are evaluated with widely diverging strategies, which adds to the intrinsical difficulties—that is, related to the variability typically observed in response to dietary exposures—met in establishing intake requirements. The individual variability in the response to dietary exposures likely reflects the genomics of the individuals as well as their responses to various insults such as bacteria, viruses, environmental pollutants, excess calories, and multiple nutrient—nutrient interactions (Figure 21.1). Palou et al. (2009) proposed strategies to achieve an integration of food risk/benefit analysis—whether the food is provided as such or as a dietary supplement and potentially also including bioactive food components—to accurately predict food-related outcomes. They introduced the concept of a window of benefit assessment to define specific ranges of intakes, that is, the range of intakes sufficient to prevent deficiency while avoiding toxicity, and ranges of intakes for additional benefit so that a food intake within the range defined by the lower and the upper

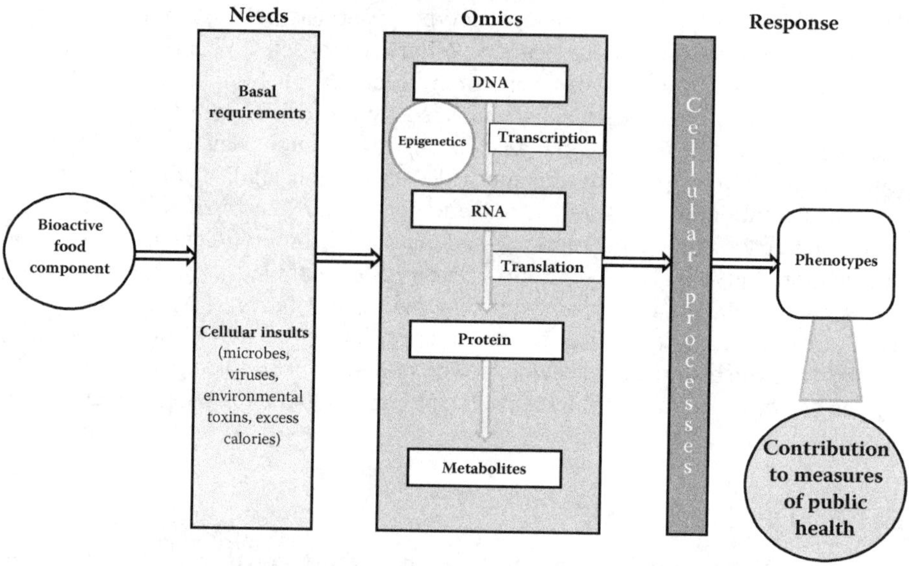

FIGURE 21.1 The dynamic interrelationship between the needs for bioactive food components for promoting a disease-free phenotype as influenced by their requirements for normal growth and development, cellular stressors (excess calories, environmental toxins/contaminants, viruses, and bacteria), and cellular processes as influenced by the individual genes and associated "omics."

levels of the additional benefit range for that food should be protective against a specified health or nutritional risk of public health relevance. At the present time, the strategic rationale of nutrigenomics relies on the identification of markers of susceptibility and/or of early stage development of diet-related diseases. If a marker is identified at this pre-disease or early disease stage, the extent of an individual's susceptibility to the disease might be measured and personalized dietary recommendations can be developed. This nutritional intervention will then prevent either the development or the progression of diet-related diseases. Of course, the nutrigenomics' identification of specific markers for susceptibility to chronic complex diseases is on the same timescale as the identification of the genetic variations associated with these diseases by genomic research.

Another goal of nutrigenomics is to study the effects of bioactive food components and of "health food" on people's health and the eventual development of functional food designed specifically for a person's needs and that will keep this person healthy (Eussen et al., 2011; van Boekel et al., 2010). Noncommunicable chronic diseases of major concern today are multifactorial in origin. Effective strategies to prevent and manage common multifactorial chronic diseases will likely need both a pharmaceutical approach and a nutritional approach that complement each other.

The increased number of functional foods and dietary supplements that, each with their own health implications, are marketed worldwide must be considered to be positioned between traditional foods and medicines. The expanded use of functional foods and of dietary supplements may offer opportunities to reduce health risk factors and even the risk for specific diseases and, in combination with prescription drugs, may have a role in the treatment and management of diseases. Nevertheless, the potential side effects associated with the use of these products, for example, interactions with prescription drugs, self-medication, and possibly a decrease in compliance with standard medical care, must be considered and studied. As this area grows, there will be increasing pressure to measure the cost-effectiveness of using foods or drugs or their combination in disease prevention and management.

Obesity is an important example of the potential role of nutrigenomics in public health prevention (Lillycrop and Burdge, 2011b). The fat mass and obesity-associated (FTO) gene is expressed prevalently in the cells of the brain and of the pancreatic islets (Frayling et al., 2007). Ten SNPs located in the first intron of the FTO gene—and all correlated with each other—have been found to be associated with type-2 diabetes and with increased body mass index (BMI). However, after adjusting for BMI, the association with diabetes disappeared, indicating that the FTO SNPs increased the susceptibility for diabetes only through their effect on body mass. The rs9939609 SNP is the SNP that has been studied in greatest detail. The A allele, which occurs at a frequency of 39% in the large European population studied, was associated with increased BMI. Homozygous carriers of the A allele had higher BMI than heterozygotes. The A allele was associated with increased risk for both being overweight (BMI >25 kg/m^2) and obese (BMI >30 kg/m^2). This allele was not associated with body weight at birth, but it was associated with increased BMI by age 7, and still at age 11 and 14 years in different populations (Frayling et al., 2007).

Highly prevalent celiac disease (Fasano et al., 2003; Mustalahti et al., 2010; Myléus et al., 2009) is another example for which nutrigenomics can have an important role in its prevention, diagnosis, and treatment. It is also a good example of the complexity of translating nutrigenomic research into public health practice.

People with this debilitating autoimmune disease produce antibodies against gluten, a protein present in a large variety of foods. The subsequent immune reaction causes chronic inflammation and leads to pathological alterations of the intestinal mucosa. If untreated, the disease may progress to produce severe malabsorption. There is no pharmacological treatment for celiac disease; however, changes in the daily diet allow patients to conduct a normal and productive life (Green and Cellier, 2007). Twins have approximately a 75% concordance (Greco et al., 2002) and a genetic component is well documented. Multiple genes appear to be involved; however, the most important genetic risk factor is the presence of the HLA-DQ genotype and in particular HLA-DQ2 and/or HLA-DQ8, which are necessary but not sufficient to produce celiac disease (Wolters and Wijmenga, 2008). The occurrence of not yet determined gene–environment interactions—in addition to exposure to gluten—is necessary for the development of celiac disease, and these interactions could account for the unexpected variability in the prevalence of celiac disease in different European countries (Mustalahti et al., 2010). HLA-DQ2 is associated with a higher risk for celiac disease than HLA-DQ8. DQ is an αβ heterodimer of the major histocompatibility complex class II. The β-subunit is associated with over 99% of the HLA-DQ genotype total risk for celiac disease, but the α subunit is also associated with an increased risk (Celiac-Disease.com, 2012; Hadithi et al., 2007; Megiorni et al., 2009; Sollid et al., 1989; Wolters et al., 2008). In addition, all the remaining

HLA-DQ genotypes, except for HLA-DQ4/DQ4, appear to be associated with an increased risk for sensitivity to gluten in the absence of celiac disease (Fine, 2008). More recently, non-celiac gluten sensitivity has been identified as a different anatomopathological disease (Sapone et al., 2011) and, with celiac disease, is considered part of a spectrum of gluten-related disorders (Ludvigsson et al., 2013; Sapone et al., 2012). Genetic tests for the HLA-DQ genotype are available and in certain instances their cost is covered by health insurance. Those laboratories performing a complete analysis of the HLA-DQ genotype can provide accurate information about the risk for celiac disease and for non-celiac gluten sensitivity. Genetic risk profiles for celiac disease would be helpful in clinical practice for predicting disease susceptibility and progression (Megiorni et al., 2008, 2009; Wolters and Wijmenga, 2008).

While foods and their components can present both positive and negative attributes, these are typically evaluated in largely separate evaluation strategies. Palou et al. (2009) proposed an integrated evaluation of risk and benefit of foods, and potentially for evaluating all bioactive food components, whether provided as a food or a dietary supplement. They suggest the recommended dietary allowance, and the tolerable upper intake level should fix the boundaries of intakes that should be considered sufficient to prevent deficiency, while avoiding toxicity. The difficulty in establishing adequacy comes from the benefit/risk that is being evaluated and the "family of curves" that are typically observed in response to dietary exposures. These "family of curves" likely reflect the genomics of the individual as well as a various insults such as bacteria, viruses, environmental pollutants, excess calories, and multiple nutrient–nutrient interactions (Figure 21.1).

TECHNOLOGY DEVELOPMENT AND THEIR USE BY THE PUBLIC

The technologies needed to achieve nutrigenomics' stated goals are still being developed and nutrigenomics has taken the path of developing genetic and screening tests that individuals take to be informed of their susceptibility to diseases and then make their own individual dietary decisions. Nutrigenomics has made significant progresses in translating the basic science of the Human Genome Project (HGP) into publicly available, commercialized product and services, a fact that remains undisputable even if the overall low quality of applied nutrigenomic sciences to the individual and the public is criticized (Haga et al., 2003). In just a few years, the strategy science-to-business evolved producing the current status of a commercial market focused on personalized nutrigenomic testing. The engine driving nutrigenomics at this time is the search for nutrient–gene associations common enough to allow the identification of groups of individuals large enough to support commercially viable companies (Castle, 2009). This approach has raised concerns in the scientific community because nutrigenomics appears focused primarily in addressing the needs of paying customers. These concerns and the determination to continue along the pathway of personalized nutrition through commercial testing have fed the debate on the incompatibility of nutrigenomics with public health—assumingly both research and practice, since a distinction is missing. We disagree with the proposition that nutrigenomics—and any other "omics"—are incompatible with public health either in research or practice. Public health practice adheres to

Hippocrates' principle *primum non nocere* to avoid harm to the patient at all costs. In other words, public health practice is the application of proven methods to maintain and improve the health of the population. The only exception to the application of proven methods in the practice of public health is the occurrence of a public health situation where public health officials must make decisions to prevent harm to the public in the absence of evidence-based knowledge and, possibly, only with preliminary and sketchy data available. In these circumstances, when not making a decision (because of the lack of evidence-based knowledge) may cause a greater harm to people, animals, and the environment, public health officials may have to adopt the precautionary principle or approach, which implies, "… a willingness to take actions in advance of scientific proof [or] evidence on the need for the proposed action on the grounds that further delay will prove ultimately more costly to society and nature, and, in the long-term, selfish and unfair to future generations" (United Nations, 1992). Canada, for example, has also specifically established a "Framework for the application of precaution in science-based decision making about risk" (Government of Canada, 2003). The application of nutrigenomics to public health under the precautionary principle has been discussed (Wilson, 2005). However, at the present time, there is not even the suggestion that not applying nutrigenomics to public health now will cause irreparable harm. Nutrigenomics will enter the sphere of public health practice once its benefits will have been proven and validated through public health research.

At the present, clinical genetic tests are available for more than 1500 diseases, several hundred additional genetic tests are used in research, and even more are in various stages of development (Genetic Alliance, 2007). In the United States, the Food and Drug Administration (FDA) regulates test kits (i.e., just a handful of the genetic tests available), and laboratories offering genetic testing must be compliant with the Clinical Laboratory Improvement Amendment of 1988. Usually, clinical genetic tests are available to individuals through their health-care providers. However, many genetic tests and nutrigenomic screening tests are available directly to consumers (DTC) through the Internet. Some of the DTC genetic tests are developed in-house (i.e., by the laboratory actually performing the tests) and escape FDA regulations; they may also escape quality controls. In nutrigenomics, what is usually proposed is the screening for mutations (i.e., genetic variation) of a specified number of genes along major biochemical pathways, for example, the methylation pathway. The resulting nutrigenomic panel or profile indicates whether or not genetic variation along the tested metabolic pathway(s) is present; it includes information about the association of the genetic profile with the efficiency with which the individual's body metabolize certain food and nutrients, or with a decreased resistance to environmental assaults, or with an increased risk for several chronic diseases, and it usually includes recommendations (usually generic) about appropriate nutrition and lifestyle choices.

The unregulated commercialization of nutrigenomic screening tests, which may suffer poor quality control, greediness in the commercialization of supplements, wrong and potentially dangerous health-related advice, illegal genetic testing, and the sharing of confidential genetic information with third parties are issues that affect the health of the public. In 2006, congressional investigators of the U.S. Government and Accountability Office (GAO) posed as fictitious consumers and exposed the malpractice of certain companies offering nutrigenomic screening tests. The GAO, the Federal Trade Commission, the FDA, and the Centers for Disease Control and Prevention called for improved regulatory oversight of the production and marketing of genetic tests (and specifically for closing the gap of genetic tests developed in-house) and explicitly warned individuals considering "at home" genetic testing of the associated risks (Federal Trade Commission, 2006). Unfortunately, there have been no nationwide changes to improving the regulation of genetic tests marketed DTC. Furthermore, genetic tests can be objectively difficult to interpret requiring a level of specialized knowledge that not even many physicians have. Taking celiac disease again as an example, some of the laboratories performing genetic tests for celiac disease may test for the whole DQ genotype (DQ1–DQ9) and for both subunits α and β; others may test for both subunits α and β but only for DQ2 and DQ8 genotype; still other laboratories will perform testing only for the subunit β of DQ2 and DQ8. The actual result of the genetic test will look complicated (Megiorni et al., 2008, 2009) and is complicated to interpret and, usually, the laboratory will provide the reading of the results as testing positive or negative for celiac disease and/or for non-celiac gluten sensitivity. Testing only for the subunit β of DQ2 and DQ8 is quite frequent since it is technically easier, less expensive, and over 99% of the risk is associated with subunit β. However, in this case, when the laboratory will provide the results as negative for genetic risk, such results will be at all effect misleading (at least for that number of people whose susceptibility is associated with subunit α). Furthermore, no information will be provided to the customer with respect to non-celiac gluten sensitivity. When genetic testing for celiac disease is prescribed by a health professional, the actual limits of the test and of its results are known (or expected to be known) by the prescriber, not so for individuals that have no biomedical education.

At the present date and current stage of genomic and nutrigenomics research, it is difficult to envision an "individualistic" research path—of developing nutrigenomic tests to be used by individuals—to be in conflict with public health research. Putting aside for a moment the enormous ethical, social, and legal issues associated with genetic testing in general and with nutrigenomic testing in particular, at the present stage, the research pathway of developing genetic tests for individuals is a realistic endower that has the potential of collecting useful information on genetic polymorphism and gene expression that are influenced by eating behaviors.

RESEARCH VERSUS PRACTICE

Public health practice and public health research are not synonymous. They appear alike because they have common characteristics: both may entail the collection and assessment of individually identifiable health information about living individuals; both may involve actual or potential risks to participants; e.g., privacy violation, discrimination, injuries, coercion, and anxieties; both may be justified as laudable, communal activities that further the public good; and both use the same disciplines—epidemiology and biostatistics—to assess and evaluate. However, distinguishing between public health research and public health practice is very important because the two have different goals. Public health practice is the application of proven methods to monitor and preserve the health status of the population, including by implementing preventive control measures based on the current understanding within public health sciences (Hodge and Gostin, 2004). Public health research, instead, involves testing hypotheses and entails designing a study to test new, unproven interventions, treatments, or strategies that are not known to be efficacious or effective and where there is rigorous monitoring of potential adverse, unexpected consequences to the human subjects selected for testing new unproven interventions.

Distinguishing public health practice from public health research is critical to public health researchers and practitioners since laws, rules, and regulations are significantly different. For example, identifiable health data may be collected for public health practice without informed consent and outside of federal and state human subjects' research provisions. Instead, the collection of identifiable health data for public health research occurs under a different social construct. Public health researchers, as any researcher conducting research on human subjects, must adhere to the regulations designed to protect the safety, welfare, dignity, and privacy of anyone who volunteers to participate in a research study. Similar protections of individual interests may underlie public health practice, of course, but they stem from different legal requirements. The current definitions of research and of human subjects are set in the Federal Policy for the Protection of Human Subjects (the "Common Rule"), codified under the Department of Health and Human Services (DHHS) regulations at 45 C.F.R., part 46, subpart A. In 1996, Congress passed the Health Insurance Portability and Accountability Act (HIPAA) in part to standardize the communication systems among various health-care agencies. Congress failed to pass the national health information privacy legislation pursuant to HIPAA; however, the DHHS was authorized to promulgate the first systematic national privacy protection regulations in the form of the HIPAA Privacy Rule, which was implemented in 2003. Public health researchers, including federal public health agencies, are subjected to the HIPAA Rule, while public health practitioners are not. Often, federal and state agencies while involved in the practice of public health may also engage in public health research. In these cases, the research component is subjected to all of the same regulations governing human subject research.

Distinguishing public health practice from public health research when discussing about the application of nutrigenomics—and genomics—to improving the health of human beings may facilitate at least the conceptual integration of nutrigenomic (and genomic) research with public health research, instead of carrying out a debate that is mostly theoretical. For example, in the biomedical research literature, genetic screening is considered a potential mean for achieving the application of nutrigenomic to public health (practice) even while recognizing that genetic screening presents "some unique challenges in the public health context," such as demonstrating that the test is accurate according to preestablished criteria and the test should lead to a "clinically validated outcome" (Burke et al., 2001; Castle, 2009; Hodge, 2004).

As of today, nutrigenomics screening is not even close to the meaning that screening has in public health practice. Public health screening for a disease (or secondary prevention) follows the rigorous principles established by the World Health

Organization (WHO) in 1968 in response to the increasing incidence, and public health burden, of chronic complex diseases in the Western world (Wilson and Jungner, 1968). These 10 principles were established to guide the planning of case finding for the disease of interest. It is worth briefly mentioning them in this context to provide a public health practice dimension to emerging requests from researchers to make genetic screening a public health strategy and to show that they are still very current in their protection of individuals' rights and interests as well as in the planning of the prudent use of financial resources for medical care. By definition, screening for a disease as a public health intervention is done in all people at risk for the disease (i.e., *only* on healthy asymptomatic subjects that are *not* affected by the disease) and it should follow the following principles: (1) the condition sought should be an important health problem; (2) there should be an accepted treatment for patients with recognized disease; (3) facilities for diagnosis and treatment should be available; (4) there should be a recognizable latent or early symptomatic stage; (5) there should be a suitable test or examination; (6) the test should be accepted by the population; (7) the natural history of the condition, including development from latent to declared disease, should be adequately understood; (8) there should be an agreed policy on whom to treat as patients; (9) the cost of case finding (including diagnosis and treatment of patients diagnosed) should be economically balanced in relation to possible expenditure on medical care as a whole; and (10) case finding should be a continuing process and not a "once and for all" project.

A brief comment on the first two principles guiding public health screening is provided. First, a disease does not need to have a high degree of prevalence to be considered an important health problem (even if that is the usual case). Rather, under the WHO principles, the importance of the health problem needs to be considered from the point of view both of the individual and of the community. In fact, there are extremely uncommon diseases, for example, phenylketonuria, that warrant screening despite their rarity because of the very serious consequences on the individual if not discovered and treated very early in life. On the contrary, certain conditions (e.g., overweight) are mild at the individual level, but have serious consequences for the community (overweight and obesity in a population) if not discovered early and treated, thus, warranting screening on these grounds. The second principle is considered the most important of the principles guiding public health screening, and it establishes that when screening for a disease is undertaken, the ability to adequately treat the disease, when discovered, must be present. Furthermore, treatment at the presymptomatic stage of a disease identified by screening should be associated with a better prognosis and that this is indeed the case should be verified with experimental surveys and clinical trials carried out independently from case finding/screening and well in advance of the main body of medical opinion (to guarantee unbiased data collection). Unless early detection of a disease is associated with response to treatment and better prognosis, there is no benefit, and actual harm can instead be done, in alerting people to a condition for which early detection does not change the course or the prognosis of the disease.

Considering again celiac disease as an example, genetic risk profiles for celiac disease would be helpful in clinical practice for predicting disease susceptibility and progression (Megiorni et al., 2008, 2009; Wolters and Wijmenga, 2008) and, as we have mentioned, genetic tests for the HLA-DQ genotypes are available. However, currently, there is no screening (either serological or genetic) for celiac disease as a public health intervention (i.e., mass screening). Even people at high risk for the disease* (Green and Cellier, 2007) may or may not be screened and with different protocols. Many scientific and medical authorities have expressed opinion for and against mass screening (Evans, 2009; Fasano, 2009; Hoffenberg, 2005; Kumar, 2003; Logan, 1996; Mearin and Ivarsson, 2005; Rosén et al., 2011). However, as also clearly explained by Rosén (2011), mass screening for celiac disease meets several of the public health principles for screening intervention (Wilson and Jungner, 1968), but not all. There is not enough evidence that the potential benefits will outweigh the harm and the costs for involved individuals and society. Thus, public health research continues on multiple fronts: several nations have issued joint position statements and reports to prioritize research on celiac disease prevention, diagnosis, and treatment (Troncone et al., 2008) and have joined efforts to study possible primary prevention interventions (Hogen Esch et al., 2010). The impact of missed diagnosis (Hoffenberg, 2005), of integrating genetic and serological screening (Bonamico et al., 2006; Chang and Green, 2009), of the long-term health and quality-of-life consequences of mass screening for childhood celiac disease (van Koppen et al., 2009), and of the perspective of newly diagnosed adolescents as a consequence of screening (Rosén et al., 2011) are just a few of the public health research areas for celiac disease, which we have used as example in this chapter to present the challenges of translating sciences into public health practice.

Nutrigenomics is expected to clarify how individual genetic differences can affect the way we respond to nutrients in the foods we eat and possibly the health benefits obtained through dietary changes. Nutrigenomics has the potential to have impacts on society and on public health practices (from clinical medicine to dietary and agricultural practices, and to social and public health policies). By building up knowledge in this area, it is hoped that nutrigenomics will foster a better understanding of how nutrition influences metabolic pathways and homeostatic control. As nutrigenomic science matures and knowledge accumulate, new information about the intersection of genetics and nutrition of individuals and groups will become available. Knowledge gained from comparing diet–gene interactions in different populations, through public health research, may provide information needed to address the larger problem of disease and global malnutrition.

The development and progression of multifactorial complex diseases, including cancer, is likely to be influenced by nutrition (Agelli, 1998; Ho et al., 2011; Kontou et al., 2011; Tan et al., 2011). Just before the publication of the human genome sequences draft (Venter, 2001), some authors expressed their hope that the HGP would help move human genetics from single-gene diseases into focusing on gene–environment interactions that have a public health impact (Khoury et al., 2000).

Despite deviations in one direction or another and the hype on personalized medicine and nutrition, biomedical research is a continuous fluid process, from the cell

* Factors increasing the risk of celiac disease include having one or more relatives diagnosed with celiac disease, being diagnosed with an autoimmune disease or disorder, for example, rheumatoid arthritis, systemic lupus erythematosus, Sjögren's syndrome, type 1 diabetes and autoimmune thyroid disease, Down's syndrome, Addison's disease, lactose intolerance, intestinal cancer, and intestinal lymphoma. White race and female sex are also associated with an increased risk for celiac disease.

to the individual (clinical medicine) to the population and back, where each step contributes to the formulation of research hypothesis in the preceding and following step (Potter, 2005). Nutrition is obviously a major determinant of health, and public health measures can may, and do, focus on changing dietary patterns, with or without a genetic component. To efficaciously and effectively apply nutrigenomics to public health (i.e., to "prevent chronic disease in more susceptible individuals"), population-based studies will need to be done to identify individuals and subpopulations at increased risk because of certain specific polymorphisms that can be targeted to increase the effectiveness and the efficiency of the dietary recommendations (Darnton-Hill et al., 2004).

Public health interventions and measures attempt to improve the quality of life and longevity of a population by reducing incidence of disease, injury, and disability and by making treatments and prevention practices more effective and accessible. The concept of genome stability through nutrition is appealing and the underlying concepts—that genetic damage occurs throughout the entire lifetime of an individual and that nutrition plays a role in providing micronutrients necessary for DNA repair (thus contributing to genome stability)—are supported by the accumulating evidence that chronic complex diseases are multifactorial and by experimental data, respectively (Fenech, 2002, 2005a, 2005b).

Already in 2005, a path for the integration of genomics into public health was pointed out by some authors that advocated integrating family history data—a routine aspect of medical consultations—into genomic databases and the development of population-based databases for genomic and public health research. Population-based genomic and public health research would provide population prevalence data needed to evaluate the potential impact of modifying environmental factors to reduce risk, and it would also be predictive because the genomic and pedigree data could be used in risk algorithms. The authors reminded us that genomic applications in public health practice should have an evidence base for health promotion and disease prevention and advocated the development of the institutional capacity and of human competence building without which no public health application of genomics/nutrigenomics will succeed (Foster et al., 2006; Institute of Medicine, 2003; Khoury and Mansah, 2005; Lampe, 2006).

For effective translation of genomics into public health, three important messages need to be clearly communicated to the public: (1) disease is really a function of gene–environment interactions; (2) population research is crucial to demonstrate clinical validity and utility of genetic testing; and (3) genetic information supports targeted use of interventions (Foster et al., 2006; Khoury and Mansah, 2005; Lampe, 2006).

COMMUNICATING THE CONCEPT

Another important issue to consider in looking at the application of nutrigenomics/genomics in public health practice is effective communication of risk reduction, which is never an easy concept to explain, but that is downright complicated in the face of genetic susceptibility. Understanding how to safely and effectively communicate risk reduction in the presence of genetic susceptibility will require additional research in risk communication and behavioral sciences (Khoury et al., 2000).

The management of risk is another communication challenge in the presence of susceptibility to chronic diseases. Public health researchers, in agreement with the principles guiding public health screening, have concluded that without interventions "available for any given genetic trait the identification of genetic susceptibility may do more harm than good" (Khoury et al., 2000; Rosén, 2011). Thus, as previously pointed out, the application of genomics to public health practice (i.e., systematic interventions on populations and communities to prevent the development of chronic diseases) needs to be validated by public health research.

CONCLUSIONS

Overall, this review presents the potential of applying nutrigenomics and associated technologies to public health, but it also recognizes the infancy of nutrigenomics and the long pathway before its application to public health practice. Undeniably, there are exciting opportunities for the integration of nutrigenomics into public health as well as numerous hurdles. Despite the numerous hurdles, the social impact will likely be enormous.

REFERENCES

Agelli M. (1998). Polyunsaturated fatty acids (PUFA) as steroid-sparing agents in the treatment of rheumatic polymyalgia. Personal Communication. International Congress of Rheumatology, Rome, Italy.

Agelli M. (2010). Nutrigenomics: ethic, social and public health issues. Nutrition and Cancer Prevention Research Practicum, National Cancer Institute, Bethesda, Maryland (oral presentation).

Balasubramanian S, Lee K, Adhikary G, Gopalakrishnan R, Rorke EA, Eckert RL. (2008). The Bmi-1 polycomb group gene in skin cancer: regulation of function by (-)-epigallocatechin-3-gallate. *Nutr Rev*. 66(Suppl 1):S65–S68.

Beaglehole R, Bonita R, Magnusson R. (2011). Global cancer prevention: an important path way to global health and development. *Public Health*. 125:821–831.

Bell, J. (2004). Predicting disease using genomics. *Nature*. 429:453–456.

Bonamico M, Ferri M, Mariani P, Nenna R, Thanasi E, Luparia RP, Picarelli A et al. (2006). Serologic and genetic markers of celiac disease: a sequential study in the screening of first degree relatives. *J Pediatr Gastroenterol Nutr*. 42:150–154.

Burdge GC, Hanson MA, Slater-Jefferies JL, Lillycrop KA. (2007). Epigenetic regulation of transcription: a mechanism for inducing variations in phenotype (fetal programming) by differences in nutrition during early life? *Br J Nutr*. 97:1036–1046.

Burdge GC, Lillycrop KA. (2010). Nutrition, epigenetics, and developmental plasticity: implications for understanding human disease. *Annu Rev Nutr*. 30:315–339.

Burke W, Pinsky TE, Press NA. (2001). Categorizing genetic tests to identify their ethical, legal and social implications. *Am Med Genet*. 106:233–310.

Castle D. (2009). The personal and the public in nutrigenomics. In: *Nutrition and Genomics: issues of ethics, law, regulation and communication* (D. Castle and N.L. Ries, Eds.) pp. 245–262. Academic Press, Amsterdam.

Celiac-Disease. (2012). Celiac News and Gluten-Free Diet Resources. Available at http://celiac-disease.com (accessed on April 2013).

Chang M, Green PH. (2009). Genetic testing before serologic screening in relatives of patients with celiac disease as a cost containment method. *J Clin Gastroenterol*. 43:43–50.

Chartoumpekis DV, Zaravinos A, Ziros PG, Iskrenova RP, Psyrogiannis AI, Kyriazopoulou VE, Habeos IG. (2012). Differential expression of microRNAs in adipose tissue after long-term high-fat diet-induced obesity in mice. *PLoS One*. 7(4):e34872.

Childress JF and Bemheim RG. (2003). The liberal and communitarian impasse: a framework and vision for public health. Fla Law Rev 55:1191–1219.
Darnton-Hill I, Margetts B, Deckelbaum R. (2004). Public health nutrition and genetics: implications for nutrition policy and promotion. *Proc Nutr Soc*. 63:173–185.
Davis CD, Milner JA. (2011). Nutrigenomics, vitamin D and cancer prevention. *J Nutrigenet Nutrigenomics*. 4:1–11.
Dolinoy DC, Weidman JR, Waterland RA, Jirtle RL. (2006). Maternal genistein alters coat color and protects Avy mouse offspring from obesity by modifying the fetal epigenome. *Environ Health Perspect*. 114:567–572.
Eussen SR, Verhagen H, Klungel OH, Garssen J, van Loveren H, van Kranen HJ, Rompelberg CJ. (2011). Functional foods and dietary supplements: products at the interface between pharma and nutrition. *Eur J Pharmacol*. 668(Suppl 1):S2–S9.
Evans KE, McAllister R, Sanders DS. (2009). Should we screen for coeliac disease? No. *BMJ*. 339:b3674.
Fasano A. (2009). Should we screen for coeliac disease? Yes. *BMJ*. 339:b3592.
Fasano A, Berti I, Gerarduzzi T, Not T, Colletti RB, Drago S, Elitsur Y et al. (2003). Prevalence of celiac disease in at-risk and not-at-risk groups in the United States: a large multicenter study. *Arch Intern Med*. 163:286–292.
Federal Trade Commission. (2006). At-Home Genetic Tests. Available at http://www.consumer.ftc.gov/articles/0166-home-genetic-tests (accessed on April 2013).
Fenech M. (2002). Micronutrients and genomic stability: a new paradigm for recommended dietary allowances (RDAs). *Food Chem Toxicol*. 40:1113–1117.
Fenech, M. (2005a). The genome health clinic and genome health nutrigenomics concepts: diagnosis and nutritional treatment of genome and epigenome damage on an individual basis. 20:255–269.
Fenech, M. (2005b). Low intake of calcium, folate, nicotinic acid, vitamin E, retinol, b-carotene and high intake of pantothenic acid, biotin and riboflavin are significantly associated with increased genome instability—results from a dietary intake and micronucleus index survey in South Australia. *Carcinogenesis*. 26:991–999.
Fine KD. (2008). *HLA-DQ phenotype and non-celiac gluten intolerance*. The Intestinal Health Institute, Dallas, TX. Unpublished observations.
Foster MW, Royal CDM, Sharp RR. (2006). The routinisation of genomics and genetics: implications for ethical practice. *Med Ethics*. 32:635–638.
Frayling TM, Timpson NJ, Weedon MN, Zeggini E, Freathy RM, Lindgren CM, Perry JR et al. (2007). A common variant in the FTO gene is associated with body mass index and predisposes to childhood and adult obesity. *Science*. 316:889–894.
Genetic Alliance. (2007). Eyes on the prize: truth telling about genetic testing. Available at http://www.geneticalliance.org/issues.testing (accessed on April 2013).
Genetic Association Information Network (GAIN). (2006). Available at http://www.genome.gov/19518664 (accessed on April 2012).
Gerard S, Hayes M, Rothstein MA. (2002). On the edge of tomorrow: fitting genomics into public health policy. *Law Med Ethics*. 30(Suppl):173–176.
Glanz K, Bader MD, Iyer S. (2012). Retail grocery store marketing strategies and obesity: an integrative review. *Am J Prev Med*. 42:503–512.
Gonzalez CA, Riboli E. (2010). Diet and cancer prevention: contributions from the European Prospective Investigation into Cancer and Nutrition (EPIC) study. *Eur J Cancer*. 46(14):2555–2562.
Government of Canada. (2003). The Application of Precaution—A Framework for the Application of Precaution in Science-Based Decision-Making about Risk. Available at http://www.pco-bcp.gc.ca/docs/information/publications/precaution/Precaution-eng.pdf (accessed April 2013).

Greco L, Romino R, Coto I, Di Cosmo N, Percopo S, Maglio M, Paparo F et al. (2002). The first large population based twin study of coeliac disease. *Gut*. 50:624–628.

Green PH, Cellier C. (2007). Celiac disease. *N Engl J Med*. 357:1731–1743.

Hadithi M, von Blomberg BME, Crusius JBA, Bloemena E, Kostense PJ, Meijer JWR, Mulder CJJ, Stehouwer CDA, Peña AS. (2007). Accuracy of serologic tests and HLA-DQ typing for diagnosing celiac disease. *Ann Int Med*. 147:294–302.

Haga SB, Khoury MJ, Burke W. (2003). Genomic profiling to promote a healthy lifestyle: not ready for prime time. *Nat Genet*. 34:347–350.

Hardy TM, Tollefsbol TO. (2011). Epigenetic diet: impact on the epigenome and cancer. *Epigenomics*. 3:503–518.

Ho E, Beaver LM, Williams DE, Dashwood RH. (2011). Dietary factors and epigenetic regulation for prostate cancer prevention. *Adv Nutr*. 2:497–510.

Hodge JG Jr. (2004). Ethical issues concerning genetic testing and screening in public health. *Am Med Genet*. 125C:66–70.

Hodge JG and Gostin IO. (2004). Public Health Practice vs. Research: A Report for Public Health Practitioners Including Cases and Guidance for Making Distinctions. (Council of State and Territorial Epidemiologists, Eds.). Available at http://www.cste2.org/webpdfs/CSTEPHResRptHodgeFinal.5.24.04.pdf (accessed on April 2013).

Hoffenberg EJ. (2005). Should all children be screened for celiac disease? *Gastroenterology*. 128(Suppl 1):S98–S103.

Hogen Esch CE, Rosen A, Auricchio R, Romanos J, Chmielewska A, Putter H, Ivarsson A et al. (2010). The PreventCD study design: towards new strategies for the prevention of coeliac disease. *Eur J Gastroenterol Hepatol*. 22:1424–1430.

Institute of Medicine. (2003). *Who will Keep the Public Healthy? Educating Public Health Professionals for the 21st Century*. National Academies Press, Bethesda.

Jackson AA, Burdge GC, Lillicrop KA. (2010). Diet, nutrition and modulation of genomic expression in fetal origins of adult disease. *J Nutrigenet Nutrigenomics*. 3:192–208.

Joven J, Espinel E, Rull A, Aragonès G, Rodríguez-Gallego E, Camps J, Micol V et al. (2012). Plant-derived polyphenols regulate expression of miRNA paralogs miR-103/107 and miR-122 and prevent diet-induced fatty liver disease in hyperlipidemic mice. *Biochim Biophys Acta*. 1820:894–899.

Kaati G, Bygren LO, Edvinsson S. (2002). Cardiovascular and diabetes mortality determined by nutrition during parents' and grandparents' slow growth period. *Eur J Hum Genet*. 10:682–688.

Kaati G, Bygren LO, Pembrey M, Sjöström M. (2007). Transgenerational response to nutrition, early life circumstances and longevity. *Eur J Hum Genet*. 15:784–790.

Kaput J. (2008). Nutrigenomics research for personalized nutrition and medicine. *Curr Opin Biotechnol*. 19:1–11.

Khoury MJ, Mensah GA. (2005). Genomics and the prevention and control of common chronic diseases: emerging priorities for public health action. *Prev Chronic Dis*. 2:A05.

Khoury MJ, Thrasher JF, Burke W, Gettig EA, Fridinger F, Jackson R. (2000). Challenges in communicating genetics: a public health approach. *Genet Med*. 2:198–202.

Kontou N, Psaltopoulou T, Panagiotakos D, Dimopoulos MA, Linos A. (2011). The mediterranean diet in cancer prevention: a review. *J Med Food*. 14:1065–1078.

Kumar PJ. (2003). European and North American populations should be screened for coeliac disease. *Gut*. 52:170–171.

Lampe JW. (2006). For debate: investment in nutrigenomics will advance the role of nutrition in public health. *Cancer Epidemiol Biomarkers Prev*. 15:2329–2330.

Lander ES, Linton LM, Birren B, Nusbaum C, Zody MC, Baldwin J, Devon K et al. (2001). Initial sequencing and analysis of the human genome. *Nature*. 409:860–921.

Last J. Ed. (1998). *Public health and human ecology*. 2nd Edition. McGraw-Hill Co., New York.

Li Z, Heber D. (2012). Sarcopenic obesity in the elderly and strategies for weight management. *Nutr Rev*. 70:57–64.

Lillycrop KA, Burdge GC. (2011a). The effect of nutrition during early life on the epigenetic regulation of transcription and implications for human diseases. *J Nutrigenet Nutrigenomics*. 4:248–260.

Lillycrop KA, Burdge GC. (2011b). Epigenetic changes in early life and future risk of obesity. *Int J Obes (Lond)*. 35:72–83.

Lin M, Aquilante C, Johnson JA, Wu R. (2005). Sequencing drug response with HapMap. *Pharmacogenomics J*. 5:149–156.

Liu T, Johnson JA, Casella G, Wu R. (2004). Sequencing complex diseases with HapMap. *Genetics*. 168:503–511.

Logan RF. (1996). Screening for coeliac disease—has the time come for mass screening? *Acta Paediatr Suppl*. 412:15–19.

Ludvigsson JF, Leffler DA, Bai JC, Biagi F, Fasano A, Green PH, Hadjivassiliou M et al. (2013). The Oslo definitions for coeliac disease and related terms. *Gut*. 62:43–52.

Mearin ML, Ivarsson A. (2005). Coeliac disease: is it time for mass screening? *Best Pract Res Clin Gastroenterol*. 19:441–452.

Megiorni F, Mora B, Bonamico M, Barbato M, Montuori M, Viola F, Trabace S, Mazzilli MC. (2008). HLA-DQ and susceptibility to celiac disease: evidence for gender differences and parent-of-origin effects. *Am J Gastroenterol*. 103:997–1003.

Megiorni F, Mora B, Bonamico M, Barbato M, Nenna R, Maiella G, Lulli P, Mazzilli MC. (2009). HLA-DQ and risk gradient for celiac disease. *Hum Immunol*. 70:55–59.

Mocchegiani E, Giacconi R, Costarelli L. (2011). Metalloproteases/anti-metalloproteases imbalance in chronic obstructive pulmonary disease: genetic factors and treatment implications. *Curr Opin Pulm Med*. 16 (Suppl 1):S11–S19.

Mustalahti K, Catassi C, Reunanen A, Fabiani E, Heier M, McMillan S, Murray L et al. (2010) The prevalence of celiac disease in Europe: results of a centralized, international mass screening project. *Ann Med*. 42:587–595.

Myléus A, Ivarsson A, Webb C, Danielsson L, Hernell O, Högberg L, Karlsson E et al. (2009). Celiac disease revealed in 3% of Swedish 12-year-olds born during an epidemic. *J Pediatr Gastroenterol Nutr*. 49:170–176.

Ng SF, Lin RC, Laybutt DR, Barres R, Owens JA, Morris MJ. (2010). Chronic high-fat diet in fathers programs β-cell dysfunction in female rat offspring. *Nature*. 467:963–966.

Palou A, Pico C, Keijer J. (2009). Integration of risk and benefit analysis—the window of benefit as a new tool? *Crit Rev Food Sci Nutr*. 49:670–680.

Penders B, Horstman K, Saris WHM, Vos R. (2007). From individuals to groups: a review of the meaning of 'personalized' in nutrigenomics. *Trends Food Sci Technol*. 18:333–338.

Potter JD. (2005). Epidemiology informing clinical practice: from bills of mortality to population laboratories. *Nat Clin Pract Oncol*. 2:625–634.

Rajendran P, Ho E, Williams DE, Dashwood RH. (2011). Dietary phytochemicals, HDAC inhibition, and DNA damage/repair defects in cancer cells. *Clin Epigenetics*. 3:4. doi: 10.1186/1868-7083-3-4.

Rosén A, Emmelin M, Carlsson A, Hammarroth S, Karlsson E, Ivarsson A. (2011). Mass screening for celiac disease from the perspective of newly diagnosed adolescents and their parents: a mixed-method study. *BMC Public Health*. 11:822.

Ross SA. (2010). Evidence for the relationship between diet and cancer. *Exp Oncol*. 32:137–142.

Sapone A, Bai JC, Ciacci C, Dolinsek J, Green PH, Hadjivassiliou M, Kaukinen K et al. (2012). Spectrum of gluten-related disorders: consensus on new nomenclature and classification. *BMC Med*. 10:13. doi: 10.1186/1741-7015-10-13.

Sapone A, Lammers KM, Casolaro V, Cammarota M, Giuliano MT, De Rosa M, Stefanile R et al. (2011). Divergence of gut permeability and mucosal immune gene expression in two gluten-associated conditions: celiac disease and gluten sensitivity. *BMC Med.* 9:23.

Silverton L, Dean M, Moitra K. (2011). Variation and evolution of the ABC transporter genes ABCB1, ABCC1, ABCG2, ABCG5 and ABCG8: implication for pharmacogenetics and disease. *Drug Metabol Drug Interact.* 26:169–179.

Simopoulos AP. (1999). Genetic variation and nutrition. *Nutr Rev.* 57:10–19.

Sollid LM, Markussen G, Ek J, Gjerde H, Vartdal F, Thorsby E. (1989). Evidence for a primary association of celiac disease to a particular HLA-DQ alpha/beta heterodimer. *J Exp Med.* 169:345–350.

Tan AC, Konczak I, Sze DM, Ramzan I. (2011). Molecular pathways for cancer chemoprevention by dietary phytochemicals. *Nutr Cancer.* 63:495–505.

Tourlouki E, Matalas AL, Panagiotakos DB. (2009). Dietary habits and cardiovascular disease risk in middle-aged and elderly populations: a review of evidence. *Clin Interv Aging.* 4:319–330.

Troncone R, Ivarsson A, Szajewska H, Mearin ML, Members of European Multi stake holder Platform on CD (CDEUSSA). (2008). Review article: future research on coeliac disease - a position report from the European multistakeholder platform on coeliac disease (CDEUSSA). *Aliment Pharmacol Ther.* 27:1030–1043. United Nations. (1992). Rio Declaration on Environment and Development. United Nations Environment Programme. Available at http://www.unep.org/documents.multilingual/default.asp?documentid=78&articleid=1163 (accessed onApril 2013).

van Boekel M, Fogliano V, Pellegrini N, Stanton C, Scholz G, Lalljie S, Somoza V, Knorr D, Jasti PR, Eisenbrand G. (2010). A review on the beneficial aspects of food processing. *Mol Nutr Food Res.* 54:1215–1247.

van Koppen EJ, Schweizer JJ, Csizmadia CG, Krom Y, Hylkema HB, van Geel AM, Koopman HM, Verloove-Vanhorick SP, Mearin ML. (2009). Long-term health and quality-of-life consequences of mass screening for childhood celiac disease: a 10-year follow-up study. *Pediatrics.* 123:e582–e588.

Venter JC, Adams MD, Myers EW, Li PW, Mural RJ, Sutton GG, Smith HO et al. (2001). The sequence of the human genome. *Science.* 291:1304–1351.

Wellcome Trust Case Control Consortium. (2007). Genome-wide association study of 14,000 cases of seven common diseases and 3,000 shared controls. Nature. 447:661–678.

Wellcome Trust Case Control Consortium (WTCCC). (2013). Available at http://www.wtccc.org.uk/ (accessed on April 2013).

Wilson JMG and Jungner G. (1968). Principles and practice of screening for disease. Public Health Paper No. 34, World Health Organization, Geneva.

Wilson, K. (2005). Risk, causation and population: understanding policy-making regarding public health risks. In *Public Health and Policy in Canada* (T.M. Bailey, T. Caufield and N.M.R. Ries, Eds.), LexisNexis, Markham.

Winslow CEA. (1920). The untilled fields of public health. *Science.* 51:23–33.

Wilson K. (2005). Risk, causation and precaution: understanding policy-making regarding public health risks. In *Public Health Law and Policy in Canada* (Bailey TM, Caufield T and Ries NMR, Eds.), LexisNexis, Markham.

World Health Organization. (1946). Preamble to the Constitution of the World Health Organization as adopted by the International Health Conference. Available at http://www.who.int/bulletin/archives/80(12)981–984.pdf (accessed on April 2013).

Wolters VM, Wijmenga C. (2008). Genetic background of celiac disease and its clinical implications. *Am J Gastroenterol.* 103:190–195.

Index

D

H

I

M

N

Q

R

S

T

U

V

W

X

Z

CPSIA information can be obtained
at www.ICGtesting.com
Printed in the USA
BVHW04*0552240918
527235BV00017B/137/P

9 781439 876800